MECHANISMS OF TOXICITY AND HAZARD EVALUATION

DEVELOPMENTS IN TOXICOLOGY AND ENVIRONMENTAL SCIENCE

Volume 8

Volume 1	Clinical Chemistry and Chemical Toxicology of Metals S.S. Brown editor, 1977
Volume 2	Progress in Genetic Toxicology D. Scott, B.A. Bridges and F.H. Sobels editors, 1977
Volume 3	Chemical Toxicology of Food C.L. Galli, R. Paoletti and G. Vettorazzi editors, 1978
Volume 4	Toxicology and Occupational Medicine W.B. Deichmann organizer, 1979
Volume 5	Estrogens in the Environment J.A. McLachlan editor, 1980
Volume 6	The Scientific Basis of Toxicity Assessment H.R. Witschi editor, 1980
Volume 7	Progress in Environmental Mutagenesis M. Alačević editor, 1980
Volume 8	Mechanisms of Toxicity and Hazard Evaluation B. Holmstedt, R. Lauwerys, M. Mercier and M. Roberfroid editors, 1980

MECHANISMS OF TOXICITY AND HAZARD EVALUATION

Proceedings of the Second International Congress on Toxicology held in Brussels, Belgium, July 6-11, 1980

Editors
B. HOLMSTEDT
R. LAUWERYS
M. MERCIER
M. ROBERFROID

1980

Elsevier/North-Holland Biomedical Press
AMSTERDAM · NEW YORK · OXFORD

ISBN for this volume: 0-444-80293-2
ISBN for the series: 0-444-80013-1

Published by:
Elsevier/North-Holland Biomedical Press
335 Jan van Galenstraat, P.O. Box 211
Amsterdam, The Netherlands

Sole distributors for the USA and Canada:
Elsevier North Holland Inc.
52 Vanderbilt Avenue
New York, N.Y. 10017

Library of Congress Cataloging in Publication Data

International Congress on Toxicology, 2d, Brussels, 1980.
Mechanisms of toxicity and hazard evaluation.

(Developments in toxicology and environmental science ; v. 8)
Bibliography: p.
Includes indexes.
1. Toxicology--Congresses. 2. Toxicity testing--Congresses. I. Holmstedt, Bo. II. Title. III. Series. [DNLM: 1. Toxicology--Methods--Congresses. W1 DE993T v.8 / QV 602 I61 1980m]
RA1191.I6 1980 615.9'07 80-24719
ISBN 0-444-80293-2

Printed in the Netherlands

PREFACE

Already during the First International Congress on Toxicology held in Toronto in 1977, the need was felt for a follow-up and the city of Brussels was selected as an appropriate location for the Second Congress, the results of which are presented in this volume. Furthermore, during the three years which have elapsed, international toxicology has been formalized through the creation of an International Union of Toxicology (IUTOX) which took place in Brussels on July 10, 1980.

Five symposia covering a wide variety of topics currently of great importance were selected by the programme committee of the Second International Congress on Toxicology. Several free communications to a large extent related to the themes of the symposia were also presented.

The expanding field of toxicology is well documented by the fact that, at the First International Congress, 100 papers from 28 nations were presented whereas at the present congress 500 papers from 40 countries were submitted. The many interesting papers received have caused no small editorial problems to the local scientific committee. Thus, the majority of the contributions of the host country were deliberately deleted from the proceedings for lack of space.

It is hoped that the present volume will serve a useful purpose to experienced scientists, government officials and all interested in mechanisms of action and hazard evaluation of chemicals. The editors of the proceedings want to acknowledge the great help of the members of the programme committee and the local scientific committee.

B. Holmstedt, R. Lauwerys, M. Mercier, M. Roberfroid.

CONTENTS

EARLY CHANGES IN CHEMICAL CARCINOGENESIS

LONG-TERM EXPOSURE TO OCCUPATIONAL INTOXICANTS

CLINICAL TOXICOLOGY

RECENT DEVELOPMENTS IN MECHANISMS OF NEUROTOXICITY

Symposium chairmen: B. Holmstedt, P.S. Spencer and J. Willems

Mechanisms of Toxicity and Hazard Evaluation
B. Holmstedt, R. Lauwerys, M. Mercier, M. Roberfroid eds

RECENT MORPHOLOGICAL STUDIES OF TOXIC NEUROPATHY

PETER S. SPENCER and HERBERT H. SCHAUMBURG
Institute of Neurotoxicology, Albert Einstein College of Medicine, Bronx, New York, U.S.A.

INTRODUCTION

A substantial amount of progress has been made in recent years in understanding the morphological substrate of toxic neuropathies.[1] This has been achieved by applying modern methods of tissue examination to study in detail the pathological effects of a number of toxic chemicals that seemed to exert their effects on the peripheral nervous system. It has become clear from these observations that toxic neuropathies: (a) commonly have both central and peripheral nervous system components, and (b) represent a heterogeneous collection of diseases which, at the present time, are most conveniently grouped according to the likely cellular target of the toxin, *viz.* the neuronal perikaryon (*neuronopathy*); the axon (*axonopathy*), and the Schwann cell or its myelin sheath (*myelinopathy*). Examples of each type of toxic neuropathy, their identification and causation, together form the subject of this paper.

THE ROLE OF METHODOLOGY

The Examination of Animal Tissue

Application of methods of tissue fixation and examination originally intended for transmission electron microscopy has been a major factor in illuminating the different types of toxic neuropathy. The central and peripheral nervous systems (and other organs) are prepared for examination by systemically perfusing the anesthetized animal with a dilute solution of glutaraldehyde carried in a vehicle balanced for tissue pH and osmolality. This method kills the animal instantly and painlessly, and fixes the tissues without trauma or postmortem change. After perfusion, the animal is dissected and the nervous system thoroughly sampled. Postfixation in dilute, buffered osmium tetroxide, and stepwise dehydration in ascending concentrations of ethanol, prepares the fixed tissue samples for embedding in liquid epoxy resin.

Three techniques are widely used to examine peripheral nervous tissue prepared by this method: (a) microdissection of nerve fibers, (b) preparation of one-micrometer thick epoxy sections (by microtomy) for examination by light microscopy, and (c) preparation of ultrathin sections (by ultramicrotomy) for study in the transmission electron microscope.

Microdissection involves removing the connective tissue sheath surrounding a nerve trunk and teasing apart individual nerve fibers with the aid of mounted sewing needles and a binocular microscope. Light-microscope inspection of a normal myelinated fiber reveals uniform lengths (internodes) of densely-stained myelin interrupted by short, unstained nodes of Ranvier. Each segment of myelin is the territory of a single Schwann cell whose nucleus resides outside the myelin sheath in the center of the internode. The myelin sheath is interrupted periodically by Schmidt-Lanterman incisures, each a biconical cellular channel of Schwann cell cytoplasm, which are visualized in teased fibers as pairs of diverging dense lines. Abnormal nerve fibers can display a variety of changes such as: segmental ballooning and loss of myelin (demyelination), short internodes of thin myelin intercalated between internodes of normal length and thickness (remyelination), corrugated and infolded myelin (axonal atrophy), chains of myelin beads (axonal or Wallerian degeneration), or consecutive lengths of thinly-myelinated and foreshortened internodes (axonal regeneration and myelination). The pattern of pathological change found in teased nerve fibers thus provides a rapid method of tentatively assessing the nature of toxic injury. For example: (a) the presence of extensive segmental demyelination and remyelination in the absence of axonal degeneration suggests damage to the Schwann cell or myelin sheath (myelinopathy); (b) a preponderance of Wallerian degeneration is compatible with neuronal damage (neuronopathy), and (c) a clustering of axonal and myelin abnormalities is suggestive of an axonopathy.

Light-microscope inspection of one-micrometer epoxy sections is a second important method of examining nervous tissue for pathological changes. For this purpose, blocks of embedded tissue hardened by heat are cut with glass knives mounted in ultramicrotomes, and the sections immersed in a general tissue stain such as toluidine blue. Bright-field examination of stained sections reveals a wealth of cytological detail resolvable to approximately 0.2 micrometers, the width of an individual axonal mitochondrion. This extraordinary resolution makes possible a detailed morphological description which may obviate the need for subsequent study with the electron microscope. Cross-sections of nerves provide information on the number, size and condition of nerve fibers and may reveal special pathological patterns not visible in teased nerve fibers. Longitudinal sections are more useful for examining the architecture of nodes of Ranvier, Schmidt-Lanterman incisures, and Schwann cell cytoplasm.

Examination with the electron microscope of thin sections stained with uranyl acetate and lead citrate provides more detailed information about the state of nerve tissue, and is an absolute requirement for a description of the condition of unmyelinated nerve fibers and nerve terminals. Ultrastructural examination is also needed to identify abnormal organelles and aberrant cytological associations.

The Use of Organotypic Tissue Cultures

Tissue culture provides a unique method to observe and photograph sequentially the reaction of living nerve tissue to toxic agents, to identify the locus of initial pathological response and to describe the type of change produced. The organotypic tissue culture system developed by Peterson and Murray --- a structurally and functionally coupled *in vitro* facsimile of spinal cord and peripheral neuromuscular tissue --- has proved especially useful for the experimental study of toxic neuropathy. Because these culture systems can be maintained for many months, it has been possible to reproduce *in vitro* the spatial-temporal pattern of pathological events seen in chronically intoxicated animals and man.[2,3]

PATHOLOGICAL CHANGE AND NEUROTOXIC CAUSATION

Modern methods of tissue examination are so sensitive that it is relatively easy for the inexperienced observer to ascribe pathological significance to aberrant structures which actually represent normal findings, spontaneous changes or preparative artefact.[4]

Preparative Artefact

Preparative artefacts commonly encountered in teased nerve fibers include: paranodal myelin splits attributable to non-optimal fixation, traumatized fiber ends caused by tissue excision, tissue pallor from inadequate osmication, and fractures at incisures produced by stretching during dissection. Thick sections may display central areas of poor osmication, tissue shrinkage from drying during dissection or dehydration, structural damage to nerve fibers restricted to traumatized foci of the nerve, enlarged blood vessels from excessive perfusion pressure, and a variety of sectioning and staining artefacts. Most commonly ascribed pathological significance are fixation artefacts found with the electron microscope such as vacuolated mitochondria, split myelin, edematous axons and cellular processes, and discontinuous plasma membranes.

Spontaneous Changes

Spontaneous changes in peripheral nerves are uncommonly encountered. Rarely, the sciatic nerve of a rat may show extensive damage unilaterally. Nerve fibers prepared by teasing occasionally display thickened paranodal myelin, and the endoneurial connective tissue separating nerve fibers is sometimes edematous.

Age-related Changes

It is essential in long-term toxicity studies to isolate normal structural changes acquired with advancing age from an induced neurotoxic lesion. This task presents special difficulties not only because few contemporary papers address the subject of age-related changes, but also because these changes often resemble those induced by toxic chemicals.

Advancing age is associated with the following pathological appearances:[5,6] (a) widespread neuronal pigmentation --- the progressive accumulation of cytoplasmic lipofuscin granules, (b) scattered neuronal degeneration, (c) Wallerian-like degeneration of a few nerve fibers, (d) massive bubbling of the myelin sheath of isolated fibers, most commonly encountered in spinal roots, (d) scattered remyelination, and (e) swollen axon terminals. The plantar nerves of aged members of some species often display spectacular changes: many axons are packed with metachromatic, spherical structures that, on electron microscope examination, are seen to be composed of clusters of glycogen granules surrounded by a single membrane; some axons may be swollen and/or demyelinated; other fibers contain accumulations of axonal organelles, some of which may be sequestered by invaginations from the inner compartment of the Schwann cell. Some of these pathological findings seem to spread proximally with advancing age and thereby affect the tibial and sciatic nerves. Pathological changes are also consistently encountered in the gracile nucleus of the medulla oblongata which, although strictly part of the central nervous system, houses the terminal regions of axons emanating from peripheral sensory neurons. Affected regions of axons are massively swollen and contain densely-packed accumulations of smooth tubulo-vesicular profiles.

THE MORPHOLOGICAL SUBSTRATE OF TOXIC NEUROPATHIES

Three groups of toxic "neuropathy" are presently recognized. (a) Neuronopathies are rather rare disorders associated with primary damage of the peripheral sensory neuron; toxic motor neuronopathies have not been recognized. (b) Axonopathies are divided into the common type that affects distal axons of long and large fibers in the CNS and PNS (central-peripheral distal axonopathy), and the type where damage occurs first in the proximal axon (proximal axonopathy). A central distal axonopathy, in which only the central processes of peripheral sensory neurons undergo degeneration, is seen in experimental clioquinol intoxication. (c) Myelinopathy refers to diseases in which there is primary damage to the Schwann cell or myelin sheath, with the axon remaining largely intact.

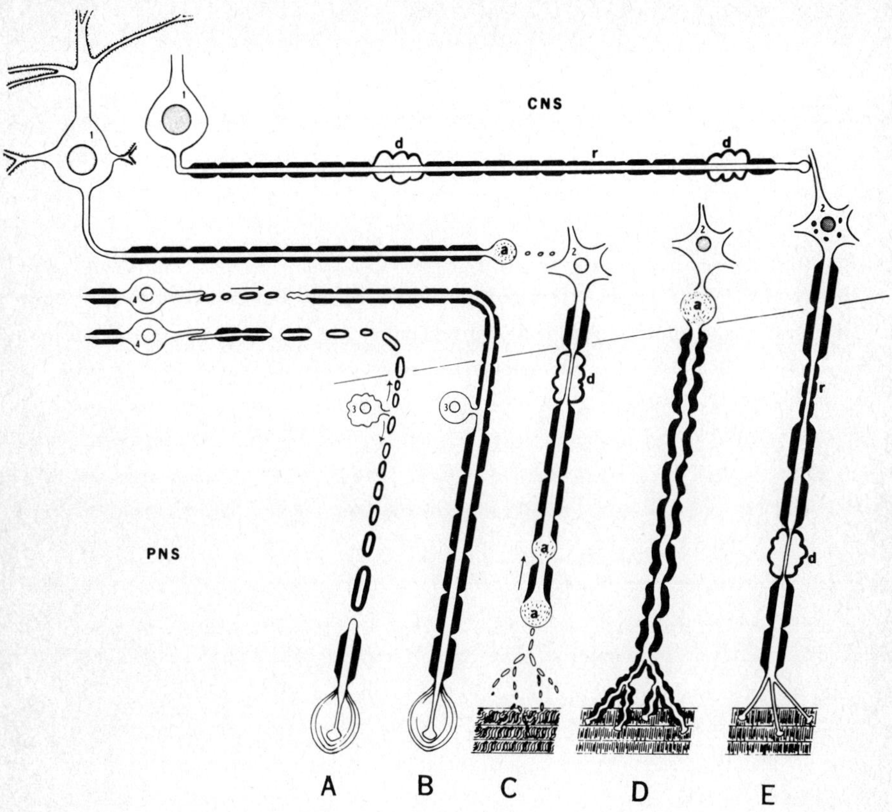

Figure. Types of cellular response to neurotoxic compounds illustrated by upper (1) and lower (2) motor neurons, dorsal root ganglion cells (3), and second-order sensory neurons (4) in the gracile nucleus of the medulla oblongata. The sloping horizontal line divides the central (CNS) and peripheral nervous system (PNS). The peripheral receptors on fibers A and B are Pacinian corpuscles. Fibers C-E innervate extrafusal muscle fibers. A: Neuronopathy, e.g. Doxorubicin; B: Central distal axonopathy, e.g. clioquinol; C: Central-peripheral distal axonopathy, e.g. n-hexane; D: Proximal axonopathy, e.g. IDPN; E: Myelinopathy, e.g. AETT. d: demyelination; r: remyelination. Arrows indicate temporal progression of degeneration. Modified from figure 7.1, Experimental and Clinical Neurotoxicology, eds. P.S. Spencer & H.H. Schaumburg, Williams & Wilkins, 1980.

Sensory Neuronopathies

The peculiar vulnerability of peripheral sensory neurons to certain neurotoxins is believed to be associated with the special permeability of their associated intraneural blood vessels. Tracer studies with horseradish peroxidase have demonstrated that blood-borne materials normally have intimate access to sensory neurons in dorsal root and autonomic ganglia.[7] It is surprising, therefore, that toxic sensory neuronopathies have only been recognized in relationship to mercury,[7] doxorubicin, and pyridoxine intoxication.

Doxorubicin (Adriamycin). This antineoplastic glycosidic anthracycline antibiotic induces a progressive limb ataxia in the rat beginning 11 d following a single intravenous injection of 10 mg/kg.[8] Morphological studies have demonstrated that doxorubicin, which blocks DNA-dependent DNA and RNA synthesis, binds to neuronal nuclei in dorsal root ganglia within one minute of injection[9] and, by three hours, causes focal clearings to develop in certain neuronal nuclei. During the following days, affected neurons undergo nuclear and cytoplasmic disruption which culminates in neuronal degeneration.[8] The axon, which is totally dependent on the neuronal perikaryon for metabolic maintenance, rapidly degenerates in an anterograde fashion.[9]

Pyridoxine Megavitaminosis. Large (300 mg/kg) daily oral doses of this essential, water-soluble vitamin (pyridoxol hydrochloride) causes Beagles to develop a swaying gait after 4-9 days of treatment. By 10-30 d, the animals display frank limb ataxia and eventually are unable to walk. Pathological studies demonstrate changes restricted to dorsal root and Gasserian ganglia, and their processes. Membrane-bound vacuoles develop in the neuronal cytoplasm and eventually fuse to form large hydropic cavities. Prolonged treatment leads to the formation of necrotic neurons and nodules of Nageotte. As with doxorubicin, neuronal breakdown is associated with Wallerian-like degeneration of sensory axons throughout the length of the dorsal roots, dorsal columns of the spinal cord, and peripheral nerves.[10] The etiology of this lesion is unknown.

Axonopathies

Central-peripheral distal type.[11] Numerous chemicals and drugs induce distal, retrograde axonal degeneration in long and large fiber pathways in the central and peripheral nervous systems. The majority of compounds (eg. n-hexane, acrylamide, carbon disulfide, zinc pyridinethione) requires repeated administration to induce this type of symmetrical sensorimotor neuropathy, while many organophosphorus compounds can induce this change in fowl with a single dose. Unlike the sensory neuronopathies, animals developing central-peripheral distal axonopathy progress from ataxia to frank weakness, usually evident distally in the hindlimbs before the forelimbs. Morphological studies demonstrate that changes begin distally and multifocally, and are often associated with abnormal focal accumulations of organelles. With n-hexane and its metabolic relatives (e.g. 2,5-hexanedione), 10-nm neurofilaments accumulate proximal to nodes of Ranvier whereas, with zinc pyridinethione, smooth tubulo-vesicular profiles first appear terminally.[9] Such accumulations of organelles are variably associated with abnormalities in the axonal transport systems, thus raising the possibility of a causal relationship between transport abnormalities and axonal breakdown. In the case of acrylamide and n-hexane, both of which are associated with focal abnormalities of fast anterograde transport in the swollen regions,[12,13] the distal axon breaks down in a Wallerian-like pattern. With time and continued intoxication, the degenerative process moves retrogradely along the fiber. This results in a characteristic distribution of distal degeneration in long peripheral nerves, and in long ascending and descending spinal cord tracts. Distal regions of shorter nerve fiber pathways, such as the optic nerve, may become involved later in the disease process. The neuronal perikaryon does not degenerate and is therefore able to sustain axonal regeneration after intoxication.

Studies with diisofluorophosphate,[14] disulfiram[15] and 2,5-hexanedione[16] have suggested that these compounds induce distal axonopathy by direct toxic action on the nerve fiber. For example, when 2,5-hexanedione is applied directly to a nerve trunk, giant axonal swellings filled with 10-nm neurofilaments ---the hallmark of the systemic disease, develop beneath the position of application. By contrast, 2,4-hexanedione, a diketone unable to induce neuropathy by systemic administration, fails to induce this characteristic pattern of axonal damage.[16]

Central Distal Axonopathy. Clioquinol, an intestinal amebicide implicated as the causative agent in the Japanese epidemic of "subacute myelo-optico neuropathy," seems to induce in experimental animals a typical pattern of distal axonopathy which is restricted to the central nervous system . Beagles daily intoxicated with 400 mg/kg develop an ataxic, stiff-legged gait after approximately 20 d, but fail to show signs of peripheral neuropathy such as footdrop, muscle atrophy, or impaired motor nerve conduction. Neuropathological examination reveals distal axonal degeneration only in the gracile, optic and corticospinal tracts, and no sign of peripheral nerve degeneration.[17] Why only central axonal processes are vulnerable to clioquinol is unknown.

Proximal Axonopathy. β,β'-Iminodipropionitrile (IDPN) administration to experimental species causes the formation of giant axonal swellings in the proximal part of the axon. The swollen regions are filled with 10-nm neurofilaments which appear to accumulate during their anterograde passage along the axon.[18] Indeed, Griffin and colleagues[19] demonstrated a blockade in the proximal axon of the slowly transported triplet polypeptides believed to constitute neurofilaments. However, these investigators found no abnormalities of the fast axonal transport system, a feature which may explain why there is sparse axonal degeneration in this model. Instead, the axon distal to the giant axonal swellings undergoes atrophy, suggesting that neurofilaments play a role in the maintenance of normal axonal caliber.[19]

Myelinopathies

Some neurotoxic compounds specifically damage the myelin sheath of peripheral nerve fibers and leave the axon largely intact. Hexachlorophene, triethyl tin, certain halogenated salicylanilides, and acetyl ethyl tetramethyl tetralin (AETT) belong to this group. The latter compound, once widely used as a fragrance, induces large-diameter fibers to undergo segmental demyelination after weeks of daily topical administration of 10 mg/kg. Demyelination is preceded by an increase in the number of Schmidt-Lanterman incisures per internode. The damaged myelin is removed by hematogenous phagocytes, and daughter Schwann cells remyelinate the denuded axon. AETT has no morphological effect on the remyelination process, or on the behavior of Schwann cells during Wallerian degeneration or regeneration. This suggests that AETT or its metabolite acts directly on the myelin sheath rather than on the Schwann cell perikaryon.[20] Cammer[21] has recently demonstrated that AETT and its putative diacetyl metabolite share with other demyelinating toxins the property of uncoupling mitochondrial respiration *in vitro*, but a causal relationship between this property and demyelination remains to be demonstrated.

RATIONALE FOR A NOSOLOGIC APPROACH TO TOXIC NEUROPATHIES

The classification of toxic neuropathies presented here, which is based on the locus of initial pathological change identified by sensitive morphological methods, presumably reflects the different cellular targets of neurotoxic chemicals. This approach to the nosology of toxic neuropathies is useful because it allows one to predict the pattern of dysfunction and to design appropriate tests to detect subclinical deficits in the cellular systems affected. In addition, a precise understanding of the spatial-temporal pattern of pathological damage facilitates the identification of a particular organelle or system affected by the toxin, and may stimulate the investigator to develop ideas on the mechanism of pathogenesis. Such ideas may then form the basis for biochemical investigations that identify the molecular locus of toxic action.

ACKNOWLEDGEMENTS

Ms. Monica Bischoff is thanked for preparing the figure and Ms. Laurell Edwards for typing the manuscript.

Studies conducted by the author were supported by the following grants: NSF PFR 78-12701, NIOSH OH 00535, ES-02168 and NIOSH OH-00851.

REFERENCES

1. Spencer, P.S. and Schaumburg, H.H. (1980) Experimental and Clinical Neurotoxicology. Williams and Wilkins, Baltimore, Md.
2. Veronesi, B.V. et al. (1980) in Experimental and Clinical Neurotoxicology, Spencer, P.S. and Schaumburg, H.H., eds., Williams and Wilkins, Baltimore, Md., pp. 863-871.
3. Yonezawa, T. et al. (1980) in Experimental and Clinical Neurotoxicology, Spencer, P.S. and Schaumburg, H.H., eds., Williams and Wilkins, Baltimore, Md., pp. 788-802.
4. Spencer, P.S. and Bischoff, M.B. (in press) in Target Organ Toxicity: The Nervous System, Mitchell, C.L., ed., Raven Press, New York.
5. Spencer, P.S. and Ochoa, J. (in press) in Aging and Cell Structure, J. Johnson, ed., Plenum Press, New York.
6. Grover-Johnson, N. and Spencer, P.S. (in press) J. Neuropathol. Exp. Neurol.
7. Jacobs, J.M. (1980) in Experimental and Clinical Neurotoxicology, Spencer, P.S. and Schaumburg H.H., eds., Williams and Wilkins, Baltimore, Md., pp. 102-117.
8. Cho, E.S. et al. (1980) Neurotoxicol. 1, 583.
9. Mendell, J.R. and Sahenk Z. (1980) in Experimental and Clinical Neurotoxicology, Spencer, P.S. and Schaumburg H.H., eds., Williams and Wilkins, Baltimore, Md., pp. 139-160.
10. Krinke, G. et al. (1980) Neurotoxicol. 2.
11. Spencer, P.S. and Schaumburg, H.H. (1976) in Progr. Neuropathol. III, Zimmerman, H., ed., Grune & Stratton, pp. 253-295.
12. Griffin, J. et al. (1977) J. Neuropathol. Exp. Neurol. 36, 603.
13. Chretien, M. et al. (1978) Neurosci. Lett., S9.
14. Lowndes, H.E. and Baker, T. (1980) in Experimental and Clinical Neurotoxicology, Spencer, P.S. and Schaumburg H.H., eds., Williams and Wilkins, Baltimore, Md., pp. 193-205.
15. Zuccarello, M. and Anzil, A.P. (1979) Exp. Neurol.
16. Politis, M.J., Pellegrino, R.G. and Spencer, P.S. (in press) J. Neurocytol.
17. Schaumburg, H.H. and Spencer, P.S. (1980) in Experimental and Clinical Neurotoxicology, Spencer, P.S. and Schaumburg H.H., eds., Williams and Wilkins, Baltimore, Md., pp. 395-406.
18. Chou, S.M. and Hartmann, H.A. (1965) Acta Neuropathol. 4, 590.
19. Griffin, J. and Price, D.L. (1980) in Experimental and Clinical Neurotoxicology, Spencer, P.S. and Schaumburg, H.H., eds., Williams and Wilkins, Baltimore, Md.., pp. 161-177.
20. Spencer, P.S. et al. (1980) in Experimental and Clinical Neurotoxicology, Spencer, P.S. and Schaumburg, H.H., eds., Williams and Wilkins, Baltimore, Md., pp. 296-307.
21. Cammer, W. (1980) Biochem. Pharmacol. 29, 1531.

© 1980 Elsevier/North-Holland Biomedical Press
Mechanisms of Toxicity and Hazard Evaluation
B. Holmstedt, R. Lauwerys, M. Mercier, M. Roberfroid eds

AXONAL FLOW AND TOXIC NEUROPATHIES

BERNARD DROZ and MONIQUE CHRETIEN
Département de Biologie, Commissariat à l'Energie Atomique, Centre d'Etudes Nucléaires de Saclay, B.P. n°2, 91190 Gif sur Yvette (France)

INTRODUCTION

Today it is common knowledge that the nerve cell bodies exert a trophic influence upon their axons and myelin sheaths. Growth and maintenance of nerve fibres in peripheral and central nervous system depend indeed on the supply of macromolecules originating from the neuronal perikaryon in which the synthetic machinery is enclosed. On the basis of experiments on compressed nerves, Weiss and Hiscoe[1] proposed the theory of perpetual growth of the axonal process from the neuronal perikaryon. The advent of radioactive precursors and of high resolution radioautography permitted to visualize the migration of proteins from the cell bodies into and along the axons of intact nerve fibres[2]. Migration rates of 0.6-2.5 mm per day corresponded to slow axoplasmic transport of proteins. The transported labeled proteins were found to be associated with microtubules and neurofilaments in electron microscope radioautographs[3] and with "soluble" proteins in nerve extracts[4]. In contrast most labeled "particulate" fractions which contain membranous proteins, were found to move at rates of 200-400 mm per day with fast axonal transport[4, 5, 6]. Reverse movement, which sends back molecules from axon terminals to neuronal cell bodies at rates of 150-250 mm per day, was referred to as retrograde axonal transport[7, 8].

METHODS FOR INVESTIGATING AXONAL FLOW

Light microscope examination of living nerve fibres combined with time-lapse cinematography permits to study motion of large organelles such as mitochondria and vacuoles [9]. A higher resolution can be achieved by the use of radioactive precursors. Labeled macromolecules traveling along intact axons can be identified by biochemical analysis and located in situ by light and electron microscope radioautography[6, 10, 11] (Figs. 1 and 3). Presynaptic uptake of exogenous markers such as horseradish peroxidase, labeled toxins or lectins is mainly used to trace retrograde axonal transport from the nerve endings to the cell bodies [12, 13].

A different approach consists in interrupting the axonal traffic by nerve section, compression, local coooling or application of antimitotic alkaloids. Under these conditions, axonally transported material accumulates in nerve segments immediately above or below the block [8, 14-16]. The early rates of accumulation of enzymes, or more precisely of the various molecular forms of acetylcholinesterase (AChE)[16], can provide an estimate of the amount of material transported per unit of time with fast orthograde and retrograde transport.

PHENOMENOLOGICAL AND PHYSIOLOGICAL ASPECTS OF AXONAL FLOW

In the course of the past ten years, conjugationof biochemical and ultrastructural data led to the concept that axonally transported macromolecules are enclosed within specific compartments of the axon[17] and move therefore as part of cytological structures[18].

Axoplasmic proteins and slow axonal transport. The axoplasm forms a huge compartment which extends from the cell body to the nerve endings. Most axoplasmic proteins contribute to build up the elements of the axonal cytoskeleton (microtubules, neurofilaments and microfilaments) and to a lesser degree, a variety of soluble enzymes controling energetic metabolism and biosynthesis of the neurotransmitters (e.g. choline acetyltransferase or tyrosine hydroxylase). Kinetic analysis of the labeled axoplasmic proteins reveals that they are transported along the axons at different velocities[11, 18, 19]. Tubulin and neurofilament triplet proteins proceed at rates not exceeding 2 mm per day, whereas actin, myosin and soluble enzymes move at rates of about 4 mm per day.

In young growing animals, perikaryal synthesis of the axoplasmic protein is enhanced as compared with mature animals. Moreover a two- or three-fold acceleration of the migration rates is observed in peripheral axons[3]. When nerves are transsected, regrowth of the regenerating proximal segments is probably limited by slow axoplasmic transport which carries most constituentsrequired for axonal repair and sprouting. Thus the role of slow axoplasmic flow consists mainly in supplying the axonal process with large amounts of proteins required not only for growth and regeneration but also for maintenance of the nerve fibres.

Intraaxonal mitochondrial movements. Microcinematography of living nerve fibres[9] clearly shows that axonal mitochondria are animated by brief and swift motions. In the course of their back and forth shuttle, fusion and fission of the organelles can be occasionally observed. Furthermore net displacements of the axonal mitochondria occur at rates as high as 10 mm per day or more[6, 10]. Study of movements of labeled mitochondria is rendered difficult by the fact that these organelles can incorporate labeled proteins and phospholipids transferred from the smooth endoplasmic reticulum[17, 20]. Thus, transfer of molecular constituents as well as axonal transport of the organelles contribute to rejuvenate the mitochondrial population which produces most of the energy expended by the axon.

Smooth endoplasmic reticulum and fast axonal transport. The use of 1-2μm thick sections impregnated with heavy metals makes it possible to visualize directly the continuous arrangement of the intraaxonal smooth endoplasmic reticulum (SER)[17, 21]. Conventional or high-voltage electron microscope reveals indeed a loosely interconnected system of flattened cisternae and elongated tubules running parallel to the long axis of the nerve fibre. Tubules and cisternae are frequently disposed underneath the axolemmal membrane. In the terminal part of cholinergic axons, small and short tubules which evolve from the SER network are often terminated by small vesicles resembling synaptic vesicles. In neurosecretory and monoaminergic neurons, the continuous network of the SER as well as large granules would contribute to fast axonal transport of macromolecules[22, 23]. Electron microscope radioautography points to the SER as the most radioactive organelle found in the axon when the front wave of labeled glycoproteins or phospholipids shifts rapidly along the axons[21]. Afterwards part of the axonally transported glycoproteins and phospholipids are stored in subaxolemmal tubules and cisternae prior to be incorporated in the axolemma[24]. Contrary to glycoproteins which are strongly anchored in the axolemmal membrane, cholinephosphoglycerides may be transferred from the axon to the adjacent Schwann cells and incorporated into the inner myelin layers[20]. Another part of the axonally transported glycoproteins and phospholipids reaches the axon terminals with the SER and ensures the renewal of membrane constituents in the presynaptic plasmalemma, synaptic vesicles and mitochondria[10, 25].

Thus fast axonal transport dispatches at rates of 200-400 mm per day membrane associated macromolecules from their sites of synthesis to their sites of utilization, in the axolemma or in the specific presynaptic structures. Such a selective distribution of fast axonally transported molecules is remarkably illustrated by the kinetic analysis of the heavy molecular forms of AChE (20 S and 11 S) in chicken sciatic nerve : the 20 S form is entirely mobile and transported to the nerve terminals whereas only 20% of the 11 S form is actually in transit along the axons; the other 80% are immobilized, probably in the axolemma[16, 25].

Membranous bodies and retrograde transport. Recent electron microscopic studies have revealed that the axon possesses independent membranous organelles distinct from the continuous network of the SER[21]. These ovoid or oblong-shaped organelles contain retrogradely transported material[26, 27]. The largest ones may be seen to move backward in living nerve fibres[9]. Retrograde axonal transport drives back mainly membrane-associated macromolecules from the presynaptic nerve endings at rates of 150-250 mm per day. Once sent back to the cell body, retrogradely transported material may be broken down by the lysosomes. There, catabolic products can be recycled and reincorporated into new macromolecules. Other molecules could inform the cell body on the nature, amount and turnover of membrane constituents in nerve terminals and hence influence regulation of macromolecular biosynthesis[13].

Molecular mechanisms of axonal motility. Among the various mechanisms proposed to explain slow axoplasmic transport, passive diffusion of the proteins can be ruled out[18]. The forces propelling slowly the axoplasmic constituents could be generated by either peristalsis of the nerve fibre[28] or actin-myosin interactions[11].

Although the organelles responsible for fast orthograde and retrograde transport are distinct, these two systems of membrane-associated transport have in common physiological characteristics[29]. These rapid displacements are sensitive to temperature. They continue after nerve interruption. These bidirectional movements depend on the Ca^{++}concentration and the production of ATP by mitochondria. Both are more efficiently impeded by batrachotoxin than by antimitotic alkaloids[30]. Yet the molecular mechanisms ensuring bidirectional transport of membrane-associated material are still conjectural. The interaction of myosin and actin microfilaments, by giving rise to activated actomyosin, could indeed generate intraaxonal movements.However axonal motility could also result from sudden assembly and disassembly of actin filament bundles. Rapid polymerisation of actin filament into a meshwork would produce a local and transitory high viscosity of the axoplasm. Conversely rapid disintegration of actin into disperse monomers would increase the axonal fluidity. Thus different modes of axoplasmic motility could coooperate to ensure the traffic of molecules and organelles along the axons[31].

NEUROTOXIC AGENTS AND AXONAL TRANSPORT

Various neurotoxic agents have long been suspected to give rise to peripheral and central neuropathies by altering axonal transport[32]. Prior to demonstrate the involvement of axonal flow in toxic neuropathies, it is important to estimate to what extent other parameters could be altered : perikaryal synthesis of macromolecules, distribution of the axonally transported material, removal and turnover of axonal and synaptic constituents. In other words, it is required to compare the amount and the type of macromolecules transported per unit of time in control and intoxicated animals before the onset of axonal degeneration.

Acute intoxication with antimitotic drugs such as colchicine, vinblastine, vincristine, podophyllotoxin or nocodazole produces an effective block of axonal transport, presumably by acting upon tubulin[33-36]. Yet drugs which are not known to interfer with tubulin assembly such as colchiceine[37] or batrachotoxin[38] are even more potent inhibitors of axonal transport.

Chronic intoxication with industrial substances may give rise to various neuropathies in which axonal transport was investigated.

In neurofibrillary degenerations experimentally induced by aluminium salts, axonal transport was reported to be unchanged[39]. Intoxication by $\beta\beta$'iminodipropionitrile produces axonal swellings in the initial portion of the axon. These enlargements are filled with neurofilaments which accumulate in the proximal segments whereas more distal segments of the axon are atrophied[40]. After the intraspinal injection of ^{35}S-methionine, the analysis of the distribution of labeled cytoskeletal proteins transported along the sciatic nerve shows that most neurofilament triplet proteins are arrested in the proximal portions of the axons and that the axoplasmic convection of tubulin and actin is markedly slackened down in $\beta\beta$'iminodipropionitrile treated animals[41]. In contrast, fast orthograde and retrograde transport are not affected. From this remarkable study,it is concluded that the traffic of the slowly transported axoplasmic proteins, is, to a large extent, halted by $\beta\beta$' iminodipropionitrile. This early arrest of neurofilament triplet proteins could be responsible for proximal axonal balloons[40, 41].

In dying back neuropathies produced by toxic n-hexacarbon compounds, great accumulations of neurofilaments are observed in the enlarged parts of the distal axons[42]. Investigations on axonal flow of labeled proteins shows that the rate of fast transport is more reduced in sensory than motor nerve fibres of severely paralyzed rats previously exposed to n-butyl-ketone[43]. The impediment of fast axonal transport could result from a focal clogging of the axons with neurofilaments. In rats intoxicated with 2,5 hexanediol, electron microscope radioautography indicates that axonally transported labeled proteins pile up in axonal swellings in which they are mainly associated with mitochondria and SER underneath the axolemma[44]. On the basis of these results, it is postulated that fast transported proteins slow down when they pass through axonal swellings.

Other dying back neuropathies give rise to early accumulations of tubulovesicular profiles, referred to as local retentions of the SER[45]. Pioneer studies of Pleasure et al[46] drew attention on the fact that slow axoplasmic flow of proteins persists in cats intoxicated with tri-orthocresylphosphate (TOCP). According to Bradley and Williams[47], TOCP would reduce the "crest" velocities of fast and slow

waves of transported proteins. Intoxication with zinc-pyridinethione produced neuropathies characterized by the early increase of branched tubulovesicular profiles in the terminals, then in the distal portions of motor nerves[48].
In both sensory and motor nerve fibres, the velocity of fast transported proteins is slowed down and retrograde transport of material is delayed and reduced in amount. It is assumed that a failure occurs in the turn-around process taking place in the distal axons of intoxicated rats[49].

The investigation of axonal transport in the genesis of dying back neuropathies resulting from acrylamide intoxication[50] gives rise to conflicting results. Decreased rates of protein synthesis in nervous tissue are reported as results from acute or chronic effects[51-53]. Slow axoplasmic transport of proteins is found to be more frequently interrupted in sensory than in motor nerves[46]; yet other studies[47, 56-58 (55)] do not confirm a clear impairment of slow axoplasmic flow but point to an altered behavior of fast axonally transported proteins such as reduced velocities[47, 55], focal retention of membrane-associated components in distal axons [25,56, 50], lack of utilization or removal of fast transported material[51]. The wide spectrum of the administered doses, the variable exposures to the toxic agent, the species and the age of the intoxicated animals, the clinical severity of the neuropathy, the type of nerve selected and the methods used to estimate axonal transport hightlight "the complexity of investigations of axoplasmic flow in neuropathies"[47]. There is therefore a need to investigate axonal transport in a homogeneous population of nerve fibres at the very early stages of acrylamide neuropathy. For this purpose, forty chickens were given 8 intraperitoneal injections of acrylamide (100 mg per kg body weight) every two days. ^{3}H-lysine was intracerebrally injected to label proteins transported along cranial nerves. The distal portion of the preganglionic axons of the ciliary ganglion were not or hardly affected. Light microscope radioautographs made 7 days after the injection of ^{3}H-lysine showed that the amount of slowly transported proteins was slightly reduced in 40% of the intoxicated chickens[58].
By 3 hours after the injection of ^{3}H-lysine, labeled proteins transported with fast axonal flow were found to pile up in a few axons (compare Fig. 2 with Fig. 1). Electron microscopy allowed us to specify that the clustered labeled proteins were confined to axonal periphery which was occupied by focal accumulations of SER and mitochondria (compare Fig. 3 with Fig. 4). Thus early and discrete disorganization of the axonal SER (Fig. 5 and 6) precedes the onset of the axonal disintegration. The focal arrest of fast transported proteins en route to the presynaptic endings is probably responsible for the diminution of fast transported proteins arriving at nerve endings in about 25% of the axon terminal population.

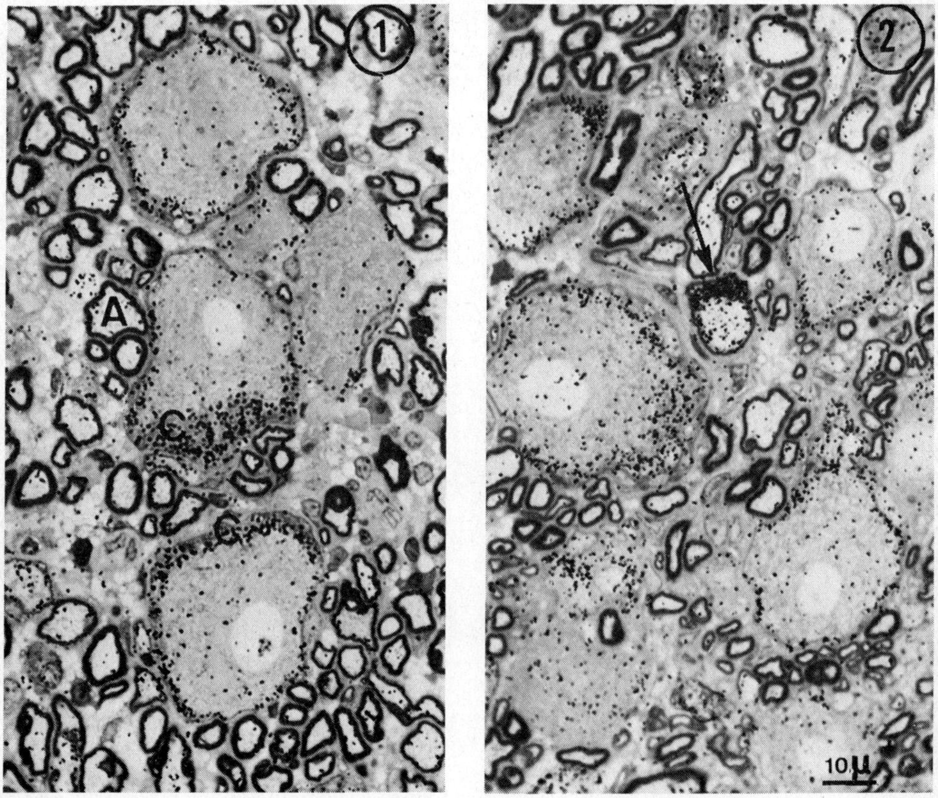

Figs. 1 and 2 Light microscope radioautographs of ciliary ganglia 3 hr after the intracerebral injection of ^{3}H-Lysine in control (Fig. 1) and in acrylamide treated chickens (Fig. 2). In control chickens (Fig. 1), the preganglionic axons (A) are poorly labeled as compared to the giant caliciform nerve endings (C). In acrylamide treated chickens (Fig. 2) the labeling of most preganglionic axons and nerve endings does not differ from control; however a few axons display a focal and intense labeling at their periphery (arrow) whereas some calices show a depressed radioactivity.

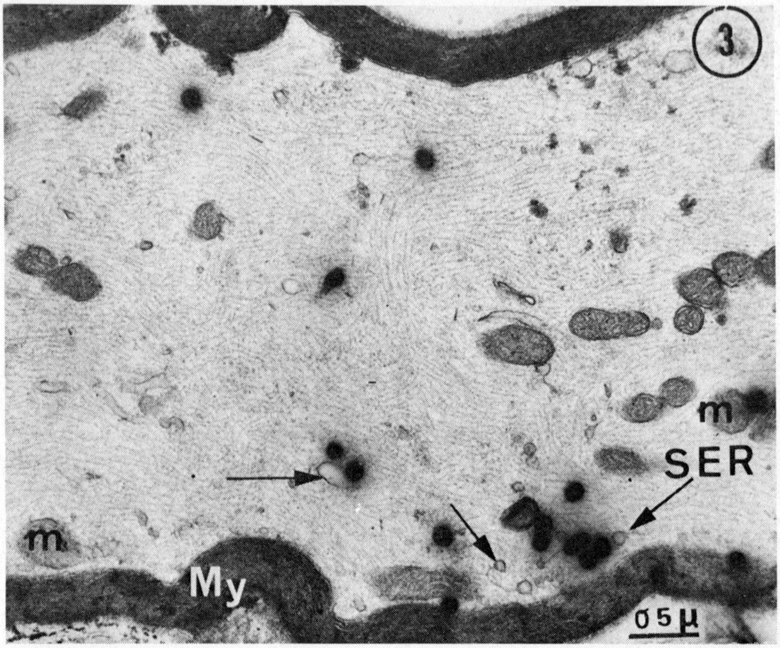

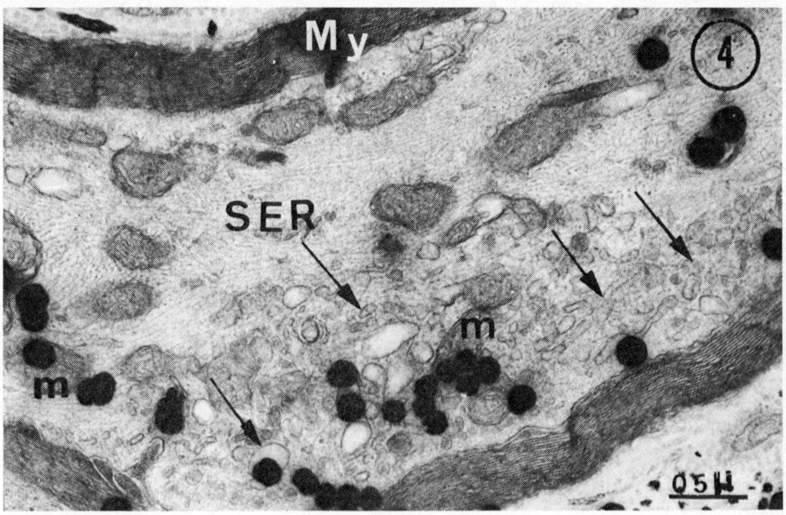

<u>Figs. 3 and 4</u> - Electron microscope radioautographs of preganglionic axons 3 hr after intracerebral injection of ^{3}H-lysine. Fig. 3, control chicken : few silver

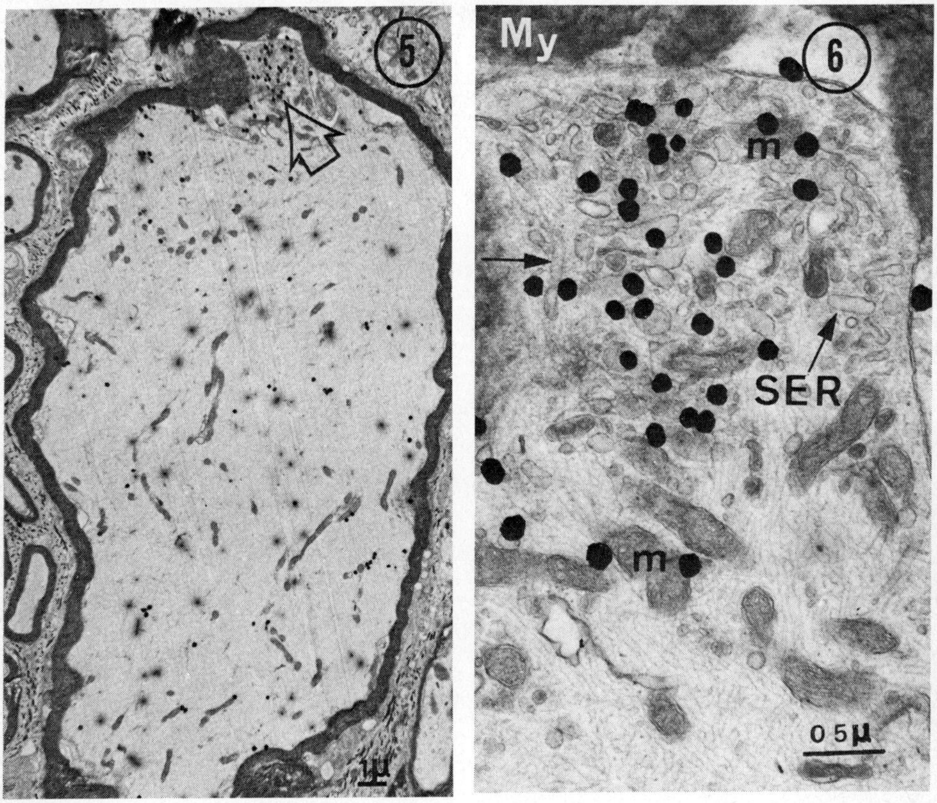

grains are chiefly encountered at the vicinity of S.E.R. tubular and vesicular profiles located underneath the axolemma (oblique arrow) or in the core of the axon (horizontal arrow). Some silver grains are also observed over mitochondria (m). Fig. 4., Acrylamide treated chicken : in an axon which does not show any sign of swelling, silver grains are concentrated at the periphery of the axoplasm, in an area containing abnormal accumulation of tubulo-vesicular profiles of the S.E.R. (arrows) and mitochondria (m). My, myelin.

Figs. 5 and 6. Electron microscope radioautograph of a ballooned myelinated preganglionic axon 3 hr after intracerebral injection of ^{3}H-lysine in acrylamide treated chicken. At a low magnification (Fig. 5), this swelled axon displays a small area in which are accumulated labeled proteins (large arrow). At a high magnification (Fig. 6), the radioactive area shows clumps of silver grains associated with mitochondria (m) and with numerous tubular or vesicular profiles of the S.E.R. (arrows). My, myelin.

When axonal transport was studied by measuring the accumulation of AChE in the sciatic nerve of acrylamide intoxicated rats[15] or chickens[25], the amount of

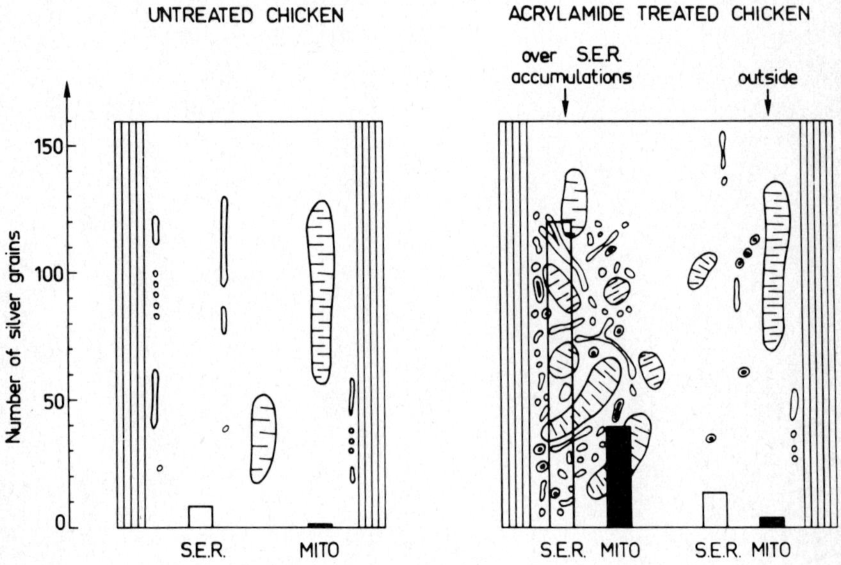

Fig. 7 Relative labeling of S.E.R. profiles and mitochondria in axons of untreated chickens and in highly labeled axons of acrylamide treated chickens.

enzyme transported per unit of time was slightly decreased. Analysis of the molecular forms of AChE allowed Di Giamberardino and Couraud[25] to specify that most of the 20 S form was in fact immobilized in the intoxicated nerves instead of being entirely in transit. It may be concluded that the local retention of fast transported proteins in the disorganized SER of distal axons impedes distribution of membrane components to the terminal part of the axons. By unbalancing the dynamic state of preterminal axons, this defect would contribute to enhance the further axonal and myelin breakdown[57].

In conclusion, the axons behave as dynamic structures and are continuously run by a complex traffic of macromolecules. In well developed neuropathies, great abnormalities of the nerve fibres can impair or interrupt axonal transport. More interestingly, it is important to determine whether axonal transport is altered or not at the very early steps of the toxic neuropathy, that is when the axon displays no or extremely discrete lesions. However, even at these initial stages of the pathological evolution, it is often difficult to decide whether an alteration of axonal transport is the cause or the effect of the developing neurotoxic process.

REFERENCES

1. Weiss, P. and Hiscoe, H. (1948) J. exp. Zool., 107, 315-395.
2. Droz, B. and Leblond, C.P. (1962) Science, 137, 1047-1048.
3. Droz, B. (1965) Symp. Intern. Soc. Cell Biol., 4, 159-173.
4. McEwen, B.S. and Grafstein, B. (1968) J. Cell Biol., 38, 494-508.
5. Lasek, R.J. (1966) Anat. Rec., 154, 373-374.
6. Schonbach, J. and Cuénod, M. (1971) Acta neuropath., Suppl. 5, 153-161.
7. Kristensson, K. and Olsson, Y. (1971) Brain Res., 21, 363-365.
8. Lubinska, L. (1971) Acta Neuropath., Suppl. 5, 136-143.
9. Forman, D.S. Padjen, A.L. and Siggins, G.R. (1977) Brain Res., 136, 197-213.
10. Koenig, H.L., Di Giamberardino and Bennett, G. (1973) Brain Res., 62, 413-417.
11. Lasek, R.J. and Hoffman, P.N. (1976) Cell Motility, Vol. 3, Cold Spring Harbor Laboratory, New York, pp. 1021-1049.
12. Lavail, J.H. and Lavail, M.M. (1974) J. comp. Neurol., 157, 303-358.
13. Thoenen, H., Otten, U. and Schwab, M. (1979) The Neurosciences Fourth Study Program, The M.I.T. Press, Cambridge, Mass., pp. 911-928.
14. Brimijoin, S. and Duck, P.J. (1979) Exp. Neurol., 66, 467-470.
15. Rassol, C.G. and Bradley, W.G. (1978) J. Neurochem., 31, 419-425.
16. Di Giamberardino, L. and Couraud, J.Y. (1978) Nature, 271, 170-172.
17. Droz, B. (1975) The Nervous System, Vol. 1, Raven Press, New York, pp. 111-127.
18. Lasek, R.J. (1980) Trends in Neurosciences, 3, 87-91.
19. Willard, M., Cowan, W.M. and Vagelos, P.R. (1974) Proc. Nat. Acad. Sci. (U.S.A.), 71, 2183-2187.
20. Droz, B., Brunetti, M., Di Giamberardino, L., Koenig, H.L. and Porcellati, G., Soc.,Neurosci. Symp., 4, 344-360.
21. Rambourg, A. and Droz, B. (1980) J. Neurochem., 35, 16-25.
22. Alonso, G. and Assenmacher, I. (1979) Cell Tissue Res., 199, 414-429.
23. Schwartz, J.H. (1979) Ann. Rev. Neurosci., 2, 467-504.
24. Markov, D., Rambourg, A. and Droz, B. (1976) J. Microsc. Biol. Cell., 25, 57-60.
25. Droz, B., Koenig, H.L., Di Giamberardino, L., Couraud, J.Y., Chrétien, M. and Souyri, F. (1979) Progr. Brain Res., 49, 23-44.

26. Tsukita, S. and Ishikawa, H. (1980) J. Cell Biol., 84, 513-530.

27. Lavail, J.H., Rapisardi, S. and Sugino, I.K. (1980) Brain Res., 191, 3-20.

28. Weiss, P. (1974) Actual. Neurophysiol., Vol. 10, Masson, Paris, pp. 91-98/

29. Ochs, S. (1975) The Nervous System, Vol. 1, Raven Press, New York, pp. 137-146.

30. Chan, S.W., Worth, R. and Ochs, S. (1980) J. Neurobiol., 11, 251-264.

31. Lazarides, E. (1976) J. Cell Biol., 68, 202-219.

32. Cavanagh, J.B. (1964) Intern. Rev. Exp. Pathol., 3, 219-267.

33. Kreutzberg, G.W. (1969) Proc. Nat. Acad. Sci. (U.S.A.) 62, 722-728.

34. Flament-Durand, J. and Dustin, P.C. (1972) , Z. Zellforsch., 130, 440-452.

35. Paulson, J.C. and McClure, K.O. (1973) Mol. Pharmacol., 9, 41-50.

36. Samson, F.E. (1976) Ann. Rev. Pharmacol. Toxicol., 16, 143-159.

37. Schönarting, M., Breer, H., Rahmann, H., Siebert, G. and Rösner, H. (1977) Cytobiol., 16, 106-117.

38. Ochs, S. and Worth, R. (1975) Sciences, 187, 1087-1089.

39. Liwnicz, B.H., Kristensson, K., Wieniewski, H.M., Shelanski, M.L. and Terry, R.D. (1974) Brain. Res., 80, 413-420.

40. Clark, A.W., Griffin, J.W. and Price, D.L. (1980) J. Neuropath. Exp. Neurol. 39, 42-55.

41. Griffin, J.W., Hoffman, P.N., Clark, A.W., Carroll, P.T. and Price, D.L. (1978) Science 202, 633-635.

42. Spencer, P.S. and Schaumburg, H.H. (1977) J. Neuropath. Exp. Neurol., 36, 276-299.

43. Mendell, J.R., Sahenk, Z., Saida, K., Weiss, H.S., Russel, S. and Couri, D. (1977) Brain Res., 133, 107-118.

44. Griffin, J.W. and Price, D.L. (1977) J. Neuropath. Exp. Neurol., 36, 603.

45. Jacobs, J.M., Miller, R.H., Whittle, A. and Cavanagh, J.B. (1979) Acta Neuropath., 47, 85-92.

46. Pleasure, D.E., Mishler, K.C. and Engel, W.K. (1969) Science, 166, 524-525.

47. Bradley, W.G. and Williams, M.H. (1973) Brain, 96, 235-246.

48. Sahenk, Z. and Mendell, J.R. (1979) J. Neuropath. Exp. Neurol. 38, 532-550.

49. Sahenk, Z. and Mendell, J.R. (1980) Brain Res., 186, 343-353.

50. Cavanagh, J.B. (1979) Arch. Path. Lab. Med., 103, 659-664.

51. Hashimoto, K. and Ando, K. (1973) Biochem. Pharmacol., 22, 1057-1066.

52. Asbury, A.K., Cox, S.C. and Kanada, D. (1973) Neurology, 23, 406.

53. Schotman, P., Gipon, L., Jennkens, F.G.I. and Gispen, W.H. (1978) J. Neuropath. Exp. Neurol. 37, 820-837.

54. Griffin, J.W., Price, D.L. and Drachman, D.B. (1977) J. Neurobiol., 8, 355-370.

55. Sumner, A., Pleasure, D. and Ciesielka, K. (1976) J. Neuropath. Exp. Neurol., 35-319.

56. Chrétien, M., Souyri, F. and Patey, G. (1979) C.R. Acad. Sci. (Paris) série D, 288, 689-692.

57. Droz, B., Souyri, F., Chrétien, M. and Brunetti, M. (1970) Abstr. First Europ. Neuropath. Meet., Wien, p. 19.

58. Souyri, F., Chrétien, M. and Droz, B. (1980) Brain Res., in press.

59. Chrétien, M., Patey, G., Souyri, F. and Droz, B. (1980) Brain Res., in press.

© 1980 Elsevier/North-Holland Biomedical Press
Mechanisms of Toxicity and Hazard Evaluation
B. Holmstedt, R. Lauwerys, M. Mercier, M. Roberfroid eds

DELAYED NEUROTOXICITY INDUCED BY ORGANOPHOSPHORUS COMPOUNDS - AREAS OF UNDERSTANDING AND IGNORANCE

M.K. JOHNSON
Biochemical Mechanisms Section, Toxicology Unit, Medical Research Council Laboratories, Carshalton, Surrey, United Kingdom.

INTRODUCTION

Many organophosphorus esters inhibit the activity of the enzyme acetylcholinesterase. The acute toxic effects of organophosphorus pesticides and the so-called nerve agents arise from this inhibition[1]. However, some esters produce a different toxic effect not related to any ability to inhibit acetylcholinesterase. This is delayed neurotoxicity. Anticholinesterase activity ranges from high to negligible among the large number of neurotoxic esters which are now known. The review[2] lists over 200 esters which had been screened up to that time and includes compounds produced as potential plasticisers, flame-proofers and hydraulic fluids as well as candidate pesticides. Extensive clinical, pathological and experimental descriptions of the syndrome have been published; these reports have been summarised and reviewed[3,4,31]. The essential features are as follows.

Neurotoxic effects are not seen until 8-14 days after ingestion of the toxic agent, but then ataxia and weakness in the lower limbs develops. This progresses to paralysis, which in severe cases affects the upper limbs also. Children and young animals are less severely affected than adults and recovery is slow and seldom complete in adults. Cats, hens and a number of larger species are affected by a single dose[5]. Repeated dosing does not reduce the delay in onset to less than 8 days from the first dose. It is difficult to produce delayed neurotoxic effects in rodents even by repeated dosing, and hens have become the species of choice in laboratory tests. Early histological examinations used methods showing predominantly degeneration of the fatty myelin sheath surrounding long nerve axons and names such as Organophosphate Demyelinating Disease are still erroneously used, in spite of later work which showed that the nerve axon itself was primarily affected and damage to myelin was secondary[6]. Recent studies[7] have shown that degeneration is a multi-focal process commencing in the distal region of some long axons. It is therefore not strictly analogous to Wallerian degeneration. Although the abnormalities seen in the distal region are different, the pattern is similar to that described as central-peripheral distal axonopathy by Spencer & Schaumberg[8] in their account of hexacarbon neuropathy.

KNOWN STEPS IN THE BIOCHEMICAL MECHANISM

1. Phosphorylation of neurotoxic esterase. Until recently the first indicator of neurotoxic potential in an unfamiliar organophosphate was a positive chronic abnormality of gait observed in clinical tests; this may be detected before any histological signs are visible. Although there are degrees of severity of ataxia the test gave essentially all-or-none results. Repeated dosing schedules revealed that some compounds were neurotoxic, although not in a single dose[9,10]. There was, however, no way of deciding whether any compound was genuinely non-neurotoxic. Aldridge[11] pointed out that neurotoxic organophosphorus esters either inhibit esterases directly or are metabolized in vivo to form inhibitory products. Guesses have been made over many years suggesting that a particular esterase was the initial target for neurotoxic compounds. Each guess has been disproved by a programme of testing[12,13].

Since neurotoxic compounds such as DFP (di-isopropyl phosphorofluoridate) and Mipafox do not last more than a few hours in the body it seemed reasonable to look for an early reaction which would initiate a series of events culminating in ataxia. The proposition was made that phosphorylation of a protein in the central nervous system is an essential prerequisite for the development of the lesion[14]. Analytical methods have been developed to measure only a selected few of all the proteins in normal brain that can react with a radio-labelled neurotoxic agent, $DF^{32}P$. Using this analytical method the brains of chickens treated with neurotoxic and non-neurotoxic organophosphorus compounds were examined; neurotoxic compounds reduced appreciably the phosphorylation of the selected site by $DF^{32}P$, whereas non-neurotoxic compounds had little effect[14]. During the course of this investigation compounds were found that produced significant reduction in labelling, but which had been classified by previous workers as non-neurotoxic; a reinvestigation with multiple dosing showed that a typical delayed neurotoxicity was produced. For neurotoxic effects to be produced, more than 70% of the "neurotoxic protein" must be phosphorylated shortly after dosing.

The fact that the "neurotoxic protein" is an esterase was shown as follows. It is known that the rate of phosphorylation of an esterase by an organophosphorus compound is greatly reduced when an appropriate substrate is present. Numerous esters were therefore examined for their influence on the rate of phosphorylation of the "neurotoxic protein". Only phenyl phenylacetate significantly diminished the rate and the "neurotoxic protein" was subsequently shown to hydrolyse this ester[15]. Active brain enzymes hydrolysing this ester had previously been identified but they were very sensitive to some non-neurotoxic inhibitors such as paraoxon and TEPP[16] and these enzymes were shown not to be associated with delayed neurotoxicity[13]. The presence of the esterase activity of the "neurotoxic protein" can therefore be detected only after selective inhibition of the similar but irrelevant enzymes. This particular esterase activity was shown to be inhibited in vivo by neurotoxic compounds and not inhibited by non-neurotoxic compounds[15, 17,2]. The enzyme is now referred to as neurotoxic esterase (NTE) and its substrate and inhibitor specificity in vitro has been described in detail[18]. There is an excellent correlation between blocking of the labelling site by a wide variety of compounds both in vivo and in vitro and inhibition of NTE activity[17]. For routine assay of NTE phenyl valerate is a more convenient substrate in terms of both sensitivity and specificity: the optimum assay conditions are described by Johnson[19] but 6 mg of brain tissue are required, not 0.6 as erroneously stated there. Under these conditions NTE hydrolyses about 2400 nmoles of substrate/min/g brain while the rates in spinal cord and sciatic nerve are about 550 and 100 respectively. The proportion of NTE to total paraoxon-resistant esterases is about 65, 45 and 30% respectively in these tissues so that the differential assay is essential in each case and the precision of assays with hen peripheral nerve is poor.

2. "Aging" of inhibited NTE. The intoxication process is unusual in that the metabolic disturbance depends on the nature of the chemical group which becomes bound to the esteratic site of NTE: it does not depend on the loss of catalytic activity per se[17,20]. Thus inhibitors of NTE can be divided into 2 groups: those in Group A (phosphates, phosphonates and phosphoramidates) are neurotoxic while

those in Group B (carbamates, sulphonyl fluorides and phosphinates) are not only not neurotoxic but prior administration of Group B inhibitors to hens protects them from the neurotoxic effects of challenge doses of Group A compounds. For neurotoxic effects to occur, inhibition of NTE is the first of 2, or possibly 3, essential steps. Step (2) is conversion of the inhibited enzyme to a modified form bearing an ionised acidic group on the phosphorus atom (analogous to "aging" of inhibited cholinesterase). Reaction (2) could not happen after inhibition by Group B compounds (see Fig.1). For NTE inhibited by a variety of OP esters the aging process has proved to be extraordinarily rapid[21,22] and the molecular basis of this reaction is being

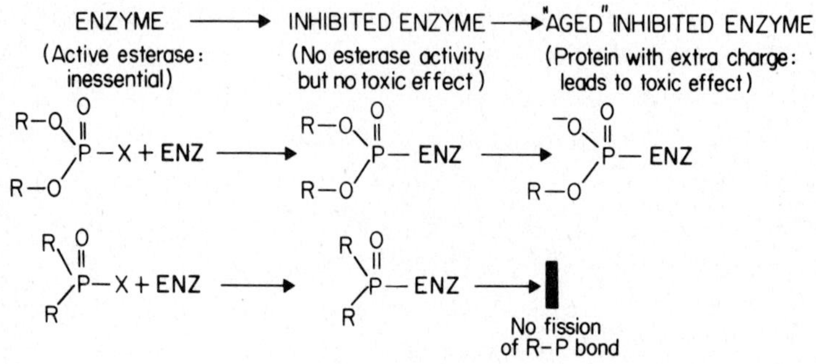

Fig. 1. Contrast of the events following the inhibiton of NTE by (a) A phosphate (Group A, neurotoxic) and (b) A phosphinate (Group B, protective).

investigated. One conclusion from the discovery of rapid aging is that prospects for therapy using rationally designed oximes to attack the phosphorylated site seem doomed to failure since nucleophilic reactivators are unable to regnerate active esterase from aged enzymes.

I proposed that nerve degeneration ultimately occurs because of the formation of the charged group attached to the NTE molecule proposing that this charge upsets a normal physiological process of the neurone[20,23]. However, the possibiliy that Reaction (3) (below) is the significant event must now be considered.

3. <u>Transfer to a secondary site of group lost during aging</u>. During the aging of NTE which had been inhibited by either tritiated DFP

or di-n-pentyl 2,2-dichlorovinyl phosphate it was found that the label associated with the alkoxy groups which were removed from phosphorus was not liberated into solution but became attached to another macromolecular site[21,22]. This was in contrast to the liberation of small molecular-weight products in solution after inhibition of brain cholinesterases[21]. Without a complete range of radio-labelled neurotoxic esters it is impossible to show whether this efficient transfer occurrs when every variety of chemical group takes part in the aging reaction. My view has been that this is unlikely for, say, phosphoramidates or for phenoxy substituents. However, if Reaction (3) does occur when NTE is inhibited by any neurotoxic ester then modification of the receiving site could be proposed as the event which precipitates neuropathy rather than formation of the charged group on the aged enzyme. Recent studies in our laboratory using a phosphonodifluoridate to generate phosphonofluoro-inhibited NTE which could only liberate fluoride ion if it aged, appear to give indirect support to this alternative mechanism. The compound is protective in vivo like inhibitory phosphinates. However, we do not yet know whether the inhibited NTE obtained with this compound does actually age.

PHYSIOLOGICAL DISORDERS FOLLOWING ATTACK ON NTE - AN AREA OF IGNORANCE.

Inhibition by benzyl sulphonyl fluoride or by some phosphinates has been maintained by repeated dosing during 2 weeks with no overt toxic effect[17,20] so if the esteratic activity of NTE has a role in normal physiological processes this role is not vital. No observation has been made on hens kept for a lifetime with NTE inhibited by a protective compound. Clearly the typical neuropathy will not occur but whether any disorder of the neuron might ultimately develop is not known. It follows from the absence of neuropathic effects of the protective NTE inhibitors above that searching for the normal physiological substrate of NTE, if indeed one exists, will not help explain the disorder.

In 1975 I discussed several areas (protein and lipid metabolism, copper metabolism, axonal flow) which had been explored without discovery of any insight into mechanism of neuropathy[5]. A recent paper[24] claims effects on axonal flow in the optic nerve have been seen shortly after intraocular injection of tri-ortho-cresyl phosphate. The experiments seem to appear to suffer from such major defects in design that the result should be treated with caution especially since better-designed experiments (see refs 128-130 of Ref 5) have previously shown nil effects. Thus (a) substantial volumes of organophosphate in solvent were injected which must have produced abnormally high local concentrations, (b) the compounds used all require metabolic activation before they exert their toxic effect but the extent (if any) of such activation in the eye was not evaluated and (c) the species chosen was the rat which is not susceptible to organophosphate-induced neuropathy.

A number of experiments have been done dosing hens with altered immune status or injecting nervous tissue from ataxic hens into other hens[25]. No evidence was obtained of an involvement of the immune system in the genesis of neuropathy.

The idea[20,23] that the negative charge on aged inhibited NTE disrupts processes normally controlled by cAMP-modulated protein kinases has found no support. I have found[26] no influence of ATP ± cAMP on the rate of phosphorylation of NTE by [^{32}P]-DFP and Alexander & Rodknight[27] using radio-labelled ATP found that preincubation with DFP did not affect labelling of certain cyclic-nucleotide sensitive sites in brain.

NEUROTOXIC ESTERASE - ITS LOCATION AND BEHAVIOUR

NTE is widely distributed in the nervous system and not localised in any specialised region[28]. In hen brain it is firmly bound to small membranes in sub-cellular fractions[29] but the source of these membranes is not clear. The possibility that they are synaptic remains but is less attractive now that it has been shown[7] that degeneration of neurones commences in the distal region but not actually at the terminus of an affected axon.

NTE can hydrolyse a wide variety of ester but not amide substrates[18]. K_m for phenyl phenylacetate is about 0.1mM (Johnson, previously unpublished) so that the use of phenyl valerate (K_m about 10 mM) as substrate of choice reflects no special affinity but the more selective response with this substrate in assays where NTE is mixed with a number of other esterases. It is a pity that the selectivity of thiophenyl, naphthyl, umbelliferyl, etc. esters is so poor[18] that histochemical procedures cannot aid in determining the regional or intracellular distribution. There has been some progress in attempts to solubilise active NTE[30] and to purify radio-labelled inhibited NTE (by Dr. D.G. Williams in my laboratory). There is therefore a growing possibility of preparing an antibody to NTE and of using this in distribution studies.

NTE appears more stable to extremes of pH than are the other brain esterases and, again in contrast to the other esterases, the pH/activity, pH/inhibition and pH/aging profiles are all remarkably flat with only modest decline over the range pH 8 down to 5.2 (Johnson, previously unpublished and Ref.21).

NEUROTOXICITY TESTING - EXPLOITING UNDERSTANDING

The performance of tests. The chronic lesion can now be assessed in terms of an acute event, inhibition of NTE. Moreover this acute event can be measured quantitatively and neurotoxic potential can be graded on the basis of an assay of NTE activity in brain tissue taken from hens one day after dosing[15,2]. The gain over the previous all-or-none three-week observation test is obvious. It must be realised, however, that measurements of NTE inhibition do not correlate with the clinical state of dosed birds ON THE DAY OF ASSAY but with their state 7-14 days later. Also during the delay period resynthesis of NTE is considerable[20] so that with single-dose experiments it is possible to have ataxic hens whose brain and cord NTE activity is not highly inhibited at that time[44]. Inhibition of at least 70% of NTE is a prerequisite to development of frank neuropathy 1-2 weeks later so that estimates of safety margin can often be made on the basis of the degree of NTE inhibition observed at doses producing no overt effect. Many examples of dose/response data are available in Ref. 2 and the absolute non-neurotoxicity of triphenyl phosphate and symmetrical meta-substituted phenyl phosphates has been demonstrated by nil response in the dose/assay test[2,32,33].

In the case of chronic dosing where compound is administered daily until neuropathy develops the situation is complex since the final 5-10 doses have probably not contributed to the severity of the clinical state which is being viewed on any particular day. This problem confounds attempts to calculate the effective cumulative dose. The problem is most marked in those experiments where ataxia is seen comparatively early so that the 7-14 day lag period is an appreciable proportion of the total dosing period. It is, of course, also necessary, if assays of NTE and clinical assessment are to be correlated, that observation of dosed birds should be continued for 3 weeks after administration of compounds has been halted.

It is now clear that in a chronic dose situation inhibition of NTE and resynthesis of enzyme brings about an equilibrium point of residual activity. The equilibrium point and the time needed to come to it will depend on the dose (as a fraction of a single effective dose) and the persistence of active material in the body. Monitoring of NTE levels of both brain and spinal cord once a week during a chronic dosing regime supplies much information as to the prospective clinical effect and, as with single-dose experiments, provides quantitative data for the situation of a nil clinical response. Most multi-dose studies reported so far[34-39] with a variety of neurotoxic esters indicate that clinical neuropathy was only seen when a high-point of inhibition was obtained. When daily dosing was maintained for 3-10 weeks the threshold of persistent NTE inhibition which correlates with clinical neuropathy seems to be about 50% in spinal cord or 60% in brain[34,35]. This is not far short of the inhibition needed to cause neuropathy after a single dose. Out of 5 different reported studies only one[39] claims that neuropathy can be associated with prolonged low levels of inhibition. I was unable to reproduce this result[34] and it is hoped that the Round Table Discussion on Neurotoxicity Testing at this International Congress may illuminate this discrepancy. Strain differences in the hens do not seem to account for it.

Paper predictions of neurotoxicity. Much data on the response of NTE in vivo to adminstration of test compounds has been assembled and structure-activity relationships have been worked out in more detail than has been possible hitherto[2,18]. Some clear principles of prediction of delayed neurotoxicity potential from inspection of structural formula have been enumerated[2,33]. For triaryl phosphates the original reference[2] should be consulted but for potential pesticides the essentials are repeated below. The principles do not indicate the effective dose or rank compounds according to potency in mg/kg but indicate the likelihood of a delayed neurotoxic effect at the LD_{50}. If we consider the spectrum of OP esters $R^1R^2P.(O \text{ or } S).X$ then:

(A) Factors which INCREASE delayed neurotoxicity potential more than acute toxicity are:

(1) Choice of phosphonates rather than analogous phosphates.

(2) Increase in chain-length or hydrophobicity of R^1 and R^2.

(3) A leaving group X which does not sterically hinder approach to the active site of NTE.

(B) Factors which DECREASE the comparative potential are:

(1) The converse of (A) 1-3.

(2) Choice of R or X groups which are very bulky (naphthyloxy) or non-planar.

(3) Choice of a nitrophenyl group at X (? a steric effect).

(4) Choice of comparatively more hydrophilic X groups (oximes or heterocyclics).

(5) Choice of thioether linkages at X.

Considering these factors we can see why Malathion and Diazinon are both far below the neurotoxicity hazard line; why, in its homologous series, only dichlorvos is not neurotoxic at LD_{50}; why EPN, a phosphonothioate with a hydrophobic phenyl group at R^1 is neurotoxic even with a 4-nitrophenyl leaving group and why it is not surprising that other phenylphosphonothioates such as Desbromoleptophos or Cyanofenphos are also neurotoxic. The apparent non-neurotoxicity of the ethyl analogue of Leptophos[40] seems to contradict (A.2) above but when we consider such a molecule has two bulky aromatic groups attached to phosphorus (one directly and one through oxygen) then factor (B.2) suggests that although the methoxy group of Leptophos oxon may permit a "fit" at the active site the greater congestion with an ethoxy analogue hinders access markedly.

Monitoring Leucocyte NTE. The detection of low levels of "NTE-like" activity in lymphocytes and platelets[45,46] raised hopes that man and/or animals could be monitored easily for exposure to neurotoxic agents. However the response of this activity to chronic dosing bears no relation to nervous tissue NTE response[35].

EXTRAPOLATION TO MAN

We have characterised NTE in a number of human post-mortem nervous tissue samples[28,41]. It responds to inhibitors rather similarly to the hen brain enzyme but I_{50}s may vary over a 3-fold range and the ratio $I_{50}^{AChE}/I_{50}^{NTE}$ varies over an 8-fold range for the 2 species when a wide variety of inhibitors are studied. There is a remarkable similarity of the ratio $I_{50}^{AChE}/I_{50}^{NTE}$ and the ratio LD_{50}/ Neurotoxic dose when values obtained with hens are compared[41]. Certain caveats are attached to this statement which interested readers may study in the original article. However, we did conclude that these in vitro ratios derived from appropriate active inhibitors (i.e. NOT thionates) could be used predictively as a guide to say whether or not a new compound would be neurotoxic below the LD_{50}. We still do not know why EPN oxon (resolved isomers) does not fit this simple relationship[26]. We also pointed out that human sensitivity to neurotoxic effects compared with sensitivity to lethal effects might be more or less in man than in hen according to which way the ratio varied. There is no direct way of assessing whether the threshold of 70% inhibiton found in hen pertains also to man. If post-mortem brain and spinal cord samples could be obtained in any regrettably successful suicide case involving ingestion of OP pesticides it might be possible to assess the degree of inhibition of NTE compared with that of AChE (the latter presumably very high in such a case) and to compare this with the inhibitory powers measured in vitro.

CONCLUSION

It is only recently that the benefits to toxicology of detailed mechanistic studies have begun to be appreciated. This paper has illustrated these benefits by reference to dose/response evaluation, to assessing the hazard of repeated dosing by means of extrapolation from the NTE response to a single dose, and to relating hen and human enzymic data.

As an esterase NTE is interesting for the unique facility of the aging reaction after inhibition by OP esters. The ability to assay it is proving valuable in toxicity testing but we are still a long way from understanding either the normal function of the protein or the processes which follow after aging and which lead to axon degeneration. NTE itself deserves more study and we must refine our procedures and hope both to purify NTE and to locate it precisely within neurons before we can advance much further along the pathway of understanding. The question as to whether all the pathological events occur within the axon near the site of degeneration or whether degeneration is a response to events in the neuronal cell body is entirely open although the work of Lowndes and Riker[42,43] who succeeded in producing a (very mild) unilateral neuropathy in one leg of cats injected intra-arterially with DFP suggests that the former possibility may be true.

REFERENCES

1. Heath, D.F. (1961) Organophosphorus poisons. London: Pergamon Press.
2. Johnson, M.K. (1975a) Arch. Toxicol., 34, 259-288.
3. Davies, D.R. (1963) Neurotoxicity of organophosphorus compounds. Handbuch der experimentellen Pharmakologie, Erganzungswerk, vol.XV (ed. G.D. Koelle), pp.860-882. Berlin-Heidelberg-New York: Springer.
4. Cavanagh, J.B. (1973) Crit. Rev. Toxicol., 2, 365-417.
5. Johnson, M.K. (1975b) Crit. Rev. Toxicol., 3, 289-316.
6. Cavanagh, J.B. (1954) J. Neurol. Neurosurg. Psychiat., 17 163-172.
7. Bouldin, T.W. and Cavanagh, J.B. (1979) Amer. J. Path., 94, 241-252 and 253-270.
8. Spencer, P.S. and Schaumberg, H.H. (1976) In Progress in Neuropathol. (Ed. H.M. Zimmerman). Greene & Stratton, New York 252-295.
9. Henschler, D. and Bayer, H.H. (1958) Naumyn-Schmiedebergs Arch. exp. Path. Pharmak., 233, 512-517.
10. Bondy, H.F., Field, E.J., Worden, A.N. and Hughes, J.P.W. (1960) Brit. J. industr. Med., 17, 190-200.
11. Aldridge, W.N. (1954) Biochem. J., 56, 185-189.
12. Davison, A.N. (1953) Brit. J. Pharmacol., 8, 212-216.
13. Aldridge, W.N. and Barnes, J.M. (1966) Biochem. Pharmacol., 15, 541-548 and 549-554.
14. Johnson, M.K. (1969a) Biochem. J., 111, 487-495.
15. Johnson, M.K. (1969b) Biochem. J., 114, 711-717.
16. Poulsen, E. and Aldridge, W.N. (1964) Biochem. J., 90, 182-189.
17. Johnson, M.K. (1970) Biochem. J., 120, 523-531.
18. Johnson, M.K. (1975c) Biochem. Pharmacol., 24, 797-805.
19. Johnson, M.K. (1977) Arch. Toxicol., 37, 113-115.
20. Johnson, M.K. (1974) J. Neurochem., 23, 785-789.
21. Clothier, B. and Johnson, M.K. (1979a) Biochem. J., 177, 549-558.
22. Clothier, B. and Johnson, M.K. (1980) Biochem. J., 185, 739-747.
23. Johnson, M.K. (1976a) Fed. Proc. 35, 73-74.
24. Reichert, B.L. and Abou-Donia, M.B. (1980) Molec. Pharmacol., 17, 56-60.

25. Watanabe, P.G. and Sharma, R.P. (1977) Arch. env. Contam. Toxicol. 6, 233-240

26. Johnson, M.K. (1980) In Progress in Neurotoxicology. (Eds. L. Manzo, Lery, N., Lacasse, Y. and Roche, L.) Pergamon Press, Oxford. pp. 223-236.

27. Alexander, D.R. and Rodknight, R. (1974) Biochem. J., 137, 253-262.

28. Lotti, M. and Johnson, M.K. (1980) J. Neurochem., 34, 747-749.

29. Richardson, R.J., Davis, C.S. and Johnson, M.K. (1979) J. Neurochem., 32, 607-615.

30. Davis, C.S. and Richardson, R.J. (1980) Toxicol. app. Pharmacol., 53, A147 (Abstr. 441).

31. Bradley, W.A. (1976) In Pesticide-induced delayed neurotoxicity. (Ed. R.L. Baron: EPA-600/1-76-025), U.S. E.P.A. Office of Res. & Dev. N.C., U.S.A. pp. 84-101.

32. Wills, J.H., Barron, K., Groblewski, G.E., Benitz, K.F. and Johnson, M.K. (1979) Toxicol. Lett., 4, 21-24.

33. Johnson, M.K. (1976b) In Pesticide-induced delayed neurotoxicity. (Ed. R.L. Baron: EPA-600/1-76-025), U.S. E.P.A. Office of Res. & Dev. N.C., U.S.A. pp. 70-83.

34. Johnson, M.K. and Lotti, M. (1980) Toxicol. Lett., 5, 99-102.

35. Lotti, M. and Johnson, M.K. (1980) Arch. Toxicol. In the press.

36. Hussain, M.A. and Oloffs, P.C. (1979) J. env. Sci. Hlth., B14, 367-382.

37. Sprague, G.L. and Castles, T.R. (1979) Fed. Proc., 38, 679. (Abstr. 2378) and private communication.

38. Ohkawa, H. Private communication.

39. Olajos, E.J., DeCaprio, A.P. and Rosenblum, I. (1978) Ecotoxicol. env. Safety, 2, 383-399.

40. Hollingshaus, J.G., Sameer, A-E-H. and Fukuto, T.R. (1979) J. ag. Fd. Chem., 27, 1197-1201.

41. Lotti, M. and Johnson, M.K. (1978) Arch. Toxicol., 41, 215-221.

42. Lowndes, H.E., Baker, T. and Riker, W.F.Jr.(1974) Eur.J.Pharmacol., 29, 66-73.

43. Glazer, E.J., Baker, T. and Riker, W.F.Jr.(1978) J. Neurocytol., 7, 741-758.

44. Johnson, M.K. (1978) Arch. Toxicol., 41, 107-110.

45. Dudek, B.R., Barth, M., Gephart, L., Huggins, J. and Richardson, R.J. (1979) Toxicol. app. Pharmacol., 48, A198.

46. Dudek, B.R. and Richardson, R.J. (1980) Toxicol. app. Pharmacol., 53, A145 (Abst. 433).

Mechanisms of Toxicity and Hazard Evaluation
B. Holmstedt, R. Lauwerys, M. Mercier, M. Roberfroid eds

CLINICAL AND EXPERIMENTAL WORK IN NEUROTOXICITY

A. Bischoff
Dept. of Neurology, Univ. of Berne Med. School, Inselspital, CH 3010 Berne (Switzerland)

INTRODUCTION

Two models of diseases of the nervous system due to toxic substances with similarity between their clinical features and striking differencies in their morphologic reaction are demonstrated. Although in both conditions the common pathological effect is axonal degeneration, high resolution studies of peripheral nerve tissue by electron microscopy reveal evident differentiation of the pathogenetic mechanisms.

TRI-ORTHO-CRESYL PHOSPHATE INTOXICATION

Clinical Picture. In 1940, a group of 89 soldiers of the Swiss army was involved in an outbreak of intoxication related to the consumption of cooking oil which by an accident was contaminated with machine-gun oil containing tri-ortho-cresyl phosphate (TOCP). TOCP, an aryl phosphate that is derived from phosphorylation of phenols, is a small molecule with a molecular weight of 368 which is soluble in lipids and lipid solvents. (Fig. 1)

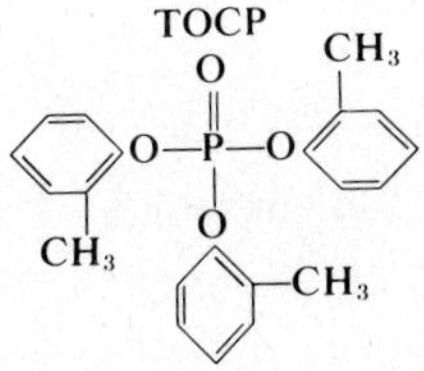

Fig. 1. Chemical formula of tri-ortho-cresyl phosphate.

TOCP is a component of industrial tri-cresyl phosphate which contains about 30 per cent of TOCP. Tri-cresyl phosphate today has a wide variety of uses in the industry, particularly as a plasticizer and as a high temperature lubricant. It shows the same chemical base as organophosphorus compounds employed as insecticides.

As it has been evaluated by Staehelin[1], who first examined the diseased soldiers, intoxication was produced by only 0.12 g of TOCP, i.e. approximately by 2 mg per kilogram body weight. A severe neurological disorder developed after ingesting various amounts between at least 0.5 g and 35 g. 95 per cent of the soldiers who consumed the contaminated cookies were affected.

The clinical course, according to a careful review of all case histories, was strikingly uniform. (Fig. 2).

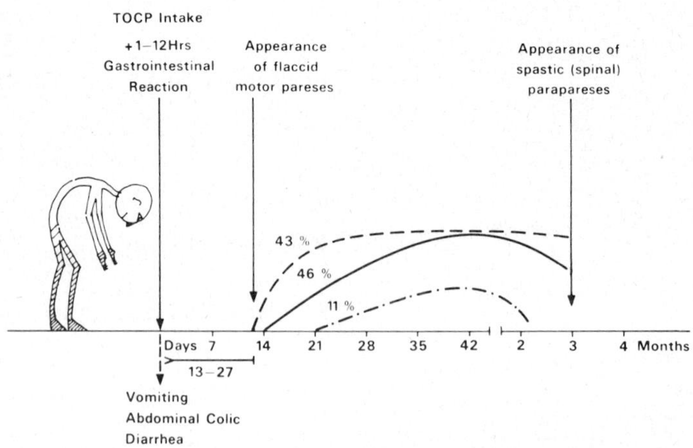

Fig. 2. Diagram of the clinical course of tri-ortho-cresyl phosphate intoxication in 89 young men.

After a lapse of time of 1 to 12 hours after the intake of the toxic substance, gastrointestinal disturbances were experienced by all patients. Vomiting was present in 90 per cent of the affected subjects. It made it difficult to obtain a correlation between the calculated intake of TOCP and the severity of the neurotoxic reaction. Abdominal cramps and diarrhea were also frequent. They lasted for 24 to 36 hours. Then, after a latency of 13 to 27 days, initiated one to two days before by muscle cramps and painful paresthesias in the legs, a flaccid paresis developed distally in the legs, involving first the toes and the foot extensor muscles. In 11 per cent of the cases, who showed as a whole the longest latency, functional defects remained restricted to the slight distal pareses. In 46 per cent of the cases the motor weakness spread to the intrinsic muscles of the hands, and in 43 per cent to the thighs and the muscles of the pelvic girdle. A marked atrophy of the intrinsic muscles of the hand and feet became apparent. The ankle jerk was absent in all patients with neurological signs, but sensory functions remained almost intact, and cranial nerves were also spared. Many patients showed marked vasomotor disturbances with coolness of the feet, as well as sweating abnormalities. In 26 per cent there was a paresis of the urinary bladder, and a certain number of patients complained of transient impotence. Blood examination and kidney and liver function showed the results within normal limits.

The maximum of pareses was reached after 3 to 4 weeks. Then, remission of the peripheral neuropathy occurred. After three months, however, signs of spinal cord damage, such as spasticity and ataxia became apparent in many cases.

10 patients with slight pareses recovered completely, 52 patients retained a walking disability invalidating the more severely affected men by 50 per cent and more.

Experimental Pathology. Since pathologic studies on patients had not clarified the site and nature of the structural damage produced by TOCP, experimental investigations into various animals like chicken, cats, baboons, squirrel monkeys were performed by many investigators (Barnes and Denz[2], Beresford and Glees[3], Cavanagh[4], Cavanagh and Patangia[5], Hern[6]). In previous own studies (Bischoff [7, 8]), TOCP intoxication was produced in chicken. 1.5 ml per kilogram body weight of pure industrial TOCP was administered by a stomach tube in a single dose. After a regular interval of 10 to 12 days a distal paresis became manifest which was apparent by an unstable gait and the tendency to sit down on the heel for pecking at the food. Already one day after the appearance of the earliest clinical signs, histologic abnormalities in the sciatic nerve were visible. They were confined to single nerve fibres and appeared as focal ballooning and disruption of the axon. (Fig. 3.). The histologic feature definitely could be discerned as representing axonal degeneration. Demyelination could not be observed.

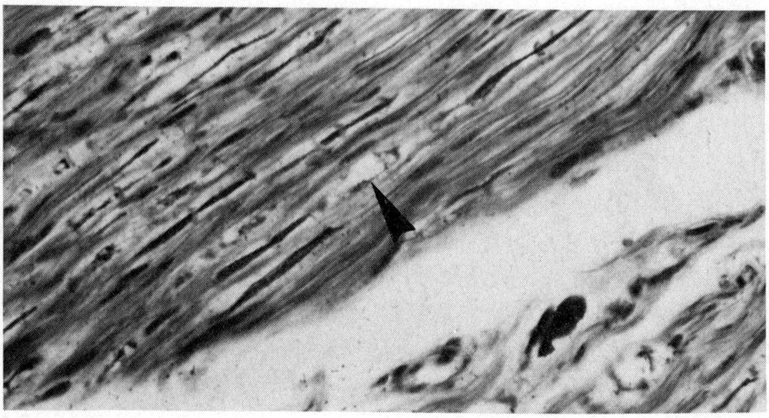

Fig. 3. Chicken sciatic nerve showing axonal degeneration in single nerve fibres characterized by focal ballooning of the axon (arrow). Silver staining x 400

By electron microscopic analysis the axonal degeneration (Fig. 4) showed a characteristic feature indicated by an accumulation of vesicular and tubular profiles coinciding with a desintegration of the normal filamentous organelles (Bischoff[7], Prineas[9]).

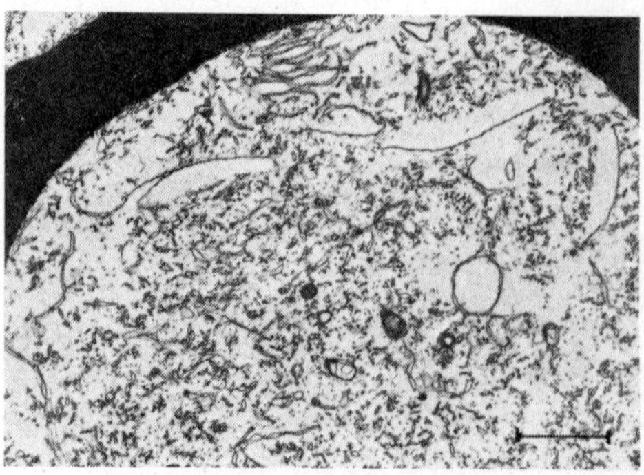

Fig. 4. Transverse section througha myelinated nerve fibre showing an increase of vesicular and tubular elements of the endoplasmic reticulum.

Similar changes could be observed also in the long tracts of the lumbar spinal cord already by the second day after the appearance of clinical paresis. Here, the accumulation of membraneous and granular pathological material was strikingly predominating in distended distal endings of the central axon (Bischoff[8]). Figs. 5 and 6.

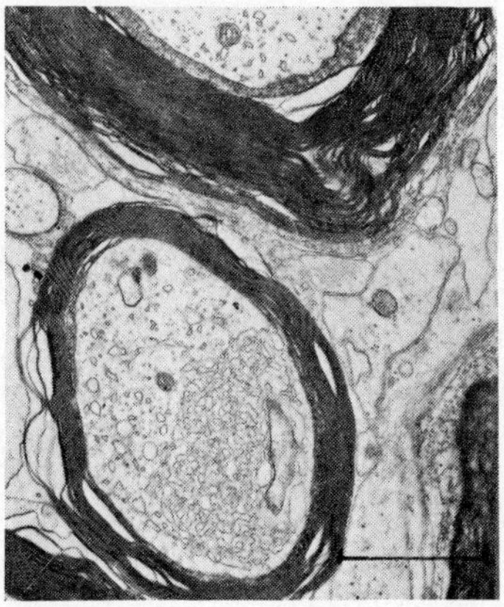

Fig. 5. Transverse section through the ventromedial tract in chicken spinal cord showing single nerve fibre degeneration.

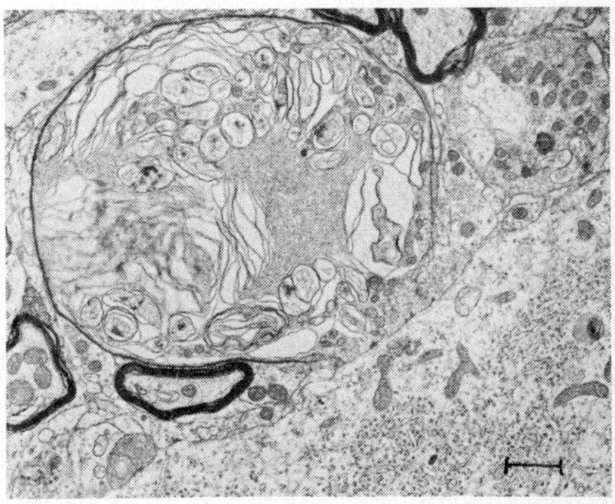

Fig. 6. An axonal ending shows marked extension and accumulation of membraneous and granulear material.

In the axon endings within the lumbar spinal cord anterior grey column, as a very striking pathological reaction, in approximately 10 to 20 per cent of the axosomatic synaptic structures, a marked swelling and partial dissolution of the synaptic vesicles was evident (Bischoff[10]). The alteration was confined to one type of nerve terminals with spherical vesicles (S type) and did not involve the other one with flattened vesicles (F type). Since the first type functionally corresponds to excitatory synapses, the structural abnormality, in terms of pathophysiology, is indicative of the suggestion of a primary defect of excitatory neurotransmitter effects, and otherwise means an exaggerated inhibitory influence on the motoneuron which itself showed only minor structural abnormality. (Fig. 7).

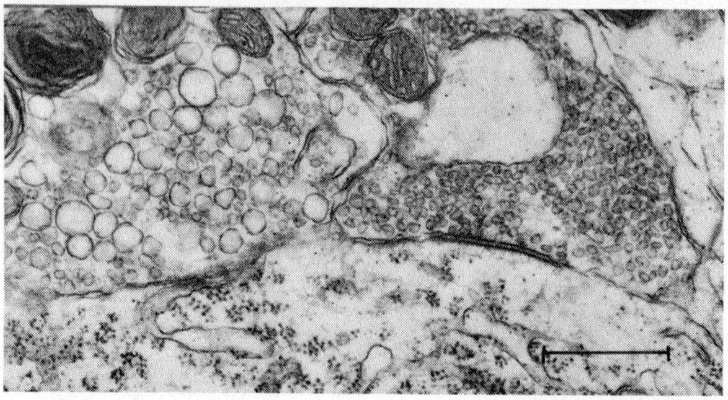

Fig. 7. Axosomatic synaptic knobs of the type with spherical vesicles which are markedly inflated (left) and of the type with flattened vesicles (right) which are preserved.

Isotope Studies. There exist some reports on investigations into the phosphorus metabolism of TOCP- poisoned animals that were substantiated by studies of the incorporation of radioactive tracers, particularly of ^{32}P [11, 12, 13]. They concentrated on the problem of whether TOCP causes abnormalities of the biosynthesis rates of labelled precursors into the phospholipid compound of the nervous tissue. They failed to bring any evidence of inhibition of the uptake of ^{32}P in the intoxicated animals in either spinal cord or nerves [11, 12, 13]. With regard to in vivo phosphorus incorporation into normal chicken phospholipid the results suggested that this is slow, and that the rate of incorporation of the isotope into chicken sciatic nerve was faster than into the spinal cord.

In order to study the fate of TOCP in experimental animals we investigated the in vivo-incorpation of $TOC^{32}P$. Oral administration of tri-(ortho-cresyl-T(G) phosphate (0.5 mC for every 2 ml TOCP per kilogram body weight) was carried out on adult chickens. The animals were sacrificed at 2, 6, and 10 days after administration of the labelled substance. Samples of the spinal cord, sciatic nerve, and other tissues such as liver and spleen were prepared by dissolution in chloroform methanol and by freezing and homogenizing. The activity of ^{32}P was determined by liquid scintillation counting. (Fig. 8).

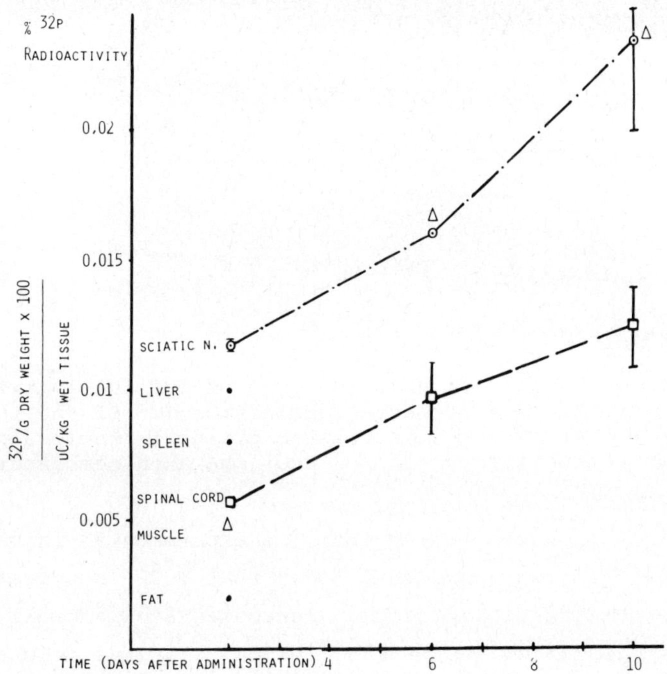

Fig. 8. Diagram of incorporation of TOC^{32}P into sciatic nerve and spinal cord following administration of the isotope in adult chicken.

The accumulation rate of ^{32}P in the lipid fraction of the examined spinal cord and sciatic nerve shows a gradual rise in concentration during the first 10 days. The increase in radioactivity turned out to be greater in the sample of chicken sciatic nerve than in spinal cord. The rates of uptake of ^{32}P expressed as relative specific activities are in remarkable agreement with those for the incorporation of non-toxic phosphates with the isotope ^{32}P as reported by Webster[13].

Audioradiography. In order to localize the isotope at the histological level, the incorporation of TOC^{32}P was investigated also by autoradiography. In 10 μ thick sections of the lumbar spinal cord and sciatic nerve of chicken, stained with Hemalaun, 10 days after administration of TOC^{32}P, reduced grains of emulsion can be recognized over single nerve fibers. They show a preponderant accumulation in relation to the surface of the axon, i.e. the axon membrane. (Fig. 9).

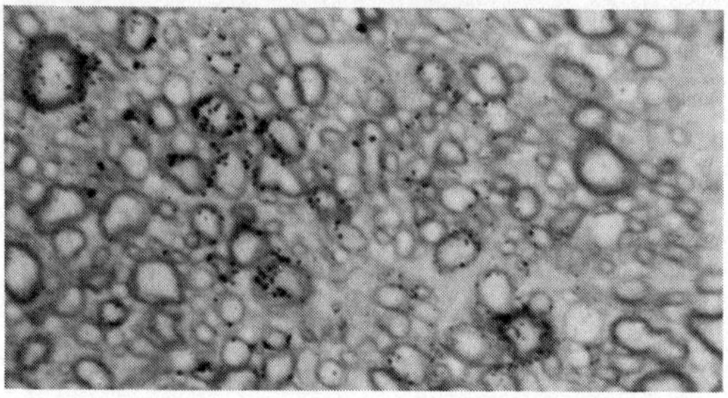

Fig. 9. Autoradiography of sciatic nerve of chicken intoxicated with $TOC^{32}P$ at the 10th day after administration of the toxic radioactive tracer. The reduced silver grains of the emulsion are located in single nerve fibres near the axon membrane.

Conclusion. As a conclusion from the experimental animal studies, there is wide agreement today that TOCP intoxication affects the peripheral and central nervous system as well, and that in both instances the primary lesion is axonal degeneration. As evidenced from examination of the lumbar spinal cord the pathologic alterations are confined mainly to the longest tracts, and initially the nerve endings, i.e., the presynaptic nerve terminals seem to be particularly affected. As a most striking feature, an abnormality of the synaptic vesicles which is confined to the excitatory axosomatic synapses, is visible.

The obvious inflation of the synaptic vesicles with indication of a disruption of their membrane strongly indicates an abnormality of the biophysical properties of the vesicle membrane. Analogous changes seem to occur in the axonmembrane and membraneous organelles of the axonplasm.

The suggestion of a membraneous abnormality is consistent with the biochemical findings as presented by Johnson ([14, 15, 16]), indicating that TOCP by phosphorylation of a specific membrane-bound nervous system esterase, from which a charged negative group has split away, produces a pathological alteration of membrane function.

As to the delayed neurotoxic effect of TOCP, it is commonly assumed that the compound is passing into a conversion system in the liver and that neurotoxicity is caused by its metabolites. The present isotope and autoradiographic studies show that the labelled phosphorus molecule is incorporated in the phospholipids of the central and peripheral nervous system. The rate of incorporation is suggestive of the hypothesis that only after accumulation of a certain amount of the compound which contains ^{32}P, the neurotoxic effect appears.

CHLOROQUINE INTOXICATION

Introduction. Chloroquine, one of a large series of 4-aminoquinolines, is a drug that has been proved to be one of the most effective and less toxic of the quinoline derivatives in the treatment of malaria, rheumatoid arthritis, lupus erythematosus and hepatic amebiasis. Minor and reversible side effects and adverse reactions were commonly experienced. Only after prolonged administration of a daily dose of more than 250 mg, more serious reactions like optic nerve atrophy, perceptive deafness and cardiovascular collapse may occur (Klinghardt [17]).

Clinical findings. A 65 year old woman had suffered for two years from polyarthralgia had been treated continously during five months with chloroquine phosphate in a dose of 250 mg a day (Fig. 10). Three months after beginning of the therapy she developed a progressive weakness of the thighs with difficulties in walking and getting out of chairs. Moderate paresthesias and a sensation of numbness in the feet did also occur. By examination a marked flaccid paresis of the proximal parts of the legs was found, in association with absend tendon reflexes and reduction of vibration perception in the feet. A discrete paresis of the shoulder girdle was also present.

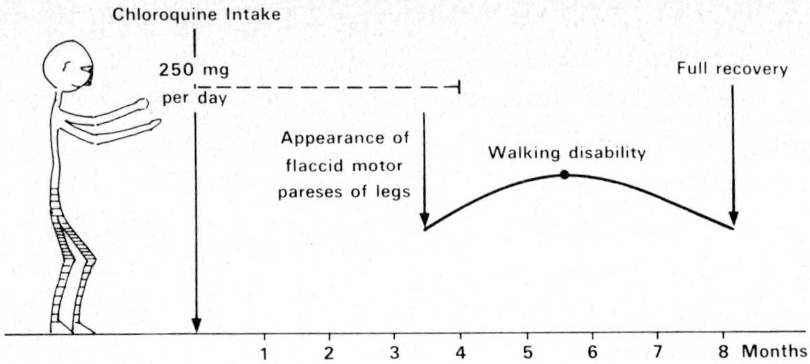

Fig. 10. Diagram of the clinical course of chloroquine neuropathy.

The electromyogram showed a neurogenic pattern of muscular dysfunction. Nerve conduction velocity measurement indicated a distinct reduction of distal transmission in both sensory and motor nerves. Apart from the neurological abnormalities all other findings were normal.

Pathology. A muscle biopsy revealed no significant pathological changes. A sural nerve biopsy was performed two months after onset of clinical neuropathy. By light microscopy, in the transverse section, a distinct loss of myelinated nerve fibers of all caliber sizes was striking. Some obviously collapsed myelin sheaths indicating axon shrinkage and a few clusters of small myelinated nerve fibers suggestive of nerve fiber regeneration were also apparent. By histometry the numerical decrease of myelinated nerve fibers by 24 % was evident, with the more prominent defect of the thick myelinated ones.

Electron microscopic analysis revealed two clear-cut findings:

- Axonal degeneration, evidenced by the accumulation of membraneous organelles, and
- the occurrence of pathological inclusions within the axon and the cytoplasm of the Schwann cells (Fig. 11).

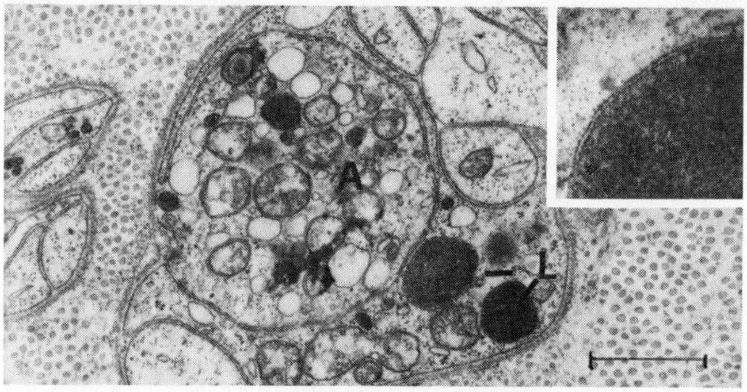

Fig. 11. Electronmicrograph of the biopsied sural nerve showing axonal degeneration (A) as well as proliferation of pathologic lysosomes (L). Insert: by high resolution.

Already by low resolution, different features of inclusion bodies are visible: dark homogeneous and concentric-multimembraneous bodies. By high resolution the inclusions appear to be bound by a single membrane surrounding a paracrystalline-structured compound.

Comment. The present findings correspond to the results of experimental intoxication of dorsal root ganglia which were exposed to chloroquine by Klinghardt[17] and Tischner[18]. These authors interpreted their findings as indicative of a drug induced lysosomal abnormality. Thus, they could demonstrate by autoradiographic analysis that chloroquine accumulates in lysosomal organelles within the ganglion cell and in Schwann cells, - that the lipid content within the lysosomes shows a two- to three-fold increase of a mixture of gangliosides, as an evidence of an insufficiency of a lysosomal enzyme, a gangliosidase - that this lipid storage process can be visualized and identified by electron microscopic analysis - and that by pathogenetical considerations the axonal degeneration is suggested to represent the secondary consequence of the primary neuronal abnormality.

As to the effect of the drug on the lysosomal organelle, chloroquine is one of the best investigated substances in the group of lysosomotropic chemotherapeutic agents. In particular, its therapeutic effect on malaria plasmodia has been extensively studied.

Three main pharmacokinetic mechanisms have been proposed:

- An inhibition of lysosomal enzymes due to its capacity to bind to DNA and by that to inhibit protein synthesis and DNA-dependent nucleic acid polymerase reactions (Davies et al.[19])
- by the accumulation of the drug in lysosomes and by its convertion by the acid pH to a lipid insoluble form to interfere with lysosomal enzyme activities (Homewood et al.[20])
- by the effect of the drug on lysosomal membranes to alter permeability so that ingested lipids cannot be digested further (Abraham et al.[21]).

Regardless this controversy of the pharmacodynamics, chloroquine neuropathy represents a unique well defined condition caused by a drug in which the pathogenetic neurotoxic as well as the therapeutic effect depend on its sufficiently documented lysosomotropic properties.

REFERENCES

1. Staehelin, R. (1941) Schw. med. Wschr., 71, 1-5
2. Barnes, J.M. and Denz, F.A. (1953) J. Pathol. Bacteriol., 65, 597-605
3. Beresford, W.A. and Glees, P. (1963) Acta Neuropathol. (Berl.), 3, 108-118
4. Cavanagh, J.B. (1954) J. Neurol. Neurosurg. Psychiatry, 17, 163-172
5. Cavanagh, J.B. and Patangia, G.N. (1965) Brain, 7, 165-180
6. Hern, J.E.C. (1967) Nature, 215, 963
7. Bischoff, A. (1967) Acta Neuropathol. (Berl.), 9, 158-174
8. Bischoff, A. (1970) Acta Neuropathol. (Berl.), 15, 142-155
9. Prineas, J. (1969) J. Neuropathol. Exp. Neurol., 28, 571-597
10. Bischoff, A. (1977) Neurotoxicology, Raven Press, New York pp. 431-441
11. Majno, G. and Karnovsky, M. (1961) J. Neurochem., 8, 1-16
12. Porcellati, G. and Mastrantonia, M.A. (1964) Ital. J. Biochem., 13, 332-352
13 Webster, G.R. (1954) Biochem. J., 57, 153-158

14. Johnson, M.K. (1969) Br. Med. Bull., 25, 231-235

15. Johnson, M.K. (1972) Proc. Roy. Soc. Med., 65, 195-196

16. Johnson, M.K. (1976) Fed. Proc., 35, 73-74

17. Klinghardt, G.W. (1977) Neurotoxicology, Raven Press, New York, 371-380

18. Tischner, K. and Fischer, H.A. (1975) Acta Neuropathol. (Berl.), 32, 353-357

19. Davies, E.E., Howells, R.E., Peters, W. (1971) Ann. Trop. Med. Parasitol., 65, 461-464

20. Homewood, C.A., Warhurst, D.C., Peters, W. (1972) Nature, 235, 50-52

21. Abraham, R., Hendy, R. and Grasso, S. (1968) Exp. Mol. Pathol., 9, 212-229.

Mechanisms of Toxicity and Hazard Evaluation
B. Holmstedt, R. Lauwerys, M. Mercier, M. Roberfroid eds

SAFETY EVALUATION OF FOUR BICYCLIC MUSK FRAGRANCE-CHEMICALS RELATIVE TO THE NEUROTOXIN, ACETYL ETHYL TETRAMETHYL TETRALIN (AETT)

YALE GRESSEL, WILLIAM R. TROY, G. V. FOSTER
Avon Products, Inc., Suffern, New York 10901 (U.S.A.)

INTRODUCTION

Acetyl Ethyl Tetramethyl Tetralin (AETT), a synthetic musk, had been widely used as a fragrance fixitive in cosmetic, toiletry and soap products until industry scientists reported that it produced neurotoxicity and blue discoloration of internal organs[1,2,3,4]. This was followed by a voluntary discontinuance of use by industry and a search for substitutes that would closely duplicate AETT's odor and functional properties while being devoid of its neurotoxic and tissue discoloration liabilities. Chemicals suggested as possible replacements (Figure 1) were acetyl methyl tetramethyl tetralin (Tonalid), hexahydro hexamethylcyclopenta benzpyran (Galaxolide), acetyl tertiary butyl dimethyl indan (Celestolide), and acetyl hexamethyl indan (Phantolid).

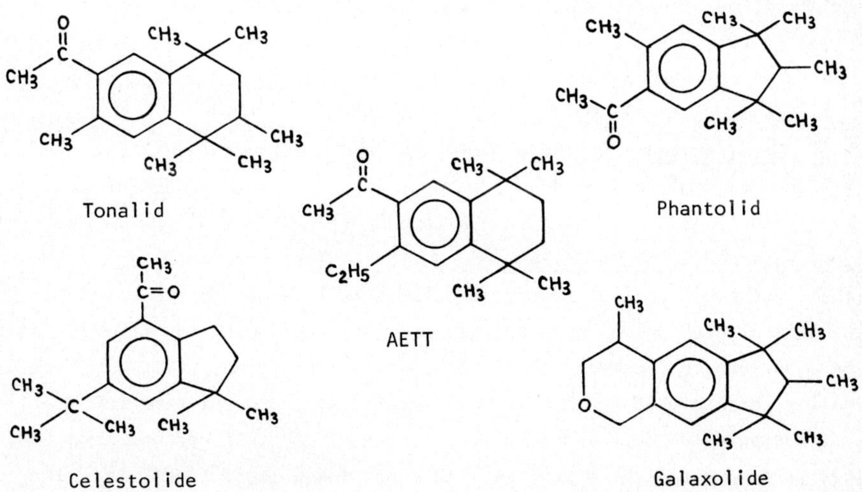

Fig. 1 Chemical Structures

Although these chemicals had been utilized for many years with apparent safety, none had been evaluated for their potential to cause cumulative systemic toxic effects. Furthermore, their structural similarity to AETT gave added impetus to evaluating their neurotoxic potential prior to their substitution for AETT. The present study was therefore undertaken to evaluate the cumulative systemic toxic potential of each of the four "substitutes" relative to the neurotoxin AETT and in addition, to better define the no effect level for AETT.

MATERIALS AND METHODS

Experimental animals. Female albino rats of the Crl: COBS CD(SD) BR strain from Charles River Breeding Laboratories, Inc., Wilmington, Mass. were employed. They ranged in weight from 156-232 g. Animals were housed individually and given food and water *ad libitum*.

Test materials. The test chemicals, received from the Givaudan Corp., were analyzed for purity by means of gas chromatography, infrared spectroscopy and nuclear magnetic resonance. The purity of AETT, Celestolide and Tonalid was each found to be approximately 99.9%. Purity of the Phantolid sample was approximately 88% and that of the Galaxolide sample was 50% in a solvent consisting primarily of diethyl phthalate.

For dosing purposes, ethanol dilutions of each material, with the exception of Celestolide, were prepared weekly. Celestolide dilutions were prepared daily because of a tendency to precipitate on standing for more than 24 hours.

Experimental design. At the end of a two week acclimation period, animals were randomly assigned to treatment groups. Table 1 summarizes the test conditions.

Exposure schedule and clinical observations. Test materials were applied by gentle inunction to the anterior dorsal (scapular region) shaved skin of each animal once daily, seven days per week. No attempt was made during the treatment period to preclude ingestion.

Animals were weighed on the first treatment day and weekly thereafter, doses being adjusted correspondingly. Throughout the test period, observations were made daily for any specific overt toxicologic signs, including mortality, general appearance, and condition of the skin at the site of application. Once weekly, each animal was further examined with particular attention being paid to any changes in behavioral and motor function.

TABLE 1
TEST CONDITIONS

Test Material	Conc. %	Dose (mg/kg)	No. of Rats	Exposure Duration(Wks.)
Untreated control	-	-	15	13
Untreated control	-	-	20	26
Ethanol control	100	-	15	13
Ethanol control	100	-	20	26
Tonalid	1	100,10,1	15 ea.	13
Tonalid	1	36,18,9	20 ea.	26
Galaxolide	2	100,10,1	15 ea.	13
Galaxolide	2	36,18,9	20 ea.	26
Celestolide	1	100,10,1	15 ea.	13
Phantolid	1	100,10,1	15 ea.	13
AETT	1	36,18,9	20 ea.	26
AETT	10	100,30	10 ea.	13
AETT	1	10,3,1	10 ea.	13
AETT	0.1	0.3,0.1	15 ea.	13

Hematology and serum chemistry. During the seventh and thirteenth weeks of treatment, for animals on the thirteen week exposure regimen, five rats from each group were selected at random and fasted overnight (16 hours). The following morning, blood samples were obtained from each rat, under light ether anesthesia, by means of orbital sinus puncture. All animals on the twenty six week exposure regimen had blood samples drawn one week prior to their scheduled interim (week 13) or terminal (week 26) necropsy. The following parameters were evaluated: hematocrit, hemoglobin, red blood cell count, mean corpuscular volume, fasting blood glucose, urea nitrogen, glutamic-oxaloacetic transaminase, glutamic-pyruvic transaminase and alkaline phosphatase.

Pathology. Two animals from each group on the 13 week exposure regimen were selected for special neuropathological examination based on a consistent display of clinical signs of neurotoxicity. In the absence of such signs, animals were randomly selected. At the interim sacrifice of the 26 week study, two animals each from the ethanol control, and 36, 18 and 9 mg/kg AETT groups, were selected for special neuropathological examination. In addition, at the terminal sacrifice, two animals from each group (except untreated controls) were similarly chosen. All other animals at all sacrifice points were subjected to routine necropsy.

For the routine interim and terminal necropsies, animals were fasted overnight, anesthetized with ether and then exsanguinated. The adrenals, brain, heart, kidneys, liver, lungs, spleen and uterus were removed and weighed. The following tissues were fixed in 10% neutral buffered formalin, paraffin embedded, and sectioned and stained with hematoxylin and eosin for microscopic examinations: brain, spinal cord, sciatic nerve, liver and kidney. Animals selected for special neuropathologic examination were anesthetized with sodium barbital and perfused *in situ* through the heart with 4% paraformaldehyde followed by 5% buffered glutaraldehyde solution. Brain, spinal cord and peripheral nerves were then stained with osmium tetroxide, embedded in epoxy resin, sectioned and stained with toluidine blue.

RESULTS

Clinical changes. Two treatment related deaths occurred and both were in the 100 mg/kg AETT treatment group. The first was after 28 doses and the second after 69 doses. Both animals suffered severe weight loss and exhibited the blue tissue discoloration and histopathologic changes in the central nervous system characteristic of AETT toxicity[3,4]. High dose (100 mg/kg) animals in the 13 week exposure regimen from the AETT, Tonalid and Phantolid groups, as well as the 30 mg/kg AETT group, exhibited a significant depression in body weight gain compared to controls. A similar effect was seen at both interim and terminal sacrifice in the 26 week study for animals treated with 36 mg/kg of AETT, Tonalid and Galaxolide, as well as with 18 mg/kg AETT. By 26 weeks, the 9 mg/kg AETT group also had reduced body weight gain.

Behavioral treatment-related changes were noted only among animals given 30 mg/kg AETT or higher. These changes consisted of hyperexcitability, aggressive and irritable behavior, and impaired motor function, the latter characterized by ataxia, wobbly gait and hind limb weakness.

Hematology and serum chemistry. In the 13 week regimen, a significant depression in hemoglobin, hematocrit and red blood cell count was observed for animals given 100 mg/kg of Tonalid or Phantolid. Tonalid at 36 mg/kg also produced a depressed hemoglobin level and red blood cell count.

Serum chemistry changes considered to be clinically significant were observed only for Tonalid and Phantolid at the 100 mg/kg dose level (13 week regimen). Both produced elevated serum alkaline phosphatase levels. In addition, Phantolid treated animals exhibited elevated fasting glucose.

Pathology. On gross examination, liver discoloration was observed in animals treated for 13 weeks with 100 mg/kg of Phantolid or Tonalid. Prominent liver lobular patterns were also observed in the latter group. Similar observations were made in the 36 mg/kg Tonalid treatment group after 26 weeks of treatment. At all AETT dose levels down to 9 mg/kg, the characteristic blue discoloration of brain, spinal cord, peripheral nerves, subcutaneous tissues and internal organs was observed. No discoloration was observed at the lower dose levels even after 26 weeks of treatment.

The only significant organ weight changes after 13 weeks of treatment were relative and absolute liver weight increases in the 100 mg/kg Tonalid, Galaxolide, Celestolide and Phantolid treatment groups. After 26 weeks, animals treated with Tonalid at 36 and 18 mg/kg also demonstrated elevated liver weights.

Microscopically, animals treated for 13 weeks with 100 mg/kg of Tonalid or Phantolid exhibited liver changes consisting of minimal to moderate degrees of hepatocytomegaly and minimal to moderate deposition of an iron positive pigment. A similar, but less pronounced effect, was observed in animals treated for 26 weeks with Tonalid at 36 mg/kg.

No microscopic changes were observed in the nervous tissues of animals treated with Tonalid, Galaxolide, Celestolide or Phantolid at any of the dose levels employed. Animals treated with AETT at levels of 100 or 10 mg/kg for 13 weeks, and those treated for 26 weeks at levels of 36, 18 or 9 mg/kg, exhibited the previously reported changes in nervous system tissues[3,4]. These consisted of vacuolation of brain, spinal cord and peripheral nerves as well as neuronal demyelination and granule deposition.

DISCUSSION

This study demonstrated no clinical or histopathological changes indicative of neurotoxicity in rats treated for 13 weeks with Tonalid, Galaxolide, Celestolide or Phantolid at levels of 1, 10 and 100 mg/kg/day or for 26 weeks with Tonalid and Galaxolide at levels of 9, 18 and 36 mg/kg/day. In contrast, rats treated with AETT exhibited dose-related behavioral and neuropathalogic changes at levels as low as 9 mg/kg/day.

Rats treated with AETT at levels of 3, 1, 0.3 and 0.1 mg/kg/day did not exhibit neurotoxic effects.

While not neurotoxic, Phantolid at 100 mg/kg/day and Tonalid at 36 and 100 mg/kg/day produced biological changes suggestive of a potential cytotoxic effect on red blood cells with secondary involvement of the liver. This consisted of a significant depression of several red blood cell parameters with an accompanying histopathologic picture of iron pigment deposition in the liver. In addition, liver weights were elevated, serum alkaline phosphatase activity was elevated, and microscopic evaluation revealed hepatocytomegaly.

Finally, in terms of the safety of Tonalid, Phantolid, Celestolid and Galaxolide as substitutes for AETT, the no effect levels determined in this study represent safety factors of at least 100 fold over levels commonly employed in consumer products. Based on this criterion, these compounds are considered to be acceptable substitutes for AETT.

ACKNOWLEDGMENTS

The authors gratefully acknowledge the valuable technical assistance provided by Roger J. Minner and Stephen C. Pennisi of the Avon Products, Inc. Toxicology Department.

REFERENCES

1. Spencer, P.S., *et al.* (1979) Science, 204, 633-635.
2. Opdyke, D.L.J. (1979) Fd. Cosmet. Toxicol., 17, 357-360.
3. Spencer, P.S., *et al.* (1979) Neurotoxicology, 1, 221-237.
4. Spencer, P.S., *et al.* (1980) Experimental and Clinical Neurotoxicology, Williams and Wilkins, Baltimore, in press.

© 1980 Elsevier/North-Holland Biomedical Press
Mechanisms of Toxicity and Hazard Evaluation
B. Holmstedt, R. Lauwerys, M. Mercier, M. Roberfroid eds

BRAIN SLICES, ASSAY SYSTEMS FOR THE NEUROTOXICITY OF ENVIRONMENTAL POLLUTANTS AND DRUGS ON MAMMALIAN CENTRAL NERVOUS SYSTEM

Yoichiro KURODA
Department of Neurochemistry, Tokyo Metropolitan Institute for Neurosciences, 2-6, Musashidai, Fuchu-shi, Tokyo 183 (Japan)

INTRODUCTION

There is an increasing number of patients suffering from neurological diseases by environmental toxicants (for example, Minamata disease by methylmercury[1]) and by secondary effects of drugs (for example, subacute myelo-optico neuropathy; SMON by chinoform[2]). To prevent such tragedies, it is fundamentally necessary to examine the neurotoxicity of agents before we take them up into our body. Although the intoxication often became a serious social problem, very little has been studied to get appropriate nerve preparations of mammals for examining the neurotoxicity which is closely related to the human diseases.

For testing the neurotoxicity of various compounds quickly and accurately, *in vitro* nerve preparations have several advantages;

1) We can observe direct effects on the site of action without considering the absorption processes such as blood-brain barrier and get accurate dose-response relationships at the site of action.
2) For screening, we can apply an agent at different doses, or even different agents one by one, on the same preparation when the previous one can be washed out without remaining apparent effects.
3) We can investigate the mechanism of action at the cellular level.

Olfactory cortex slices of guinea pigs are one of the *in vitro* brain preparations in which we can study the effects of various agents on neural functions and metabolism both by electrophysiological and biochemical methods[3]. Inhibitory action of adenosine on the synaptic transmission and its molecular mechanism have been investigated using the slices[4].

MATERIALS AND METHODS

Olfactory cortex slices were prepared from guinea pig brain by the method of Yamamoto and McIlwain[5]. After preincubation at 38°C for at least 20 min in the standard Krebs-bicarbonate-glucose medium gassed with a mixture of 95% O_2 and 5% CO_2, the slice was transferred to a stimulating and recording chamber and monitored for the amplitude of postsynaptic potentials (PSP), which were evoked by stimulating the frontal end of the lateral olfactory tract (LOT) with rectangular pulses of 10 V in strength and 0.1 msec in duration at 2 cycles/sec. After checking the stability of PSP, the original amplitude of the PSP was recorded. The medium was then replaced by a fresh one with or without test agents, and the slice was further incubated. At various times after the replacement of the medium, the amplitude of PSP was recorded again on an oscilloscope and the change was calculated in relation to the original amplitude.

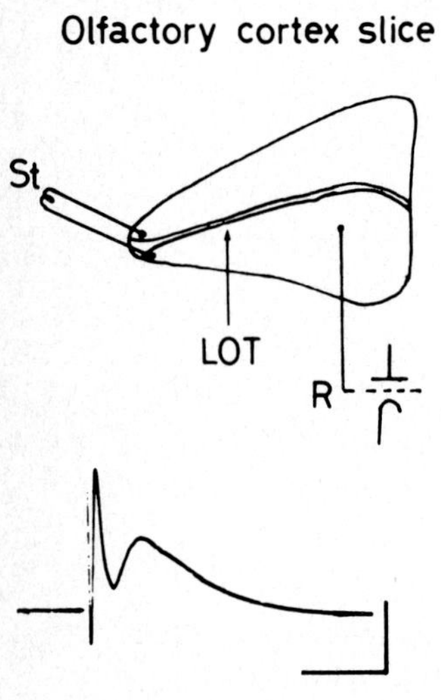

Fig. 1. PSP from olfactory cortex slices.

RESULTS AND DISCUSSION

Recording of PSP and its stability. Electrical stimulation of LOT evokes synchronous PSP in a number of the pyramidal neurons located in the superficial layer of the slices. Thus the summation of the PSPs is easily recorded from the surface of the slices as field potentials. When the recording electrode is positioned at R (Fig. 1, upper part), two responses are recorded; the first one is presynaptic axon potential and the second one is the evoked PSPs (Fig. 1, lower part). The shape and amplitude of the PSPs depends on the position of the recording electrode. However, they are stable for several hours (sometimes up to 16 hrs) when the slice was properly prepared and incubated under enough supply of oxygen. After some practice, even beginners will be able to record 0.5- 3 mV of PSPs which is enough to analyze the change of PSPs quantitatively.

Application of typical neurotoxicants. DDT (1,1,1-trichloro-2,2-bis-(4-chlorophenyl)ethane) and toluene were applied in the incubation medium and the change of PSP was observed. DDT ($5x10^{-4}$M) caused a slow decrease of the PSP amplitude up to 70% inhibition within 60 min. Additional 40 min incubation did not change the amplitude. During the incubation, presynaptic axon potentials did not show any considerable changes, suggesting that DDT acts primarily on the process of synaptic transmission, not on the propagation of impulses along the axon (Fig. 2).

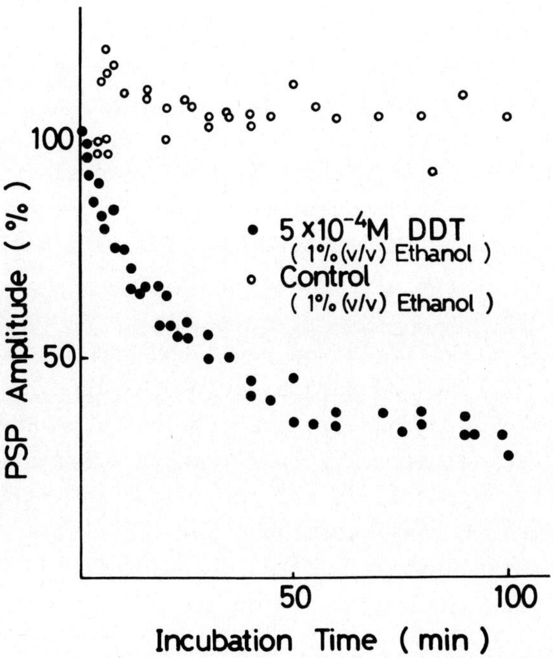

Fig. 2. Effect of DDT on the evoked PSP.

Low dose of toluene (0.005%,v/v) had no effect, but 0.01% and 0.02% of toluene caused 10% and 70% inhibition respectively, after the 10 min incubation. Toluene suspension (0.03%) completely diminished the PSP within 5 min. Toluene decreased the amplitude of presynaptic axon potentials in parallel with that of PSP, indicating it primarily inhibits the propagation of impulses along the axon.

A screening system for the toxicity on neurotransmission in mammalian brain. The present results show that olfactory cortex slices will be useful for the screening of neurotoxic compounds. The slices are relatively easy to handle and a large number of agents can be tested in a reasonably short period of time.

Comparing to other in vitro assay systems, this system has some advantages and disadvantages.

Advantages;

1) More general screening by electrophysiological observation.

A number of experiments have been investigated biochemically, for example, organophosphate insecticides using the inhibition of cholinesterase[6]. However, this type of approach is very limited for general screening since those neurotoxicants which do not affect such enzymatic system never give a positive result. In contrast, electrophysiological method is expected to pick up any agents blocking even a process of many which are necessary to synaptic transmission. In other words, it is possible to detect a new type of neurotoxicants which inhibit unknown but essential process of neurotransmission, a fundamental function of nervous system. Electrophysiological observation also provides information on the site or mechanism of action of toxicants.

2) More related to human brain.

It is suggested that neurotoxicity of an agent changes depending on animal species and on types of nervous system. Narahashi's group has developed several *in vitro* nerve preparations from invertebrates to test insecticidal activity, for example crayfish abdominal cord[7]. Olfactory cortex slices are one of the *in vitro* brain preparations, on which we can investigate the electrical activity, is suitable for the purpose of testing the toxicity on mammalian brain which is closely related to the human brain.

Disadvantage;

3) Only for short-term effects.

Practically, it is difficult to see the effect of agents for longer than a few hours, this slice system is not suitable for testing long-term effects. Whether we can predict the long-term effects from the results of the short-term test is a very important point and open to further investigation.

REFERENCES

1. Takeuchi,T. and Eto,K. (1977) Minamata disease, methylmercury poisoning in Minamata and Niigata, Japan. Ed. Tsubaki,T. and Irukayama,K., Kodansha, Tokyo pp103-141.
2. Tsubaki,T. et al. (1971) Lancet, 1, 696.
3. Kuroda,Y. et al. (1976) Brain Res. 109, 196-201.
4. Kuroda,Y. (1978) J. Physiol. Paris, 74, 463-470.
5. Yamamoto,C.and McIlwain,H. (1966) J. Neurochem. 13, 1333-1343.
6. Fukuto,T.R. (1971) Bull. W.H.O. 44, 31.
7. Narahashi,T. (1979) Neurotoxicology of Pheromones and Insecticides. Ed. Narahashi,T., Plenum, New York, pp211-243.

Mechanisms of Toxicity and Hazard Evaluation
B. Holmstedt, R. Lauwerys, M. Mercier, M. Roberfroid eds

INHIBITOR CHARACTERISTICS OF NATIVE, SOLUBILIZED, AND LIPID-RECONSTITUTED NEUROTOXIC ESTERASE

C.S. DAVIS, M.L. BARTH, B.R. DUDEK, and R.J. RICHARDSON
Toxicology Research Laboratory, Department of Environmental and Industrial Health, School of Public Health, The University of Michigan, Ann Arbor, MI 48109, U.S.A.

INTRODUCTION

The earliest known biochemical event in organophosphorus-induced delayed neuropathy is inhibition of neurotoxic esterase (NTE)[1]. NTE is membrane-bound[2], but can be solubilized with detergent[3]. By including asolectin in the solubilization procedure, any loss of NTE during solubilization can be prevented[3]. It was important to determine if NTE retained its definitive inhibitor characteristics during solubilization, so complete inhibitor titration curves were determined for the enzyme under different solubilization conditions. A titration curve was also done for NTE immobilized on DEAE-Sephacel.

MATERIALS AND METHODS

Female, white Leghorn chicks (*Gallus domesticus*) were obtained from Napoleon Hatchery, Napoleon, OH.

Phenyl valerate and mipafox were synthesized as previously described[4]. Paraoxon, Triton X-100, and sodium cholate were purchased from Sigma Chemical Company, St. Louis, MO. Asolectin was from Associated Concentrates, Woodside, NY. DEAE-Sephacel and Sephadex G-25 were obtained from Pharmacia, Piscataway, NJ. All other chemicals were of analytical reagent grade or the highest grade commerically available. All water was distilled and deionized.

Preparation and Solubilization of Microsomes. Whole brain homogenates and microsomes were prepared according to Richardson *et al.*[2]. Microsomal pellets, containing approximately 20 mg protein, were hand homogenized in 11 ml of an appropriate detergent suspension until a homogeneous dispersion was obtained. For sodium cholate, a suspension of 1% (w/v) detergent in 50 mM Tris, 2 mM EDTA, pH 8.0, was used for solubilization. For Triton X-100, a suspension of 0.1% (w/v) detergent was used. The microsomal-detergent suspension was then centrifuged at 100000 x g for 60 min (r avg) in the Beckman Model L5-75 ultracentrifuge. The supernatants (soluble NTE) were carefully pipetted off and

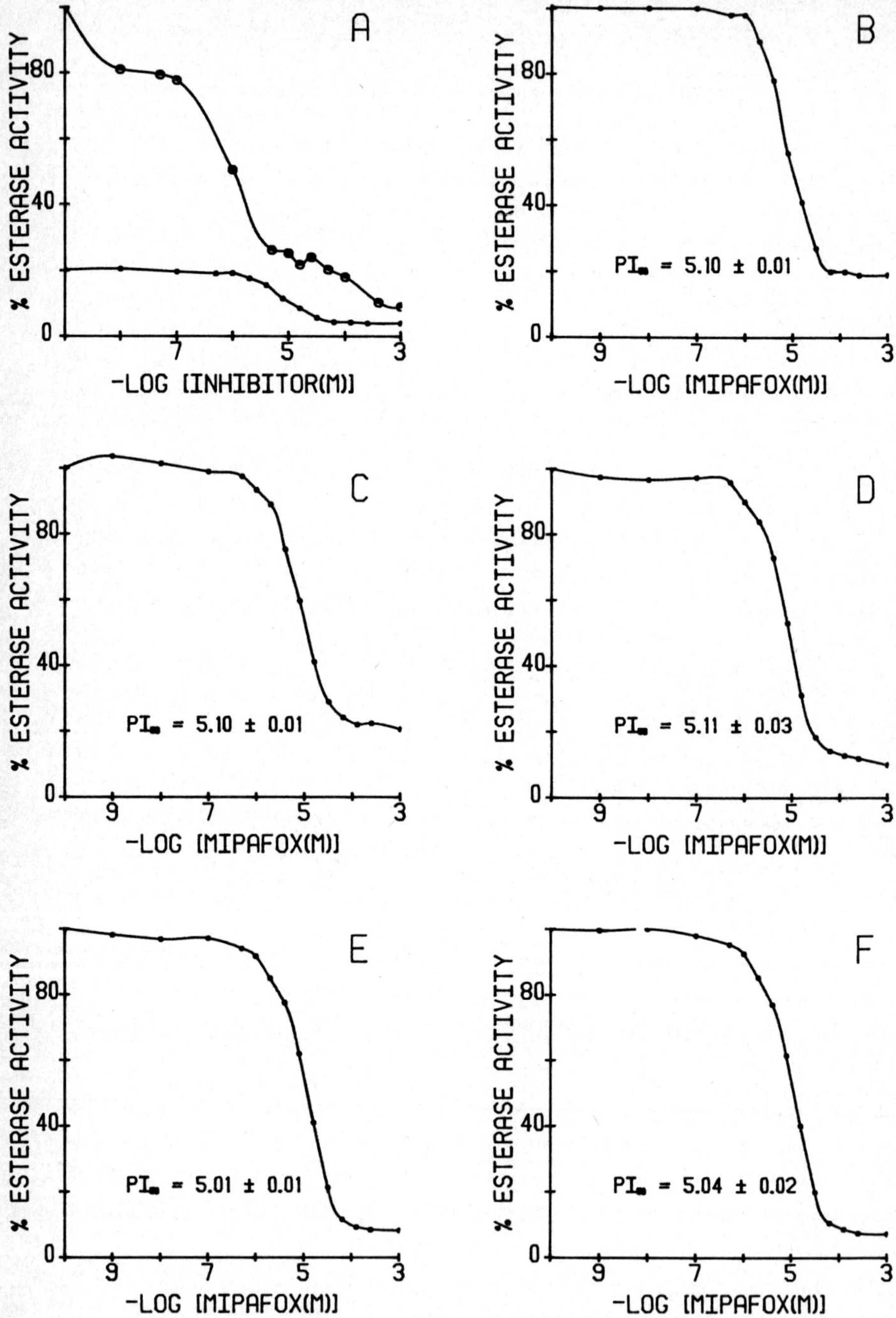
A
% ESTERASE ACTIVITY
80
40
0
7
5
3
-LOG [INHIBITOR(M)]
B
% ESTERASE ACTIVITY
PI = 5.10 ± 0.01
-LOG [MIPAFOX(M)]
C
% ESTERASE ACTIVITY
PI = 5.10 ± 0.01
-LOG [MIPAFOX(M)]
D
% ESTERASE ACTIVITY
PI = 5.11 ± 0.03
-LOG [MIPAFOX(M)]
E
% ESTERASE ACTIVITY
PI = 5.01 ± 0.01
-LOG [MIPAFOX(M)]
F
% ESTERASE ACTIVITY
PI = 5.04 ± 0.02
-LOG [MIPAFOX(M)]

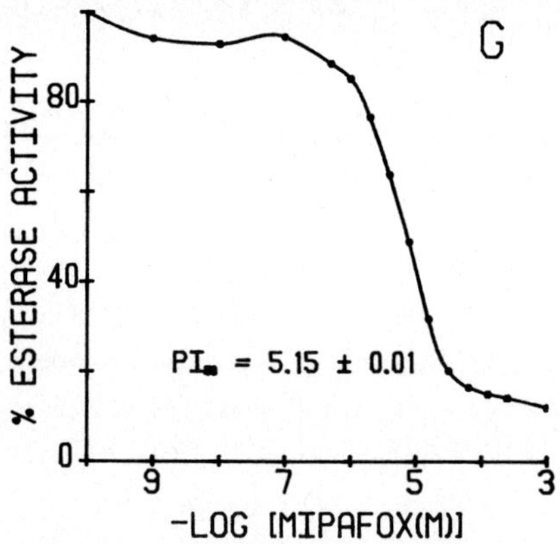

Figure 1. Titration curves for various forms of NTE. Each point is the mean of 3 separate experiments. o--o paraoxon inhibited esterase activity. ●--● mipafox plus constant paraoxon (100 μM) inhibited esterase activity. pI_{50}'s are the mean of 3 experiments ± standard error. A. Whole brain homogenate NTE. B. Whole brain homogenate NTE, mipafox curve with expanded scale. C. Triton X-100 solubilized NTE. D. Sodium cholate solubilized NTE. E. Sodium cholate + asolectin solubilized NTE. F. Sodium cholate + asolectin solubilized NTE with detergent removed. G. Immobilized NTE.

used for determining titration curves or for immobilization.

When asolectin was included in the solubilization procedure, 4 mg/ml was added to the sodium cholate-buffer mixture before homogenization with microsomes.

Titration Curve. The hydrolysis of phenyl valerate was monitored colorimetrically as described by Johnson[4], over a range of inhibitor concentrations.

Removal of Detergent. Sodium cholate was removed by passing the solubilized NTE preparations through a Sephadex G-25 column (26 by 65 mm). The column was eluted with 50 mM Tris, 2 mM EDTA, pH 8.0.

Immobilization of NTE. DEAE-Sephacel™ was adjusted to approximately pH 7.0 by the dropwise addition of 1 N NaOH, and then washed twice with water.

Triton-solubilized NTE was used for immobilization with approximately 100 to 300 nmol/min of NTE activity per ml of unwashed gel suspension. The gel-NTE mixture was stirred for 1 hr in an ice bath and then allowed to stand at 4°C overnight. The gel was washed 3 times with water to remove unbound enzyme. The washed pellet was resuspended in water, and aliquots of the gel suspension were taken for titration with paraoxon and mipafox.

RESULTS

A typical titration experiment can be represented by two curves: the first showing the inhibition of esterases by paraoxon (a non-neurotoxic inhibitor) and the second showing the inhibition of neurotoxic esterase by mipafox (a neurotoxic inhibitor) at constant paraoxon concentration (Fig. 1-A). The esterase activity that cannot be inhibited by either paraoxon or mipafox at $\geq 10^{-3}$ M has been called inhibitor-resistant esterase or IRE[2].

The titration of mipafox-sensitive activity at constant paraoxon concentration can also be shown with an expanded scale, as in Figure 1-B. Expanded mipafox titration curves with calculated pI_{50}'s for various solubilized NTE preparations and immobilized NTE are shown in Figure 1-C through 1-G.

It is notable that all of the mipafox titration curves are of a similar shape with pI_{50}'s between 5.01 and 5.15. The results indicate that the initial steps of NTE purification can be performed without the loss of definitive inhibitor characteristics.

ACKNOWLEDGEMENTS

This work was sponsored, in part, by research grants R-805339030, USEPA, and 5 R01 ES01611, NIEHS. CSD is a recipient of a Monsanto Fund Postdoctoral Fellowship in Toxicology.

REFERENCES

1. Johnson, M.K. (1975) Critical Review in Toxicology, 3, 289-316.
2. Richardson, R.J., Davis, C.S. and Johnson, M.K. (1979) Journal of Neurochemistry, 32, 607-615.
3. Davis, C.S. and Richardson, R.J. (1980) Toxicology and Applied Pharmacology, in press (abstract).
4. Johnson, M.K. (1977) Archives of Toxicology, 37, 113-115.

© 1980 Elsevier/North-Holland Biomedical Press
Mechanisms of Toxicity and Hazard Evaluation
B. Holmstedt, R. Lauwerys, M. Mercier, M. Roberfroid eds

NEUROTOXICITY OF LEAD IN RABBITS

EINO HIETANEN[1], JUKKA KILPIÖ[2], ULLA KOIVUSAARI[3], TIMO NEVALAINEN[3], MATTI NÄRHI[3], HEIKKI SAVOLAINEN[2] and HARRI VAINIO[2]
Department of Physiology, University of Turku[1], SF-20520 Turku 52, Department of Physiology, University of Kuopio[3], SF-70101 Kuopio 10 and Institute of Occupational Health[2], SF-00290 Helsinki 29 (Finland)

INTRODUCTION

Lead enters the body in the inspired air and in food[1] and forms an environmental and occupational problem[2]. The effects of lead as an inhibitor of Δ-aminolevulinic acid dehydrogenase are well known impairing thus the heme synthesis[2]. The inhibition can be detected already at lead concentrations of 1 μmol/l which may represent the concentration found in environmental lead exposure[3,4]. Lead is also a potent inhibitor of adenyl cyclase activity in the central nervous system[2]. Acute high dose lead exposure in drinking water increases the brain lead content in rats in a linear ratio to the blood concentration[5]. We have earlier shown in a cross-sectional study that lead decreases peripheral motor nerve conduction velocity along with increased lead levels[6].

In the present study we have evaluated the effect of the lead exposure in drinking water on the motor nerve conduction velocity and on tissue and blood lead concentrations. The effect of simultaneous zinc administration on the accumulation of lead was also studied.

MATERIALS AND METHODS

Twentyfive adult male Californian rabbits were fed *ad lib*. The sole source of drinking water was either 0.2 % lead solution (as lead acetate), 0.5 % zinc (also as acetate), both combined or 0.2 % sodium (acetate) solution. The solutions containing lead were buffered to pH 6.5. Before the beginning of the experiment rabbits were weighed and divided into 4 groups mentioned above. The motor nerve conduction velocity was measured before the administration of metals in drinking water and after 2 and 4 weeks when also blood, brain and sciatic nerve samples were taken for metal analyses. The motor conduction velocity was measured in sciatic nerve, which was stimulated with a bipolar skin electrode half way between hip and knee joints[7]. The muscle response was picked up by means of a needle electrode inserted in the gastrocnemius muscle. The lead and zinc contents were analyzed with an atomic absorption spectrophotometer[5].

RESULTS

The weight gain of the metal exposed rabbits was slower than that of the controls (Table 1). The drinking rate was lower in the rabbits exposed to zinc alone or in combination with lead than in the lead exposed or control rabbits. Therefore, the cumulative lead dose as combined to zinc was lower than in the sole lead exposure (Table 1).

TABLE 1

BODY WEIGHTS AND METAL INTAKE

	Body Weight			Daily Metal Intake (mg)	
Exposure	0 (n=6-7)	2 (n=3)	4 Weeks (n=3)	Pb	Zn
Pb	2442 ± 148[a]	2895 ± 189	2590 ± 95	448 ± 26	-
Pb/Zn	2525 ± 96	3035 (n=2)	2550 (n=2)	231 ± 6	576 ± 15
Zn	2458 ± 121	2673 ± 52	2337 ± 38	-	483 ± 49
Controls	2379 ± 108	2955 ± 159 (n=7)		-	-

[a]Mean ± SEM.

The metal contents of blood and nervous tissues are shown in Table 2. The blood lead content increased 15-fold after a 2-wk lead administration as compared to the controls but further administration did not increase blood lead concentration. However, both in the cerebrum and cerebellum the lead content doubled between weeks 2 and 4 (Table 2). Although the blood zinc concentration increased 13-fold after a 2-wk zinc administration and after a 4-wk administration even more, there was only rather low, but significant, increase in the cerebral and cerebellar zinc concentrations after the 4-wk exposure although sciatic zinc concentration increased 2-4-fold. When both lead and zinc were administered to rabbits for 2 or 4 weeks the blood zinc level was maximal after a 2-wk exposure while the lead concentration increased between weeks 2 and 4 (Table 2). The brain lead contents were significantly lower in those rabbits having both zinc and lead after a 2-wk exposure than in lead exposed rabbits.

When the motor nerve conduction velocity was analyzed there was a significant decrease in lead exposed rabbits as compared to the controls (Table 3). When zinc was administered together with lead in the drinking water the conduction velocity was at the same low level as in lead exposed rabbits (Table 3).

TABLE 2

METAL CONTENTS IN TISSUES

Metal Exposure	Blood Zinc	Blood Lead	Cerebrum Zinc	Cerebrum Lead	Cerebellum Zinc	Cerebellum Lead	Sciatic Nerve Zinc	Sciatic Nerve Lead
Controls	66±0.9	0.3±0.02	188±5	0.4±0.03	172±4	0.8±0.1	67±7	0.7±0.1
Lead								
2 Weeks	58±2.7	4.5±0.7***	179±6	2.1±0.5***	178±6	3.0±0.6***	59±10	4.0±0.7***
4 Weeks	61±3.0	4.3±0.7***	193±6	4.2±0.9***	175±3	4.5±0.8***	68±12	5.7±0.6***
Zinc								
2 Weeks	883±156***	0.2±0.03	212±9*	0.3±0.1	191±11	0.9±0.2	129±18**	0.8±0.2
4 Weeks	1069±155***	0.2±0.03	226±6***	0.4±0.1	219±7***	0.8±0.1	213±14***	0.6±0.2
Zinc/Lead								
2 Weeks	422±76***	5.1±0.4***	181±6	1.2±0.2***	181±2	1.0±0.1	89±29	3.1±0.9**
4 Weeks	289±66**	11.3±3.0***	207±13	2.7±0.6***	238±7***	4.2±0.6***	112	4.0

Metal contents are as nmol/g, mean ± SEM are shown. Statistical significances (Student's t-test) are shown as follows: *: $P < 0.05$; **: $P < 0.01$; ***: $P < 0.001$.

TABLE 3

THE MOTOR NERVE (SCIATIC) CONDUCTION VELOCITY (m/s).

Exposure	Pre-exposure	Weeks 2	Weeks 4
Lead	49.5 ± 6	13 ± 3***	7 ± 0***
Zinc	43.0 ± 7	34 ± 1	27 ± 16
Zinc/Lead	39.5 ± 5	11 ± 1***	12 ± 2**
Controls	35.5 ± 4	32 ± 8	43 ± 7

DISCUSSION

Interestingly, the lead concentration in the blood from rabbits exposed to both lead and zinc in their drinking water was considerably higher than in the blood of rabbits having lead alone despite lower cumulative dose. Zinc possibly induced protein which binds lead in the circulation. However, this is not reflected in the tissue lead contents. In rabbits having only lead there was a clearcut increase in the brain lead content from 2 to 4 weeks of exposure despite very small changes in the blood content.

The zinc contents of the brain were quite nonresponsive to the administration of zinc in the drinking water despite marked changes in the blood and sciatic zinc concentrations. The blood zinc concentration was even 5-fold in comparison with the brain although in controls a reverse was true. However, zinc apparently decreased the lead accumulation in the brain. This well agrees with previous data suggesting that zinc stabilizes membranes and may thus protect the cells[8-10]. The motor nerve conduction velocity was highly responsive to the lead content of the peripheral nervous tissue suggesting that motor conduction velocity might be among the first toxic signs of lead exposure. There was no significant decrease in the peripheral lead content in zinc exposed rabbits and zinc did not protect from the decrease in the conduction velocity in the sciatic nerve.

ACKNOWLEDGEMENTS

This study was supported by grants from NIH (R01 ES 01684) and J. Vainio Foundation. Ms. A. Grundström provided the superb technical assistence in metal determinations.

REFERENCES

1. Fishbein, L. (1976) J. Toxicol. Env. Hlth., 2, 77-109.
2. Eisinger, J. (1978) Quart. Rev. Biophys., 11, 439-466.
3. Hernberg, S. and Nikkanen, J. (1972) Prakov. Lek., 24, 77-83.
4. Roels, H.A., Buchet, J.P. and Lauwerys, R.R. (1974) Int. Arch. Arbeitsmed., 33, 277-284.
5. Savolainen, H. and Kilpiö, J. (1977) Scand. J. Work Environ. Hlth., 3, 104-107.
6. Hietanen, E., Kilpiö, J., Närhi, M., Savolainen, H. and Vainio, H. (1980) Arch. Environ. Cont. Toxicol., 9, 351.
7. Seppäläinen, A.M. and Linnoila, J. (1975) Scand. J. Work Environ. Hlth., 1, 178-183.
8. Chvapil, M. (1973) Life Sci., 13, 1041-1049.
9. Early, J.L. and Schnell, R.C. (1978) Res. Commun. Chem. Path. Pharmacol., 19, 369-372.
10. Levander, O.A. (1978) Environ. Health Perspect., 25, 77-80.

Mechanisms of Toxicity and Hazard Evaluation
B. Holmstedt, R. Lauwerys, M. Mercier, M. Roberfroid eds

NEUROPATHOLOGICAL CHANGES CAUSED BY TRIALKYLLEAD COMPOUNDS IN THE RAT

A.A. SEAWRIGHT, A.W. BROWN, W.N. ALDRIDGE, R.D. VERSCHOYLE and B.W. STREET
Toxicology Unit, Medical Research Council Laboratories, Carshalton, Surrey, United Kingdom.

INTRODUCTION

Recently, low levels of organic lead (possibly trialkyllead) of unknown significance have been reported in the brains of people dying from natural causes in an urban environment[1]. Trialkyllead compounds are formed from the ingested or inhaled tetraalkyllead by the microsomal monooxygenases in the liver from which they are transported to the brain where they exert toxic effects[2,3].

In the present investigation the proximately toxic trialkyllead metabolites were dosed to rats and the brain lesions resulting were studied in semi-serial paraffin sections from perfusion fixed tissue.

MATERIALS AND METHODS

Animals. Female rats of 40 to 50g and of 120 and 150g body weight were used. These were fed on the MRC 41B cubed diet and given tap water *ad libitum*.

Experimental procedures. The rats were dosed by gavage after overnight fasting with either trimethyl-(TML) or triethyllead acetate (TEL) dissolved in distilled water. For pathological examination of the brains, the animals were anaesthetised and killed by cardiac perfusion with FAM following clamping of the thoracic aorta[4]. The brains were embedded in paraffin wax and each 20th section stained with haematoxylin and eosin, cresyl violet, Luxol fast blue and cresyl violet, and phosphotungstic acid haematoxylin for histological examination.

Triethyllead concentrations in blood and brains of a separate group of rats dosed with TEL acetate were measured using a modification of the method of Bolanowska[5] (Street, B.W. unpublished).

RESULTS

Single dose TEL acetate. The clinical signs of toxicity following 20mg/kg TEL acetate in both weanling and 120-150g rats after over night fasting were similar in that no changes were apparent until the second day when the animals became hyperexcitable, lost weight and showed whole body fine tremor. On the third day all animals became aggressive with continuous crying out, sparring and fighting and had to be separated to prevent mortality. This state persisted for a further five days during which most rats had impaired balance when standing on the hind legs and some died in convulsions, paralysis or coma. Behaviour in surviving rats was normal again by about ten days when growth was resumed.

Significant pathological changes were confined to the brain. Microscopically on the first day there was sporadic necrosis of neurones in the pyriform cortex characterised by nuclear pyknosis or karyorrhexis with shrunken eosinophilic cytoplasm. By the second day necrotic neurones were present as well in the retrohippocampal and entorhinal cortex, the fascia dentata and regions h3-5 of the antero-dorsal hippocampus. On the third day there was extensive necrosis in the postero-ventral region of the fascia dentata and chromatolysis of most other neurones of the hippocampus. Later, sporadic neuronal necrosis was present in the neocortex and accompanied neuronal chromatolysis and fragmentation in various brain stem nuclei, the septum, amygdaloid nuclei, caudate nucleus and thalamus. Progressive levels of TEL in the blood and brain of intoxicated 150g rats are set out in Table 1.

TABLE 1.

MEAN LEVELS OF TEL (nmoles/g wet weight) IN BLOOD AND BRAIN OF FEMALE RATS DOSED WITH 20mg/kg TEL ACETATE BY THE ORAL ROUTE.

	Day 1[a]	Day 2	Day 3	Day 4	Day 5	Day 10
Blood	83.25(4)[b]	142.10(8)	89.21(9)	89.23(8)	59.81(7)	13.23(8)
Brain	34.50(4)	52.41(8)	35.73(9)	40.89(8)	33.76(7)	15.99(7)

[a]Day 1 means 24 hours after dosing
[b]Numbers of animals in parenthesis

The highest level of TEL in both blood and brain occurred on the second day after dosing (Table 1). High levels were still present on the fifth day but were much lower by 10 days by which time the animals did not show behavioural abnormalities and aggression. In contrast to trimethyltin[6], no correction for blood content in brain is required. The minimal levels of trimethyltin in brain tissue producing neuronal damage is 8.6 nmoles/g wet weight[6]; this is much less than the results shown for triethyllead in Table 1.

In rats dosed with 36 mg/kg TML acetate, the clinical syndrome was similar but lesions in the brain stem, neocortex, and hippocampus were more diffuse.

Multiple doses of TEL acetate. Rats of 150g body weight were dosed with 10 mg/kg of TEL acetate weekly to effect. Typical signs of intoxication appeared on the 3rd day after the 4th dose. All rats then recovered during 2 weeks when dosing was resumed. In all, some 120 mg/kg total of TEL acetate were dosed to these rats over 19 weeks during which similar episodes of toxicity followed by recovery occurred 5 times. Notwithstanding this treatment the rats had reached the same weight as undosed controls and appeared normal at the time of necropsy.

Neuropathological examination of the brains of these animals after 3 and 5 episodes of non fatal intoxication revealed moderate to extensive loss of neurons in h3-5 of the hippocampus and in the pyriform cortex. Occasional necrotic neurones were also observed in nuclei of the medulla oblongata.

In a further experiment, 120g rats were dosed with 5 mg/kg of TEL acetate approximately twice weekly for 29 doses giving a total intake of TEL of 145 mg/kg. No clinical signs of typical TEL toxicity occurred but final weight of the animals was only about 2/3 that of undosed controls. No neuropathological changes could be observed in these animals examined at the conclusion of the experiment.

DISCUSSION

The behavioural changes, toxic effects and distribution of neuropathological lesions found in rats dosed with LD_{50} doses of TEL and TML were similar to, but less severe than, those described in rats intoxicated with trimethyltin chloride[6,7], suggesting a common mechanism of injury. However, in the trialkyllead intoxications, lesions were not restricted mainly to elements of the limbic system as with trimethyltin but extended to various brain stem nuclei, particularly the red nucleus, vestibular nucleus and nuclei of the reticular formation. The concentration of neuronal injury in the rats in TEL intoxication is of interest and may indicate their particular susceptibility to the toxin and/or the local concentration of the toxin itself. There is no evidence for the latter in trimethyltin intoxication[7].

Blood and brain levels of TEL persist for several days after dosing[8,9] (cf. Table 1). No significant signs of toxicity occurred for 24 hours despite the fact that brain levels of the compound were already high and necrosis of neurones observed. Moreover, while brain levels of TEL were highest 2 days after dosing, major behavioural changes and toxic effects were not present until 3 days. Blood and brain levels of TEL were low by 10 days after dosing when the behaviour had returned to normal.

The results of multiple dosing with subsequent multiple episodes of toxicity confirms that in the rat at least, substantial loss of neurones may occur in the hippocampus and other centres without apparent neurological deficit[6,10]. The outcome of the present multiple dose study in the rat resembles the clinical picture in an adolescent subject addicted to sniffing leaded gasoline[11] in whom death occurred after several bouts of encephalopathy. In the latter and other studies[12,13] the distribution of cerebral lesions was stated to be non-specific but extensive loss of neurones from regions h3-5 of the hippocampus was a feature of the neuropathology. The present studies indicate, however, that under controlled experimental conditions of intoxication with TEL and TML, the distribution of lesions in the CNS is in fact characteristic and resembled that seen in trimethyltin toxicity in the rat[6].

REFERENCES

1. Nielsen, T., Jansen, K.A. and Grandjean, P. (1978) Nature, 274, 602-603.
2. Cremer, J.E. (1959) Br. J. industr. Med. 16, 191-199.
3. Cremer, J.E. and Callaway, S. (1961) Br. J. industr. Med. 18, 277-282.
4. Brown, A.W. and Brierley, J.B. (1968) Br. J. exp. Path. 49, 87-106.
5. Bolanowska, W. (1967) Chemia analit. 12, 121-129.
6. Brown, A.W., Aldridge, W.N., Street, B.W. and Verschoyle, R.D. (1979) Am. J. Path. 97, 59-76.
7. Street, B.W., Verschoyle, R.D. and Aldridge, W.N. (unpublished information)
8. Bolanowska, W. (1968) Br. J.industr. Med. 25, 203-208.
9. Hayakawa, K. (1972) Japn. J. Hyg. 26, 526-534.
10. Bullock, J.D., Uley, R.J., Zaia, J.A., Zarembok, I. and Schroeder, H.A. (1966) Arch. Environ. Health, 13, 21-22.
11. Valpey, R., Sumi, S.M., Copass, M.K. and Goble, G.J. (1978) Neurobiology, 28,507-510.
12. Davis, R.K., Horton, A.W., Larson, E.E. and Stemmer, K.L. (1963) Arch. Environ. Health, 6, 473-479.
13. Schepers, G.W.H. (1964) Arch. Environ. Health, 8, 277-295.

© 1980 Elsevier/North-Holland Biomedical Press
Mechanisms of Toxicity and Hazard Evaluation
B. Holmstedt, R. Lauwerys, M. Mercier, M. Roberfroid eds

METHYLMERCURY POISONING IN MOTHERS AND THEIR SUCKLING INFANTS

LAMAN AMIN-ZAKI, S.B. ELHASSANI, M.A. MAJEED, University of Baghdad, Baghdad, Iraq, T.W. CLARKSON, R.A. DOHERTY, M.R. GREENWOOD, Environmental Health Sciences Center, University of Rochester School of Medicine, Rochester, New York 14642, USA

INTRODUCTION

Probably the most catastrophic outbreak of methylmercury poisoning took place in rural Iraq in the winter of 1971-72. The rural families prepared and consumed contaminated bread from seed wheat treated with a methylmercury fungicide for a period of 1-3 months[1]. Thus, all ages and both sexes were exposed to highly neurotoxic methylmercury compounds. Infants who were born shortly before their mothers consumed the contaminated bread and were exposed exclusively through their mothers' milk are the subjects of this and previous reports[2,3].

In rural Iraq, infants are breast fed almost exclusively for one year and often throughout the second year. In the second year of life solids, in the form of bread, may be given to the infant to suck. Thirty infant-mother pairs were observed and followed over a period of five years (1972-1977) in order to detect neurological, mental, or other adverse health effects of methylmercury.

RESULTS AND COMMENTS

Mothers. Signs and symptoms in the mothers is typical of methylmercury poisoning in adults[4,5,6]. Sensory, visual, motor and cerebellar dysfunction dominated the clinical picture. The mothers were classified into three groups: 1)asymptomatic (no signs or symptoms); 2) symptoms only; 3) signs and symptoms. Mothers having only subjective complaints (symptoms only) would correspond to the "mild" category and those who had both signs and symptoms would correspond to the "moderate" to "very severe" category as proposed by Damluji for classifying Iraqi cases of methylmercury poisoning[6].

The concentration of total mercury in blood at the time the first sample was collected shows wide individual variations (Fig. 1A). In general, a downward trend is apparent in samples collected later in the year (1972). This is to be expected since, in most cases, intake of contaminated bread had ceased about the middle of January and no new cases of poisoning were reported after March 1, 1972[7]. The severity of poisoning, as indicated by the three groups defined above, showed no relationship to current blood mercury levels.

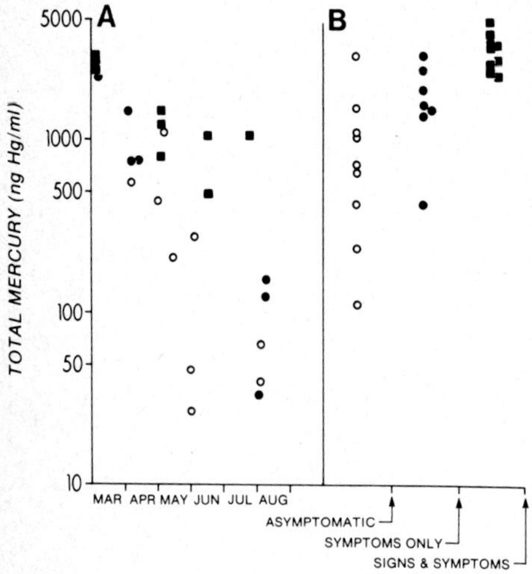

Fig. 1. Blood concentrations at (A) the time of sampling and (B) extrapolated to the estimated value on March 1 are given in relation to date of sampling and severity of poisoning. The symbols are: ○ Asymptomatic; ● Symptoms only; ■ Signs and symptoms.

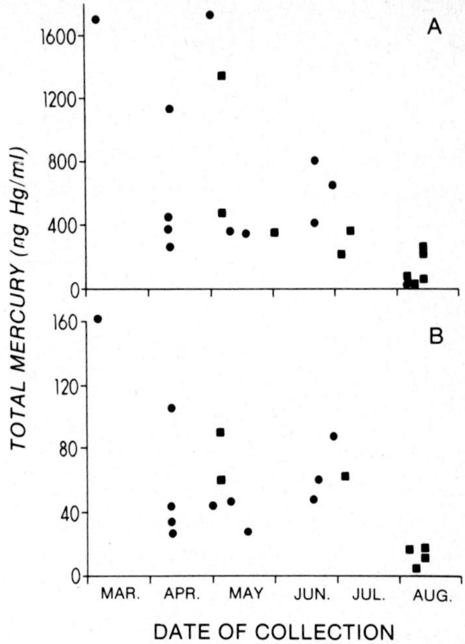

Fig. 2. Concentrations of samples of infant blood (A) and maternal milk (B) plotted according to date of collection. Each point is from one infant. In most cases the blood and milk sample was collected on the same date. The infants are divided into two groups: those fed solely on breast milk (●) (group I), and those who may have ingested some additional methylmercury from contaminated bread (■) (group II).

Since the clinical effects were persistent, whereas the blood concentrations were changing, it was decided to make the clinical comparison with blood levels estimated to exist immediately following the outbreak. For those patients from whom a sufficient number of samples had been collected, the biological half-time in blood estimated for each individual, was used to extrapolate the blood concentration back to March 1, 1972. Adequate data were available for 10 mothers. In cases where only one or two samples of blood had been collected (16 mothers), the average biological half-time in blood (45 days) collected for the ten mothers was used to make this extrapolation. The estimated half-times are typical of the short biological half-times reported previously in lactating women[8].

When blood concentrations are corrected to March 1, 1972 a wide range is still seen within each clinical group (Fig. 1B). Nevertheless, the group with the most severe poisoning (signs and symptoms) has an average mercury concentration significantly higher than either the milder (symptoms only) or the asymptomatic group.

The mercury concentrations reported in Fig. 1 are total mercury. However, organic mercury (identified as methylmercury[1]), accounted for most of the mercury in blood.

Infants. The concentrations of total mercury in infant blood and in milk of their mothers decreased with time (Fig. 2). Some of the infants observed had blood concentrations well in excess of the minimum toxic range (200-500 ng/ml) estimated for adults by a WHO expert committee[9]. Infants who were nine months of age or younger at the earliest date the mother consumed the contaminated bread are depicted as group I. These infants consumed only their mothers' milk. Group II infants were older and may have sucked and eaten some contaminated bread. However, there were no striking differences in blood concentrations between the two groups indicating that even in group II the predominant route of intake of mercury was breast milk.

As is the case of maternal blood, the organic fraction is large, accounting for an average of 86% of the total mercury in infant blood. However, maternal milk had a much lower fraction of organic mercury, about 60% of the total.

The 11 male and female infants ranged from 1 to 20 months of age at the time of exposure. On first examination, the only evidence of effect on the central nervous system was the excessively brisk deep tendon reflexes which did not seem at the time to interfere with motor function. The remaining 19 cases were free from clinical manifestations of methylmercury poisoning. The children were old enough to have acquired such skills as sitting without support, crawling and even walking before the exposure. Yet on follow-up, over a five year period, the development of these infants apparently slowed down. In at least 5 of the infants who were not old enough to walk during the outbreak, walking was delayed beyond two years of age.

Language development seemed to be specifically affected. Mothers voluntarily stated they had noticed and worried about delay of speech in these children before the authors questioned them about possible delay. Hearing did not seem to be affected as judged by the children's ability to hear ordinary spoken words. Therefore, the delay in language development is considered a part of the development disorder found in these children. Language development correlates with intelligence and children of subnormal intelligence (I.Q. 50-70) usually exhibit relatively severe speech and language deficiences when compared with children of normal intelligence[10].

The combination of delay in motor development, language development, and toilet training, together with brisk deep tendon reflexes and sometimes a bilaterally positive Babinski's reflex, were interpreted to indicated damage to the central nervous system. The mothers of these infants had noticed their impairment and they described their infants: "They are like needles blunted by the poison."

ACKNOWLEDGEMENTS

We should like to thank the Universities of Baghdad, Iraq and Rochester, USA for sponsoring the study. This work was supported by the National Institute of Environmental Health Sciences, Grant No. ES 01247 and ES 01248.

REFERENCES

1. Bakir, F., Damluji, S.F., Amin-Zaki, L., Murtada, M., Khalidi, A., Al-Rawi, N.Y., Tikriti, S., Dhahir, H.I., Clarkson, T.W., Smith, J.C. and Doherty, R.A. (1973) Science, 181, 230-241.
2. Amin-Zaki, L., Elhassani, S., Majeed, M.A., Clarkson, T.W., Doherty, R.A. and Greenwood, M.R. (1974) J. of Pediatrics, 85, 81-84.
3. Amin-Zaki, L., Elhassani, S.B., Majeed, M.A., Clarkson, T.W., Doherty, R.A. and Greenwood, M.R. (1976) Am. J. Dis. Child., 130, 1070-1076.
4. Tsubaki, T., Shirakawa, K. (1969) Science, 13, 85-88.
5. Rustam, H. and Hamdi, T. (1974) Brain, 97, Part III, 499-510.
6. Damluji, S.F. and the Clinical Committee on Mercury Poisoning (1974) Bull WHO Suppl 53, 65-81.
7. Al-Tikriti, L. and Al-Mufti, A.W. (1974) Bull WHO, Suppl 53, 15-21.
8. Greenwood, M.R., Clarkson, T.W., Doherty, R.A., Gates, A.H., Amin-Zaki, L., Elhassani, S.B., Majeed, M.A. (1978) Environ. Res. 16, 48-54.
9. WHO Criteria Document on Mercury (1977), WHO, Geneva, Switzerland.
10. Nelson, W.E., Vaughan, V.C. and McKay, J. (1969) Textbook of Pediatrics. W.B. Saunders Co., Philadelphia, p. 106.

Mechanisms of Toxicity and Hazard Evaluation
B. Holmstedt, R. Lauwerys, M. Mercier, M. Roberfroid eds

THE EFFECT OF THE GASTROINTESTINAL FLORA ON TISSUE CONTENT OF MERCURY AND ORGANOMERCURIAL NEUROTOXICITY IN RATS GIVEN METHYLMERCURIC CHLORIDE.

I.R. Rowland, M.J. Davies and J.G. Evans.
The British Industrial Biological Research Association, Woodmansterne Road, Carshalton, Surrey. SM5 4DS. Gt. Britain.

INTRODUCTION

We have previously demonstrated [1] that the human and rat gut microfloras can metabolise methylmercury in vitro to metallic mercury and to a sulphur derivative of methylmercury - later shown to be bis (methylmercuric) sulphide [2]. In view of the great differences in biological activity and toxicity of the different forms of mercury [3] it is possible that these bacterial biotransformations of methylmercury could significantly affect the toxicity of the ingested mercurial. In the present communication we have assessed the influence of the gut flora on the in vivo metabolism, excretion, tissue content and toxicity of methylmercuric chloride, by using conventional rats and rats treated with antibiotics to eliminate their intestinal bacteria.

MATERIALS AND METHODS

Accumulation of mercury by rats. Of two groups of 7 male Wister rats (135-150g), one group ('conventional') was given water and autoclaved Spratt's Laboratory Animal Diet No. 1 ad lib. The other group was given the autoclaved diet and water containing bacitracin, neomycin sulphate and streptomycin sulphate each at 2 mg/ml. The faeces were found to be free of bacteria after 3 days of the antibiotic regimen and remained so until the end of the experiment.

On days 4-8 and 11-14, the rats were given, by gastric intubation, 13 µg $CH_3{}^{203}HgCl$ in saline (0.5 ml; 0.03 µc/rat/day). In other experiments doses of 1µg/day were given. 18 hours after the last dose of $CH_3{}^{203}HgCl$ the rats were killed and the amount of radioactivity in the blood, kidney, liver, lung, brain, skeletal muscle and faeces was measured. The proportion of methylmercury in the homogenised tissues was determined by extraction with benzene [4] and then chromatography of the benzene extract on thin layer plates of silica gel G using chloroform-n-hexane (9:1 vol/vol)

Although the organ weights of the antibiotic-treated animals were lower, the total mercury content of the whole organs of these animals was significantly greater than in the conventional rats, except in the case of the liver. Similar results were obtained in rats given 1μg CH_3HgCl per day although the increase in mercury content of tissues in the antibiotic treated animals was smaller (20-30%). The proportion of mercury present in the methylated form in the different tissues varied considerably (Table 1), being highest in brain, muscle and lungs, whereas in liver, blood and kidney a substantial part of the mercury was apparently present in an inorganic form. In the kidney, but not in any other organ studied, the proportion of mercury present as methylmercury was significantly higher in the rats without a gut flora than in the conventional animals (Table 1).

The faecal mercury concentration in the conventional rats was five times that of the antibiotic treated group and the total faecal excretion of mercury over 24 hours, which compensates for the greater faecal bulk of the latter animals, was two fold higher in the conventional rats. Thus it would appear that the elimination of the intestinal flora of the rat leads to an increase in the amount of mercury in tissues, reduces the excretion of mercury in faeces and results in a greater proportion of methylmercury in the kidneys and faeces.

When rats in which the gut flora had been eliminated were treated with high doses of CH_3HgCl (10mg/kg/day) for 5 days), they gained less weight over the experimental period (35 days) than did conventional rats given the same dose of alkylmercurial (Table 2). Four out of five rats given CH_3HgCl with antibiotics developed signs of neurological toxicity and furthermore, histological examination of three of the clinically affected rats revealed damage in the granular layer of the cerebellum, consisting of large numbers of pyknotic nuclei with some reduction in numbers of neurones (Table 2).

In contrast, only one of five conventional rats given CH_3HgCl developed signs of neurological damage.

The results indicate that the gut flora of the rat plays a protective role by effectively reducing the toxicity of ingested CH_3HgCl.

as developer [5].

Neurotoxic effects and cerebellar lesion induced by methylmercuric chloride

Conventional and antibiotic-treated rats were given 5 oral doses of CH_3HgCl (10mg/kg/day) in 50% aqueous polyethylene glycol 400. Crossing over of hind limbs when the rat was suspended by its tail was taken as a sign of neurological damage. Thirty days after the last dose 3 rats from each group were subjected to whole body perfusion [6] using the fixative formalin-glacial acetic acid-methanol (10:10:80). Sections of cerebellar tissue were prepared and stained with Ehlichs haemotoxylin and eosin.

RESULTS & DISCUSSION

In rats given 13 µg $CH_3{}^{203}HgCl$ per day, the concentration of mercury in kidney, blood, muscle, brain and lung was significantly higher (by 30-40%) in the antibiotic-treated animals than in the conventional group (Table 1).

TABLE 1

TISSUE CONCENTRATION AND FORM OF MERCURY IN RATS GIVEN $CH_3{}^{203}HgCl$ (13 µg/day for 9 days)

Values shown are the means ± standard error of mean for 7 rats and those marked with asterisks differ significantly from controls (Wilcoxon rank sum test. $*P < 0.05$; $**P < 0.01$

Tissue	Conventional rats		Antibiotic-treated rats	
	ng Hg/g	% extracted by benzene	ng Hg/g tissue	% extracted benzene
Kidney	1720 ± 70	58.6 ± 1.3	2450** ± 110	66.4* ± 1.0
Blood	1530 ± 70	53.0 ± 2.2	2060** ± 180	51.5 ± 1.7
Liver	430 ± 30	61.8 ± 2.5	410 ± 30	54.8 ± 1.9
Lung	360 ± 20	72.9 ± 1.4	480** ± 40	82.8 ± 1.2
Muscle	320 ± 30	85.9 ± 3.0	450** ± 20	83.8 ± 1.5
Brain	110 ± 10	82.8 ± 1.0	140 ± 10	82.3 ± 1.0

TABLE 2.

INFLUENCE OF INTESTINAL FLORA ON INDUCTION OF NEUROLOGICAL SYMPTOMS AND CEREBELLAR DAMAGE BY CH_3HgCl IN RATS.

Treatment	Body weight		No. of rats with neurotoxic symptoms[d]	No. of rats with cerebellar damage[e]
	initial	final[c]		
Untreated	141 ± 6	349 ± 6	0/5	0/3
Antibiotics[a]	139 ± 5	340 ± 20	0/5	0/3
CH_3HgCl[b]	140 ± 6	276 ± 33	1/5	1/3
Antibiotics[a] + CH_3HgCl[b]	141 ± 5	221 ± 18	4/5	3/3

[a] 5 daily doses of 10mg/kg by stomach tube.
[b] Bacitracin, neomycin, streptomycin each at 2mg/ml in drinking water.
[c] 35 days after start of experiment.
[d] Crossing over of hind limbs when rats was held vertically.
[e] Pyknotic nuclei in granular layer (3 rats from each group studied)

ACKNOWLEDGEMENT

This work forms part of a research project sponsored by the UK Ministry of Agriculture Fisheries and Food to whom our thanks are due. The results of the research are the property of the Ministry and are Crown Copyright.

REFERENCES

1. Rowland, I.R., Davies, M.J. and Grasso, P. (1978) Xenobiotica 8, 37-43.

2. Craig, P.J., and Bartlett, P.D. (1978). Nature (London) 275, 635-637

3. Friberg, L. and Vostal, J. (1972) Mercury in the Environment, CRC Press, Cleveland, Ohio.

4. Westöö, G. (1966) Acta Chem. Scand. 28, 2131-2137.

5. Snyder, D.R. and Braun, J.J. (1977) Toxic. appl. Pharmac. 41, 277-284.

6. Glauert, A.M. (1974). Practical Methods in Electron Microscopy 3, p.82 North Holland/American Elsevier.

Mechanisms of Toxicity and Hazard Evaluation
B. Holmstedt, R. Lauwerys, M. Mercier, M. Roberfroid eds

EFFECTS OF XYLENE AND ALCOHOL ON HUMAN VISUAL EVOKED POTENTIALS

ANNA MARIA SEPPÄLÄINEN, KAI SAVOLAINEN and TERO KOVALA
Institute of Occupational Health, Haartmaninkatu 1, SF-00290
Helsinki 29 (Finland)

INTRODUCTION

Changes in visual evoked potentials (VEP) of the brain have been described in connection with experimental human exposure to methylene chloride[1]. Industrial workers, who are occupationally exposed to solvents, may simultaneously consume alcohol or come to work with some alcohol still prevailing in the blood after drinking the day before. We have studied the effect of an industrial solvent - m-xylene - and alcohol, each alone and also in combination, upon visual evoked potentials.

MATERIALS AND METHODS

Subjects. The subjects of this study were 8 healthy male volunteers, 21 - 26 yr of age. All had normal physical findings in medical examination, their electroencephalograms (EEG) were normal as well.

Exposures. Four persons at a time were exposed to m-xylene in a 15 m^3 exposure chamber with a dynamic controlled environment. The exposures were performed for four hours once a week over nine consecutive weeks. The experiments were single-blind and the subjects acted as their own controls. As exposures were used about 150 ppm (700 mg/m^3) and 300 ppm (1200 mg/m^3) of xylene alone or in combination with a single dose of alcohol 0.8 g/kg body weight, and single doses of alcohol 0.4 g/kg and 0.8 g/kg. During the first, 5th and 9th experimental days the subjects stayed for four hours in the exposure chamber without any exposure, the first experimental day served as an adaptation day, the other nonexposure days were used as controls. The peak blood alcohol concentrations of about 0.3 and 0.7 g/l were measured 60 min after ingestion of the alcohol and the concentration had decreased to 0.03 and 0.25 g/l at the time of electrophysiological tests.

Visual evoked potentials (VEP) were recorded in a semidark room with a midoccipital electrode 5 cm above the inion and the reference electrode on the earlobe. Responses to 50 flashes of 0.2 J were averaged. The main components of the VEPs were identified from plotted analog recordings and the exact latencies and peak-to-peak amplitudes were taken from a digital computer print-out.

The recordings took place in the mornings before the subjects entered the exposure chamber and before they were given the alcoholic (or nonalcoholic control) drink, and in the afternoons 15 - 30 min after stopping the exposure.

For statistical comparisons of the results the differences in the latencies and amplitudes were calculated between the morning and evening recordings in each day. The within-day differences were used in statistical analysis when comparing VEPs during various exposure conditions. As the reference values we used the means of respective values in experimental days 5 and 9 (control days). Wilcoxon Matched-Pairs Signed-Ranks Test was applied for testing the significance of differences.

RESULTS

Seven peaks were identified in the VEPs. The interindividual variation in the latencies was of the order of 10 %, in the amplitudes there was a slightly greater interindividual variability. The intraindividual variability of morning registrations was small in the latencies and slightly larger in the amplitudes.

During the control days nearly all the latencies were a little shorter in the afternoon registrations. The peak-to-peak amplitudes of P29-N40, N60-P115, P115-N155 and N155-P205 were slightly higher in the afternoons of the control days. Alcohol dose of 0.8 g/kg increased the latencies of P50, N60, P115 and N155.[x] The effect of alcohol 0.4 g/kg was smaller, but concerning the latency of P50 the difference in comparison to the control day was statistically significant ($p<0.5$).

When the subjects were exposed to xylene alone or in combination with alcohol, the latencies often were shorter in the after-

---

[x], concerning the latter three latencies the difference was statistically significant ($p<0.05$).

noons than in the mornings, and the magnitude of the change was similar to that in the control days. The latencies tended to be longer, when the subjects had ingested 0.8 g/kg alcohol and had been exposed to 150 ppm of xylene.

The changes in the amplitudes were not great, and alcohol alone did not decrease the amplitude significantly. Figure 1 represents actual VEPs of a subject in a control day afternoon as well as after exposure to xylene and alcohol. Exposure to 300 ppm of xylene in combination with prior ingestion of alcohol 0.8 g/kg decreased significantly ($p<0.05$) the amplitude of N60-P115. The effect of this exposure was of similar direction upon the amplitude of P115-N155. The effects of xylene 150 ppm with alcohol and that of xylene 300 ppm alone were towards similar direction, but without statistical significance. 150 ppm of xylene did not have any effect on the amplitudes of the VEP components.

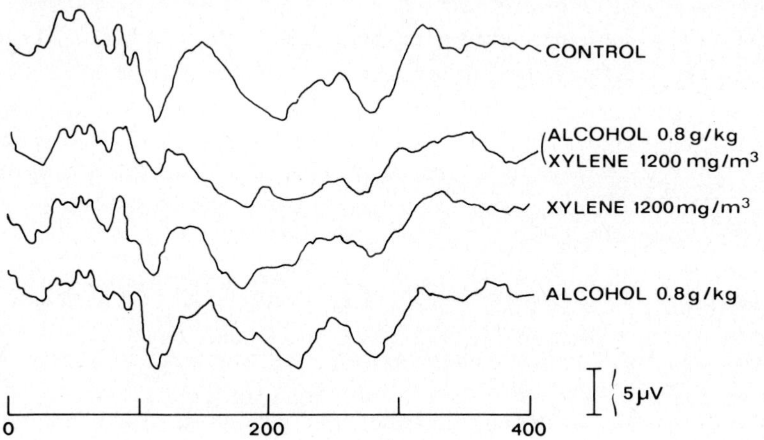

Fig. 1. VEPs of a healthy person during a control day afternoon and after exposures to xylene and alcohol

DISCUSSION

In the afternoons of the control days the latencies were slightly shorter and amplitudes slightly higher, perhaps reflecting a higher level of arousal. Alcohol, especially the higher dose, increased the latencies, but did not affect the amplitudes of VEP. Xylene had no effect on the latencies and counteracted in this regard the effect of alcohol. The combined effect of xylene and alcohol decreased the amplitude of major VEP components and exposure to 300 ppm of xylene alone tended to have a similar effect. All the latencies increased and amplitudes decreased belong to the components originated in the cerebral cortex[2]. The minor changes noted in VEPs after exposure to xylene or alcohol could be explained by variations in the arousal level as suggested by Kalant[3], although Obitz et al.[4] argued that alcohol-induced increases in the latencies of VEP components could reflect a direct cortical depression.

Thus, even after 4h had passed since ingestion of alcohol and while the actual blood alcohol concentrations were very low, changes could be noted in VEPs. In certain aspects, changes could be noted after combined exposure to xylene and alcohol, although xylene alone had no significant effect. The combined effects of certain solvents and alcohol may be more deleterious than exposure to a single agent.

REFERENCES

1. Stewart, R.D., Fischer, T.N., Hosko, M.J., Peterson, J.E., Baretta, E.D. and Dodd, H.C. (1972) Arch.Environ. Health, 25, 343-348.
2. Allison, T., Matsumiya, Y., Goff, G.D. and Goff, W.R. (1977) Electroenceph. Clin. Neurophysiol. 42, 185-197.
3. Kalant, H. (1978) Advances in Pharmacology and Therapeutics. vol. 8, Pergamon Press, Oxford, pp. 199-209.
4. Obitz, F.W., Thodes, L.E. and Creel, D. (1977) J. Studies on Alcohol, 38, 2057-2064.

© 1980 Elsevier/North-Holland Biomedical Press
Mechanisms of Toxicity and Hazard Evaluation
B. Holmstedt, R. Lauwerys, M. Mercier, M. Roberfroid eds

SENSITIVITY OF RAT BRAIN SYNAPTOSOMAL ATPases TO SEVERAL STRUCTURALLY RELATED ORGANOCHLORINE COMPOUNDS

D. DESAIAH, C. H. TROTTMAN* AND S. K. BANSAL

Department of Neurology, University of Mississippi Medical Center, and Veterans Administration Medical Center, Jackson, Ms. 39216 and *Department of Chemistry, Jackson State University, Jackson, Ms. 39217 (U.S.A.)

INTRODUCTION

In recent years several organochlorine compounds were extensively investigated to elucidate their mechanism of action without much success. However, several laboratories have shown that ATPase activities are sensitive to many of these compounds.[1-10] The sensitivity of specific enzymes differ depending on the structure of the compound used. For example, DDT (Tri-chloro, bis (P-chlorophenyl) ethane) inhibited the oligomycin-sensitive Mg^{2+} ATPase more than it did other ATPases.[1-4] Chlordecone (decachlorooctahydro-3,4-methano-2H-cyclobuta (cd) pentalen-2-one) inhibited both Na^{+} - K^{+} and oligomycin-sensitive Mg^{2+} ATPases but had no inhibitory effect on oligomycin-insensitive Mg^{++} ATPase.[6,7,9,10] Mirex (dodecachloropentacyclodecane), a close structural analog of chlordecone, did not inhibit any of the ATPases tested.[6,7]

In the present investigation an attempt was made to compare the sensitivity of Na^{+} - K^{+} and Mg^{2+} ATPases to six structurally related organochlorine compounds whose structures are shown in Figure 1. Also, we have attempted to elucidate the mechanism of enzyme inhibition by means of kinetic evaluation of the effects of these compounds on rat brain synaptosomal ATPases.

MATERIALS AND METHODS

Male Sprague-Dawley rats (200g) obtained from Charles River Company, Wilmington, Ma., were used. Chlordecone was kindly supplied by Allied Chemical Company, Morristown, N.J. Mirex and its photoproducts were donated by the late Dr. B. R. Layton of Mississippi State University. All other chemicals used for enzyme assay were purchased from Sigma Chemical Company, St. Louis, Mo.

Rat brain synaptosomal fractions were prepared using a discontinuous Ficoll - sucrose gradient method.[10] ATPase activities were measured by the coupled enzymatic method.[7-10] Protein content was determined by the method of Lowry et al.[11] Kinetic analysis of the effect of the test compounds on various substrate activation was done as reported.[12]

Double reciprocal plots of kinetic data were constructed according to the method of Lineweaver and Burk,[13] Data were subjected to regression analysis and regression lines plotted for best straight-line fit. Km and Vmax values were read from the graphs and tabulated. Student's t test was employed to calculate the significance ($P < 0.05$ or better). Each assay was done using four different brain preparations and each preparation was repeated two or more times.

RESULTS AND DISCUSSION

Rat brain synaptosomal Na^+ - K^+ and oligomycin-sensitive Mg^{2+} ATPase activities were in general inhibited by all the compounds tested in a concentration-dependent manner (Figs. 1-2). However, the degree of inhibition of these enzyme activities varied dramatically. For example, 100% inhibition of both enzyme activities were obtained by 10 μM chlordecone as compared to 10% inhibition by mirex at the same concentration. The photo-mirex derivatives inhibited both the enzyme activities. However, the monohydro derivatives were less effective as compared to the dihydro derivatives (Figs. 1-2). A similar response was observed in other tissue fractions.[5]

TABLE 1

EFFECT OF ORGANOCHLORINE COMPOUNDS ON THE RAT BRAIN SYNAPTOSOMAL ATPases' KINETIC PARAMETERS

Compound (μM)		Na^+ - K^+ ATPases						Mg^{2+} ATPases	
		ATP		Na^+		K^+		ATP	
		Km	Vmax	Km	Vmax	Km	Vmax	Km	Vmax
Control		0.14	28.6	3.5	35.7	1.1	34.5	0.08	17.2
Mirex	(20)	0.13	25.0	3.1	30.3	1.4	31.3	0.08	15.6
8-monohydro	(20)	0.11	25.0	3.1	30.3	1.1	30.3	0.07	14.7
10-monohydro	(20)	0.14	23.3	4.5	25.0	1.3	27.0	0.07	13.0
5, 10-dihydro	(20)	0.08	24.4	5.6	28.6	1.4	27.0	0.09	14.9
2, 8-dihydro	(20)	0.13	24.4	3.1	30.3	1.1	31.3	0.08	15.4
Chlordecone	(0.5)	0.14	22.7	3.4	25.0	1.2	26.3	0.07	10.6
Chlordecone	(2.0)	0.13	17.9	3.7	19.2	1.5	17.5	0.06	8.8

Km = mM; Vmax = μmoles Pi/mg protein/hr.

Activation of the Na^+ - K^+ and Mg^{2+} ATPases at low affinity nucleotide-directed sites by ATP was demonstrated by varying ATP concentrations in the presence and absence of the organochlorine compounds (Figs. 3-4 and Table 1). The kinetic data obtained showed a reduction in the Vmax without any significant changes in Km. These results suggested that the effects of the compounds tested on the enzyme activities were independent of substrate ATP and thus of a non-

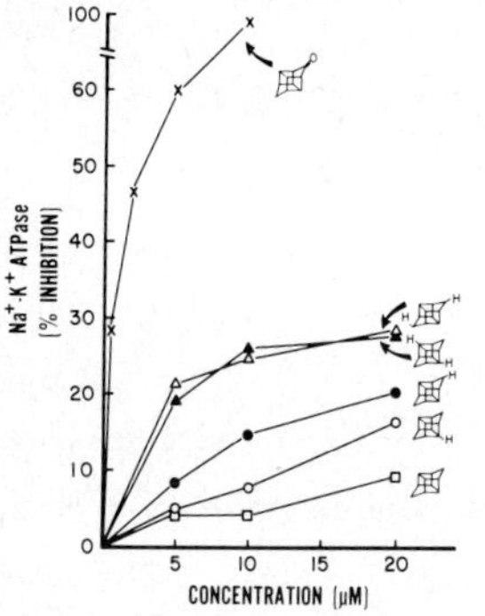

Fig 1. Percent inhibition of Na^+ - K^+ ATPase activity by organochlorine compounds.

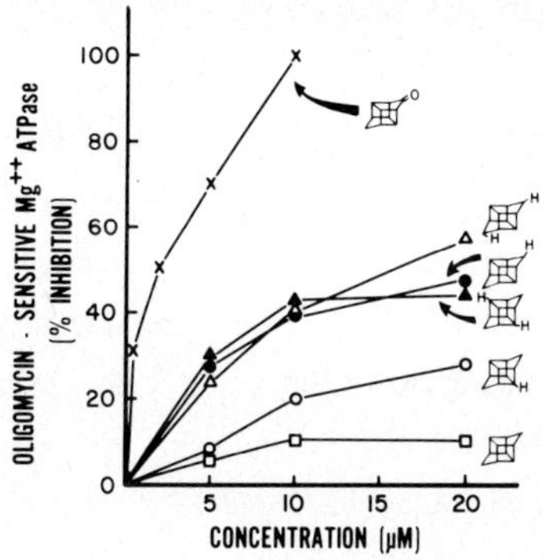

Fig 2. Percent inhibition of Mg^{2+} ATPase activity by organochlorine compounds.

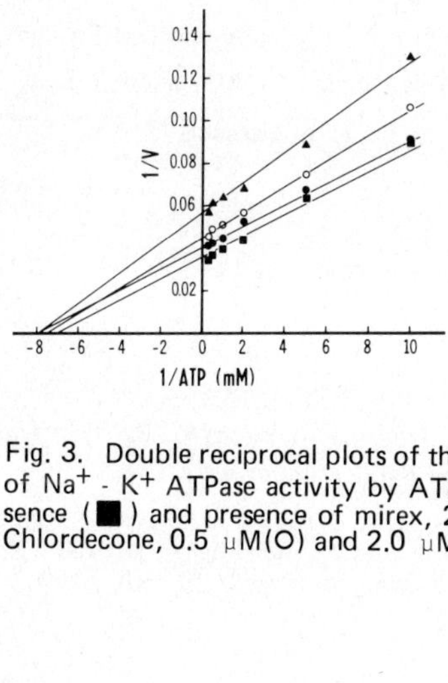

Fig. 3. Double reciprocal plots of the activation of Na^+ - K^+ ATPase activity by ATP in the absence (■) and presence of mirex, 20 μM(●); Chlordecone, 0.5 μM(O) and 2.0 μM(▲).

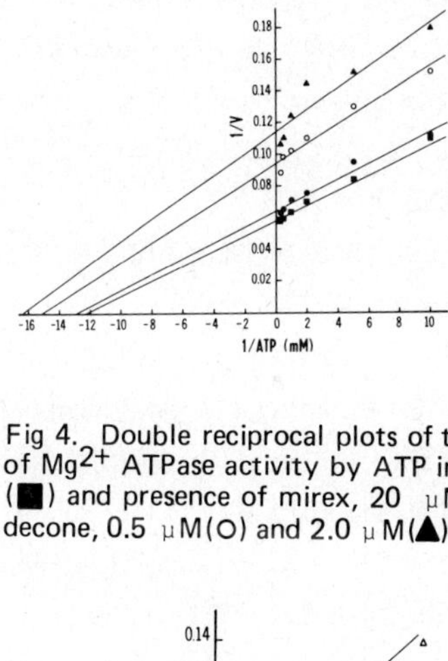

Fig 4. Double reciprocal plots of the activation of Mg^{2+} ATPase activity by ATP in the absence (■) and presence of mirex, 20 μM(●); Chlordecone, 0.5 μM(O) and 2.0 μM(▲).

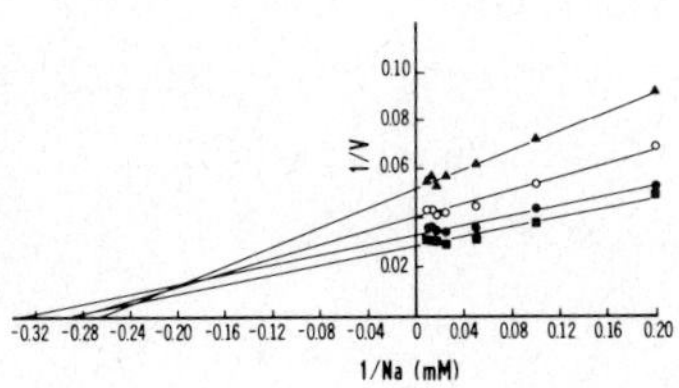

Fig. 5. Double reciprocal plots of the activation of Na^+ - K^+ ATPase by Na^+ in the absence (■) and presence of mirex, 20 μM(●); Chlordecone, 0.5 μM(O) and 2.0 μM(▲).

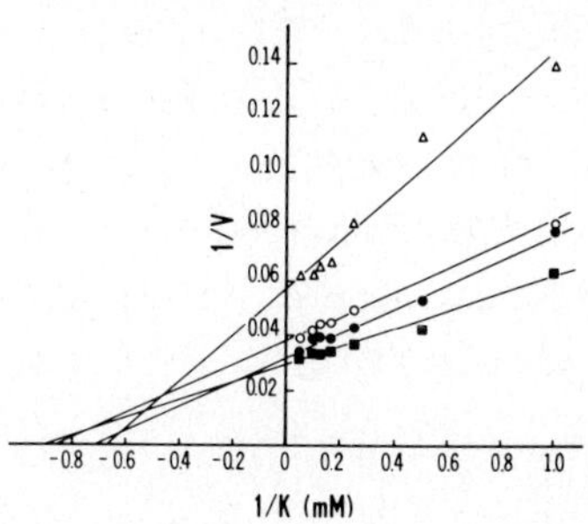

Fig 6. Double reciprocal plots of the activation of Na^+ - K^+ ATPase by K^+ in the absence (■) and presence of mirex, 20 μM(●); Chlordecone, 0.5 μM(O) and 2.0 μM(▲).

competitive nature.

Activation of Na^+ - K^+ ATPase by Na^+ and K^+ was demonstrated by varying the concentrations of Na^+ and K^+ in the absence and presence of the test compounds (Figs. 5-6 and Table 1). The kinetic data obtained showed a reduction of Vmax without any significant changes in Km suggesting a non-competitive type interaction. However, 10-monohydro and 5, 10-dihydro mirex altered the Km as well as Vmax values (Table 1).

The present results indicate that the inhibition of Na^+ - K^+ and Mg^{2+} ATPase activities varies with the structure of the compound. Chlordecone, a polar compound, exhibited the highest inhibitory effect as compared to mirex, a non-polar compound. Similarly, the monohydro derivatives are less effective as compared to the dihydro derivatives thus suggesting that the polarity of these compounds play a major role in the inhibition of ATPase systems.

ACKNOWLEDGEMENTS

This work was supported in part by NIH/MBS Grant RR08047-10 (awarded to C.H.T.) and in part by a grant from the Mississippi Heart Association (awarded to D. D.). We wish to thank the Government of India for providing a post-doctoral fellowship to Dr. S. K. Bansal.

REFERENCES

1. Koch, R.B. (1969) J. Neurochem., 16, 145.
2. Matsumura, F. and Narahashi, T. (1971) Biochem. Pharmacol., 20, 825.
3. Davis, P.W. and Wedemeyer, G.A. (1971) Comp. Biochem. Physiol., 40B, 823.
4. Desaiah, D., Cutkomp, L.K. and Koch, R.B. (1974) Pestic. Biochem. Physiol., 4, 232.
5. Desaiah, D. and Koch, R.B. (1975) J. Agr. Food Chem., 23, 1216.
6. Desaiah, D. and Koch, R.B. (1975) Bull. Enviorn. Contam. Toxicol., 13, 153.
7. Dessaiah, D., Ho, I.K. and Mehendale, H.M. (1977) Toxicol. Appl. Pharmacol., 39, 219.
8. Trottman, C.H. and Desaiah, D. (1979) J. Environ. Sci. Hlth., B. 14, 393.
9. Desaiah, D. (1980) J. Environ, Pathol. Toxicol. (In press).
10. Desaiah, D., Gilliland, T., Ho, I.K. and Mehendale, H.M. (1980) Toxicol. Letters (In press).
11. Lowry, O.H., Rosebrough, N.J., Farr, A.L. and Randall, R.J. (1951) J. Biol. Chem., 193, 265.
12. Phillips, T.D., Hayes, A.W., Ho, I.K. and Desaiah, D. (1978) J. Biol. Chem., 253, 3487.
13. Lineweaver, H. and Burk, D.J. (1934) J. Amer. Chem. Soc., 56, 658.

© 1980 Elsevier/North-Holland Biomedical Press
Mechanisms of Toxicity and Hazard Evaluation
B. Holmstedt, R. Lauwerys, M. Mercier, M. Roberfroid eds

EFFECTS OF LONG TERM EXPOSURE TO TRICHLOROETHYLENE ON LEARNING BEHAVIOUR IN RATS

TOSHIKO IKEDA, REIKO KISHI and HIROTSUGU MIYAKE
Department of Public Health, Sapporo Medical College, S.1, W.17, Chuo-ku, Sapporo 060, Japan

INTRODUCTION

Effects of *long term* exposure to *trichloroethylene*(TCE) on *learning* in rats were investigated in a dose-effects relationship through operant behaviour(FR30, DRL12 sec).

METHODS

The procedure consisted of four parts:(1)selection of rats based on body weight and test battery(CRF and FR30 for learning ability, activity wheel test for spontaneous activity and open field test for emotional response);(2)exposure(2,600, 5,000 and 8,000ppm for 30min/day,6days/week, for 80days);(3)retests about 2 weeks later from the final exposure;(4)acquisition on the DRL12 sec. Forty of 60 naive male Wistar rats were selected on the basis of performance and body weight at 6th months of age. They were then divided into 4 groups each of 10rats:cont.,I(2,600ppm),II(5,000ppm) and III(8,000 ppm).

RESULTS

(1)Before exposure, significant difference was not found among 4 groups except for ambulation between cont. and III(Table 1).(2)All exposed rats recovered from the acute effects of exposure within 10 min after being removed from the chamber.(3)After exposure, any effects on body weight, spontaneous activity and emotional response were not detected except for ambulation of I(Table II).(4)On the retention score of the 1st session of relearning of FR30, difference was not observed between cont. and exposed groups. At the 2nd and later sessions, the responses of the cont. group immediately recovered to the level of responses performed before exposure. On the contrary the responses of the all exposed groups generally did not recover. This result was obvious in inferior rats, expressed by

TABLE 1
RESULTS OF THE TEST PERFORMED BEFORE EXPOSURE

items	group			
	control	I	II	III
(1) Continuous-reinforcement (CRF)[a]	94± 11	97± 17	89± 12	90± 14
(2) Fixed-ratio 30 (FR 30)[b]	287±204	283±199	272±203	279±194
(3) Spontaneous activity and Emotionality				
1. Activity Wheel[c]	619±295	736±282	716±329	713±273
2. Open field test[d]				
A) Ambulation	48± 11	51± 13	47± 13	37± 5
B) Rearing	9± 5	11± 3	11± 5	12± 5
C) Defecation	0.7±1.2	0.7±1.0	0.6±1.0	0.5±1.1
(4) Body weight[e]	311± 24	316± 22	314± 22	309± 24

All figures are given by M±S.D.. (n=10)
a, b : numbers of response/10 min
c : numbers of revolution/30 min, d : counts/2 min, e : gram

TABLE II
RESULTS OF THE TEST PERFORMED AFTER EXPOSURE

items	group			
	control	I	II	III
(1) Continuous-reinforcement (CRF)[a]	98± 14	99± 15	94± 27	96± 13
(2) Fixed-ratio 30 (FR 30)[b]	Retention, Relearning and Extinction			
(3) Spontaneous activity and Emotionality				
1. Activity Wheel[c]	769±423	863±301	914±532	681±280
2. Open field test[d]				
A) Ambulation	45± 17	71± 24*	53± 19	44± 9
B) Rearing	9± 5	11± 5	9± 7	13± 5
C) Defecation	0.6±0.9	0.9±1.6	0.2±0.3	0.9±1.0
(4) Body weight[e]	313± 25	317± 21	310± 23	306± 25

All figures are given by M±S.D.. (C, I, III : n=10, II : n=9)
a, b : numbers of response/10 min
c : numbers of revolution/30 min, d : counts/2 min, e : gram
* : $P<0.05$ (between control and I)

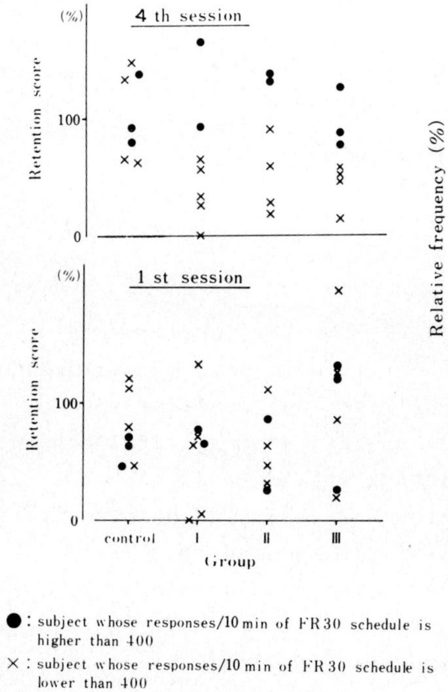

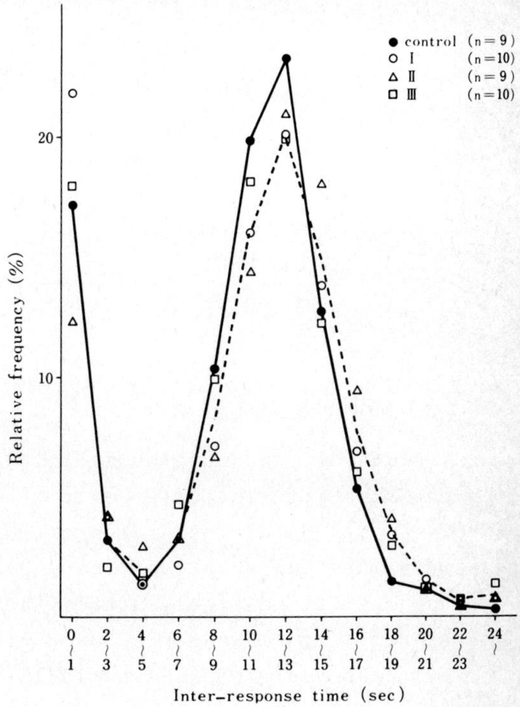

(Fig.2)

(Fig.1)

Fig.1. Retention and relearning of FR30 schedule.(Retention score means responses after exposure/responses before exposure).

Fig.2. Relative frequency of IRT of the 25th-27th sessions of DRL 12 sec schedule.

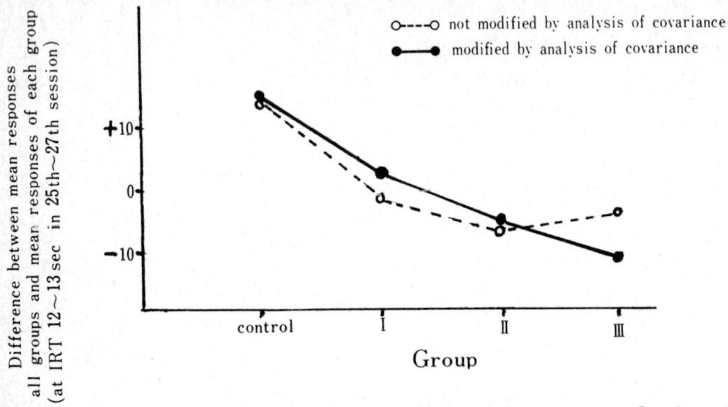

Fig.3. Responses at IRT 12-13 sec of the 25th-27th sessions, modified by analysis of covariance.

cross mark,of exposed groups(Fig.1).(5)Levels of performance on CRF ,which was performed after extinction of FR30, were equal in all groups(Table II)(6)Acquisition of DRL12 sec was observed for 27 sessions. In the relative frequency of IRT(per cent total responses) of the 25-27th sessions, longer intervals than 12-13 sec were significantly high in every exposed groups(Fig.2). And position of peak of exposed groups, especially of III shifted from 12-13 sec to showter or longer intervals. Dose-effects relationship of the relative frequency of IRT was revealed by analysis of covariance, where covariate was ambulation before exposure(Fig.3)(7)On the pathological examination, any change was not detected.

CONCLUSION

Exposed rats were inferior in the relearning of FR30 and the acquisition of DRL12 sec. Retention of FR30 and CRF, spontaneous activity, emotional response and body weight were not influenced. These results suggest impairment of the CNS which was caused by long term exposure to TCE. We propose that learning behaviour(acquisition) is a sensitive measure for adverse effects of environmental neurotoxicants on the CNS.

ACKNOWLEDGEMENTS

We wish to thank Dr.T.Iwamoto,Dept. of Psycol,Hokkaido Univ.,N. Takahashi,Hokkaido Inst. of Technol. for helpful advice on behavioral technique and Dr.T.Okuyama,Dept. of Pathol.,Higashinihon Univ..

© 1980 Elsevier/North-Holland Biomedical Press
Mechanisms of Toxicity and Hazard Evaluation
B. Holmstedt, R. Lauwerys, M. Mercier, M. Roberfroid eds

NEUROLOGIC RESPONSE TO WHITE SPIRIT EXPOSURE

KARL-HEINZ COHR[a], JENS STOKHOLM[a], & PETER BRUHN[b]
Danish National Institute of Occupational Health[a] and University Hospital[b], Copenhagen, Denmark

INTRODUCTION

In Denmark symptoms from the mucosae in the respiratory tract and the nervous system have been described among house painters during the past ten years[1,2,3]. Recently, reports on house painters having presenile dementia and cerebral atrophia have occured in Denmark[4,5]. A swedish investigation described psychological function changes among house painters[6], and in male students exposed through a breathing mask to 4000 mg/m^3 for 50 minutes simple reaction time was significantly prolonged and short-term memory was significantly reduced[7].

In order to investigate acute effects on the human nervous system from white spirit we conducted a series of seven hours exposures to different concentrations of white spirit in a controlled environment exposure chamber. The effects on the nervous system were observed by symptom registration, clinical neurological observations and neuropsychological testing.

MATERIALS AND METHODS

Experimental conditions. In a 15.4 m^3 large controlled environment chamber two groups of male volunteers were exposed to white spirit containing 17% of aromatic hydrocarbons. Group 1 consisted of students with a mean age of 23 years and group 2 consisted of house painters with a mean age of 49 years. The two groups were divided into subgroups of three persons each. The exposure sequence was partially balanced using a block design. Group 1 was exposed to 0, 34, 100, 200 and 400 ppm. Group 2 was exposed to 0, 50 and 100 ppm. The concentrations were within $\pm$ 10% during the seven hours of exposure. The odour of the white spirit was masked with a perfume.

---

a Arbejdsmiljøinstuttet, Baunegaardsvej 73, DK-2900. Hellerup, Denmark

b Rigshospitalet, afsnit N 2084, Blegdamsvej 9, DK-2100 Copenhagen Ø, Denmark

Symptom registration. The symptom registration was performed through self-administered questionnaires: One concerning symptoms during exposure at 0.25, 1, 3.5, 5 and 6.5 hours and one concerning symptoms at 0-1, 1-3, 3-8 hours after exposure, during the night, and the next morning. Questions were asked about mucosal, gastro-intestinal and neurological symptoms.

Clinical neurological observations. Clinical neurological signs were observed before exposure and just after exposure.

Neuropsychological functions. The neuropsychological functions were tested with a battery of four tests, which were relevant for workplace performance. The total test sequence durated 25 minutes and was performed four times a day: before exposure and during exposure at 1, 3.5 and 6.5 hours. The following tests were used:

Simple continuous reaction time (CRT). One hundred visual stimuli were presented to the volunteers. Reaction times were measured electronically. The most sensitive test variable was 90-10 percentile difference.

Paced auditory serial addition test (PASAT). Sixty numbers from one to nine were presented randomized to the volunteers through earphones. The numbers should be added one to the next. The results were said loud and noticed. Three series of numbers with the time intervals 2.4, 2.0 and 1.6 seconds were used consecutively in each sequence. The most sensitive test variable was the total number of mistakes, i.e. missed and wrong results.

Verbal learning and memory test (MT). Ten nouns with 1-2 syllables were presented with five seconds interval to the volunteers through earphones. Immediately after presentation the remembered nouns should be written down within one minute. The test variable for short-term memory was the number of right nouns. Half an hour after exposure the volunteers should write down within five minutes as many of the forty nouns they remembered. The number of right nouns was the test variable for long-term memory.

Purdue pegboard test (PPT). Twentyfive steel pegs were taken from a reservoir one by one and placed in the pegboard holes. First with the dominant hand and then with the non-dominant hand. Time to finish the row was the test variable for both hands.

RESULTS

Symptom registration

Mucosal symptoms. The questions were about: Smarting eyes, watering eyes, smarting nose or throat, pain in the throat, running nose, dryness in mouth or throat, strange taste, coughing, pressure on the breast and breathlessness.

Only the symptoms smarting eyes, smarting nose or throat and running nose were significantly increased in course of seven hours of exposure (table 1). The symptoms smarting eyes, smarting nose or throat, running nose and strange taste exhibited significantly frequency after seven hours of exposure (table 2).

Gastro-intestinal symptoms. The questions were about: Sickness, nausea, rumble in the stomach, air in the stomach, belch and bad appetite.

Only a few of these symptoms were noticed and none could be related to exposure.

TABLE 1

SYMPTOM REGISTRATIONS

Symptoms which increased significantly during seven hours of exposure at the concentrations shown.

Group	Concentration	Symptom	p-value
1	200 ppm	Smarting eyes	$\leq$ 0,05
	400 ppm	Smarting eyes	$\leq$ 0,05
	400 ppm	Smarting nose/throat	$\leq$ 0,05
	200 ppm	Tired etc.	$\leq$ 0,05
	400 ppm	Headache	$\leq$ 0,01
	400 ppm	Tired etc.	$\leq$ 0,001
	400 ppm	Giddy	$\leq$ 0,05
2	100 ppm	Smarting eyes	$\leq$ 0,01
	100 ppm	Smarting nose/throat	$\leq$ 0,05
	100 ppm	Running nose	$\leq$ 0,05
	100 ppm	Headache	$\leq$ 0,05
	100 ppm	Tired etc.	$\leq$ 0,05
	100 ppm	Giddy	$\leq$ 0,05

<u>Neurological symptoms.</u> The questions were about: peripheral nervous system (trembling or vibration of hands or body, reduced muscle strength in extremities, reduced control of extremities, and prickling or tingling in extremities) and central nervous system (headache; giddy; dizzy; tired, blunt, faint or indisposed; feeling of drunkenness; and visual disturbances).

Only few symptoms from the peripheral nervous system were noticed and none could be related to exposure. From the central nervous system the symptoms tired etc., headache and giddy were significantly increased in course of seven hours of exposure (table 1). The same symptoms showed a dose-related significant increase after seven hours of exposure (table 2). In group 1 headache was the only symptom which persisted significantly after exposure (table 2).

TABLE 2

SYMPTOM REGISTRATION AND CLINICAL NEUROLOGICAL OBSERVATIONS

Symptoms observations which showed a dose-related significant increase after seven hours of exposure.

Group	Symptom/observation	p-value	Remarks
1	Smarting eyes	$< 0,001$	
	Smarting nose/throat	$\leq 0,05$	
	Headache	$\leq 0,05$	
	Tired etc.	$\leq 0,01$	
	Giddy	$\leq 0,01$	
	Headache	$\leq 0,05$	0-1 hour after exposure
	Walk with dozed eyes	$\leq 0,01$	
	Romberg	$\leq 0,01$	
2	Smarting eyes	$\leq 0,01$	
	Running nose	$\leq 0,05$	
	Strange taste	$\leq 0,05$	
	Headache	$\leq 0,1$	
	Romberg	$\leq 0,05$	

Clinical neurological observations. The observations were conducted in accordance with clinical practice. The following signs were observed: Walk with open eyes, walk with closed eyes, Romberg, finger/nose trial, knee-heel trial, diadokinesis, eye movements, pupil observation, tremor, discriminative sensibility, muscle reflexes, muscle strength, joint kinestesia, touch reflexes. The only clinical neurological observations which exhibited a dose-related reduced performance due to seven hours of exposure were walk with closed eyes and Romberg (table 2).

TABLE 3
NEUROPSYCHOLOGIC RESPONSE
Neuropsychological performances, which were significantly decreased during seven hours of exposure.

Group	Concentration	Test	p-value
1	100 ppm	CRT	$\leq$ 0,01
	100 ppm	PASAT	$\leq$ 0,05
	200 ppm	CRT	$\leq$ 0,05
	200 ppm	PPT (non-dominant)	$\leq$ 0,05
	400 ppm	CRT	$\leq$ 0,05
	400 ppm	PASAT	$<$ 0,001
	400 ppm	PPT (non-dominant)	$\leq$ 0,1
2	50 ppm	MT (short-term)	$\leq$ 0,05
	100 ppm	MT (short-term)	$\leq$ 0,05

Neuropsychologic functions. In table 3 are shown the different exposure levels at which the volunteers through seven hours of exposure had significantly reduced performance in one or more of the neuropsychologic tests.

Tabel 4 shows the neuropsychologic tests in which the volunteers had a dose-related significantly reduced performance due to seven hours of exposure.

TABLE 4
NEUROPSYCHOLOGIC RESPONSE
Neuropsychological performances, which showed significant dose-related decrease after seven hours of exposure.

Group	Test	p-value
1	CRT	$\leq$ 0,01
	PASAT	$\leq$ 0,01
	MT (long-term)	$\leq$ 0,05
	PPT (dominant)	$\leq$ 0,05
	PPT (non-dominant)	< 0,001
2	MT (short-term)	< 0,001

CONCLUSIONS

Sensory irritants have trigeminus stimulating effect with symptoms from the nasal mucosa, decreased respiration rate and puls, as well as an increase in systolic blood pressure[8]. We found dose-related increases in symptoms from mucosae in eye and upper respiratory tract, which points at white spirit containing 17% aromatic hydrocarbons as a weak trigeminus stimulating agent.

In workplace investigations, symptoms from the central and the peripheral nervous system, as well as from the vegetative nervous system were observed[3]. In our exposure experiments only symptoms from the central nervous systems were significantly increased. Headache, tiredness etc. and giddyness were significant in the painters group at 100 ppm and at higher concentrations in the students group. Headache persisted after exposure.

The clinical neurological observations showed that the vestibular-cerebellar reflex path was affected. The signs "walk with closed eyes" and Romberg were significantly affected in the students group, whereas the painters group only showed an affected Romberg. This difference can be explained with the difference in maximal exposure level between the two groups.

Vigilance (CRT) and attention function (PASAT) were significantly affected at 100 ppm in the students group, whereas the painters group showed no significant effect on vigilance and attention function related to exposure level. Vigilance was significantly affected in the painters group when related to the calculated retention of white spirit (500-1499 mg). This is in accordance with previous observations[7]. The PASAT test was difficult to the elder painters. This might explain why no effect on attention function was seen in the painters group.

The manual dexterity (PPT) was only affected in the students group at 200 and 400 ppm. This is in accordance with previous findings[9].

Short-term memory function (MT) in the painters group was affected already at 50 ppm, whereas long-term memory function in general was so poor, that the response could not be evaluated. In the students group short-term memory function was not significantly affected and the long-term memory function was only affected at 400 ppm. The poor long-term memory function in the painters group and the significant effect in the students group points at an affected information transfer from the learning area to the storage area of the memory or a loss of information from the storage area[9].

The effect on short-term memory function in the painters group at low exposure levels could be a result of age-dependent reduced memory function, of age-dependent sensitivity or of occupation-dependent sensitivety of the type found with presenile dementia.

One may conclude, that exposure to white spirit containing 17% aromatic hydrocarbons stimulates the trigeminus nerve and affects the central nervous system. Whether these acute effects are warnings about more severe chronic effects, as the ones reported in Denmark previously[4, 5], is not known. The effects appear at lower exposure levels in elder house painters with at least 10 years of occupational exposure as compared to younger students with no previous exposure. The reasons for this difference could be age- or occupation-dependent. In both cases it should be taken into account when setting a value for acceptable exposure level for white spirit.

ACKNOWLEDGEMENTS

Supported by grants from the Danish medical research council (512-3895, 512-7298 and 512-8517).

The authors are grateful to mrs. Mona Groth for her skillful help with the manuscript.

REFERENCES

1. Andersen, S. et al (1972) Malerrapport København 1972, Malernes Fagforening, Copenhagen, pp. 1-92.
2. Arbejdsmiljøgruppen (1974) Rapport nr. 2. Arbejdsmiljøundersøgelsen, Arbejdsmiljøgruppen af 1972, Copenhagen, pp. 1-199.
3. Lajer, M. (1976) Ugeskr. Laeg. 138, 1225-1230.
4. Gregersen, P. et al (1978) Ugeskr. Laeg. 1401638-1644.
5. Arlien-Søborg, P. et al (1978) Ugeskr. Laeg. 140, 1645-1649.
6. Hane, M. et al (1977) Scand. J. Work Environ. Health 3, 91-99.
7. Gamberale, F. et al (1975) Scand. J. Work Environ. Health 1, 31-39.
8. Alarie, Y. (1973) CRC Crit. Rev. Toxicol. 2, 299-363.
9. Miller, E. (1971) Neuropsychologia 9, 75-81.

SHORT-TERM TESTS FOR PREDICTING LONG-TERM EFFECTS

Symposium chairmen: L. Golberg and A. Leonard

© 1980 Elsevier/North-Holland Biomedical Press
Mechanisms of Toxicity and Hazard Evaluation
B. Holmstedt, R. Lauwerys, M. Mercier, M. Roberfroid eds

APPRAISAL OF THE MERITS AND SHORT COMINGS OF TESTS OF MUTAGENIC POTENTIAL

I F H PURCHASE
Imperial Chemical Industries Limited, Central Toxicology Laboratory,
Alderley Park, Cheshire, UK.

In the last decade many tests capable of detecting phenotypic events caused by mutation of the genomes have been developed. Large numbers of chemicals have been tested in a variety of these tests and in some cases the exact lesion produced by the chemical on DNA identifed and its consequences on the phenotype understood. It is against this background that in the late 1970s various countries introduced draft legislation aimed at controlling the potentially harmful effects of mutagenic chemicals on man. These regulatory initiatives have brought into sharp focus the two scientific disciplines which are directly involved in genetic toxicology, namely the science of genetics and toxicology. It is the interplay between these two disciplines which has revealed much of interest in recent years and will be the subject of this paper.

This paper is limited to mutagenicity *per se* and does not consider the use of mutagenicity assays in predicting carcinogenic potential.

THE GENETICIST'S APPROACH TO GENETIC TOXICOLOGY

> "It is remarkable that a bacterium low on the organismic scale should code for its protein with the same code words used by the cells of the Nobel prize winners who broke the code"[1].

Genetic toxicology is a unique branch of toxicology. It is based on a long history of observation and experimentation in genetics from Mendel onwards. There is a firm theoretical background supported by a vast amount of observation on the behaviour of organisms, of biochemical and chemical understanding of DNA and the way it behaves. This breadth of information is unequalled in any other branch of toxicology.

Observations in man confirm the presence of mutation and diseases which are the direct consequence of mutation in both adults and children.

From experimental observations of the effects of chemicals on lower organisms it is reasonable to assume that man will suffer from chemically-induced mutation. Because of the long generation time and the high and variable incidence of mutation in man chemically-induced mutations are likely to be difficult to observe. Hence, strategies for the protection of man must be based on testing of chemicals in mutation assays based on lower organisms.

The logic which leads the genetic toxicologist to testing strategies for detecting mutagenic chemicals is very complex. The discussion which follows is based on two sets of guidelines produced over the last few years. The first of these are the guidelines produced by the Environmental Protection Agency of the US government which were published as a discussion document in August of 1978[2]. The second document is a consultative document by the Committee on Mutagenicity of Chemicals in Food, Consumer Products and the Environment, set up by the Department of Health and Social Security within the United Kingdom[1]. Although there are differences in the final recommendations made in these two sets of guidelines there are fundamental similarities in the thinking which leads to the selection of various test systems. In summary, the fundamental building blocks of the strategy for testing chemicals for mutagenicity are as follows:

(i) All organisms (with the exception of a few RNA viruses) have DNA as the genetic material.

(ii) The subunits of DNA are chemically identical in all species.

(iii) There is a remarkable universality in the DNA code which appears to be the same in all organisms.

(iv) The essential features of gene replication are the same in all organisms.

(v) DNA replicates faithfully unless there is a mutation. This replication occurs in each generation for unicellular organisms and in somatic and germ cells for multicellular organisms.

(vi) Chemicals can react with the DNA (or alter the quantity per cell following cell division).. If this damage is repaired properly no mutation occurs. If the damage is not repaired or if the repair results in an error prior to replication the alteration in the DNA may result in a mutation.

(vii) Although some mutations can be expected to be beneficial to the organism, in general mutations are expected to have an harmful overall effect on an organism which is well adapted to its environment.

(viii) A single lesion in DNA may result in a mutation.

(ix) All tests for chemically-induced mutation are basically the same. They only differ in the phenotypic marker and organism which is used to reveal the underlying damage to the genetic material. Hence, cells from all species can be used to detect and predict genetic changes in the cells of other species.

(x) Although from the genetic point of view the organism is irrelevant there are different types of damage to DNA which are easily recognised and which require different markers and organisms for their detection.

(xi) Many chemicals must be converted into reactive metabolites and hence there is a need to take into account the metabolism of mammals in the selection of mutation assays.

(xii) Because of the variability in test execution and the type of damage which may be produced to DNA more than one test should be used for the detection of mutagenic effects.

As a consequence of these fundamental statements regarding genetic events two sets of recommendations with certain similarities have been produced. In the draft statement by the EPA a battery of eight different kinds of tests is required[2]:

<u>(i) For detecting gene mutations</u>. A minimum of three tests with no more than one selected from any of the following kinds of tests:

(A) Bacteria, with and without metabolic activation:

(B) Eukaryotic micro-organisms, with and without metabolic activation:

(C) Insects (eg, sex-linked recessive lethal test):

(D) Mammalian somatic cells in culture, with and without metabolic activation: and

(E) The mouse specific locus test.

<u>(ii) For detecting chromosomal aberrations</u>. A minimum of three tests with no more than one selected from any of the following four kinds of tests:

(A) *In vivo* cytogenetic tests in mammals:

(B) Insect tests for heritable chromosomal effects:

(C) Dominant lethal effects in rodents: and

(D) Heritable translocation tests in rodents.

<u>(iii) For detecting primary DNA damage</u>. A minimum of two tests with no more than one selected from any of the following four kinds of tests:

(A) DNA repair in bacteria (including differential killing of DNA repair-defective strains) with and without metabolic activation:

(B) Unschedudled DNA repair synthesis in mammalian cells, with and without metabolic activation:

(C) Mitotic recombination and/or gene conversion in yeast, with and without metabolic activation: and

(D) Sister-chromatid exchange in mammalian cells, with and without metabolic activation.

The proposed guidelines procede further by recommending criteria for classifying substances with respect to mutagenicity or non-mutagenicity. These criteria are:

(i) Valid negative results in each of the eight tests performed in accordance with the proposed guidelines would be considered sufficient to define operationally that the substance is a non-mutagen.

(ii) A compound would be considered mutagenic if any of the following minimum criteria were satisfied:

(a) positive results in two different kinds of tests for demonstrating gene mutations (other than the mouse specific locus test),

(b) a positive result in a mouse specific locus test, or

(c) a positive result in any chromosomal test.

(iii) Ambiguous result such as suspicious negative result, a marginally positive result at very high doses, a positive result in a single point mutational test other than the mouse specific locus test, any positive DNA damage test or positive result in any valid mutagenicity test which was not included in the battery of tests in the proposed guidelines shall suggest the need for additional tests beyond the minimum eight and a review by an expert advisory committee or both.

The UK guidelines proposed a basic package of four tests for screening chemicals for mutagenic properties. These tests are:

Test 1 A test designed to demonstrate the induction of point mutations (base pair change and frame shift mutations) in established bacterial test systems such as *Salmonella typhimurium*, *Escherichia coli* or *Bacillus subtilis*. The tests should be conducted with and without the use of appropriate metabolic activation systems.

Test 2 A test designed to demonstrate the production of chromosome damage in appropriate mammalian cells grown *in vitro* with and without the use of appropriate metabolic activation systems.

Test 3 The induction of mutations in mammalian cells grown *in vitro*.

or

Tests designed to induce recessive lethals in *Drosophila melanogaster*.

Test 4 A test designed to demonstrate the induction of chromosomal damage in the intact animal using either the micronucleus test or preferably the metaphase analysis of bone marrow or other proliferative cells.

or

The induction of germ cell damage as demonstrated by the dominant lethal test in the rat or mouse.

There is a basic similarity between the EPA and UK guidelines. In the UK guidelines two tests for point mutations are required; first (Test 1) the induction of point mutations from bacteria and the second (Test 3) point mutations in mammalian cells for *Drosophila*. Two tests for demonstrating chromosome damage are also required; the first in appropriate mammalian cells *in vitro* (Test 2) and the second, chromosomal damage in intact animals (Test 4). There is no clear indication in the UK guidelines about the decision criteria which would be used for judging the results of the four tests selected. Presumably an extra committee would be required to review the information on any particular chemical and assess the likely consequences of the results.

In both guidelines there is room for the use of tests in addition to the ones nominated in the guidelines provided sufficient evidence is given to support the selection of that particular test.

From the point of view of the practical application of these regulatory strategies there is very little experience available to those outside the regulatory authorities in judging whether they are effective and suitable. It is only when the strategies have been in use for some time that it will be possible to decide whether they provide a suitable means of controlling mutagens in the environment.

THE TOXICOLOGIST'S APPROACH TO GENETIC TOXICOLOGY

The theoretical background to mutation and its phenotypic expression applies to so many different organisms that it is inevitable that when we know enough man will be found to suffer from mutations that are induced by defined chemical or physical events. It is therefore our duty as toxicologists to use our knowledge of genetics and toxicology to reduce or prevent such mutational events occurring in man.

Toxicology is essentially pragmatic in approach trying first of all to understand observations made in the target organism and secondly to build models of those observations using laboratory organisms. Once these models have been properly developed and understood they can in turn be used for understanding the observations made in the target organism and for extrapolating information to man. In taking this deliberately pragmatic approach there are a number of questions which the toxicologist would wish to ask:

(1) What Evidence is there of Induced Mutations in Man?

It is now well established that man suffers from a number of diseases which are the result of mutations. These can be point mutations such as sickle-cell anaemia, or chromosal level events such as is seen in Down's syndrome. The study of abortuses and children with malformation has indicated that a large number of abortions and malformations can be the consequence of genetic diseases. The precise cause of the mutations leading to genetic disease which the human population carries is not known.

By studying genetic toxicology from the point of view of the chemical or physical agent which causes genetic damage it might be possible to determine whether specific insults can result in mutation in man.

Cigarette Smoking

Bridges, Clemmesen and Sugimura[3] have recently reviewed the evidence of the mutagenic effects of cigarette smoking in man. There is no doubt that mutagens are present in cigarette smoke and that as cigarette smoke has such an intimate contact with the lungs that many of these mutagenic substances would be absorbed by the lungs into the systemic circulation. It is not surprising, therefore, that certain genetic events can be observed in smokers. The best documented effects which are considered to be genetic or closely related to genetic events are: (a) Cigarette smoking associated with an increase in the number of morphologically abnormal sperm. This effect was seen to be more pronounced in smokers who had been smoking for more than ten years when compared with those who had smoked for shorter periods. (b) There is an increase in the frequency of sister-chromatid exchanges in the peripheral lymphocytes of smokers. (c) From a cytogenetic study of peripheral lymphocytes of smokers it was found that there is an increase in exchange-type aberrations amongst heavy smokers. (d) There is an increase in perinatal mortality amongst the children of smoking fathers. (e) There is an increase in the number of major congenital malformations amongst the children of smoking fathers and this appears to increase with an increase in the number of cigarettes smoked per day. These observations are consistent with a dominant mutation being produced by cigarette smoking although observations on sperm abnormalities and chromosomes of peripheral lymphocytes are not evidence of heritable changes. The observations as they currently stand do not establish causality and can be considered only to indicate a preliminary correlation between cigarette smoking and these events which needs further confirmation.

Vinyl Chloride

Infante and co-workers[4] reported an increase an foetal wastage amongst workers exposed to vinyl chloride. This was observed by comparing pre- and post-employment reproductive history and by comparison of vinyl chloride workers with workers in other parts of the chemical industry. Observations of an increase in foetal wastage are compatible with the suggestion that vinyl chloride can produce chromosomal level aberrations which in turn can lead to dominant lethal mutations. In considering these observations on vinyl chloride workers and their families it is worthwhile noting that the study has certain deficiencies. In the first place no exposure history was available and therefore no dose-effect relationship was established. The survey was carried out as a consequence of questioning the fathers, a system which is unlikely to provide particularly accurate data on reproductive history. Similarly, the data were corrected for paternal age when it is known that maternal age is the feature which has the biggest effect on foetal wastage. Finally, the number of workers who were actually interviewed formed a low percentage of the total number of workers available for interview. These criticisms suggest that the observations on the effect of vinyl chloride on foetal wastage will need to be confirmed before they can be considered as definitive. In considering this information and comparing it with other available information on the effects of vinyl chloride there are certain incompatibilities which would also need to be explained. Although vinyl chloride produces chromosome abberations it does not produce dominant lethal effects in mice. If vinyl chloride was producing the increase in foetal wastage it might be expected that congenital malformations would also increase but this is not the case. In conclusion, observations of an increase in foetal wastage would be consistent with the dominant chromosomal effect but currently it is by no means proven that vinyl chloride is causally associated with such effects in man.

Other Occupational Exposures

Exposure to lead and to anaesthetic gases has been reported to increase the abortion rate in wives of exposed workers. In both cases the evidence cannot yet be considered to be conclusive.

The four chemicals considered - cigarette smoke, vinyl chloride, lead and anaesthetic gases - are the best documented examples of potential mutagenic effects in man. In none of them is there unequivocal evidence of a heritable genetic effect being produced. This probably reflects more on the difficulty of establishing a cause effect relationship in this difficult area than it does an absence of induced mutations caused by these chemical influences. In particular, recessive mutations can occur at high frequency in an outbred population without being expressed. Nevertheless, there are insufficient established effects in man against which to judge the validity of laboratory screening tests.

(2) What Laboratory Models are Available for Screening Chemicals for Mutagenic Effects?

There is no shortage of laboratory methods for detecting genetic events caused by chemicals. These have been the subject of extensive review and cover a range of genetic end points (including point mutation, chromosomal level effects, DNA damage, non-disjunction and various other end points) and a variety of organisms (including many prokaryotic systems and eukaryotic systems on yeasts, mammalian cells in culture and whole mammalian systems). Because there is such a wide variety of test systems available and because it is not possible to validate these tests systems against mutational events in man the toxicologist is in the difficult position in knowing how to select assay systems.

(3) How Should the Appropriate Assay System be Selected?

Mutation-based assay systems are used for screening chemicals for potential carcinogenicity and within this context it has been possible to validate such mutation assays. However, this should not be confused with the use of these same assay systems for screening chemicals for possible mutagenic effects in man. As has been pointed out earlier, there is insufficient evidence to enable us to validate mutation-based assays.

Hence, the concept of a validated mutational assay for detecting potential human mutagens is not achievable.

Because of these considerations alternative approaches must be used for the selection of appropriate test systems. In the first place, it is possibly helpful to select the test systems from the point of view of the way in which they perform with chemicals rather than considering them solely as genetic systems. When viewed from this point of view it is clear that a number of factors are likely to influence the outcome of the test results and to produce different results between different organisms. Many of these factors are well documented and, indeed, are mentioned in the guideline documents produced by the EPA and the UK committees.

(i) Differences in metabolism.

There are vast differences in the metabolic capability of eukaryotes and prokaryotes and single cell organisms and multicellular mammals. The use of the S-9 mix, although proving remarkably good for the detection of potential carcinogens, cannot be considered entirely satisfactory to represent a whole mammalian metabolic capability in all situations. From the study of _in vitro_ systems there are already a large number of known effects which can confound the interpretation of results which include different inducers, the effect of separation of the S-9 fraction from the rest of the liver homogenate, the presence or absence of co-factors, the time and temperature at which the S-9 is stored, whether the incubation is carried out under anaerobic or aerobic conditions, the balance of detoxification and toxification pathways with no excretory pathways available to _in vitro_ systems, and the close contact which it is possible to achieve between direct acting agents and the DNA. The toxicologist would normally view these differences in metabolic capability between organisms and assay systems as extremely important in contributing to the likely outcome of an assay on a particular chemical.

(ii) Differences in organisms

The similarity in the DNA, the types of damage which can occur to DNA and the mechanisms which organisms have for repairing it have led to the view that is expressed earlier in this paper, namely that genetic events seen in any organism can be useful in extrapolation to any other organism. In spite of this there are enormous differences in the arrangement and organisation of the genetic mechanisms of cells which should be taken into account.

Major differences occur in the arrangement of the genome. The simple classification of prokaryotes and eukaryotes is based on the absence of the organisation of DNA into a nucleus in prokaryotes. In addition, there are major differences in the process of cell division, differences in the quantity of DNA, in the organisation of the DNA into chromosomes, in the proteins associated with the DNA in the formation of chromosomes, and in the gene control and regulation. These major differences, whilst they may not affect the expression of genetic damage in a measurable phenotypic marker, may well have profound effects on the way in which the cell responds to the damage produced by different chemicals.

There are also major differences which are recognised in the DNA repair processes between the various organisms used for mutation assays. Some of the prokaryotic assay systems have specific repair deficiences inserted into them. Even without the introduction of repair deficiences it is now recognised that repair in prokaryotic systems is less efficient than in mammalian systems. In addition to that, mammalian cells are recognised as having a more efficient DNA repair system than do rodent cells. These considerations lead the toxicologist to the conclusion that there are profound differences in the DNA repair processes and their control between the different organisms. As a consequence we would expect variation in the response to a chemical by the different organisms because of the way they handle the chemical and because of the way in which they respond to it.

EXPERIMENTAL EVIDENCE WHICH ASSISTS IN THE SELECTION OF GENETIC TEST SYSTEMS

As has been mentioned above it is not possible to validate mutational assay systems. The best that can be achieved is to examine the data on the performance of these systems to establish how consistent that data is when it is derived from various different sources.

Within-test Variation

An assessment of the variation that is obtained within a test is most easily achieved by comparing the performance of two tests which independently assay the same chemical. There are three examples available of this type of study being carried out.

In the first of these[5] ninety-nine chemicals were assessed using the *Salmonella* plate incorporation assay carried out in two separate laboratories. For seventy-seven of the chemicals there was agreement between the two laboratories but in twenty-two there was no agreement.

If it is assumed that in these twenty-two cases one or other of the laboratory's results was correct this gives an error rate of approximately 11%. The differences in test results could be attributed to differences in technique, for example, the strains used or the way in which the S-9 was prepared.

The second example[6] involved the testing of twenty-three chemicals by three laboratories. In each case seven different protocols were used which were considered to be identical between the three laboratories. There were, thus, seven sets of data from twenty-three chemicals giving a total of one hundred and sixty-one data sets. There was complete agreement between the assay systems in all but twenty-three cases. Once again the error rate can be calculated as twenty-three disagreements amongst one hundred and sixty-one data sets giving a total of 7.1%.

The third set of data derives from the International Collaborative Study on Short Term Tests for Carcinogenicity. In this study there were twelve *Salmonella* plate incorporation assays which were carried out on forty-two compounds. On reviewing the data it was possible to identify twenty compounds which were considered to be bacterial point mutagens. There were two hundred and thirty-one results reported and of these two hundred and three were positive and twenty-eight negative. The error rate in this case was 12.1%. For the nineteen compounds which were agreed to be non-mutagenic there were two hundred and thirty-three results, one hundred and ninety-seven recorded as negative and thirty-six as positive. This gives an error rate of 11.7%.

In all three of these collaborative studies error rates in the region of 10% were observed when comparing the results from the *Salmonella* plate incorporation assay carried out in different laboratories. It is worth while considering the consequences of a 10% error rate when a battery of eight tests is used. If a single test is used 90% of the mutagens will be correctly identified and 90% of the non-mutagens will be correctly identified. If it is assumed that each one of the six tests provides an independent assessment of the mutagenicity of the chemical, and that the error rate of each test for both positive and negative results is 10%, six tests will identify 99.9999% of the mutagens. However, at the same time, only 53% of the non-mutagens will be negative in all six test systems.

Between-test Variation

If we consider test systems which, although they may assess the same genetic end point, use different organisms, the range of variability can be seen to be high. In the work described by Poirier and de Serres data was obtained from three assay systems. The first, the *Salmonella* plate incorporation assay, the second the pol A- assay in *E.coli* and the third a point mutational assay using *S.cerevisiae* D3. In this set of data there is agreement between the three assay systems for fifty-five chemicals (twenty-five all negative and thirty all positive). However, for forty-four there was no agreement.

The data from the International Collaborative Study provides additional information about the same points. The key features of the international study were that assay systems using a large number of different end points were used to assess the mutagenicity of the same sample. The sample was despatched to the scientists under code, a total of forty-two chemicals was assessed in this study. Although the study was designed with the specific purpose of detecting carcinogens, the same data may be used for assessing the usefulness of some of the mutational assays for the detection of mutations. A battery similar to that required by the EPA has been selected from the data sets (Figure 1). The selection was based on the largest available data base in any one assay system and was fairly straight forward with the exception of the selection of the second assay for chromosomal level events. No suitable assay was available and so the assay which detects aneuploidy in yeast was used. In all other respects the battery selected from the international study conforms with the data that would be required by the EPA.

Notes for Figure 1

a *Salmonella* plate incorporation assay
b *Yeast* forward mutation assay
c *Drosophila* sex-linked recessive lethal assay
d *In vitro* cytogenetics
e *Aneuploidy* in yeast
f Micronucleus in mice
g Rec assay in *E.coli*
h UDS in HeLa *cells* in culture
i Number positive
1 ND: Not done
2 ND/- and ND/+: Chemical not assayed in the laboratory that was selected and hence data from a similar assay carried out in another laboratory was used.
3 The number of positive results has been corrected. Thus, if 3 positives were observed in 5 assays, the corrected figure is 3/5 x 8 = 4.8, reported as 5.
4 Decision based on the criteria recommended by the EPA.
5 Selection of this assay does not comply with the criteria provided by the EPA. No other chromosomal level assay with sufficient data was available.
6 Disagreement between two laboratories.

		POINT MUTATION			CHROMOSOMAL MUTATION			DNA DAMAGE			
		a	b	c	d	e[5]	f	g	h	i[3]	4
2	3,3'-5,5'-Tetramethylbenzidine	-	-	-	-	-	-	-	-	0	-
21	Y-butyrolactone	-	-	-	-	-	-	-	-	0	-
38	Sugar	-	ND/-[2]	ND[1]	ND	-	-	-	-	0	-
10	Methyl orange	-	+	ND	-	-	-	-	-	1	?
22	Methionine	-	-	-	ND/-	+	ND/-	-	-	1	+
30	1,1,1-trichlorethane	-	-	ND	ND	-	-	+	-	1	?
35	3-Ammotriazole	-	ND/-	-	ND	-	-	-	+	1	+
5	Pyrene	+	-	-	-	-	-	-	+	2	?
7	Diethylstilboestrol	+	-	-	-	-	+	-	-	2	+
17	Diphenylnitrosamine	+	-	-	-	+	-	-	-	2	+
18	Anthracene	+	-	ND	-	-	-	+	-	2	?
19	Dinitrosopentamethylene tetramine	-	-	+	+	-	-	-	-	2	+
23	Safrole	-	+	-	-	-	-	+	-	2	?
24	Dimethylformamide	+	-	-	-	+	-	-	-	2	+
28	Isopropyl N(3-chlorophenyl)carbonate	-	ND/+	ND	-	+	ND/-	-	-	2	+
4	1-Naphthylamine	-	-	-	+	+	-	-	+	3	+
6	Chloroform	-	+	-	ND	-	ND/-	+	+	3	?
9	2-Naphthylamine	+	-	+/-[6]	+	-	-	-	+	3	+
25	DL-Ethionine	-	+	-	-	-	+	+	-	3	+
31	Urethane	+	-	ND	ND	-	+	-	-	3	+
40	Ascorbic acid	-	ND/-	ND	ND	+	-	-	+	3	+
42	Auramine	+	ND	ND	ND	-	-	-	+	3	?
20	Ethylenethiourea	-	-	-	-	+	-	+	+	3	+
3	4-AAF	+	-	ND	ND	+	-	+	-	4	+
11	Benzidine	+	-	-	+	+	+	-	-	4	+
16	HMPA	+	-	+	ND/-	-	+	-	+	4	+
1	Butter Yellow	+	-	ND	-	+	+	-	+	4	+
26	Epichlorhydrin	+	+	-	ND/+	+	-	-	-	4	+
32	Dimethylcarbamoyl chloride	+	+	-	-	+	+	-	-	4	+
27	N-nitrosomorpholine	+	+	+	-	+	+	-	-	5	+
29	B-Propiolactone	+	+	+	ND	+	-	+	-	5	+
8	4NQO	+	+	ND	+	+	-	+	+	6	+
13	Benzopyrene	+	-	-	+	+	+	+	+	6	+
14	Hydrazine	+	+	ND	-	+	ND/-	+	+	6	+
33	Azobenzene	+	ND/+	-	ND	+	+	+	-	6	+
34	Cyclophosphamide	-	ND	ND	ND	+	ND/+	+	+	6	+
39	9,10-dimethylanthracene	+	ND/+	-	ND	+	-	+	+	6	+
41	o-Toluidine	+	ND	ND	ND	+	-	+	+	6	+
36	MOCA	+	ND/-	+	ND	+	+	+	+	7	+
12	2-AAF	+	+	ND	+	+	+	+	+	8	+
15	3Me-4NQO	+	+	ND	+	+	+	+	+	8	+
37	Methylazoxymethanol	+	+	+	ND	ND	ND	+	+	8	+

Figure 1 Results from 8 assays conducted on 42 chemicals. The assay systems were selected to conform to the EPA requirements for mutagenicity testing

Once again it is possible to consider this data in two ways. In the first case the agreement between assays using the same end point can be considered. Within the point mutational assay systems there was agreement in the case of eighteen chemicals but disagreement for twenty-three. Using the chromosomal level assays there was again agreement with eighteen chemicals but disagreement in twenty-three. The chemicals in which there was agreement and disagreement within these two assay systems were not necessarily the same. When the two DNA repair assays are considered there was agreement in twenty-seven and disagreement in fifteen. It can be seen that when two or three tests using the same category of end points are used on these forty-two chemicals in approximately 50% of the cases the test systems disagree with one another.

When all eight assay systems are considered similar patterns are observed. Only three compounds produced results which were negative in all eight assays and three in which the results were positive in all assays. For thirty-six compounds there were between one and seven positive results. When considering the distribution of these results profiles there was no particular number of positive results which occurred with a greater frequency than any of the other numbers.

If the criteria used for judgement by the EPA is applied to these forty-two chemicals, three are found to be non-mutagenic, eight provide results which require additional testing or expert assessment. In the case of thirty-one chemicals, including methionine and vitamin C, they would be classified as mutagens using these criteria of judgement.

It might have been expected that a consideration of the distribution of positive and negative results would have indicated a clear separation between those chemicals which are negative and those which are positive in mutational assays. The even distribution across all eight assays and within the three assays which make up the points and chromosomal level systems indicates that these assay systems do not discriminate adequately between mutagens and non-mutagens using the criteria for judgement which have been laid out.

CONCLUSIONS

There is no doubt that mutation occurs in man and in all probability environmental factors contribute considerably to this level of mutation. As mutational diseases are a heavy burden on the human population any attempts which are aimed at reducing this burden can be considered to be advantageous. Unfortunately, there are insufficient examples of induced mutations in man with proven causality to be helpful to the toxicologist in the selection of assay systems for potential human mutagens. There are obviously important genetic similarities between the various assay systems used in genetic toxicology but equally there are significant differences between these assay systems. From the toxicological point of view these differences may be more important than are the similarities.

The strategy of using a battery of test systems reflects assumptions about similarity of tests with common genetic end points combined with a high level of uncertainty about the performance of these different test systems. The use of a battery of tests, each of which has a finite error rate, has certain consequences which we must recognise. An analysis of a limited data base indicates that current decision rules do not cope adequately with these consequences.

A consideration of genetic toxicology from the point of view of the toxicologist leads to the conclusion that more emphasis should be given to the chemical in developing a strategy for testing. The role of metabolism and the differences between organisms with the same genetic end points should be emphasised; the diversity of genetic end points should receive less emphasis because DNA damage induced by chemicals leads to both point and chromosomal mutations.

In the meantime it would be advisable to take more account of error rates in selecting the number of tests to be used. In the examples quoted, overall accuracy decreased if more than two tests were used. If more tests are deemed useful, there should be more opportunities for discussion of the results and decision making before all tests are carried out.

REFERENCES

1. Committee on Mutagenicity of Chemicals in Food, Consumer Products and the Environment (1979). A Consultative Document on Guidelines for the Testing of Chemicals for Mutagenicity, Department of Health and Social Security, London.
2. Anon (1978). Fed Register, 43, 37400-37403.
3. Bridges, B.A., Clemmesen, J. and Sugimura, T. (1979). Mutation Research, 65, 71-81.
4. Infante, P.F., Wagoner, J.K., McMichael, A.J., Waxweiler, R.J. and Falk, H. (1976). Lancet, 734.
5. Poirier, L.A. and de Serres, F.J. (1979). J. Natl. Cancer Inst., 62, 919-926.
6. Dunkel, V. (1979). J. Assoc. Off. Anal. Chem., 62, 874-882.
7. Anon (1978). Mutation Research, 54, 203-206.

© 1980 Elsevier/North-Holland Biomedical Press
Mechanisms of Toxicity and Hazard Evaluation
B. Holmstedt, R. Lauwerys, M. Mercier, M. Roberfroid eds

THE INDUCTION OF MUTATION AND DIFFERENTIATION IN MAMMALIAN CELLS BY CHEMICALS WHICH INITIATE OR PROMOTE TUMOR FORMATION

ELIEZER HUBERMAN
Oak Ridge National Laboratory, Biology Division, P. O. Box Y, Oak Ridge, TN 37830 USA

INTRODUCTION

Many industrial chemicals are introduced each year into our environment[1], yet the biological consequences of exposure to these chemicals is largely unknown. A fraction of these chemicals are suspected of being carcinogens[2]; therefore, it is essential that sensitive assays be developed which can predict the potential danger of these substances to man. While the mechanism by which chemicals induce cancer is unknown, one of the simplest explanations is that a somatic mutation resulting from the interaction of the carcinogens with cellular DNA is responsible for the initiation of cancer. Indeed, chemical carcinogens are capable of binding to DNA of susceptible mammalian cells[3-8], and may therefore induce mutations[9-10], some of which could involve the genes that control the expression of malignant transformation[11-14]. Therefore, studying the mutagenic activity of carcinogens in mammalian cells should provide an important technique for identifying cancer-causing agents, and possibly for elucidating the mechanism of carcinogenesis[14-19]. However, most chemicals encountered in the environment are chemically non-reactive and have to be enzymatically activated before they can manifest biological activity[20,21]. Furthermore, many mammalian cell lines which are suitable for mutagenesis studies are not able to metabolically activate these chemicals[22-25]. To overcome this limitation for using mutable mammalian cells in culture, such cells have to be used with an exogenous metabolic activation system. The activation systems most commonly used are subcellular fractions derived from homogenized liver cells[19,26-28]; however, subcellular fractions will not necessarily metabolize compounds in a manner analogous to that of intact cells[18,29,30].

Cell-mediated Mutagenesis. The cell-mediated mutagenesis assay that we have previously developed[17] utilizes viable cells to activate the chemicals and may thus be more useful for such studies. In this assay, Chinese hamster V79 cells, which are useful cells for mutagenesis[15] but cannot metabolize carcinogens[17,25,31], are cocultivated with lethally irradiated cells that can metabolically activate these compounds[25]. The reactive metabolites produced by the metabolizing cells are apparently transferred to the cells used for testing mutagenesis and induce mutation. In these systems, carcinogens can be tested without having to isolate the active metabolites. After cocultivation, the V79 cells are subcultured to determine cell survival and after an appropriate time of expression[32], also to determine the mutational frequencies for various genetic markers such as 8-azaguanine, 6-thioguanine or ouabain resistance[15,17,26-28,31-36] (Figure 1).

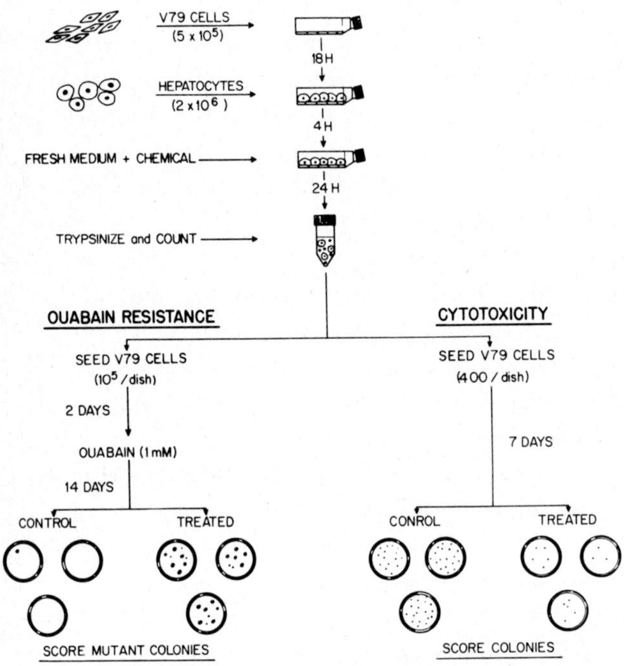

Fig. 1. Scheme for the induction of ouabain-resistant mutants in the hepatocyte-mediated assay. (From Jones and Huberman, 31).

By testing a series of polycyclic aromatic hydrocarbons with different degrees of carcinogenicity in the cell-mediated assay using hamster embryonic fibroblasts as the metabolizing cells, we have established a relationship between degree of mutagenicity and degree of carcinogenicity[17,36] (Table 1).

TABLE 1

INDUCTION OF OUABAIN-RESISTANT MUTANTS IN THE FIBROBLAST-MEDIATED ASSAY BY CARCINOGENIC POLYCYCLIC HYDROCARBONS AFTER TREATMENT WITH OR WITHOUT AMINOPHYLLINE

		No. of ouabain-resistant mutants per 10^6 survivors	
Hydrocarbon	Concentration (μg/ml)	Without aminophylline	With aminophylline
Control	0	1	1
Phenanthrene	1	1	1
Pyrene	1	1	1
Benzo(e)pyrene	1	1	NT
Benz(a)anthracene	1	2	NT
Chrysene	1	2	NT
Dibenz(a,c)anthracene	1	3	5
Dibenz(a,h)anthracene	1	4	46
7-Methylbenz(a)anthracene	1	24	NT
3-Methylcholanthrene	1	108	413
Benzo(a)pyrene	1	121	214
7,12-Dimethylbenz(a)anthracene	0.1	66	NT

Cells were treated with 0.1 mM aminophylline. The data are based on results from Huberman (10) and from Huberman and Sachs (36).

After cocultivation, four carcinogenic aromatic hydrocarbons, 7,12-dimethylbenz(a)anthracene, benzo(a)pyrene, 3-methylcholanthrene, and 7-methylbenz(a)-anthracene induced drug resistant mutants, whereas five non-carcinogenic hydrocarbons, (benzo(e)pyrene, benz(a)anthracene, phenanthrene, pyrene and chrysene), were not mutagenic. The mutagenic activities of the carcinogenic hydrocarbons were dependent on the number of metabolizing cells present, and on the concentration of the carcinogens. Dibenzo(a,c)anthracene and dibenzo-(a,h)anthracene, which have been reported to be non-carcinogenic in golden hamsters showed a weak mutagenic effect. In the presence of aminophylline, which enhances polycyclic aromatic hydrocarbon metabolism[37], there was a two- to four-fold increase in mutagenicity with benzo(a)pyrene and 3-methylcholanthrene (Table 1). Dibenzo(a,c)anthracene, which had a low degree of mutagenicity without aminophylline, showed a less than two-fold increase in mutagenicity with aminophylline. Dibenz(a,h)anthracene, which is a carcinogen for the mouse and rat, and which exhibited mutagenic activities similar to that of dibenz(a,c)anthracene without aminophylline, showed a ten-fold increase in mutagenicity with aminophylline (Table 1). These results indicate that there is a relationship between the degree of mutagenesis in the cell-mediated system and the degree of carcinogenicity of polycyclic aromatic hydrocarbons.

While fibroblasts are capable of metabolizing carcinogenic polycyclic aromatic hydrocarbons to mutagenic intermediates, they are not capable of activating some other classes of chemical carcinogens, such as those which cause cancer of the liver[38,39]. Therefore, to expand the spectrum of compounds which can be studied in the cell-mediated assay, we developed a system using primary cultures of rat hepatocytes to activate the carcinogens and V79 cells for the detection of mutagenic intermediates[31,40]. The basic procedure for the hepatocyte-mediated assay was similar to that of the fibroblast-mediated assay (Figure 1). The primary hepatocytes were obtained after enzymic digestion of perfused[41] or sliced[31,42] livers from adult rats, with the latter being more susceptible. In this liver cell-mediated assay, the mutagenicity of nitrosamines was detected at dose levels which were two-to-three orders of magnitude lower than those observed in other common short-term assays[31,43]. Furthermore, we have found that, as in the case of the polycyclic aromatic hydrocarbons, a relationship between the degree of carcinogenicity and the degree of mutagenicity can be established for nitrosamines (Figure 2).

In addition, by studying the mutagenic response of various metabolites and derivatives of a series of polycyclic aromatic hydrocarbons, such as benz(a)-anthracene[45], benzo(a)pyrene[46,47] and 7,12-dimethylbenz(a)anthracene[48,49] in the V79 cells cocultivated with or without hamster embryonic fibroblasts, we have identified the metabolic pathway that leads to the production of diol-epoxides which are presumably the ultimate mutagenic forms of these carcinogens. Other studies indicated that these metabolites are also the ones that are presumably responsible for induction of tumors in experimental animals.

Cell-mediated mutagenesis and tissue specificity. The cell-mediated mutagenesis assay has the potential to be used as a means of investigating tissue or cell type specificity of chemical carcinogens. As an initial approach to studying cell type specificity *in vitro*, we compared the abilities of rat embryonic fibroblasts (fibroblast-mediated assay) and rat hepatocytes (liver cell-mediated assay) (Figure 1) to activate benzo(a)pyrene, a potent

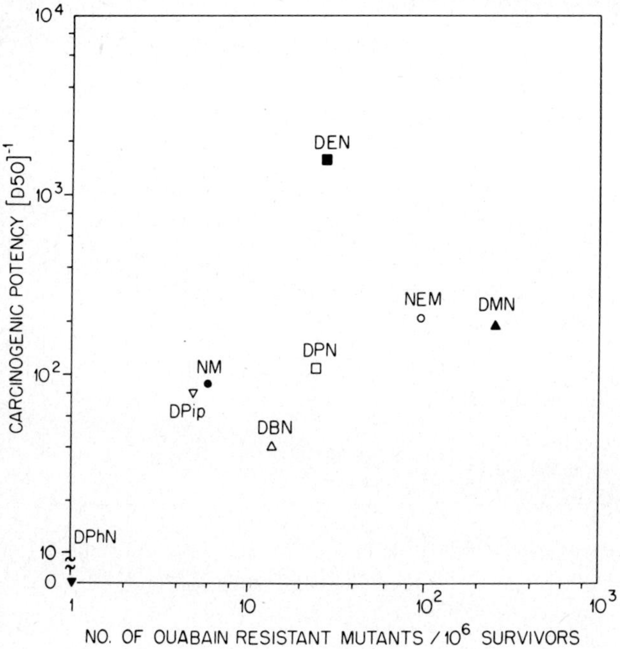

Fig. 2. Relationship between the mutagenic activity of a series of 8 nitrosamines and their carcinogenic potency. Mutagenic activity, the number of ouabain-resistant mutants obtained for 10^6 survivors following treatment with 100 μM of a nitrosamine. Carcinogenic potencies were calculated according to the method of Bartsch et al. (43) using the carcinogenesis data in rats of Druckery et al. (44). DMN, N-nitrosodimethylamine; NPip, 1-nitrosopiperidine; DBN, N-nitrosodibutylamine; DPN, N-nitrosodipropylamine; DPhN, N-nitrosodiphenylamine; NM, N-nitrosomorpholine; NEM, N-nitrosoethylmethylamine; DEN, N-nitrosodiethylamine. (From Jones and Huberman, 31).

skin and lung carcinogen, which can induce fibrosarcoma, and aflatoxin B_1, a potent liver carcinogen, to metabolites which are mutagenic to V79 cells[50]. In agreement with the in vivo activities of these two carcinogens, benzo(a)-pyrene exhibited a mutagenic response in the fibroblast-mediated assay, but not in the hepatocyte-mediated assay, while aflatoxin B1 exhibited an inverse situation (Table 2).

TABLE 2
FIBROBLAST- AND HEPATOCYTE-MEDIATED MUTAGENESIS OF V79 CELLS BY THE CARCINOGENS BENZO(a)PYRENE AND AFLATOXIN B_1

Metabolizing cell type	Compounds	
	Benzo(a)pyrene	Aflatoxin B_1
	(Number of ouabain resistant mutants per 10^6 survivors)	
None	1	1
Fibroblast	50	2
Hepatocyte	2	41

The concentration of the carcinogens was 3 μg/ml. The data are based on results from Langenbach <u>*et al*</u>. *(50).*

We have further established that the absence of mutagenicity of aflatoxin B_1 in the fibroblast-mediated assay was due to the inability of the fibroblasts to metabolize this liver carcinogen. In the case of benzo(a)pyrene, both fibroblast and hepatocytes did sufficiently metabolize this carcinogen, which resulted in binding to DNA[50]; however, only the fibroblasts produced the diol epoxide adducts which are assumed to be associated with the carcinogenic and mutagenic effect of benzo(a)pyrene[51]. These results indicate that a cell type specificity in chemical carcinogenesis can be investigated by the cell-mediated assay.

In conclusion, our mutagenesis studies with mammalian cells may present a system which may (1) be predictive of carcinogenic potential, (2) be indicative of the organ specificity of a carcinogen, and (3) indicate the magnitude of potential threat posed by a particular chemical.

<u>Induction of cell differentiation by tumor promoting phorbol diesters</u>. Our present state of knowledge indicates that carcinogenesis is a multistage process that may require a step or steps beyond the initial mutational event. Thus, it is possible that many environmental causative agents may act at the later stage of the carcinogenesis process in a non-mutational mechanism similar to that of tumor promotion[52-54]. Since certain initiating agents are presumably ubiquitous in the environment, the rate limiting determinants in

cancer causation in humans may be exposure to such agents. In view of this, it is important both to elucidate the mode of action and to identify environmental chemicals which may act as tumor promoters. At the present time, the *in vivo* test which can be used to study and identify such chemicals are both time consuming and require large numbers of experimental animals. It would therefore be of importance to substitute or supplement such experimental animal systems with simple *in vitro* cell systems. However, many of the short-term assays, including Ames *Salmonella typhimurium*-S9 test[9,55] and the mammalian cell-mediated mutagenesis assay[17,31,36,50], are designed to detect carcinogens/mutagens and therefore are not suitable for studying promoting agents, many of which are devoid of mutagenic activity. Tumor promoters act most likely via an epigenetic event, presumably by altering differentiation processes[52]. Indeed, phorbol-12-myristate-13-acetate (PMA)[53], which is a tumor promoter in a two-stage skin carcinogenesis system[52-54], was recently found to alter cell differentiation in some avian and murine cells[56-61]. In our studies with PMA, we found that this chemical can also induce terminal differentiation in some human cells, including promyelocytic HL60[62] leukemia and HO melanoma cells[63]. Differentiation in the leukemia cells was determined by inhibition of cell growth, increase in the percentage of morphological mature cells, increase in phagocytosis, and lysozyme synthesis. Differentiation could be induced by PMA at doses as low as 10^{-10} molar. In the melanoma cells, differentiation was determined by an inhibition of cell growth, formation of dendrite-like structures, and melanin synthesis. As in the case of the leukemia cells, induction of differentiation could be detected at low doses. In analyzing the effect of ten phorbol esters, we found that their ability to induce terminal differentiation in the HL60 leukemia cells was correlated with the tumor promoting activity in mouse skin (Figure 3). Similar results were found also in the case of the HO melanoma cells. These results suggest that alteration of cell differentiation characteristics in some cultured cells may represent an approach by which environmental tumor promoting agents can be studied and perhaps detected. Thus, future developments in cultured mammalian cells, including human cells, may allow us to study and to identify chemicals with a potential to initiate and/or promote tumor formation in experimental animals and humans.

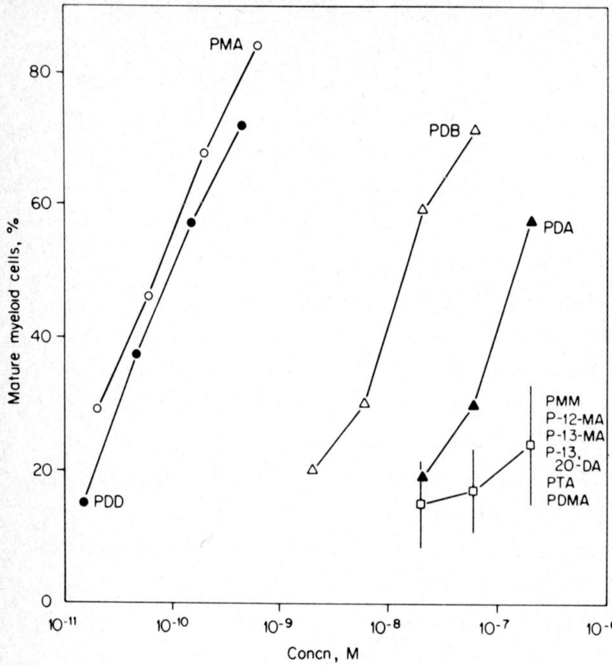

Fig. 3. Differentiation in the HL60 cells 2 days after treatment with various concentrations of the phorbol esters. The percent of mature myeloid cells was determined after cells were stained with Wright/Giemsa. The control cultures contained about 15% mature myeloid cells. O, PMA; O, phorbol-12,13-didecanoate; Δ, phorbol-12,13-dibutyrate; Δ, phorbol-12,13-diacetate; □, phorbol-12-monomyristate, phorbol-12-monoacetate, phorbol-13-monoacetate, phorbol-13,20-diacetate, phorbol-12,13,20-triacetate, and phorbol-20-oxo-20-deoxy-12-myristate-13-acetate. (From Huberman and Callaham, 62).

SUMMARY

A cell-mediated mutagenesis assay was developed to predict the potential carcinogenic hazard of some environmental chemicals. In this assay, cells with appropriate markers for mutagenesis, such as the Chinese hamster V79 cells, are co-cultivated with cells capable of metabolizing chemical carcinogens. Use of this assay made it possible to demonstrate a relationship between the degree of carcinogenicity and mutagenicity of a series of polycyclic hydrocarbons, nitrosamines and aflatoxins, and to establish means to study organ specificity of some chemical carcinogens. However, most short-term *in vitro* assays are designed to detect mutagenic activity and therefore do not detect tumor promoting agents which are devoid of this activity. By analyzing various markers of terminal differentiation in cultured human melanoma and myeloid leukemia cells, we have established a relationship between the activity of a series of tumor promoting phorbol diesters in the mouse skin and their ability to induce terminal differentiation. We suggest that measuring alterations in the differentiation characteristics of some cultured cells may represent an approach by which environmental tumor promoting agents can be studied and detected.

ACKNOWLEDGEMENTS

Research sponsored jointly by the National Cancer Institute under Interagency Agreement 40-636-77, the Environmental Protection Agency under Interagency Agreement 79-D-X0533, and the Office of Health and Environmental Research, United States Department of Energy, under Contract W-7405-eng-26 with the Union Carbide Corporation.

REFERENCES

1. Doll, R. (1977) Nature, 265: 589-596.
2. Hiatt, H. H., Watson, J. D., and Sinsten, J. A. (eds.) (1977) Origins of Human Cancer, Cold Spring Harbor Laboratory, Cold Spring Harbor, New York.
3. Miller, F. C. and Miller, J. A. (1966) Pharmacol. Rev. 18, 805-838.
4. Brookes, P. and Lawley, P. D. (1964) Nature 202, 781-784.
5. Kuroki, T. and Heidelberger, C. (1971) Cancer Res. 31, 2168-2176.
6. Huberman, E. and Sachs, L. (1977) Int. J. Cancer 19, 122-127.
7. Essigmann, J. M., Croy, R. G., Nadzan, A. M., Busby, W. F., Reinhold, V. N., Buchi, G. and Wogan, G. N. (1977) Proc. Natl. Acad. Sci. USA 74, 1870-1874.
8. Jeffrey, A. M., Weinstein, I. B., Jenette, K. W., Grzeskowiak, K., Nakahishi, K., Harvey, R. G., Authrup, M. and Harris, C. (1977) Nature 269, 348-350.
9. Ames, B. N. (1979) Science, 204, 587-593.
10. Huberman, E. (1978) J. Environ. Path. Toxicol. 2, 29-42.
11. Todaro, G. J. and Huebner, R. J. (1972) Proc. Natl. Acad. Sci. USA 69, 1009-1015.
12. Yamamoto, T., Rabinowitz, Z. and Sachs, L. (1973) Nature New Biol. 243, 247-250.
13. Temin, H. M. (1974) Cancer Res. 34, 2835-2841.
14. Huberman, E., Mager, R. and Sachs, L. (1976) Nature 264, 360-361.
15. Chu, E. H. Y. and Malling, H. V. (1968) Proc. Natl. Acad. Sci. USA 61, 1306-1312.
16. Kao, F. T. and Puck, T. T. (1971) J. Cell. Physiol. 78- 139-144.
17. Huberman, E. and Sachs, L. (1974) Int. J. Cancer 13, 326-333.
18. Newbold, R. F., Wigley, C. B., Thompson, M. H., and Brookes, P. (1977) Mutat. Res. 43, 101-116.
19. Clive, D., Johnson, K. O., Spector, J. F. S., Batson, A. G., and Brown, M. M. M. (1979) Mutat. Res. 59, 61-108.
20. Miller, J. A. (1970) Cancer Res. 30, 559-576.
21. Heidelberger, C. (1970) Ann. Rev. Biochem. 44, 79-121.
22. Corbett, T. H., Heidelberger, C. and Dove, W. F. (1970) Mol. Pharmacol. 6, 667-679.
23. Miller, E. C. and Miller, J. A. (1971) In Chemical Mutagens: Principles and Methods for their Detection, Vol. 1, Plenum Press, New York, pp. 83-119.
24. Gelboin, H. V., Huberman, E. and Sachs, L. (1969) Proc. Natl. Acad. Sci. USA 64, 1188-1194.
25. Huberman, E., Selkirk, J. K. and Heidelberger, C. (1971) Cancer Res. 31, 2161-2167.

26. Krahn, D. F. and Heidelberger, C. (1977) Mutat. Res. 46, 27-44.

27. Kuroki, T., Drevon, D. and Montesano, R. (1977) Cancer Res. 37, 1044-1050.

28. Abbondanolo, A., Bonatti, S., Corti, G., Fiorio, R., Loprieno, N., and Mazzaccaro, A. (1977) Mutat. Res. 46, 365-373.

29. Selkirk, J. K. (1977) J. Toxicol. Environ. Health 2, 1245-1258.

30. Bigger, C. A. H., Tomaszewski, J. E., and Dipple, A. (1978) Biochem. Biophys. Res. Commun. 80, 229-235.

31. Jones, C. A. and Huberman, E. (1980) Cancer Res. 40, 406-411.

32. Van Zeeland, A. A. and Simons, J. Y. I. M. (1975) Mutat. Res. 35, 129-138.

33. Baker, R. M., Brunette, D. M., Maknovitz, R., Thompson, L. H., Whitmore, G. F., Siminovitch, L. and Till, J. E. (1974) Cell 1, 9-21.

34. Arlett, C. F., Turnbull, C., Harcourt, S. A., Lehmann, A. R., and Collela, C. M. (1975) Mutation Res. 33, 261-278.

35. Baker, R. M., Brunette, D. M., Mankovitz, R., Thompson, L. H., Whitmore, G. F., Siminovitch, L. and Till, J. E. (1974) Cell 1, 9-21.

36. Huberman, E. and Sachs, L. (1976) Proc. Natl. Acad. Sci. USA 731, 188-192.

37. Huberman, E., Yamaski, H. and Sachs, L. (1976) Int. J. Cancer 18, 76-83.

38. Magee, P. N., Montesano, R. and Preussmann, R. (1976) In Chemical Carcinogens, C. E. Searle (Ed.), ACS Monograph 173.

39. Wogan, G. N. (1976) In Liver Cell Cancer, H. M. Cameron, D. A. Linsell, and Warwick, G. P. (Eds.), Elsevier/North-Holland Biomedical, New York, pp. 121-151.

40. Langenbach, R., Freed, H. J. and Huberman, E. (1978) Proc. Natl. Acad. Sci. 75, 2864-2867.

41. San, R. H. C. and Williams, G. M. (1977) Proc. Soc. Exp. Biol. Med. 156, 534-538.

42. Fry, J. R., Jones, C. A., Wiebkin, P., Bellemann, P. and Bridges, J. W. (1976) Analyt. Biochem. 71, 341-350.

43. Bartsch, H., Malaveille, C., Camus, A.-M., Brun, G. and Hautefeuille, A. (1979) In Short-Term Mutagenicity Test Systems for Detecting Carcinogens, K. Norpoth and C. Garner (Eds.), Springer Verlag, New York.

44. Druckery, H., Preussmann, R., Ivankovic, S. and Schmähl, D. (1967) Z. Krebsforsch. 69, 103-201.

45. Slaga, T. J., Huberman, E., Selkirk, J. K., Harvey, R. G. and Bracken, W. M. (1978) Cancer Res. 38, 1699-1704.

46. Huberman, E., Sachs, L., Yang, S. K. and Gelboin, H. V. (1976b) Proc. Natl. Acad. Sci. USA 73, 607-611.

47. Huberman, E., Yang, S. K., McCourt, D. W. and Gelboin, H. V. (1978) Cancer Lett. 4, 35-43.

48. Huberman, E. and Slaga, T. (1979) Cancer Res. 39, 411-414.

49. Huberman, E., Chou, M. W. and Yang, S. K. (1979) Proc. Natl. Acad. Sci. USA 76, 862-866.

50. Langenbach, R., Freed, H. Y., Raveh, D. and Huberman, E. (1978) Nature 276, 277-280.

51. Jones, C. A., Santela, R., Huberman, E., Selkirk, J. K. and Grunberger, D. In preparation.

52. Berenblum, I. (1969) Prog. Exp. Tumor Res. 11, 21-30.

53. Hecker, E. (1978) In Mechanisms of Tumor Promotion and Cocarcinogenesis, T. J. Slaga, A. J. Sivak, and R. Boutwell (Eds.), Raven, New York, pp. 11-49.

54. Boutwell, R. L. (1978) In Mechanisms of Tumor Promotion and Cocarcinogenesis, T. J. Slaga, A. J. Sivak, and R. K. Boutwell (Eds.), Raven, New York, pp. 49-58.

55. McCann, J. and Ames, B. N. (1977) In Origins of Human Cancer, H. H. Hiatt, J. D. Watson and J. A. Winston (Eds.), Cold Spring Harbor Laboratory, Cold Spring Harbor, New York, pp. 1431-1450.

56. Cohen, R., Pacific, M., Rubinstein, N., Biehl, J. and Holtzer, M. (1976) Nature (London) 259, 1232-1233.

57. Rovera, G., O'Brien, T. and Diamond, L. (1977) Proc. Natl. Acad. Sci. USA 74, 2894-2896.

58. Yamasaki, H., Fibach, E., Nudel, U., Weinstein, I. B., Rifkind, R. A. and Marks, P. A. (1977) Proc. Natl. Acad. Sci. USA 74, 3451-3456.

59. Ishi, D. N., Fibach, E., Yamasaki, H. and Weinstein, B. I. (1978) Science 200, 556-559.

60. Diamond, L., O'Brien, T. G. and Rovera, G. (1977) Nature (London) 269, 247-249.

61. Miao, R. M., Fieldsteel, A. H. and Fodge, D. (1978) Nature (London) 274, 271-274.

62. Huberman, E. and Calaham, M. F. (1979) Proc. Natl. Acad. Sci. USA 76, 1293-1297.

63. Huberman, E., Heckman, C. and Langenbach, R. (1979) Cancer Res. 39, 2618-2624.

© 1980 Elsevier/North-Holland Biomedical Press
Mechanisms of Toxicity and Hazard Evaluation
B. Holmstedt, R. Lauwerys, M. Mercier, M. Roberfroid eds

PROBLEMS ASSOCIATED WITH THE METABOLIC ACTIVATION OF CARCINOGENS AND MUTAGENS IN SHORT-TERM TESTS

HELMUT BARTSCH

Programme of Environmental Carcinogenesis and Host Factors, Division of Chemical and Biological Carcinogenesis, International Agency for Research on Cancer, 150 cours Albert-Thomas, F-69372 Lyon Cédex 2, France

INTRODUCTION

Extensive studies carried out to evaluate whether short-term tests for the detection of genotoxic agents are reliable indicators (predictors) of the potential carcinogenic hazard of chemicals[1-5] have revealed that apart from the indicator organism or the end points scored the metabolic activation system used is of critical importance.

The detection of electrophilic intermediates in short-term tests produced from active precarcinogens (premutagens) by metabolism[6] is a complex problem. Electrophilic ultimate carcinogenic/mutagenic metabolites are formed either directly or through one or more intermediates (proximate carcinogens) from the precarcinogens. Once formed, the ultimate carcinogen may react with target molecules like DNA in genetic indicator organisms, or be deactivated by binding with other cellular nucleophiles, spontaneous breakdown or enzymatic detoxification. Similarly, pre- and proximate carcinogens may be subject to enzymic and non-enzymic detoxification reactions. Thus, the carcinogenicity/mutagenicity of many chemicals is largely determined by competition between activation and detoxification reactions. The specificity of some chemical carcinogens/mutagens which are not active *per se* for certain animal species and organs seems in part to be determined by the concentration of reactive metabolites in target cells, which has to be sufficiently high. For all these reasons, mutagenicity assays in intact animals (like the host-mediated assay) may give false negative results; therefore *in vitro* techniques, or a combination of *in vivo*/*in vitro* methods, have been developed (Chapter C). On the other hand, an incomplete picture of the mutagenic effects of carcinogens may be obtained by *in vitro* techniques because of many exogenous and endogenous factors that affect the mammalian metabolism of foreign compounds. An ideal mutagenicity (short-term) test would therefore have to include a full metabolic competency of an intact animal, preferably human. But the self-evident difficulties of developing and applying such a system have led to the conclusion that a battery of tests is needed, whereby different metabolic activation systems are included.

In the following article, some of the metabolic systems commonly used in short-term tests for the detection of carcinogens/mutagens are reviewed, representing a summary of 2 previous publications dealing with related subjects[7,8].

ABBREVIATIONS

S9 (15), 9000 (15,000) x *g* supernatant; PMS, postmitochondrial tissue supernatant; MFO, mixed function oxidase (monooxygenase) system; PAH, polycyclic aromatic hydrocarbons

MATERIALS AND METHODS

Mutagenicity assays in bacterial and mammalian cells in the presence of microsome- or cell-mediated metabolic activation systems are commonly used for the detection of carcinogens. The following published procedures are most widely applied:

Plate incorporation assay in the presence of *S. typhimurium* (or other bacterial) tester strains[9]

The test compound, dissolved in DMSO, 0.5 ml of a mixture containing various amounts of tissue S9 (normally up to 150 μl), cofactors, Sørensen phosphate buffer pH 7.4 and a suspension containing 1-2 x 10^8 bacteria (S9 mix) are combined with 2 ml histidine-poor soft agar. The agar mixture (final volume, 2.7 ml) is poured onto plates of minimal agar; these are then incubated at 37°. The number of *his*$^+$ revertant colonies is counted, usually after incubation for 48 hr.

Pre-incubation assay[10]

Pre-incubation of S9 mix with the bacteria at 37^oC for 5-30 min prior to addition of soft agar.

Gaseous exposure assay[11]

Mutagenicity tests with compounds that are volatile or gaseous at room temperature are performed by exposing inverted petri dishes containing bacteria and the same ingredients as for the plate assay, except that DMSO and the test compound were omitted, to various concentrations of the test compound in air in 10-l desiccators for various times at 37° in the dark. The desired concentration of a gaseous compound in air is, for example, achieved by evacuating the desiccator introducing a known volume of the gas to be tested, then allowing air to enter until atmospheric pressure was reached. Mutants are scored after a total of 48 hr incubation time. Quantitation of the test compound dissolved in the aqueous phase is achieved by gas-liquid chromatography.

Liquid incubation[12]

The incubation medium (final volume, 220 µl) may contain 60 µl S9 liver supernatant, cofactors, Sørensen phosphate buffer (pH 7.4), a bacterial suspension (average 4 x 10^7 cells) and the test compound dissolved in saline or DMSO solution. The incubation is carried out at 37° for 30 min under oxygen and is stopped by dilution with ice-cold saline. The numbers of mutants and survivors are determined by plating on selective medium after appropriate dilution.

Microsome-mediated mutagenesis in mammalian cells[13]

V79 Chinese hamster cells are incubated 18-24 hr after plating in the presence of a 15,000 x *g* postmitochondrial fraction of rat liver (S15), cofactors and the chemicals to be tested, for 1-15 hr. The cells are then washed, incubated for 2-3 hr in fresh culture medium and plated for toxicity and mutagenicity. Mutations are determined by resistance to 8-azaguanine (AZA^r) 20 µg/ml and to 1 mM ouabain (OUA^r). The selective media are added 48 hr after plating and changed once 5-7 days later. The cultures are fixed and stained with Giemsa after 12 days for AZA^r and after 14 days for OUA^r. Mutation frequency is calculated per 10^5 survivors.

Cell-mediated mutagenesis

This can be measured by following the procedure described by Huberman and Sachs[14] when rat embryonic cells or other cell lines are used, and by following that of Langenbach et al.[15] when primary hepatocytes are used. V79 cells, co-cultivated with metabolic cells, were incubated for 48 hr in the presence of the chemicals to be tested before plating for toxicity and mutagenicity (AZA^r or OUA^r mutants).

RESULTS AND DISCUSSION

A number of mammalian activation systems have been developed in order to compensate for the limited capabilities of most (sub-mammalian) indicator organisms to metabolize carcinogens/mutagens. Some of the advantages and

TABLE 1

SOME METABOLIC ACTIVATION SYSTEMS COMMONLY USED TO METABOLIZE CARCINOGENS AND MUTAGENS TO THEIR REACTIVE FORM (MODIFIED FROM IARC 1980 [7])

Activation Systems	Advantages	Disadvantages
A. Cell-free systems		
1. Postmitochondrial 9000 x *g* or 15,000 x *g* supernatant fraction of rodent liver (S9 or S15)	Easily prepared, contains most of the enzymes associated with xenobiotic metabolism; large data base from previous studies. Good system for routine screening. This system favours activation of carcinogens and mutagens.	High amounts of nucleophiles may bind ultimate carcinogens and mutagens and reduce sensitivity. Difficult to identify the particular enzyme(s) involved in activation or detoxification.
2. Microsomal fraction of rodent liver	Contains high level of cytochrome P-450-dependent MFO activity; recombination with 100,000 x *g* supernatant permits partial identification of pathways of metabolism.	Preparation requires preparative ultracentrifuge and more time than S9. Cytosolic enzymes are not present.
3. Purified enzymes, e.g. monooxygenase system, epoxide hydratase, glutathione transferase(s)	Biochemically well defined; unequivocal identification of metabolites identified under same conditions which induce mutations; ratio of various enzymes easily altered.	Technical difficulty in preparing enzymes; general knowledge of each test compound's metabolic fate needed. Many important enzymes may be absent. Not suited for routine screening.
B. Mammalian cells	Cellular integrity and enzyme relationships preserved, endogenous levels of cofactors. An intermediate between cell-free and *in vivo* activation systems.	Technically difficult and limited sample throughout; more costly than cell-free systems. In some cell lines, important enzymes are present in low amounts or absent.
C. Host-mediated assay *in vivo* using micro-organisms or mammalian cell lines as indicators	Compound metabolized and tester organism mutated under *in vivo* conditions. Pharmacokinetic parameters of absorption, distribution, metabolism and excretion of compound in part accounted for.	Limited sensitivity throughout for the detection of mutagens and carcinogens. Technically more difficult than *in vitro* tests; host reaction against tester organisms. Limited sample throughout compared to *in vitro* system.

limitations of cell-free and cellular metabolic activation systems currently used in short-term tests are summarized in Table 1.

A. Sub-cellular metabolic activation systems:

1. Hepatic postmitochondrial supernatant (S9) fraction from rats

The widespread metabolic activation system used in short-term tests is liver S9 from rats pre-treated with polychlorinated biphenyls (PCB's), e.g. Aroclor 1254. A large data base and general suitability of the activating system described by Ames et al.[9] for use in conjunction with microorganisms as target cells favour its continued use in routine screening tests for detection of DNA damaging agents. The liver postmitochondrial supernatant, S9 or S15, has also been successfully used to activate different chemicals to DNA damaging products in cultured mammalian cells (see Chapter B). The efficiency for the detection of carcinogens/mutagens and the reproducibility of the results in such *in vitro* assays have been shown to be affected by several parameters, including the following:

1.1 Animal treatment by inducers/modifyers of drug metabolizing enzymes

1.2 Mode of co-incubation of the test compound and the genetic indicator with the metabolic activation system

1.3 Effect of co-factors/modifyers added to the *in vitro* activation system

1.4 Dose response relationship with S9 proteins and test compound

1.5 Effect of solvents and length of storage of tissue preparations

A few of these variables are briefly discussed below.

1.1 Effect of inducers/modifyers on drug metabolizing enzymes. Variability of liver S9 preparations among different laboratories or at different times may be related to their qualitative and quantitative extent of induction of various forms of cytochrome P450. Thus, the cytochrome P450 and protein content of each preparation should be determined and recorded in order to verify the presence and extent of induction of the MFO system. Additionally, an assay of some marker enzymic reactions, e.g. of benzo(*a*)pyrene hydroxylase and aminopyrine *N*-demethylase, will calibrate the preparation with respect to the two major forms of cytochrome P450 induced by PCB's.

Numerous studies have shown that inducers/inhibitors of hepatic microsomal monooxygenases when administered to animals alter the liver microsome-dependent mutagenicity of carcinogens/mutagens; these treatments also modify carcinogenicity *in vivo*, possibly by changing the balance between activation and detoxification reactions. Comparison of such drug-induced alterations *in vitro* and *in vivo* show in general a good but not perfect correlation[16,17]. Reasons for these discrepancies are possibly associated with the use of sub-cellular fractions which do not mimic the entire metabolic competency of an intact mammalian cell.

Furthermore, as studied in more detail with aflatoxin B_1 and Aroclor 1254, an inducer treatment of rats, the change of bacterial mutagenicity was shown to be dependent on the type of assay, the concentration of rat liver S9 and that of aflatoxin B_1 used[18]. Thus, when comparing the mutagenicity in *S. typhimurium* in assays carried out either with liver S9 from induced rats or those from untreated ones, the plate incorporation assay revealed either no change or an increased mutagenicity following inducer treatment. In contrast, in assays in liquid incubation, at all concentrations of aflatoxin B_1 and of S9 tested, Aroclor treatment caused a decrease in mutagenicity. Possible reasons for these differences have been discussed[18].

1.2 Mode of co-incubation of the test compound and the genetic indicator with the metabolic activation system. In the plate incorporation assay[9] metabolic activation of the test compound takes place in the soft agar overlay. However, certain compounds, e.g., some *N*-nitrosamines[19], are more efficiently detected as mutagens in liquid suspension. This phenomenon is probably related to the higher S9 protein concentration which can be achieved in liquid assays as compared to plate assays. For a more efficient detection of certain mutagens, the two assays can be combined by pre-incubating liver S9, co-factors and test compound with the bacteria at $37^{o}C$ for 5-30 min prior to addition of soft agar. The utility of the procedure has been demonstrated[10].

Because of loss of highly volatile test compounds during incubation in plates, procedures for testing such gaseous substrates in desiccators have been described[20,9,21].

1.3 Effect of co-factors/modifyers on *in vitro* activation reactions. NADPH (or an NADPH generating system) required for the activity of the MFO system is the only enzyme co-factor specifically added to the *Salmonella*/microsome assay described by Ames et al.[9]. However, *in vitro* addition of many other co-factors or modifyers of Phase I and II enzymes has been shown to enhance or decrease the mutagenicity of pre-carcinogens/mutagens requiring metabolic activation. Some examples include 7,8-benzoflavone, 1,1,1-trichloropropene oxide, norharman, riboflavin, glutathione, ATP, UDPGA, Vitamin A, C and E. Thus, a number of compounds have been used or proposed to optimize or increase the utility *in vitro* metabolic activation system used for short-term testing. However, at the present time an insufficient data base exists to state whether any of these factors will increase the predictive value of the short-term tests to an extent that will justify their incorporation into a standard testing protocol.

1.4 Dose response relationship with S9 proteins and test compound. A complete assessment of the compound's mutagenic (DNA damaging) activity, or lack thereof, requires for *in vitro* assays using sub-cellular tissue fractions that both the concentration of the test compound and the amount of enzymes be varied several fold. Such a protocol defines conditions for optimal (highest) mutagenic response as well as for expressing mutagenic activity both in terms of amount of test compound and of enzyme (protein) concentration needed for activation.

The actual amount of liver PMS needed for optimal (highest) mutagenesis in bacterial and mammalian mutagenicity assays *in vitro*, however, has been shown to vary widely according to the structure (lipophilic properties) and concentration of the test compound, as well as the source of the liver preparation (inducer treatment of animals)[9,18,22].

2. Species variations in hepatic metabolic activation reactions

Species differences in the activity of many of the enzymes associated with xenobiotic metabolism are pronounced[23]. As a consequence, large differences in the species capacity for activation have been observed when liver tissue from different experimental animal species were used to activate precarcinogens (Table 2). Although eventually mixtures of liver homogenates from different animal species may circumvent some of the possible metabolic limitations imposed by using only one species (e.g., rat) much interest has arisen to study these differences with the aim to reveal to what extent species variation in the carcinogenic response to chemicals may be attributable to metabolic activation (or detoxification) reactions.

Based on results from the *Salmonella*/microsome mutagenicity assay for which an increasing data base is available, it appears that the source of liver S9 from different animal species is an important factor for the efficient detection of carcinogens/mutagens (Table 2): hamster liver S9 was much more efficient to demonstrate mutagenicity for a series of *N*-nitrosamines and 2-acetylaminofluorene as compared to rat and mouse liver. Phenacetin was found only mutagenic in the presence of hamster but not of a rat liver S9. Mutagenicity of vinylidene chloride was 3 times higher in the presence of mouse

TABLE 2

SPECIES VARIATIONS IN THE CAPACITY OF LIVER TISSUE FRACTIONS FROM EXPERIMENTAL ANIMALS TO ACTIVATE SOME PRE-CARCINOGENS MEASURED BY THE *SALMONELLA* MUTAGENICITY ASSAY

Test Compound	Inducer Treatment of Rodent	Species Capacity for Activation	References
N-nitrosodimethylamine	none, PCB or PB[a]	H>M>R[b]	25
	PCB	H>M>R>GP	26
N-nitrosodiethylamine	none	H>R	11
	PB	R>H	11
N-nitroso-di-*n*-propylamine and 5 β-oxidized derivatives	PB	H>R	27
Benzo(*a*)pyrene	none	M>GP	28
	none	GP>M>H>R	26
	PCB	R>M>GP>H	26
2-acetylaminofluorene	none	H>GP>M>R	26
	PCB	H>GP>M>R	26
	none	GP>Rab>R>M	29
Phenacetin	PCB	H>R	5 26
Aflatoxin B_1	none	Duck>R>Monkey>M	24
Vinylidene Chloride	none	M>R	30

[a] PCB: polychlorinated biphenyls; PB: phenobarbitone (Aroclor 1254)

[b] M: mouse; H: hamster; R: rat; GP: guinea pig; Rab: rabbit

than of rat liver S9. Activation capacity of aflatoxin B_1 into mutagens roughly paralleled the susceptibility of these species towards the hepatocarcinogenic effect of this mycotoxin[24].

3. Carcinogen/mutagen activation by human liver (or other tissue) enzymes

In vitro short-term assays are also useful in studies in species differences in pathways or rates of carcinogen metabolism using tissue fractions or cells from different organs derived from human subjects, in most cases surgical biopsy specimens or autopsy material. Such data may be helpful for extrapolation from animal species to man when tissues or cells from human origins are qualitatively or quantitatively compared with experimental animals. An increasing number of results (for a compilation, see Bartsch et al.[8]) obtained with different classes of carcinogens (like *N*-nitrosamines, aromatic amino and nitrocompounds, PAH, halogenated olefins, naturally occurring carcinogens and miscellaneous compounds, including drugs and cigarette smoke condensate) in the presence of liver microsomes or liver S9 derived from different human subjects have been shown to be converted into electrophilic metabolites which can react with DNA of the indicator organism (in many cases *S. typhimurium* strains or V79 Chinese hamster cells). Other studies identified mutagenic metabolites in the urine of carcinogen/mutagen exposed human subjects following incubation of the urinary metabolites in the presence or absence of deconjugating enzymes with or without metabolic activation (mostly liver S9). Thus, human subjects dosed with either nitrofurantoin, niridazole, metronidazole, cyclophosphamide, 5-fluorouracil or persons smoking cigarettes contained detectable mutagenic activity in their urine.

B. Cellular metabolic activation systems

1. Cultured cells possessing metabolic activity and their use in short-term tests

Some of mammalian cells in culture contain appreciable amounts of enzymes to metabolize carcinogenic/mutagenic chemicals and they are being used for metabolic activation in various short-term tests such as DNA repair, transformation and mammalian cell mutagenesis (see Table 3). These cells include primary cultures of rat hepatocytes, liver epithelial cell lines, primary or secondary cultures of rodent embryo fibroblasts, C3H 10T 1/2 cell line and some human tissues and cells in culture.

Metabolically competent cells are being used at present in two ways in short-term tests: the activating cell can serve as the genetic target

TABLE 3

SOME CLASSES OF PRE-CARCINOGENS/MUTAGENS TESTED IN CELL-MEDIATED ASSAYS (MODIFIED FROM BARTSCH ET AL. 1980[5])

Cells	Endpoints measured	Chemicals tested	References
Primary rat hepatocytes	Mutation	NA	31 15 32 33
		AFB	15 32
		AAF	33
		PAH	33
Primary hamster hepatocytes	Transformation	NA,DAB,AAF,PAH	34
Rat liver cell lines	Mutation	PAH	Drevon et al. (unpublished)
Mouse liver cell lines	Transformation	AFB	35
Secondary culture of rodent embryo cells	Mutation	PAH	14 36 37
	Chromosomal change	PAH	38
BHK-21	Mutation	PAH	39
Human cells:			
alveolar macrophages	Mutation	PAH	40
bronchial explant	Mutation	PAH	41
epidermal keratinocytes	Mutation	PAH	Kuroki et al. (unpublished)

Abbreviations:

NA: *N*-nitrosamines; AFB: aflatoxin B_1; AAF: 2-acetylaminofluorene; PAH: polycyclic aromatic hydrocarbons; DAB: diaminoazobenzene (& its derivatives) (indicator) cell or they are co-cultured with metabolically deficient target cells (the cell-mediated assay). Some examples are listed in Table 3.

2. Evaluation of the efficiency of carcinogen/mutagen screening tests using intact mammalian cells for metabolic activation

Mammalian cells in culture have advantages and disadvantages when they are used for metabolic activation reactions *in vitro*. Cultured cells possess an intact cellular architecture and arrangement of the various enzyme systems and endogenous levels of cofactors. Thus, as compared to the reactions catalyzed by cell-free systems (e.g., S9 or microsomal fraction), metabolic pathways occurring in cells more closely resemble those occurring *in vivo*. Newbold et al.[39] demonstrated that DNA adducts produced by benzo(*a*)pyrene in the cell-mediated assay gave a very similar elution profile on LH-20 chromatography to those obtained in cultured cells, but were different from those treated in the presence of postmitochondrial fraction. Bigger et al.[42] also reported that the liver microsomal system does not always mimic the metabolic activation of benzo(*a*)pyrene which is seen in cultured cells and *in vivo* experiments.

The concentration of certain test compounds that are necessary to induce mutations are considerably lower when using intact cells. For example, the mutagenicity of dimethylnitrosamine can be detected at a 1-2 mM concentration by the hepatocyte-mediated assay[15] and at a 1-10 μM concentration by the improved hepatocyte-mediated assay[31]; whereas in the liver microsome-mediated assays, concentrations above 10 mM were required for efficient induction of mutation[13].

The use of intact mammalian cells offers yet another advantage that cell or tissue specificity in chemical carcinogenesis can be investigated. Hepatocarcinogens such as aflatoxin B_1, *N*-nitrosodimethylamine and 2-acetylaminofluorene, can be detected by the use of primary hepatocytes scoring for DNA repair, transformation and mutation, whereas benzo(*a*)pyrene was detected as a mutagen in the fibroblast-mediated assays, but not readily in the hepatocyte-mediated assays[32].

On the other hand, cell specificity in activation reactions implies that only a limited spectrum of chemicals can be metabolized; this may indicate that cellular activation systems may not be suitable as an initial screening test for carcinogens/mutagens. Furthermore, the use of intact cells is technically more difficult and limits the applicability of these assays.

C. Combination of *in vivo/in vitro* screening tests of carcinogens/mutagens - recent developments

A number of mammalian *in vivo* activation systems have been developed to compensate for the limitations imposed by the use of tissue fractions or cells to metabolize carcinogens/mutagens *in vitro*. Some of the systems currently being developed or in use utilize the metabolic competency of the intact mammalian organism but score for genotoxic effects *in vitro* following isolation of the affected target cells or tissues. However, because for most of these methods a large data base is not yet available, their use as routine screening tests for the detection of carcinogens/mutagens is limited and at present not recommended.

The classical host-mediated assay described by Gabridge and Legator[43] and Capizzi et al.[44] (in which chemicals are activated *in vivo* and the metabolites reach either the microorganisms or mammalian cell lines inoculated in the host) has been extended to allow scoring of different endpoints in target cells/organs from the treated animal. Procedures used include the isolation of mutated cells from specific target organs of carcinogen-treated rodents[45]; the estimation of unscheduled DNA repair synthesis or DNA fragmentation in target cells or tissues[46,47] by means of autoradiography or DNA alkaline elution techniques, respectively. Assays using transplacental mutagenesis, in which embryos are exposed *in utero* to the test chemical and then examined in culture for mutations (as well as for transformation and chromosomal changes) have been reported[48]. In addition, biological fluids like urine obtained from animals or man exposed to carcinogens/mutagens can also be employed as sources of metabolites[49].

In another system in which indicator organisms (bacteria or mammalian cells) are exposed to the perfusate or bile from isolated perfused rat liver, mutagenic metabolites derived from benzo(*a*)pyrene and *N*-nitrosodimethylamine have been detected[50]. This system has also made possible for the first time an estimation of the half-life of the mutagenic metabolite of *N*-nitrosodimethylamine (presumably the methylol derivative) which is of the order ≤ 5 seconds[50]. Cultured human bronchial explants cocultured with V79 Chinese hamster cells have also been used to metabolize polycyclic aromatic hydrocarbons to mutagenic products[41].

CONCLUSIONS

Many compounds require metabolic conversion to ultimately reactive intermediates before they can exert a carcinogenic/mutagenic (genotoxic) effect. Therefore, the choice of metabolizing system(s) in short-term tests for the detection of genotoxic agents has great importance for the efficiency of these tests, and is particularly important to avoid obtaining false negative results (i.e., carcinogens which are not detected in a short-term test). Numerous factors are known to influence metabolism of foreign compounds in mammals, and the results obtained in short-term tests are often greatly influenced by multiple details in selection, preparation and use of metabolizing systems. Because of such great complexity and variability, no single metabolic activation system can mimic all *in vivo* situations, not even for a single animal species. For this reason, when a compound is assayed in multiple short-term tests, different metabolic activation systems should be included. Interpretations of results of given short-term tests and their extrapolation to an intact mammalian organism should be made with caution and in context with results from other toxicological tests and information.

Nevertheless, despite these limitations imposed by the current methodologies, an increasing data base provides evidence that the use of appropriate metabolic activation systems in short-term tests has greatly contributed to their use in the prediction or confirmation of the carcinogenic effect of chemicals in animals[4,2] and man[51,52].

ACKNOWLEDGEMENTS

The author is grateful to C. Rowson for secretarial assistance. The author's research activities in this area are partly supported by Contract NO1-CP-55630 with the National Cancer Institute, NIH, Bethesda MD, USA and partly by Contract No. 190-77 ENVF with the Commission of the European Communities.

REFERENCES

1. McCann, J., Choi, E., Yamasaki, E. and Ames, B.N. (1975) Proc. Natl. Acad. Sci. USA, 72, 5135-5139.
2. Sugimura, T., Sato, S., Nagao, M., Yahagi, T., Matsushima, T., Seino, Y., Takeuchi, M. and Kawachi, T. (1976) Fundamentals in Cancer Prevention, University of Tokyo Press/University Park Press, Tokyo/Baltimore, pp. 191-215.
3. Purchase, I.F.H., Longstaff, E., Ashby, J., Styles, J.A., Anderson, D., Lefevre, P.A. and Westwood, F.R. (1978) Br. J. Cancer, 37, 873-959.

4. Hollstein, M., McCann, J., Angelsanto, F.A. and Nichols, W.W. (1979) Mutat. Res., 65, 133-226.

5. Bartsch, H., Malaveille, C., Camus, A.M., Martel-Planche, G., Brun, G., Hautefeuille, A., Sabadie, N., Barbin, A. and Kuroki, T., Drevon, C., Piccoli, C., Montesano, R. (1980) Mutat. Res., in press.

6. Miller, E.C. (1978) Cancer Res., 38, 1479-1496.

7. IARC (1980) IARC Monographs on the Evaluation of Carcinogenic Risk of Chemicals to Humans, Long-term and short-term screening assays for carcinogens: a critical appraisal, Supplement No. 2, Lyon, France.

8. Bartsch, H., Kuroki, T., Roberfroid, M. and Malaveille, C. (1980) Chemical Mutagens - Principles and Methods for Their Detection Vol. 7, Plenum Press, New York and London, in press.

9. Ames, B.N., McCann, J. and Yamasaki, E. (1975) Mutat. Res., 31, 347-364.

10. Nagao, M., Yahagi, T., Seino, Y., Sugimura, T. and Ito, N. (1977) Mutat. Res., 42, 335-342.

11. Bartsch, H., Malaveille, C. and Montesano, R. (1975b) Cancer Res., 35, 644-651.

12. Malling, H.V. (1971) Mutat. Res., 13, 425-429.

13. Kuroki, T., Drevon, C. and Montesano, R. (1977) Cancer Res., 37, 1044-1050.

14. Huberman, E. and Sachs, L. (1974) Int. J. Cancer, 13, 326-333.

15. Langenbach, R., Freed, H.J. and Huberman, E. (1978a) Proc. Natl. Acad. Sci. USA, 75, 2864-2867.

16. Bartsch, H. (1976) CNRS, 256, 255-281.

17. Sabadie, N., Malaveille, C., Camus, A.M. and Bartsch, H. (1980) Cancer Res., 40, 119-126.

18. Malaveille, C., Kuroki, T., Brun, G., Hautefeuille, A., Camus, A.M. and Bartsch, H. (1979) Mutat. Res., 63, 245-258.

19. Bartsch, H., Camus, A. and Malaveille, C. (1976) Mutat. Res., 37, 149-162.

20. Bartsch, H., Malaveille, C. and Montesano, R. (1975a) Int. J. Cancer, 15, 429-437.

21. Simmon, V.F., Kauhanen, K. and Tardiff, R.G. (1977) Progress in Genetic Toxicology, Elsevier/North-Holland Biomedical Press, Amsterdam, pp. 249-258.

22. Kuroki, T., Malaveille, C., Drevon, C., Piccoli, C., Macleod, M. and Selkirk, J.K. (1979) Mutat. Res., 63, 259-272.

23. Williams, R.T. (1971) Fundamentals of Drug Metabolism and Drug Disposition, Williams and Wilkins & Co., Baltimore, pp. 187-205.

24. Hsieh, D.P.H., Wong, J.J., Wong, Z.A., Michas, C. and Ruebner, B.H. (1977) Origins of Human Cancer, Cold Spring Harbor Laboratory, Cold Spring Harbor, pp. 697-707.

25. Prival, M.J., Sheldon, Jr., A.T. and King, V. (1979) 10th Annual Meeting of Environmental Mutagen Society, New Orleans, Louisiana.

26. Matsushima, T., Yahagi, T., Takamoto, Y., Nagao, M. and Sugimura, T. (1980) Microsomes, Drug Oxidations and Chemical Carcinogenesis, Academic Press, New York, in press.

27. Camus, A., Bertram, B., Kruger, F.W., Malaveille, C. and Bartsch, H. (1976) Z. Krebsforsch., 86, 293-302.

28. Ashby, J. and Styles, J.A. (1978) Nature, 271, 425-454.

29. Brusick, D.J. (1977) Toxicology Annual Vol. 2, Marcel Dekker Inc., New York and Basel, pp. 79-109.

30. Bartsch, H., Malaveille, C., Montesano, R. and Tomatis, L. (1975c) Nature, 255, 641-643.

31. Jones, C.A. and Huberman, E. (1980) Cancer Res., 40, 406-411.

32. Langenbach, R., Freed, H.J., Raveh, D. and Huberman, E. (1978b) Nature, 276, 277-280.

33. San, R.H. and Williams, G.M. (1977) Proc. Soc. Exp. Biol. & Med., 156, 534-538.

34. Poiley, J.A., Raineri, R. and Pienta, R.J. (1979) J. Natl. Cancer Inst., 63, 519-524.

35. Mondal, S., Lillehaug, J.R. and Heidelberger, C. (1979) Proc. Am. Assoc. Cancer Res., 20, 62.

36. Huberman, E. and Sachs, L. (1976) Proc. Natl. Acad. Sci. USA, 73, 188-192.

37. Kuroki, T. and Drevon, C. (1978) Nature, 271, 368-370.

38. Nishi, Y., Mori, M. and Inui, N. (1979) Toxicol. Lett., 4, 275-280.

39. Newbold, R.F., Wigley, C.B., Thompson, M.H. and Brookes, P. (1977) Mutat. Res., 43, 101-116.

40. Harris, C.C., Hsu, I.C., Stoner, G.D., Trump, B.F. and Selkirk, J.K. (1978) Nature, 272, 633-634.

41. Hsu, I.C., Stona, G.D., Autrup, H., Trump, B.F., Selkirk, J.K. and Harris, C.C. (1978) Proc. Natl. Acad. Sci. USA, 75, 2003-2007.

42. Bigger, C.A.H., Tomaszewski, J.E. and Dipple, A. (1978) Biochem. Biophys. Res. Commun., 80, 229-235.

43. Gabridge, M.G. and Legator, M.S. (1969) Proc. Soc. Exp. Biol. Med., 130, 831-834.

44. Capizzi, R.L., Papirmeister, B., Mullins, J.M. and Cheng, E. (1974) Cancer Res., 34, 3073-3082.

45. Dean, B.J. and Senner, K.R. (1977) Mutat. Res., 46, 403-407.

46. Stich, M.F. and Kieser, D. (1974) Proc. Soc. Exp. Biol. Med., 145, 1339-1342.

47. Petzold, G.L. and Swenberg, J.A. (1978) Cancer Res., 38, 1589-1594.

48. Inui, N. and Nishi, Y. (1978) Toxicol. Lett., 2, 277-283.

49. Legator, M.S., Truong, L. and Connor, T.H. (1978) Chemical Mutagens - Principles and Methods for Their Detection Vol. 5, Plenum Press, New York and London, pp. 1-22.

50. Jenssen, D., Beije, B. and Ramel, C. (1979) Chem.-biol. Interactions, 27, 27-39.

51. McCann, J. and Ames, B.N. (1977) Origins of Human Cancer, Cold Spring Harbor Laboratory, Cold Spring Harbor, pp. 1431-1450.

52. Tomatis, L., Breslow, N.E. and Bartsch, H. (1980) Cancer Epidemiology and Prevention, W.B. Saunders, Philadelphia, London, Toronto, in press.

© 1980 Elsevier/North-Holland Biomedical Press
Mechanisms of Toxicity and Hazard Evaluation
B. Holmstedt, R. Lauwerys, M. Mercier, M. Roberfroid eds

CELL CULTURE SYSTEMS FOR STUDYING MULTIFACTOR INTERACTIONS IN CARCINOGENESIS.

I. BERNARD WEINSTEIN
Division of Environmental Sciences and Cancer Center/Institute of Cancer Research, Columbia University, College of Physicians and Surgeons, New York, New York 10032

ABSTRACT:

Short term assays for potential carcinogenic factors must take into account the fact that carcinogenesis is usually a multistep process and that most human cancers probably result from a complex interaction between multiple factors, both environmental and endogenous. Thus, although extremely valuable, simple *in vitro* mutagenesis assays have major limitations. Cell culture studies with TPA and other phorbol esters provide clues to tumor promotion and the multistep nature of carcinogenesis. These effects can be divided into three categories: 1) mimicry of transformation in normal cells, and enhancement of transformation by chemical carcinogens or oncogenic viruses; 2) modulation (inhibition or induction) of differentiation; 3) membrane and receptor effects. Current evidence suggests that TPA acts by binding to specific high affinity cell surface membrane receptors and that this leads to alterations in the composition of membrane phospholipids. Presumably, these changes in the lipid matrix of cell membranes produce signals or mediators which lead to the subsequent cytoplasmic and nuclear effects of TPA. Thus, whereas the critical target in the action of initiating carcinogens appears to be cellular DNA, the critical target of the phorbol ester tumor promoters appears to be cell membranes. As a unifying concept of two-stage carcinogenesis, we postulate that during the initiation phase in carcinogenesis the covalent binding of carcinogens to DNA induces abberations in the commitment of the target cells. We believe that this involves highly ordered genetic events, for example, gene transpositions, rather than random point mutations. Certain oncogenic viruses achieve a similar effect thru integration of exogenous DNA sequences into inappropriate sites in the host genome. Tumor promoters, via their effects on growth, gene expression and differentiation, enhance the selective outgrowth of these initiated cells and induce them to express their newly acquired but previously dormant committed state. Rapid *in vitro* assays for the detection of the phorbol ester tumor promoters and for synergistic interactions between oncogenic viruses and chemicals now exist. However, simple assays for other classes of tumor promoters and cofactors remain to be developed.

INTRODUCTION:

I am delighted to have an opportunity to participate in this International Congress since it is apparent to many of us that the field of toxicology is undergoing an exciting renaissance. Not so many years ago, a toxicologist was called upon mainly to determine what poison someone had used to terminate their own life or that of their political enemy. With the major conquest of the epidemic infectious diseases, with the increasing concern for the role of natural and synthetic chemicals in our environment in causing the major diseases of our time (cardiovascular disease, cancer, chronic pulmonary disease, aging, etc.), and with exciting advances in molecular and cellular biology, the field of toxicology, like another renaissance that occurred about 500 years ago throughout Europe and reached great heights in Brussels, must develop entirely new concepts, methodologies and interactions with other disciplines.

The previous speakers have emphasized *in vitro* assays for potential carcinogens in which the end-point is mutagenesis. Although these assays are extremely valuable as part of a panel of screening tests, there are several reasons why it is desirable to have *in vitro* assays in which the end-point is the actual conversion of a normal cell to a tumorigenic cell. These reasons include: 1) the uncertainty at the present time as to whether or not carcinogenesis results from simple random point mutations[1]. The fact that in the intact animal, and in humans, the carcinogenic process occurs via multiple steps that extend over an appreciable period of time[2]. Therefore, an ideal *in vitro* model system should display similar multiple steps and permit the analysis of each of these steps. 3) It appears likely that in the natural host carcinogenesis results from a complex interaction between multiple factors including electrophilic carcinogens, tumor promoters and hormones, various cofactors and, in some cases, interactions between chemical and viral agents[3,4]. Thus, *in vitro* assays should be available that have the capacity to assay for these diverse factors and for these multifactor interactions.

I will now briefly review the current status of *in vitro* transformation assays for carcinogens that act as initiating agents and then spend the rest of my talk reviewing recent cell culture studies on the action of tumor promoters and on chemical-viral interactions in cell culture.

SYSTEMS FOR STUDYING MALIGNANT CELL TRANSFORMATION *IN VITRO*

Table 1 lists the major *in vitro* systems in which chemical carcinogens induce cell transformation (for a detailed review see ref. 5). These include

Table 1:

Examples of Cell Culture Systems That Can Be Transformed by Chemical Carcinogens

Type of System:		Usual Endpoint	Scoring Time
A:	Primary or Secondary Rodent Embryo Cultures		
1.	Syrian Hamster	Morphological Transformation	8-10 days
2.	Guinea Pig	Growth in Agar	4 months
3.	Rat or Mouse Infected with murine leukemia virus	Morphological Transformation	3-8 weeks
4.	Rat Infected with Adenovirus	Morphological Transformation	25-40 days
5.	Syrian Hamster Infected with Adenovirus	Morphological Transformation	25-30 days
B:	Rodent Fibroblast Cell Lines		
1.	3T3 - mouse	Morphological Transformation	10-28 weeks
2.	10T½ - mouse	Morphological Transformation	4-6 weeks
3.	BHK 21 hamster	Growth in Agar	2-4 weeks
4.	Rat Embryo	Morphological Transformation	40-43 days
C:	Epithelial Cell Cultures		
1.	Rat Liver	Growth in Agar, cytologic changes, tumorigenesis	8-36 weeks
2.	Mouse Epidermis	Growth in Agar, Morphological alterations, tumorigenesis	12-16 weeks
D:	Human SKin Fibroblasts	Morphological Transformation	7-14 weeks

For further details and specific references see 5.

mainly fibroblast rodent cultures, either primary cultures or established cell lines. You will note that with most of these systems morphologic transformation does not occur until several weeks after carcinogen exposure. Although the hamster embryo system shows morphologic transformation within 7-10 days, a lag of several more weeks of serial passage is required for the full expression of growth in agar and tumorigenicity , a process termed "malignant transformation". The *in vitro* transformation by chemical carcinogens of epithelial cells and of human fibroblasts occurs with an extremely low frequency and a very long lag, even though these cells are not more resistant to the induction of specific mutations (i.e., to drug resistance) by chemical carcinogens.

Thus, we see that the available examples of *in vitro* transformation already show aspects of a multistage process that is more complex than a simple point mutation. Data from several laboratories have indicated that the frequency of transformation of rodent cell cultures induced by radiation or carcinogens may be ten to several hundred times that obtained for the induction of mutations to specific markers such as drug resistance, even when both types of phenomena were scored in the same cell culture system[7-9]. This discrepancy is even greater when one considers the likelihood that cell transformation occurs via a multistep process which is limited, therefore, by the joint probabilities of each of the successive steps. This would suggest that the initial step induced by the carcinogen occurs with even a greater frequency than the net transformation frequency. Indeed, there is evidence that under certain conditions (i.e. the exposure of cells to chemical carcinogens[7] or radiation[9] at low cell densities) almost 100% of the originally exposed cells are capable of giving rise to progeny that are transformed. The fact that the phorbol ester tumor promoters can also enhance the transformation frequency in cultures previously exposed to chemical carcinogens or radiation[10-12], also provides evidence that we tend to underestimate the frequency of the initial event induced by chemical carcinogens or radiation. Some of the systems listed in Table 1 involve synergistic interactions between chemical agents and viruses and I will return to this aspect later.

Tumor promoters can be defined as compounds which lack significant carcinogenic activity when tested alone but markedly enhance the yield of tumors when applied after a low dose of an initiating carcinogen, for example benzo(a)-pyrene (BP). The most potent tumor promoter on mouse skin is 12-O-tetradecanoyl-phorbol-13-acetate (TPA), and related phorbol diesters[14]. Elsewhere, we have contrasted the properties of initiating agents with those of the phorbol ester tumor promoters[1,15,16]. The major difference is that whereas initiating carcinogens usually generate electrophiles that bind covalently to cellular DNA (and are, therefore, mutagenic) this is not the case for tumor promoters. The two stage mouse skin carcinogenesis system has served as paradigm for studies on the multistage aspects of carcinogenesis in several other tissues and species. Evidence that hepatocellular cancer, bladder cancer, colon cancer, and breast cancer also proceed via processes analogous to initiation and promotion has been reviewed elsewhere[3,14]. In addition, there are several recent studies indicating that the tumor promoting effect of the phorbol esters is not confined to mouse skin[16].

The cellular targets for the action of the phorbol ester tumor promoters are not known with certainty, but recent studies in cell culture systems have provided important clues. The effects can be classified into three categories (all of which conveniently begin with the letter "m"): mimicry of transformation, modulation of differentiation, and membrane effects (For recent reviews see 1,3,14,15,16).

MIMICRY OF TRANSFORMATION

TPA induces several properties in normal cells that mimic those often seen in transformed cells. This mimicry includes changes in cell morphology, growth properties, cell surface properties, induction of plasminogen activator (PA), ornithine decarboxylase and prostaglandin synthesis, decreases in growth requirements for serum and Ca^{2+}, TPA induced loss of actin cables and TPA induced loss of metabolic cooperation (for review see refs. 3,14,16). TPA can enhance the stable transformation of fibroblast cultures previously exposed to a chemical carcinogen, uv or X-irradiation[10-12], an adenovirus[4,17], or Epstein-Barr virus[18]. As described below, TPA can also induce the irreversible acquisition of anchorage-independent growth in "partially" transformed cells[19,20]. These stable or irreversible effects of TPA indicate that "initiated" cells have a qualitatively different response to TPA than normal cells.

Some of these effects, for example, the induction of PA[21] or the induction of cell adhesion[22] provide simple and rapid assays for the phorbol esters and related macrocyclic diterpenes. Detailed studies have shown a good structure-function relationship between these effects and tumor promoting activity on mouse skin [21,22], (Yamasaki, H., Weinstein, I.B and Van Duuren, B., unpublished studies).

MODULATION OF DIFFERENTIATION

Since it is likely that carcinogenesis involves major disturbances in differentiation, it is of interest that TPA is a highly potent inhibitor or inducer of differentiation in a variety of cell systems (Table 2). The examples include a variety of programs of differentiation and cells from such diverse species as avian, rodent, human and even echinoderm. It is possible that the ability of TPA to either induce or inhibit differentiation depends on the nature of membrane constituents of the target cell. Reciprocal effects of the same agent on differentiation, depending on the target cells, have been seen with other agents including glucocorticoid hormones cyclic AMP and BUdR.

We have previously emphasized that the ability of tumor promoters to

Table 2: TPA Modulation of Differentiation

Cell System:	Type of Differentiation:
Examples of Inhibition of Differentiation	
Chick Embryo Fibroblasts	Myogenesis
Chick Embryo Chondroblasts	Chondrogenesis
Chick Embryo Dorsal Root Ganglion	Neurite
Murine Erythroleukemia	Erythroid
Murine 3T3 Cell Line	Adipocytes
Murine Neuroblastoma	Neurite
Murine Melanoma	Melanogenesis
Hamster Epidermal Cultures	Keratinocytes
Mouse Epidermal Cultures	Keratinocytes
Rat Mammary Carcinoma	Dome Formation
Sea Urchin	Embryogenesis
Examples of Induction of Differentiation	
Murine Rauscher Virus Erythroleukemia	Erythroid
Human Myeloid Leukemia Cell Line	Macrophage and Granulocyte
Murine Myeloid Leukemia	Macrophage and Granulocyte
Human Melanoma Cell Line	Melanogenesis

*For refs. see 3,14,16.

inhibit terminal differentiation may be an important clue to their action as tumor promoters on mouse skin[15,16]. The basal cells in the adult epidermis are continually dividing, yet the tissue is in a state of balanced growth. Presumably, this is because of asymmetric division of stem cells. One daughter cell remains a stem cell and the other daughter cell is committed to keratinize and terminally differentiate, thus, irreversibly losing its growth potential. If an "initiated" stem cell were restrained to this mode of division, it could not increase its proportion in the stem cell pool. If, however, the stem cell division mode was interrupted by the action of a promoting agent, the initiated cell could undergo exponential division thus yielding a clone of similar cells. Since TPA can also induce phenotypic changes in cells that mimic those of transformed cells, the microenvironment of a clone of such cells might itself enhance their further outgrowth and development into a tumor. In addition, clonal expansion of the population of initiated cells would provide a larger population from which variants that have undergone progression to later stages of neoplasia might emerge.

MEMBRANE EFFECTS AND PHOSPHOLIPID METABOLISM

There is considerable evidence that the cell surface membrane may be the initial and major target of TPA action[16]. Table 3 is a list of effects of TPA on cell surfaces and membranes. Several of these effects occur within minutes after exposing cell cultures to TPA and are not blocked by inhibitors of protein or RNA synthesis, suggesting that they result from a direct action of TPA on cell membranes. This is true for the enhancement of 2-deoxyglucose uptake, altered membrane "fluidity", altered cell adhesion, the induction of phospholipid turnover and the inhibition of EGF receptor binding. TPA induces an increase in the incorporation of P^{32} or choline into membrane phospholipids, or deacylation of phospholipids and release of arachidonic acid, and increases prostaglandin synthesis[23-28].

Recently, R.A. Mufson in our laboratory has studied the release of choline metabolites from C3H10T½ cells prelabelled with (^{3}H) choline[29]. Within 5 minutes of exposure to TPA, the release of (^{3}H) choline metabolites was enhanced two-fold and by 60-120 minutes the release was 4-5 times that of vehicle controls. Choline metabolite release was concentration dependent between 10 and 100ng TPA/ml. Phorbol 12,13-didecanoate (PDD) was also active but 4 PDD, which is not a tumor promoter, was inactive. The radioactivity released by TPA was derived from phospholipids since changes in the acid soluble pool of choline metabolites were insufficient to account for the amount of material released. The released material was identified by chromatography as choline and phosphoryl choline. Neither cycloheximide (4-40μg/ml)

Table 3: Effects of TPA on Cell Surfaces and Membranes in Cell Culture

Altered Na/K ATPase
Increased Uptake 2-DG, ^{32}P, ^{86}RB
Increased Membrane Lipid "Fluidity"
Increased Phospholipid Synthesis
Increased Release Arachidonic Acid, Prostaglandins
Altered Morphology and Cell-Cell Orientation
Altered Cell Adhesion
Increased Pinocytosis
Altered Fucose-Flycopeptides
Decreased LETS Protein
"Uncoupling" of β-Adrenergic Receptors
Inhibition of Binding of EGF to Receptors
Decrease in Acetylcholine Receptors
Synergistic Interaction with Growth Factors
Inhibition of Metabolic Cooperation

For refs. see 3,14,16,33 and text.

nor cordycepin (4-40µg/ml) blocked the TPA induced release. The release was, however, temperature sensitive and did not occur at 4°C. TPA did not induce the release of (^{3}H) inositol from prelabelled cells. The calcium ionophore A23187 enhanced (^{3}H) arachidonic acid and (^{3}H) prostaglandin release. We believe that TPA induced choline release is due to activation of an endogenous phospholipase C or D. This TPA effect is similar to that of certain other agonists which also activate degradation of phospholipids, although in the latter case the target is phosphatidylinositol rather than phosphatidylcholine[30,31]. A hypothetical scheme for the effects of TPA on phospholipid metabolism is given in Figure 1. It is not known how these membrane effects

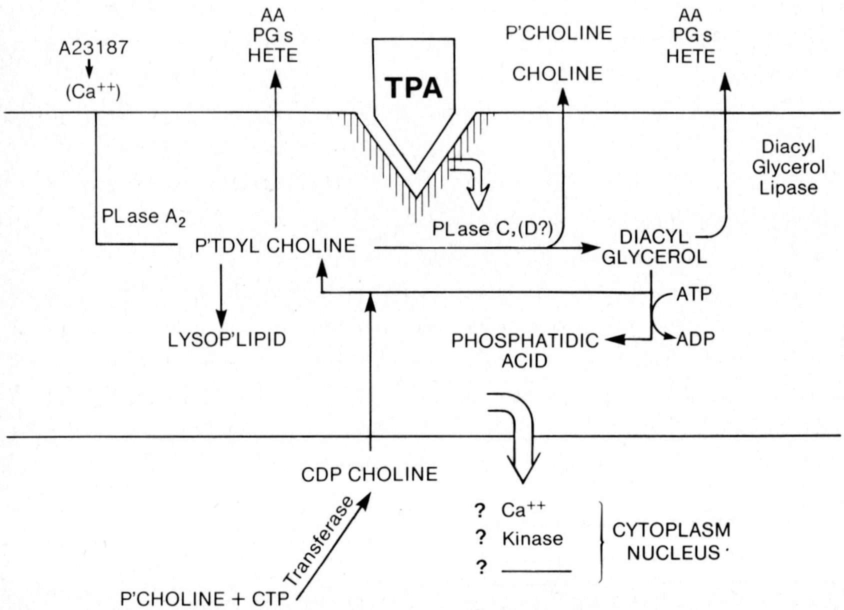

Figure 1: Schematic diagram of effects of TPA and related compounds on phosphatidylcholine turnover (29). We postulate that the binding of TPA to specific cell membrane receptors activates phospholipase (PLase) C and/or D, resulting in the conversion of phosphatidylcholine (P'TDYL Choline) to diacylglycerol plus choline. Arachidonic acid (AA) is then released by diacylglycerol lipase; prostaglandins (PG's) and other AA metabolites are also formed. AA may be released by the direct action of PLase A_2 or P'TDYL Choline. The calcium ionophore A23187 and melittin may induce AA release via the latter mechanism. P'TDYL Choline may be resynthesized via CDP choline, as shown. Presumably, during these biochemical transformations, a transmembrane signal to the cytoplasm and/or nucleus is generated, i.e., increased. Ca^{2+} uptake or redistribution, activation of a protein kinase, or some other mediator. Phosphatidic acid, serving as a Ca^{2+} ionophore (62), or some other P'TDYL Choline metabolite, may stimulate this process.

might induce signals or second messengers that mediate the subsequent cytoplasmic and nuclear events. An increase in intracellular Ca^{2+} concentration, enhanced protein kinase activity, or release of mediators remain to be explored as potential candidates for these effects.

MEMBRANE RECEPTORS FOR EGF AND TPA

TPA and EGF have similar but not identical effects on cells in culture[32-35]. We discovered that TPA causes almost an immediate inhibition of the binding of ^{125}I-EGF to cell surface receptors and that it also causes a loss of previously bound EGF from these receptors[33,35]. With a series of phorbol compounds, or chemically related macrocyclic plant diterpenes, this effect correlated quite well with the known potencies of these compounds as tumor promoters on mouse skin. An exception is the compound mezerein which, although it is equipotent to TPA with respect to several cell culture effects, and induction of ODC in mouse skin, is much weaker than TPA as a tumor promoter on mouse skin[36,37]. Recent studies suggest that tumor promotion can be divided into two phases and that mezerein acts mainly during the second phase, whereas TPA is active in both phases[37]. Studies with a variety of inhibitors[35,38], suggest that the TPA inhibition of EGF-receptor binding does not require RNA or protein synthesis, energy metabolism, or cytoskeletal changes. Thus, the effect appears to be mediated directly at the level of the plasma membrane. TPA inhibition of EGF binding is not due to increased degradation of EGF or increased internalization of the EGF-receptor complex[35]. The effect of TPA on EGF receptors is an indirect one, perhaps related to TPA induced changes in the lipid microenvironment of the EGF receptors[35,38]. Our findings on TPA inhibition of EGF binding have been confirmed and extended by other investigators[41,42].

A curious finding is that with prolonged exposure cells become refractory to TPA-induced inhibition of EGF-receptor binding[35,38]. This is consistent with evidence that following prolonged exposure cells can escape from other effects of TPA[39,40]. This phenomenon could play an important role in tissue specific and dose-scheduling effects of TPA.

The ability of TPA to inhibit the binding of EGF to its receptors, to "uncouple" the β adrenergic receptor and to cause a decrease in acetylcholine receptors in chick myoblasts (Table 3), suggest that the pleiotropic effects of TPA on cell growth, function and differentiation may relate, at least in part, to its effects on membrane receptors, thus altering the response of cells to extracellular signals. Possible affects on receptors involved in cell-cell contacts, and TPA inhibition of metabolic cooperation[43,44], could also impair cell-cell recognition in TPA exposed tissues. It appears likely that TPA exerts such effects by binding to highly specific cell surface receptors (see below), and that this then leads to multiple changes in membrane structure and function. It is perhaps for this reason that certain membrane perturbing agents like the bee venom polypeptide melittin[45], and the *Staph. aureus* polypeptide delta hemolysin[46], can induce several effects similar to those of TPA. Thus our results with TPA may relate to the action of various drugs and toxins that have as their target the cell membrane.

We have previously postulated that TPA usurps the function of a cell surface receptor whose normal function is to mediate the action of a yet to be identified growth regulator or hormone[15,33]. The postulated endogenous factor that normally utilizes the receptor system usurped by TPA could play an important role in the control of stem cell proliferation and differentiation in various normal tissues. The fact that tumor cells can make polypeptide growth factors,[47,51] suggests that changes in the function of growth factor receptors may play an important role not only in the carcinogenic process but also in maintenance of the transformed state.

Blumberg's laboratory has recently employed ^{3}H-phorbol dibutyrate (PDBu) to obtain direct evidence that the membranes of fibroblast cultures and mouse epidermal cells do contain high affinity saturable receptors for PDBu, TPA and related tumor promoting phorbol esters[48]. We have confirmed and extended this finding and developed a simple assay for these receptors using intact monolayers of rat embryo fibroblasts[49]. Although TPA does inhibit the binding of ^{125}I-EGF to its cell surface receptors, EGF does not inhibit the binding of ^{3}H-PDBu to its receptors[33,48,49]. These results provide further evidence that the receptor for the phorbol esters is distinct from that for EGF. Scatchard plots indicate that the rat embryo cells contain about 2×10^{5} high affinity PDBu receptors with a K_D of about 8nM[49]. The receptor assay for phorbol esters should prove useful in further studies on the biochemical mechanisms of action of these agents and in the search for the putative endogenous substance that normally utilizes this class of receptors.

SYNERGISTIC INTERACTIONS BETWEEN CHEMICAL AGENTS AND VIRUSES IN CELL TRANSFORMATION

There are several examples in which chemical and physical agents interact synergistically with viruses in the carcinogenic process both *in vitro* and *in vivo* (for review see refs. 4, 5,17). Indeed, it seems likely that certain human cancers may be due to interactions between chemical agents and types of viruses which alone would have little or no oncogenic potential. This is important to keep in mind in the search for viruses that might play a role in human cancer causation. These agents may not have all of the properties of oncogenic viruses seen in experimental animal systems and, when assayed alone, they may not be capable of cancer induction in the absence of chemical cofactors.

To explore these aspects of chemical-viral interactions, we have developed an *in vitro* system in which the transformation of rat embryo (RE) cells is markedly enhanced when, after infection with a mutant (H5ts125) of human adenovirus type 5, the cells are grown in the presence of TPA[17]. The presence of TPA caused an increased number of foci of transformation. Foci also appeared earlier and were larger than those obtained with adenovirus in the absence of TPA. Phorbol, 4αPDD, and 4-O-MeTPA were inactive in this system. The addition of TPA could be delayed until after viral uptake and integration of adenovirus sequences into the host genome had occurred, thus indicating that the enhancement by TPA was not exerted on these steps.

One of the best *in vitro* markers for the tumorigenicity of transformed fibroblasts or epithelial rodent cells is ancorage independence, i.e., ability to grow in agar or agarose suspension, although there are a few exceptions (for review see 4,50). We have found that although TPA does not enhance the growth in agar of normal RE cells, it does induce the growth in agar of morphologically transformed adenovirus-infected RE cells[19]. This effect appears to be inductive and not due to simple cell selection. Yet it is irreversible, since when the TPA is removed, the cells now grow in agar with a higher efficiency than prior to exposure to TPA. Certain serially passaged mouse epidermal cell cultures also undergo an irreversible increase in anchorage-independent growth when exposed to TPA[20]. This phenomenon may represent a useful *in vitro* model system for studying the process of tumor progression.

The synergistic interaction between initiating carcinogens and adenovirus was also studied in this system. If prior to infecting the cells with the virus, we exposed the cells to benzo(a)pyrene or DMBA and then within 24 hours infected the cells with adenovirus, there was an enhancement of cell transformation[17]. These results, as well as those of other investigators[52], suggest that, by damaging DNA and inducing DNA repair, initiating carcinogens increase the number of cells in a virus infected population that acquire stably integrated viral sequences[17,52,53]. The enhancement by initiating carcinogens and by tumor promoters of adenovirus transformation is additive, indicating that they occur by different mechanisms.

It seems likely that these *in vitro* interactions may be relevant to the interaction between viruses, chemical carcinogens, tumor promoters, hormones and other cofactors in the causation of specific human cancers, particularly liver cancer in Africa, Burkitt's lymphoma and possibly breast cancer[3].

MOLECULAR MECHANISM OF INITIATION AND A UNIFIED THEORY OF INITIATION AND PROMOTION

In the final analysis, the mechanism by which tumor promoters enhance the conversion of initiated cells to tumor cells must take into account the mechanism of action of initiating carcinogens. Although current evidence suggests that covalent binding of carcinogens like BP to cellular DNA is the critical event in initiation, the subsequent biochemical events that lead to establishment of the initiated cell are not known. Several possible molecular mechanisms are listed in Table 4 and have been discussed in detail elsewhere[1].

Table 4: Possible Molecular Mechanisms of Initiation of the Carcinogenic Process

A. With permanent changes in DNA sequence:
   1. Random point mutations
      a. Direct: base substitution, frame shift, deletion in structural or regulatory gene.
      b. Indirect: induction of "SOS-type" error-prone DNA synthesis.
   2. Ordered gene rearrangements: transposition, amplification, deletion, integration of exogenous sequences, (i.e. viral).

B. Without permanent changes in DNA sequence:
   altered chromatin structure, altered feedback loops, DNA methylation, etc.

For a more detailed discussion see ref. 1.

There has been a tendency to think of the initiating event in chemical carcinogenesis as a simple random-point mutation resulting from errors in replicating the damaged DNA. However, as emphasized in the Introduction, certain aspects of the carcinogenic process are not consistent with this simple mechanism. In bacteria, physical and chemical agents that damage DNA, including chemical carcinogens, induce a highly pleiotropic response called "SOS functions"[54,55], which includes induction of an error-prone DNA synthesis mechanism. Our laboratory has recently found that mutagenesis by benzo(a)pyrene diol epoxide (BPDE 1) in *E. coli* is mediated via this mechanism[56]. It is not known whether similar responses to DNA damage occur in eukaryotic cells, and if so, what the components of this response might be.

Recent studies in both prokaryotic and eukaryotic ells indicate that the linear arrangement of coding sequences in DNA may be more complex and also more plastic than previously envisioned[57-60]. It is possible, therefore, that highly specific genome rearrangements may be responsible for certain aspects of development and differentiation in eukaryotic systems, an hypothesis proposed by McClintock a number of years ago[61]. It would not be surprising if chemical modification of the DNA by carcinogens disrupted these mechanisms. One might further speculate that the "SOS" program of response to DNA damage in mammalian cells might result in transposition of specific DNA sequences. By scrambling an otherwise orderly process of genome rearrangements, carcinogens could produce distortions in cell commitment and thus initiate the carcinogenic process. Phrased in other terms, this theory postulates that during normal development, the establishment of specific populations of stem cells involves gene transpositions. By damaging DNA, initiating carcinogens induce abberant forms of gene transpostion, thus establishing aberrant stem cells. The subsequent role of tumor promoters might be to enhance the outgrowth of these cells (as discussed above), as well as "switch on" their aberrant programs of differentiation, just as normal growth factors might induce normal stem cells to express their specialized functions. Presumably, the phorbol ester tumor promoters accomplish this by binding to and usurping the function of receptors normally occupied by endogenous factors that control stem cell replication and differentiation. Following repeated exposure of initiated cells to TPA, a neoplastic population might eventually emerge which grows autonomously in the absence of TPA, perhaps due to further changes in genome structure. Several aspects of this hypothesis are currently being tested in our laboratory.

ACKNOWLEDGEMENTS:

The author gratefully acknowledges the valuable contributions made to these studies by Drs. P. Fisher, A. Horowitz, J. Laskin, Lee-Syng Lee, R. A. Mufson and H. Yamasaki. He also thanks Patricia Vickman for valuable assistance in the preparation of this manuscript, and Janet Bozzone, Ester Okin and James Chi for their valuable technical assistance.
This research was supported by National Cancer Institute Grant CA-26056 and CA-21111.

REFERENCES

1. Weinstein, I.B., Yamasaki, H., Wigler, M., Lee, L.S., Fisher, P.B., Jeffrey, A. and Grunberger, D. (1979) In: Carcinogens and Mechanisms of Action. A.C. Griffin and C.R. Shaw, (eds.) Raven Press, New York pp. 399-418.

2. Foulds, L. (1969) Neoplastic Development, Academic Press, New York.
3. Weinstein, I.B. (1980) In: Systematics of Mammary Cell Transformation, C. McGrath (eds.), Academic Press, New York, in press.
4. Fisher, P.B. and Weinstein, I.B. (1980) In: Molecular and Cellular Aspects of Carcinogen Screening Tests, R. Montesano, H. Bartsch and L. Tomatis, (eds.) IARC Scientific Publications #27, Lyon, pp. 113-131.
5. Fisher, P.B. and Weinstein, I.B. (1980) In: Carcinogens in Industry and Environment, J.M. Sontag (ed.) Marcel Dekker, in press.
6. Barrett, J.C. and Ts'o, P.O.P. (1978), Proc. Natl. Acad. Sci. USA, 75, 3761-3765.
7. Mondal, S. and Heidelberger, C. (1970) Proc. Natl. Acad. Sci. USA, 65, 219-225.
8. Han, A. and Elkind, M.M. (1979) Cancer Res. 39, 123-130.
9. Kennedy, A.R., Murphy, G. and Little, J.B. (1979), personal communication.
10. Mondal, S., Brankow, D.W. and Heidelberger, C. (1976) Cancer Res. 36, 2254-2260.
11. Kennedy, A.R., Mondal, S., Heidelberger, C. and Little, J.B. (1978) Cancer Res. 38, 439-443.
12. Mondal, S. and Heidelberger, C. (1976) Nature 260, 710-711.
13. Berenblum, I. (1975) In: Cancer, F.F. Becker (ed.), Plenum Press, New York, pp. 323-344.
14. Slaga, T.J., Sivak, A. and Boutwell, R.K. (eds.) (1978) In: Mechanisms of Tumor Promotion and Cocarcinogenesis, Vol. 2, Raven Press, New York.
15. Weinstein, I.B., Wigler, M. and Pietropaolo, C. (1977) In: Origins of Human Cancer, H.H. Hiatt, J.D. Watson and J.A. Winston (eds.), Cold Spring Harbor Conferences on Cell Proliferation IV, Cold Spring Harbor, New York, pp. 751-772.
16. Weinstein, I.B., Lee, L.S., Fisher, P.B., Mufson, A. and Yamasaki, H. (1979) Journal of Supramolecular Struct. 12, 195-208.
17. Fisher, P.B., Weinstein, I.B., Eisenberg, D. and Ginsberg, H.S. (1978) Proc. Natl. Acad. Sci. USA 75, 2311-2314.
18. Yamamoto, N. and ZurHausen, H. (1979) Nature 280, 244-245.
19. Fisher, P.B., Bozzone, J.H. and Weinstein, I.B. (1979) Cell 18, 695-705.
20. Colburn, N.H., Former, B.F., Nelson, K.A. and Yuspa, S.H. (1979) Nature 281, 589591.
21. Wigler, M., DeFeo, D. and Weinstein, I.B. (1978) Cancer Res. 36, 2254-2260.

22. Yamasaki, H., Weinstein, I.B., Fibach, E., Rifkind, R.A. and Marks, P.A. (1979) Cancer Res. 39, 1989-1994.
23. Kinzel, V., Kreibich, G., Hecker, E. and Suss, R. (1979) Cancer Res., 39, 2743-2750.
24. Suss, R., Kreibich, G. and Kinzel, V. (1972) Europ. J. Cancer, 8, 299-304.
25. Wertz, P.W. and Mueller, G.C. (1978) Cancer Res. 28, 2900-2904.
26. Levine, L. and Hassid, A. (1977) Biochem. Biophys. Res. Commun. 79, 477-483.
27. Mufson, R.A., DeFeo, D. and Weinstein, I.B. (1979) Molecular Pharmacol. 16, 569-578.
28. Yamasaki, H., Mufson, R.A. and Weinstein, I.B. (1979) Biochem. Biophys. Res. Commun. 89, 1018-1025.
29. Mufson, R.A. and Weinstein, I.B. (1980) Proc. Am. Assoc. Cancer Res. (abstracts) 21, 117.
30. Michell, R.H., Jafferji, S.S. and Jones, L.M. (1977), In: Function and Biosynthesis of Lipids, N.G. Bazaw, R.R. Brenner and N.M. Guisto, (eds.) Plenum Press, New York, pp. 447-464.
31. Salmon, D.M. and Honeyman, T.W. (1980) Nature 284, 344-345.
32. Lee. L.S. and Weinstein, I.B. (1978) Nature 274, 696-697.
33. Lee, L.S. and Weinstein, I.B. (1978) Science 202, 313-315.
34. Dicker, P. and Rozengurt, E. (1978) Nature 276, 723-726.
35. Lee, L.S. and Weinstein, I.B. (1979) Proc. Natl. Acad. Sci. USA, 76, 5168-5172.
36. Mufson, R.A., Fischer, S.M., Verma, A.K., Gleason, G.L., Slaga, T.J. and Boutwell, R.K. (1979) Cancer Res. 39, 4791-4795.
37. Slaga, T.J., Fischer, S.M., Nelson, K. and Gleason, G.L., (1980), Proc. Natl. Acad. Sci. USA 77, 3659-3663.
38. Lee, L.S. and Weinstein, I.B. (1980), submitted for publication.
39. Mufson, R.A., Fisher, P.B. and Weinstein, I.B. (1979) Cancer Res. 39, 3915-3919.
40. Diamond, L. , O'Brien, T.G. and Rovera, G. (1977) Nature 269, 247-248.
41. Brown, K.D., Dicker, P. and Rozengurt, E. (1979) Biochem. Biophys. Res. Commun. 86, 1037-1043.
42. Shoyab, M., DeLarco, J.E. and Todaro, G.J. (1979) Nature 279, 387-391.
43. Murray, A.W. and Fitzgerald, D.J. (1979) Biochem. Biophys. Res. Commun. 91, 395-401.
44. Yotti, L.P., Chang, C.C. and Trosko, J.E. (1979) Science 206, 1089-1091.

45. Mufson, R.A., Laskin, J.D., Fisher, P.B. and Weinstein, I.B. (1979) Nature 280, 72-74.

46. Umezawa, K., Weinstein, I.B and Shaw, W.V. (1980) Biochem. Biophys. Res. Commun. 94, 625-629.

47. Roberts, A.B., Lamb, L.C., Newton, D.L., Sporn, M.B. DeLarco, J.F., and Todaro, G.J. (1980) Proc. Natl. Acad. Sci. USA 77, 3494-3498.

48. Delclos, K.B., Nagle, D.S. and Blumberg, P.D. (1980) Cell 19, 1025-1032.

49. Horowitz, A., Greenebaum, E. and Weinstein, I.B., unpublished studies.

50. Montesano, R., Drevon, C., Kuroki, T., Saint Vincent, L., Handleman, S., Sanford, K.K., DeFeo, D. and Weinstein, I.B. (1977) Jl. Natl. Cancer Inst. 59, 1651-1658.

51. Fisher, P.B., Lee, L.S. and Weinstein, I.B. (1980) Biochem. Biophys. Res. Commun. 93, 1160-1166.

52. Casto, B.C., Pieczynski, W.J. and DiPaolo, J.A. (1973) Cancer Res. 33,819-824

53. Fisher, P.B., Dorsch-Hasler, K., Weinstein, I.B. and Ginsberg, H.S. (1979) Nature 281, 591-594.

54. Witkin, E.M. (1976), Bacteriol Rev. 40, 869-907.

55. Radman, M., Villani, G., Boiteux, S., Defais, M., and Caillet-Fauquet, P. (1977) In: Origins of Human Cancer, H.H. Hiatt, J.D. Watson and J.A. Winston (eds.) Cold Spring Harbor on Cell Proliferation, Cold Spring Harbor, New York, pp. 903-922.

56. Ivanovic, V. and Weinstein, I.B (1980) Cancer Res., in press.

57. Kamp, D., Kahmann, R., Zipser, D., Broker, T.R. and Chow, L.T., (1977) Nature 271, 577-580.

58. Brack, C. and Tonegawa, S. (1977) Proc. Natl. Acad. Sci. USA, 74, 5652-5656.

59. Herskowitz, I. *et al.* (1980) In: The Molecular Genetics of Development, W. Loomis and T. Leighton, (eds.) Academic Press, New York, in press.

60. Hoeijmakers, J.H.J. *et al.* (1980) Nature 284, 78.

61. Finchman, J.R.S. and Sastry, G.R.K. (1974) Ann. Rev. Genet. 8, 15-50.

62. Putney, J.W., Weiss, S.J. VanDerWalle, C.M. and Haddas, R.A. (1980) Nature 284, 345-347.

Mechanisms of Toxicity and Hazard Evaluation
B. Holmstedt, R. Lauwerys, M. Mercier, M. Roberfroid eds

IN VIVO METHODS FOR EVALUATING GENOTOXICITY

JAMES A. SWENBERG
Pathology Department, Chemical Industry Institute of Toxicology, P. O. Box 12137, Research Triangle Park, NC (USA) 27709

INTRODUCTON

The assumption that somatic mutation represents a principal mechanism for the induction of neoplasia has stimulated a renaissance in the field of mutagenesis. This renaissance is evident in the recent onslaught of "short-term tests" for predicting the carcinogenic and/or mutagenic potential of chemicals.[1,2,3,] While the majority of these assays utilize *in vitro* test systems, significant numbers of *in vivo* assays are becoming available. This paper will concentrate on mammalian test systems, reviewing the rationale for using *in vivo* assays and pointing out some of their potential pitfalls. It will briefly review available test systems and discuss some of the biochemical events involved in mutagenesis and carcinogenesis that must be considered in the interpretation of test data for risk estimation.

RATIONALE FOR IN VIVO TEST SYSTEMS

Increasing emphasis is being placed on developing as complete a "toxicologic profile" as possible on chemicals in our environment. Because a paucity of such information is available on large numbers of compounds, rapid "short-term tests" are being used to screen chemicals for genotoxic potential. The predictive potential of *in vitro* assays has steadily improved with the incorporation of various systems for metabolic activation. In spite of these changes, however, none of the *in vitro* systems can compete with the complexity of the whole animal. It is for this reason that increasing emphasis is being placed on developing and validating whole animal assays for predicting genotoxic potential.

Intact animal systems utilize routes of exposure which simulate human exposure. They also employ dose ranges which allow comparisons of test data with other toxicologic endpoints such as cell damage and necrosis. Furthermore, they take into account such important pharmacokinetic features as absorption, distribution and excretion. One of the major advantages of *in vivo* test systems is that they employ native capacities for the biotransformation of chemicals to their reactive intermediates. Lastly, whole animal systems utilize the natural homeostatic defense mechanisms for detoxification, leading to more realistic test data. By incorporating all the above features, *in vivo* assays uniquely offer the potential to predict target organs for genotoxic events and possibly for carcinogenicity.

Probably the greatest single virtue of whole animal systems, however, is their use in evaluating genotoxicity to germ cells. While germ cell assays have been available for years, the number of chemicals that have been evaluated remains low. It is important to realize, however, that none of the *in vitro* assays can accomplish this. The potential ramifications of mutations at the germ cell level include embryotoxicity, fetal malformation, a variety of genetic diseases, carcinogenesis, and the induction of recessive mutations that could become widespread throughout the human population. For these reasons, the development of a compound's toxicologic profile should include test systems for evaluating germ cell damage.

PITFALLS OF *IN VIVO* TESTS

Considering all of the advantages of *in vivo* assays, why then have they not assumed a more prominent position in screening batteries? The answer to this question really depends on the individual assay. I will try to point some of these out as I discuss each test system. Several general points can, however, be made. Different whole animal tests utilize different cells or tissues for measuring their endpoints. Just because the animal's liver is capable of metabolic activation is no guarantee that its bone marrow or spermatogonial cells can perform similarly. Thus, one must always review whole animal data from the point of view that negative results in a specific tissue don't insure that other tissues are also negative. From a more practical point of view, whole animal systems employing liver are generally predictive for many promutagens and procarcinogens.

While germ cell assays are extremely important, they frequently have the disadvantage of requiring large numbers of animals and prolonged periods of housing and/or mating. Thus, the time and expense involved greatly limits their utility.

AVAILABLE TEST SYSTEMS

Mutational End Points

Specific locus test. The most specific method for detecting mutational end points in the whole animal is the specific locus test. This assay was originally developed by Russel to measure recessive and dominant mutations at specific loci on the germ cells of mice.[4] It has not received wide-spread use, however, since it entails the use of thousands of mice. Several chemicals possessing genotoxic activity in other systems have been negative.[3,5] The specific locus test would appear to the most definitive method for evaluating the effect of specific chemicals on future populations; however, it is unlikely to be applicable as a routine method.

Spot test. The spot test measures mutational events at single gene loci in developing neural crest cells of mice following transplacental exposure to the test agent.[6,7] It is a relatively rapid test, requiring approximately 5 weeks to run, and utilizes changes in hair coat color for scoring. To date, only a small number of chemicals have been evaluated.[3]

Thioguanine resistance. A promising approach has been suggested by Dr. DeMars[8] for an *in vivo/in vitro* system which evaluates the number of thioguanine resistant lymphocytes in peripheral blood following exposure of intact animals. Future validation studies will be necessary to evaluate the utility of this method.

Clastogenic Endpoints

Somatic and germ cell cytogenetics. One of the few methods that can be applied to test animals and man is the direct analysis for chromasomal damage. Good qualitative correlations exist between clastogenic activity and mutation; however, these relationships frequently disappear when the data is examined quantitatively.[3] As with any system employing bone marrow or germ cells, the potential for false negative results due to the inability of the tissue to metabolically activate promutagens must be considered.

Micronucleus test. This technique is closely related to cytogenetics, in so far as it responds to the same group of agents over similar dose ranges.[9] It has the advantage of being much simpler to score, but shares the problems related to biotransformation.[10,11] Only 2 of 13 procarcinogens/promutagens which previously had been shown to cause DNA damage induced dose-related increases in micronuclei.[11]

Dominant lethal test. Chemical effects experienced in the dominant lethal test are thought to be due to gross chromosomal damage. Like the two previous methods, its end point is frequently negative for known genotoxic agents.[3] Negative results in a modified dominant lethal test, such as currently incorporated in Segment I reproduction study protocols, should preclude the running of a full scale test.

Sister Chromatid Exchange

An *in vivo* test system that has stimulated a great deal of recent interest is the sister chromatid exchange (SCE) assay. By differentially labeling sister chromatids with bromodeoxyuridine (BrdU), individual chromatids can be identified. Early studies on SCE were conducted *in vitro*, however, the technique has now been applied to the whole animal. BrdU is administered by repeated injection,[12] infusion[13] or subcutaneous pellet implantation.[14] Excellent dose-response relationships have been demonstrated for SCE in alveolar macrophages, bone marrow and liver of mice exposed to styrene by inhalation.[15] The method can be applied to both somatic and germ cells. While many additional chemicals and tissues still need to be examined before the method is validated, *in vivo* SCE appears to be a very promising whole animal system.

DNA Damage and Repair

Several methods are available for detecting DNA damage and repair in animals exposed to chemicals with genotoxic potential.[1,2,3] Earlier studies employed alkaline sucrose gradients to detect DNA damage and repair. These do not lend themselves to screening procedures however, since they are time consuming, variable and frequently have less than ideal recovery of applied radioactivity. Several investigators have modified the alkaline elution technique developed by Kohn et al.[16] to evaluate DNA damage and repair in a wide variety of tissues following exposure of animals to chemicals.[17,18]

DNA repair has also been demonstrated using autoradiography and primary rat hepatocytes. While most of this work has been on cells exposed *in vitro*, recent studies from our institute have demonstrated its usefulness following *in vivo* exposure.[19] At various times after exposure, the liver is perfused with collagenase and the hepatocytes placed in tissue culture medium containing ^{3}H-thymidine for 4 hours followed by a 15 hr incubation with cold thymidine. This shorter *in vitro* exposure to ^{3}H-thymidine greatly reduces the cytoplasmic background that plagues the convenional *in vitro* assay. Excellent dose-response data has been obtained for DMN and 2-AAF.

DNA repair has also been demonstrated in mouse spermatids following treatment with MMS, EMS, PMS, MNU, hycanthone, cyclophosphamide and ethylenamine.[20,21] No repair was detected when animals were treated with MNNG, DMN, DEN, benzo(a)pyrene or DMBA.

Resistant Hepatocytes

A promising *in vivo* test system which utilizes an early stage in hepatic neoplastic progression as its end point has recently been reported. Increased numbers of γ-glutamyl transpeptidase positive foci were present in the liver of rats exposed to a wide variety of chemical carcinogens and mutagens.[22]

CONCLUSIONS

While numerous test systems have been developed and are undergoing validation studies to determine their usefulness for predicting genotoxic potential, basic research on the mechanisms involved in mutagenesis and carcinogenesis continues to demonstrate the vast complexity of the problem.

Biotransformation may only occur in a single cell type, such as the hepatocyte. At low doses, small amounts of promutagenic damage may be induced and then be readily repaired in an error free manner. Conversely, greater exposure induces larger amounts of DNA damage. Some of this may be repaired in an error-free manner, while other damage could be repaired by an error-prone mechanism. The greater extent of alkylation may also cause cell death, stimulating cell replication. If such replication occurs prior to the repair of promutagenic DNA damage, a mutation will result.

Species differences, tissue differences and cellular differences in metabolic competence, DNA repair and cell replication will need to be better understood before quantitative risk estimation can be performed using mutagenesis and carcinogenesis data.

REFERENCES

1. Butterworth, B. E. (1979) Strategies for Short-term Testing for Mutagens/ Carcinogens, CRC Press, West Palm Beach, pp. 1-134.
2. Santi, L. and Parodi, S. (1979) Short-term Tests for Prescreening of Potential Carcinogens, Instituto Scientifico Per Lo Studio E La Cura Dei Tumori, Genova, pp. 1-181.
3. Hollstein, M. and McCann, J. (1979) Mutation Res., 65, 133-226.
4. Russell, W. L. (1951) Cold Spring Harbor Symp. Quant. Biol. 16, 327-336.
5. Searle, A. G. (1975) Mutation Res., 31, 277-290.
6. Russell, L. B. and Major, M. H. (1957) Genetics, 42, 161-175.
7. Fahrig, R. (1978) Chemical Mutagens: Principles and Methods for their Detection, Vol. 5, Plenum, New York, pp. 151-175.
8. DeMars, R. (1979) Mammalian Cell Mutagenesis: The Maturation of Test Systems, Cold Spring Harbor Laboratory, New York, pp. 329-340.
9. Schmid, W. (1975) Mutation Res., 31, 9-15.
10. Heddle, J. A. and Bruce, W. R. (1977) Origins of Human Cancer, Book C, Cold Spring Harbor Laboratory, New York, pp. 1549-1557.
11. Trzos, R. J., Petzold, G. L., Brunden, M. N. and Swenberg, J. A. (1978) Mutation Res., 58, 79-86.

12. Allen, J. W. and Latt, S. A. (1976) Nature (London), 260, 449-451.

13. Schneider, E. L., Chaillet, J. and Tice, E. (1976) Exp. Cell Res., 100, 396-399.

14. Allen, J. W., Shuler, C. F., and Latt, S. A. (1978) Somatic Cell Genet., 4, 393-405.

15. Conner, M. K., Alarie, Y. and Dombroske, R. L. (1980) Toxicol. Appl. Pharmacol., 54, in press.

16. Kohn, K. W., Erickson, L. C., Ewig, R. and Friedman, C. (1976) Biochemistry, 15, 4629-4637.

17. Petzold, G. L. and Swenberg, J. A. (1978) Cancer Res., 38, 1589-1594.

18. Parodi, S., Taninger, M., Santi, L., Cavanna, M., Sciaba, L., Maura, A. and Brambilla, G. (1978). Mutation Res., 54, 39-46.

19. Mirsalis, J. C. and Butterworth, B. E. (1980) The Pharmacologist, 22, #573.

20. Sega, G. A., Owens, J. G. and Cumming, R. B. (1976) Mutation Res., 36, 193-212.

21. Sega, G. A. (1978) Personal Communication.

22. Tsuda, H., Lee, G. and Farber, E. (1980) Cancer Res., 40, 1157-1164.

Mechanisms of Toxicity and Hazard Evaluation
B. Holmstedt, R. Lauwerys, M. Mercier, M. Roberfroid eds

LIMITATIONS OF METABOLIC ACTIVATION SYSTEMS USED IN SHORT-TERM TESTS FOR CARCINOGENS

C.A.H. Bigger and A. Dipple
Chemical Carcinogenesis Program, NCI Frederick Cancer Research Center, Frederick, MD 21701 U.S.A.

INTRODUCTION

In the last decade there has been a major effort to develop fast and reliable tests for the detection of chemical carcinogens and the major criteria for ranking the validity of such tests has been the degree of empirical correlation between test result and known carcinogenic activity. In our view, some alternative criteria leading to a more objective evaluation of such tests are essential. For this reason, we have chosen to investigate carcinogen-DNA adducts formed under the conditions of some short-term tests, beginning with those which employ an exogenous system for metabolic activation, and to compare these adducts with those formed in a tissue which undergoes carcinogenesis *in vivo*.

So far, our studies have been largely limited to one hydrocarbon carcinogen, 7,12-dimethylbenz[*a*]anthracene, but our findings have highlighted interesting differences between carcinogen-DNA adducts formed *in vivo* and in microsomal systems *in vitro* and suggest that this may be a valuable approach to the assessment of short-term assays for chemical carcinogens.

RESULTS AND DISCUSSION

DNA was isolated from mouse skin[1,2] and various cells in culture[1,3] exposed to [^{3}H]DMBA, or recovered from reaction mixtures containing calf thumus DNA, [^{3}H]DMBA, cofactors and Aroclor-induced rat liver microsomes[1,2] or S-9 fraction[4]. After purification, the DNA was enzymatically hydrolyzed to hydrocarbon-deoxyribonucleoside adducts and analyzed by Sephadex LH-20 column chromatography or high pressure liquid chromatography[1,4].

In an initial study[1], a comparison of the DMBA-DNA adducts isolated from mouse skin and mouse embryo cells with those generated by rat liver microsomes, showed that the adducts from mouse skin are chromatographically identical to those from mouse embryo cells. Previous analysis[5] had indicated that the mouse embryo cell adducts are formed by reaction of DNA with the "bay-region" diol-epoxide of DMBA, the metabolite which appears to be the ultimate carcinogenic form of DMBA[6]. Thus, the results suggest that DNA adducts from mouse skin, a target tissue for this carcinogen, are also formed through reaction of DNA with the "bay-region" diol-epoxide of DMBA. In contrast, the DMBA-DNA adducts generated by microsomes are different from those formed in mouse skin and elute from Sephadex LH-20 columns in coincidence with markers formed by reaction of the K-region epoxide of DMBA with DNA. Thus, rat liver microsomes do not appear to be a good model for *in vivo* activation.

However, conflicting reports in the literature on the microsomal activation of benzo[*a*]pyrene (BP), another polycyclic hydrocarbon carcinogen, led us to suspect that changes in the reaction conditions might alter the DNA-reactive metabolites generated. For example, Meehan *et al*[7] reported that in the presence of rat liver microsomes BP is exclusively bound to DNA through the "bay-region" diol-epoxide route while King *et al*[8] reported the presence of additional adducts generated by the same system. Meehan *et al*. suggested that this difference might be explained by the inclusion of magnesium ions in the reaction mixture. Other studies[9] suggested that the concentration of the carcinogen might also alter the qualitative nature of the adducts. Therefore, in a subsequent study[2], the effect of such reaction conditions on *in vitro* microsomal activation of DMBA was investigated. The results showed that the nature of the metabolites bound to DNA is not substantially affected by the presence or absence of magnesium ions but is dependent on the concentration of the hydrocarbon. At high concentrations of DMBA, activation is primarily through the K-region oxide while, at low concentrations of DMBA, activation is through other routes. When we repeated these experiments using BP as substrate for Aroclor-induced microsomal enzymes, we found a similar dose-dependent shift in the distribution of particular adducts, indicating that routes of activation of BP to DNA-reactive forms could indeed be altered by changing the concentration of the hydrocarbon.

Since rat liver S-9 fraction, rather than washed microsomes, is generally used in short-term tests, we also repeated the DMBA dose-response study with S-9 fraction. Again, the same general principle applies. The qualitative nature of the DMBA-DNA adducts changes with hydrocarbon concentration[4].

When DMBA-DNA adducts from mouse embryo cells exposed to [^{14}C]DMBA were included in the chromatograms of tritium-labeled adducts generated by microsomes[2] or by S-9 fraction[4] at low DMBA concentrations, some of the tritium-labeled adducts eluted with the carbon-14-labeled diol-epoxide adducts, indicating that these metabolic activation systems could generate the ultimate carcinogenic form of this carcinogen. However, these represented only a small fraction of the total binding. This is in contrast to the results obtained with mouse skin and mouse embryo cells where no dose-dependent qualitative changes in adducts were observed over a hundred-fold and forty-fold[2] dose range respectively.

These findings suggested that cellular integrity might be essential to the reproduction of *in vivo* activation by an *in vitro* system. To test this, we compared the binding of intact rat liver cells and human skin cells in culture with that in mouse embryo cells and found the DMBA-DNA adducts to be chromatographically identical[3]. Thus, in four intact cellular systems, mouse skin, mouse embryo cells, rat liver cells and human skin cells, activation of DMBA to a DNA-reactive species appears to occur only through the diol-epoxide route, the route apparently responsible for DMBA carcinogenesis. However, with the liver homogenates, a variety of routes of activation is available and the distribution of carcinogen over these routes is dose-dependent. This dose dependence seems to be a critical finding when one considers that it is routine practice to use dose-response curves to strengthen confidence in short-term test results. Such a procedure could be misleading since dose-related increases could reflect a change-over in the relative importance of metabolic pathways leading to DNA binding rather than a dose-related increase in metabolites involved in carcinogenesis. For example, for the carcinogens we have examined, our analysis of DNA adducts indicates that with a short-term test designed to detect carcinogens as mutagens, a dose-related increase in mutants could easily be reflecting a transition from activation by the presumed ultimate carcinogenic metabolite ("bay-region" diol-epoxide) at low doses to activation by a known mutagenic metabolite (K-region epoxide) at high doses, rather than activation by a linear increase in the "bay-region" diol-epoxide with increasing dose.

In conclusion, analysis of carcinogen-DNA adducts provides another parameter for evaluation of *in vitro* metabolic activation systems. The analyses of DMBA-DNA adducts formed in various systems presented in this paper show how this technique can reveal limitations on the use of microsomal systems as models for target tissue activation. This does not necessarily invalidate their use but obviously must be taken into consideration when interpreting results. In addition our observations that intact cells are more faithful models of target tissue activation suggests that an important task at present is the use of this methodology to identify cell-lines with appropriate metabolic capabilities which could supply activation in short-term tests.

ACKNOWLEDGEMENTS

This work was supported by Contract No. NO1-CO-75380 with the National Cancer Institute, NIH, Bethesda, Maryland 20205.

REFERENCES

1. Bigger, C.A.H., Tomaszewski, J.E. and Dipple, A. (1978) Biochem. Biophys. Res. Commun., 80, 229-235.
2. Bigger, C.A.H., Tomaszewski, J.E. and Dipple, A. (1980) Carcinogenesis, 1, 15-20.
3. Bigger, C.A.H., Tomaszewski, J.E., Dipple, A. and Lake, R.S. (1980) Science, In press.
4. Bigger, C.A.H., Tomaszewski, J.E., Andrews, A.W. and Dipple, A. (1980) Cancer Res. 40, 655-661.
5. Moschel, R.C., Baird, W.M. and Dipple, A. (1977) Biochem. Biophys. Res. Commun., 76, 1092-1098.
6. Slaga, T.J., Huberman, E., DiGiovanni, J., Gleason, G. and Harvey, R.G. (1979) Cancer Lett., 6, 213-220.
7. Meehan, T., Straub, K. and Calvin, M. (1977) Nature, 269, 725-727.
8. King, H.W.S., Thompson, M.H. and Brookes, P. (1975) Cancer Res. 34, 1263-1269.
9. Levin, W. and Conney, A.H. (1967) Cancer Res., 27, 1931-1938.

© 1980 Elsevier/North-Holland Biomedical Press
Mechanisms of Toxicity and Hazard Evaluation
B. Holmstedt, R. Lauwerys, M. Mercier, M. Roberfroid eds

EFFECT OF GLUTATHIONE AND URIDINE 5'-DIPHOSPHOGLUCURONIC ACID ON BENZO(*a*)PYRENE MUTAGENESIS IN THE *SALMONELLA*/MICROSOME ASSAY

C. MALAVEILLE, G. BRUN, A. HAUTEFEUILLE and H. BARTSCH
International Agency for Research on Cancer, 150 cours Albert-Thomas, F-69372 Lyon Cédex 2.

INTRODUCTION

Benzo(*a*)pyrene (BP) is metabolized by cytochrome P-450-dependent monooxygenases into various derivatives[1-3], among which electrophilic epoxide(s) are thought to play a major role in determining the carcinogenic and mutagenic activity of the parent compounds[4]. The electrophilic BP derivatives that damage DNA *in vivo*, or in cultivated cells, appear to be secondary metabolites[5-8], e.g., BP 7,8-dihydrodiol 9,10-oxide. However, the BP metabolites that react with exogenous DNA or bacterial DNA in the presence of a microsomal activation system *in vitro* are both primary and secondary epoxides, depending on the activity and the substrate specificity of the microsomal cytochrome P-450-dependent monooxygenases involved[9-11]. Mutagenic epoxides of BP are known to be inactivated through enzymic conjugation with glutathione (GSH)[12,13], while various phenols and diols are enzymatically conjugated with uridine 5'-diphosphoglucuronic acid (UDPGA)[14-16].

In this study we investigated the role of the conjugating enzymes, glutathione-*S*- and UDPGA-transferases, on rat liver S-9-mediated mutagenesis of BP in the *Salmonella*/microsome assay. Both enzymes may alter by their known selective conjugating activities[14,17] the pattern of, and the concentration of, mutagenic BP metabolites, thus leading to changes in the overall mutagenic activity of the parent compounds.

MATERIALS AND METHODS

Animals and liver preparation: Adult BDIV rats (120-150 g bw) were bred in the IARC laboratory and were fed on a Charles River CRF diet. Groups of 2-4 animals received 3-methylcholanthrene (40 mg/kg bw) by i.p. injection two days before they were killed. Postmitochondrial supernatants (S-9) were prepared as described[18].

Mutagenicity assays: *S. typhimurium* TA100 strain was provided by Professor B.N. Ames, Berkeley, California, USA. Plate incorporation and liquid incubation assays were carried out as described[18]; UDPGA and GSH were dissolved in 68 mM Sørensen phosphate buffer pH 7.4.

RESULTS

The effects of 2.5 mM UDPGA (concentration in the top agar) on the microsome-mediated mutagenicity of 2 and/or 5 μM BP in the plate assay in the presence of different concentrations of rat liver S-9, are shown in Fig. 1. The UDPGA-dependent reduction of BP mutagenicity was found to be related to the liver S-9 concentration: a maximal reduction (40%) in mutagenicity was obtained with an S-9 concentration of 50 μl per plate.

Similar experiments were performed using liquid assays to study the effect of UDPGA on BP mutagenesis as a function of incubation time (Fig. 2). After 20 min incubation, the addition of 2.5 mM UDPGA caused a two-fold increase in BP mutagenicity at a concentration of 40 μM BP. At a two-fold lower BP concentration (20 μM), the presence of UDPGA either did not change or decreased the mutagenicity of BP, depending on the time of incubation.

The time-dependent S-9-mediated mutagenicity of BP in the liquid assay, with or without 10 mM GSH, is shown in Figs. 3A and B. When measured after 30 min of incubation at the highest BP concentrations (20 and 40 μM), the addition of GSH to the assays decreased BP mutagenicity by 1.8- and 1.5-fold in the presence of 17.4% (Fig. 3A) and 8.7% (Fig. 3B) of liver S-9, respectively. However, for two-fold lower concentrations of BP, the addition of GSH did not alter significantly BP mutagenesis. The data reported in Figs. 3A and B are mean values of two series of experiments since, on the basis of six different experiments using four different pools of liver S-9, the change in BP mutagenicity caused by the addition of GSH was found to be related to the number of revertants obtained in the absence of GSH (Fig. 4). The GSH-dependent alteration of BP (40 μM) mutagenicity in the presence of 17.4% (v/v) liver S-9 is plotted on the abscissa and is expressed as the mutagenicity ratio (MR) (see legend to Fig. 4). The MR was inversely related to the mutagenicity of BP in the absence of GSH. Thus, both a GSH-dependent increase and a decrease of BP mutagenicity were obtained: the decrease and the increase were associated with high and low BP mutagenicity, respectively.

DISCUSSION

Our experiments revealed that UDPGA either increased or decreased BP mutagenicity, depending on the concentration of BP or the type of assay system used (Figs. 1 and 2). Such results are in keeping with data reported by Nemoto *et al.*[19] and may be explained on the basis of two reports[15,16] showing that the addition of UDPGA to the microsomal assay increased the formation of BP 7,8-dihydrodiol 9,10-oxide and the rate of oxidative BP metabolism. Thus, the

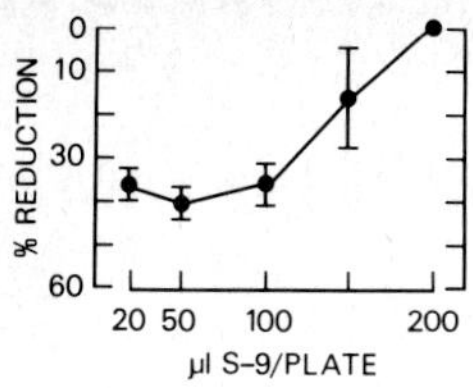

Fig. 1. UDPGA-dependent alteration of liver S-9-mediated mutagenicity of BP in *S. typhimurium* TA100 as a function of various amounts per plate of liver S-9. Percentage reduction in the presence of 2.5 mM UDPGA was calculated as follows:

$$\%\ \text{reduction} = \frac{\text{rev./pl. (-UDPGA)} - \text{rev./pl. (+UDPGA)}}{\text{rev./pl. (-UDPGA)}} \times 100$$

Before calculation, the number of revertants that occurred in the plates in the absence of BP was subtracted from each value. All assays were carried out in triplicate and each point represents the mean value ±SE of 2-4 experiments.

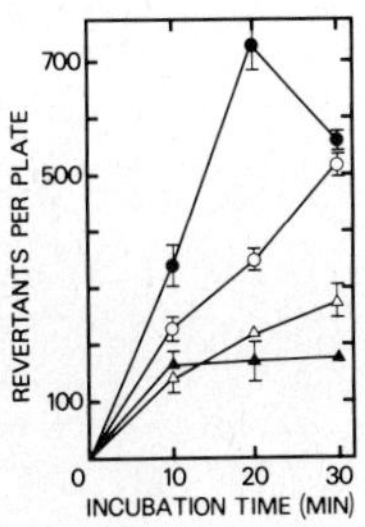

Fig. 2. Time-dependent S-9-mediated mutagenicity of BP in *S. typhimurium* TA100 using the liquid incubation assay in the absence (open symbols) or in the presence of 2.5 mM UDPGA (solid symbols). The concentration of rat liver S-9 was 17.4% v/v and those for BP were 20 μM (△,▲) and 40 μM (O,●). Each point represents the mean value ±SE of 2 experiments from which the number of revertants occurring spontaneously in the absence of BP, with or without UDPGA (70-90), has been subtracted.

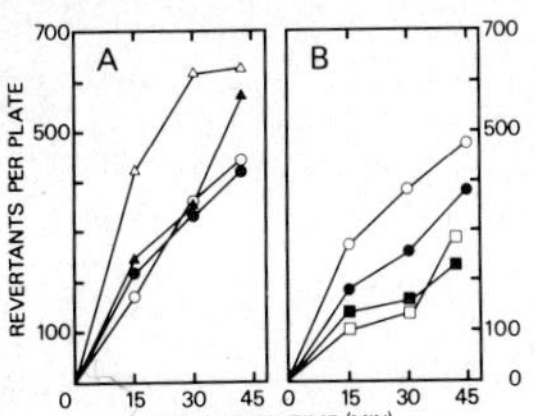

Fig. 3A, B. Time-dependent microsome-mediated mutagenicity of BP in *S. typhimurium* TA100 using the liquid incubation assay in the presence of 10 mM GSH (solid symbols) or in its absence (open symbols). The concentrations of rat liver S-9 were 17.4% and 8.7% v/v. The concentrations of BP used were 10 μM (□,■), 20 μM (O,●) and 40 μM (△,▲). Each point represents the mean value of 2 duplicate experiments from which the number of revertants occurring in the absence of BP, with or without GSH (70-90), has been subtracted.

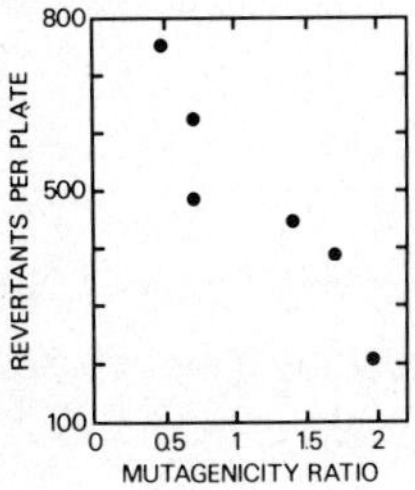

Fig. 4. Rat liver S-9-mediated mutagenicity of BP in *S. typhimurium* TA100 (ordinate) *versus* GSH-dependent alteration of BP mutagenicity (abscissa). The mutagenicity ratio (MR) was calculated by dividing the number of revertants obtained in the respective assays in the presence of 10 mM GSH by those in which GSH was omitted. Each of the 6 points corresponds to a single experiment (2-4 plates) performed in liquid medium in the presence of 17.4% (v/v) liver S-9 with 40 μM BP; incubation time was 30 min, using 4 different pools of liver S-9. The number of revertants occurring spontaneously in the absence of BP, with or without GSH (60-90), has been subtracted from the values listed.

UDPGA-dependent increase in BP mutagenicity (Fig. 2) may be associated with an increase in the formation of BP 7,8-dihydrodiol 9,10-oxide, which is more mutagenic than other BP epoxides[20]. An enhancement of oxidative BP metabolism in the presence of UDPGA, as reported elsewhere[16,21], may also be inferred from Fig. 2. At 20 μM BP the discrepancy between the two time-response curves, with respect to linearity, may be attributable to an increase in the rate of BP oxidative metabolic depletion in the presence of UDPGA. Such an effect may explain why UDPGA decreased BP mutagenicity in the plate assay with amounts of liver S-9 lower than 200 μl/plate (Fig. 1). The time during which mutagenic metabolites are formed would be longer in the absence of UDPGA than in its presence. As bacteria start to grow after plating, the number of bacteria exposed in their proliferative growth phase to mutagenic BP metabolites would be smaller in the presence of UDPGA than in its absence, thus leading to a lower number of mutants.

The modifying effect of GSH in liquid assays on BP mutagenicity was shown to be dependent firstly on the concentration of BP (Figs. 3A and B), and secondly on absolute number of revertants obtained in liquid assays with rat liver S-9 pools and BP in the absence of GSH (Fig. 4). An enhanced mutagenic effect may be attributed to an increased rate of formation of BP 7,8-dihydrodiol 9,10-oxide, which is known to be more mutagenic than simple epoxides[20]. This may result from a selective conjugation with GSH of simple oxides[17], which may compete with BP 7,8-oxide for epoxide hydratase, thus leading to a higher rate of formation of BP 7,8-diol and subsequently to a higher rate of formation of BP 7,8-dihydrodiol 9,10-oxide. A shift in metabolic pathways of BP would therefore seem to depend on (a) the balance between epoxide hydratase and GSH-transferase activities which may vary from one liver S-9 preparation to another, as both enzymes are inducible by MC-treatment[22,23], and (b) the rates of formation of both primary and secondary mutagenic BP metabolites; these in turn may be determined by the overall monooxygenase activity, by the relative proportions and substrate specificities of various forms of cytochrome P-450 and by the ratio of BP to microsomal protein concentration[9,10,24].

In conclusion, our results showed that in *in vitro* mutagenicity assays, the addition of cofactors for the conjugating enzymes, GSH- and UDPGA-transferases, can alter the metabolic activation pathways of BP and consequently *in vitro* mutagenicity.

ACKNOWLEDGEMENTS

We are grateful to Miss C. Rowson for secretarial assistance. Financial support for these studies was partly provided by the National Cancer Institute, USA, contract no. N01-CP-55630 and partly by contract no. 190-77-ENVF with the Commission of the European Communities.

REFERENCES

1. Sims, P. and Grover, P.L. (1974) Adv. Cancer Res., 20, 165-274.
2. Heidelberger, C. (1975) Ann. Rev. Biochem., 44, 79-121.
3. Selkirk, J.K., Croy, R.G., Roller, P.P. and Gelboin, H.V. (1974) Cancer Res., 34, 3473-3480.
4. Miller, E.C. and Miller, J.A. (1976) Chemical Carcinogens, ACS Monograph 173, The American Chemical Society, Washington, pp. 737-762.
5. Weinstein, I.B., Jeffrey, A.M., Jennette, K.W., Blobstein, S.H., Harvey, R.G., Harris, C., Autrup, H., Kasai, H. and Nakanishi, K. (1976) Science, 193, 592-595.
6. Vadi, H., Jernström, B. and Orrenius, S. (1976) Carcinogenesis Vol. 1, Polynuclear Aromatic Hydrocarbons: Chemistry, Metabolism and Carcinogenesis, Raven Press, New York, pp. 45-61.
7. Jernström, B., Vadi, H. and Orrenius, S. (1978) Chem.-biol. Interactions, 20, 311-321.
8. Autrup, H., Harris, C.C., Trump, B.F. and Jeffrey, A.M. (1978) Cancer Res., 38, 3689-3696.
9. Boobis, A.R., Nebert, D.W. and Pelkonen, O. (1978) Biochem. Pharmacol., 28, 111-121.
10. Oesch, F. (1979) Arch. Toxicol. Suppl. 2, 215-227.
11. Santella, R.M., Grunberger, D. and Weinstein, I.B. (1979) Mutat. Res., 61, 181-187.
12. Boyland, E. and Chasseaud, L.F. (1969) Adv. Enzymol., 32, 173-219.
13. Chasseaud, L.F. (1976) Glutathione Metabolism and Function, Raven Press, New York, pp. 77-114.
14. Nemoto, N. and Takayama, S. (1977) Cancer Res., 37, 4125-4129.
15. Nemoto, N. (1978) Conjugation Reactions in Drug Biotransformation, Elsevier/North-Holland, Amsterdam, pp. 17-27.
16. Fahl, W.E., Shen, A.L. and Jefcoate, C.R. (1978) Biochem. Biophys. Res. Commun., 85, 891-899.
17. Bend, J.R., Ben-Zvi, Z., van Anda, J., Dansette, P.M. and Jerina, D.M. (1976) Carcinogenesis Vol. 1, Polynuclear Aromatic Hydrocarbons: Chemistry, Metabolism and Carcinogenesis, Raven Press, New York, pp. 63-75.
18. Malaveille, C., Kuroki, T., Brun, G., Hautefeuille, A., Camus, A.M. and Bartsch, H. (1979) Mutat. Res., 63, 245-258.
19. Nemoto, N., Takayama, S., Nagao, M. and Umezawa, K. (1978) Toxicol. Lett., 2, 205-211.

20. Jerina, D.M., Lehr, R.E., Yagi, H., Hernandez, O., Dansette, P.M., Wislocki, P.G., Wood, A.W., Chang, R.L., Levin, W. and Conney, A.H. (1976) *In Vitro* Metabolic Activation in Mutagenesis Testing, Elsevier/North-Holland, Amsterdam, pp. 159-177.

21. Bock, K.W. (1978) Naunyn-Schmiedebergs Arch. Exp. Pathol. Pharmakol., 304, 77-79.

22. Oesch, F. (1973) Xenobiotica, 3, 305-340.

23. Mukhtar, H. and Bresnick, E. (1976) Biochem. Pharmacol., 25, 1081-1084.

24. Holder, G.M., Yagi, H., Jerina, D.M., Levin, W., Lu, A.Y.H. and Conney, A.H. (1975) Arch. Biochem. Biophys., 170, 557-566.

Mechanisms of Toxicity and Hazard Evaluation
B. Holmstedt, R. Lauwerys, M. Mercier, M. Roberfroid eds

METABOLIC INACTIVATION OF MUTAGENIC BENZO(*a*)PYRENE METABOLITES: SIGNIFICANCE TO CARCINOGENICITY AND IMPLICATIONS FOR *IN VITRO* TESTS.

H.R. GLATT, K.L. PLATT, K. VOGEL, M. BÜCKER, R. BILLINGS and F. OESCH
Pharmakolog. Institut, Universität, Obere Zahlbacher Str. 67, D-6500 Mainz FRG

INTRODUCTION AND GENERAL CONSIDERATIONS

Benzo(*a*)pyrene (BP) is one of the most thoroughly investigated carcinogens. In whole animals and tissue explants, a small number of metabolites account for most of the DNA-bound BP[1,2]. Among the many BP metabolites tested for carcinogenicity[3-8], precursors of (+)7β,8α-dihydroxy-9α,10α-epoxy-7,8,9,10-tetrahydro-BP showed activities similar to or stronger than that of BP. Most other metabolites were inactive or were much less carcinogenic than BP, although many of them readily bind to DNA[9-10] or cause mutations in bacteria[11-15] either directly or after *in vitro* metabolic activation by subcellular tissue preparations.

BP 4,5-oxide, a BP metabolite which is formed by mammalian monooxygenases and inactivated by epoxide hydrolase and glutathione (GSH) S-transferase, is a very potent ultimate mutagen in bacteria. Studies[13,16] with *S. typhimurium* TA 1537 show that BP 4,5-oxide can account for the bulk of the mutagenic effect when BP is activated by liver microsomes from mice which were not treated with enzyme inducers. However, *in vivo* it is a very weak carcinogen and it seems to account for at most a very small fraction of BP-induced effects. A few reflections may help to understand the discrepancy. In mammalian enzyme-mediated bacterial mutagenicity tests, subcellular activating systems are usually used in very dilute form compared to the liver, a point which has many grave consequences: (1) Dilution of a simple monooxygenase-epoxide hydrolase system may not change, as a first approximation, the steady state concentration of intermediary epoxides. However it extends the time required for metabolism of a given amount of BP and during this time the epoxide is present. (2) The effect of dilution is even greater with cofactor-dependent enzymes such as GSH S-transferases or NADPH-requiring monooxygenases because small amounts and low concentrations of cofactors imply a low metabolic capacity and usually a further decrease in metabolic rates. Subcellular activating systems used in short-term tests for mutagenicity and carcinogenicity are generally supplemented with NADPH, the cofactor for monooxygenases, the enzymes most often required for metabolic activation. Other cofactors are not routinely supplemented. (3) Oxidation products formed by monooxygenases from polycyclic aromatic hydrocarbons frequently can be converted by the same or other monooxygenases to secondary and tertiary oxidation products. Dilution of metabolizing systems, particularly when high concentrations of the hydrocarbon precursor are used[16], increases the relative yield of simple and decreases that of multiple oxidation products, which are metabolites of greatest importance for BP-induced effects *in vivo*. (4) It is noteworthy that dilution does not affect all balances between enzyme activities gravely. The relative amounts of a substrate metabolized by competitive enzymes may not be drastically changed when both enzymes are diluted by the same factor and conditions of activity, such as cofactor supply, do not significantly change. This may be the case with dihydrodiol dehydrogenase, an enzyme which decreases BP-induced bacterial mutagenicity under conditions favorable for dihydrodiol-epoxide formation, but not at conditions when BP 4,5-oxide seems to be the main mutagen[17]. Dihydrodiol dehydrogenase requires NADP and may therefore operate in metabolizing systems supplemented with an NADPH-generating system (although not optimally). Apart from the various effects of dilution and selective supplementation with cofactors, destruction of cell compartments and removal of some subcellular fractions are further sources of metabolic differences between subcellular *in vitro* systems and *in vivo* systems.

The simplified metabolizing system may well be a main reason for the poor quantitative correlation of mutagenicity in the Ames test and carcinogenicity with some groups of chemicals[18]. This is particularly likely with compounds such as BP with a complex metabolism involving many enzymes.

Therefore in the present study more complete metabolizing systems for the activation of BP and of premutagenic BP metabolites were used in bacterial mutagenicity tests. The activating systems were freshly isolated intact hepatocytes or homogenates of these cells supplemented with various cofactor systems.

The compounds tested were the carcinogens BP and (±)*trans*-7,8-dihydroxy-7,8-dihydro-BP (7,8-diol) and the very weak carcinogens or tumor initiators 3-hydroxy-BP (3-OH-BP), 9-hydroxy-BP (9-OH-BP) and (±)*trans*-9,10-dihydroxy-9,10-dihydro-BP (9,10-diol). All are strong mutagens in the Ames test[11-15].

MATERIALS AND METHODS

Isolation of hepatocytes. Adult male rats received a single intraperitoneal injection of 500 mg Aroclor 1254 per kg body weight 5 days before sacrifice. Hepatocytes were isolated by perfusion of the liver *in situ* with collagenase as described[19]. Part of the isolated hepatocytes were homogenized by sonicating.

Mutagenicity experiments. Reversion of *his*$^-$ *S. typhimurium* TA 100 was used for estimation of mutagenicity. Intact or sonicated hepatocytes (1.8 - 2 x 10^6

cells per incubation), bacteria (1.7 x 10^8 cells per incubation), and the indicated cofactors and metabolic modifiers were suspended or dissolved in perfusion medium containing 2.5 mM $CaCl_2$ (total 1.05 to 1.15 ml per incubation) and mixed together. After addition of the test compound in 10 µl dimethylsulfoxide, an incubation was performed in a shaking water bath at 37°C in the dark for 2 hours. Then histidine-poor top agar was added and the mixture was poured onto a petri dish with minimal agar[18]. After incubation at 37°C in the dark for 3 days, colonies (*his*$^+$ revertant) were counted.

RESULTS

Comparison of the mutagenicities with activation by intact hepatocytes or hepatocyte homogenate.

BP was not mutagenic when tested directly or in the presence of hepatocyte homogenate (data not shown). However, it became strongly mutagenic when an NADPH-generating system was added to the homogenate or when whole hepatocytes were used. The dose-response relationship differed markedly under the two situations (Fig. 1). With NADPH-fortified homogenate, BP showed strong mutagenic effects at low doses. At higher doses the number of mutants was constant over a wide dose range, probably due to limited metabolic capacity. With whole hepatocytes, the dose-response relationship was much less steep, but the mutagenic effect increased with higher doses up to a higher maximal effect than with NADPH-fortified homogenate. 3-OH-BP, 9-OH-BP and 9,10-diol were not mutagenic in the presence of homogenate. However, when an NADPH-generating system was

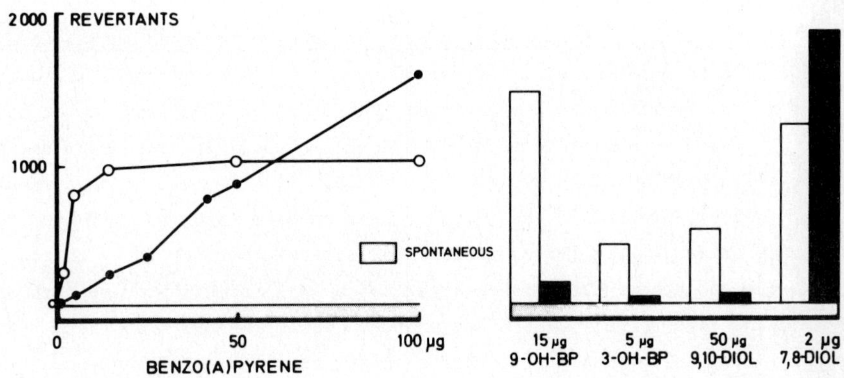

Fig. 1. Mutagenicity of BP and BP metabolites in *S. typhimurium* TA 100 in the presence of intact (dark) or homogenized (light) hepatocytes. Incubations with homogenate received 1.7 mg NADP and 1 mg glucose-6-phosphate.

TABLE 1

EFFECT OF COFACTORS FOR CONJUGATION ON HOMOGENATE-MEDIATED MUTAGENICITY

Test Compound	% Mutagenicity[a] in the presence of			
	ATP[b]	UDPGA[b]	GSH[b]	ATP+UDPGA+GSH
2 μg BP	35, 38	31, 37	53, 56	15, 23
5 μg 3-OH-BP	16, 46	22, 43	36, 37	0, 18
5 μg 9-OH-BP	84, 100	41, 45	70, 85	38, 49
0.6-1 μg 7,8-Diol	148, 166	68, 96	49, 51	55, 65
50 μg 9,10-Diol	106, 120	29, 35	18, 20	8, 14

[a] Mutants above solvent controls in the presence of cofactor expressed as percent of this value in its absence. Values represent separate experiments.
[b] Concentration of ATP 10 mM, of GSH 5 mM, of UDPGA (UDP-glucuronic acid) 10 mM. Incubations with UDPGA additionally contained 10 mM UDP-N-acetylglucosamine. All incubations received 1.7 mg NADP and 1 mg glucose-6-phosphate as well.

added with the cell homogenate, mutagenic effects were observed with all three. The mutagenic potency of 9-OH-BP was slightly stronger, that of 3-OH-BP slightly weaker and that of 9,10-diol several-fold weaker than that of BP. Intact cells also activated these three weak carcinogens. However, the mutagenic effects at all doses were weak (some data shown in Fig. 1). 7,8-Diol was activated by both homogenized or intact hepatocytes to a very potent mutagen (Fig. 1). In contrast to all other compounds, its mutagenicity was somewhat stronger with intact hepatocytes than with NADPH-fortified homogenate.

Effect of cofactors for conjugation on the homogenate-mediated mutagenicity.

Difference in metabolism is one explanation for the differences in mutagenicity of BP and BP-metabolites with intact *versus* NADPH-fortified broken hepatocytes. In order to approximate the homogenate metabolizing system to the intact hepatocytes, three cofactor systems were added: (1) ATP, which together with Mg^{2+} and sulfate present in the medium, gives rise to PAPS, the cofactor for sulfotransferases; (2) UDP-glucuronic acid, the cofactor for UDP-glucuronosyl transferase, together with UDP-N-acetylglucosamine, an activator of this enzyme; (3) GSH, the cofactor of GSH S-transferases. Table 1 shows that these cofactors strongly affected the mutagenicity of all test compounds. ATP enhanced the mutagenicity of the two dihydrodiols (by an unknown mechanism) and had little effect on the mutagenicity of 9-OH-BP. Otherwise, each cofactor reduced the mutagenicity of each test compound. All three cofactors together decreased the effects of 3-OH-BP, 9,10-diol and BP more than 80%. The least inactivation occurred with 7,8-diol.

CONCLUSIONS

The results of this study show that it is possible to activate BP and BP-metabolites to bacterial mutagens with intact hepatocytes. The mutagenicity often is weaker and the relative potencies of various compounds greatly differ from results obtained with NADPH-fortified cell homogenate. To account for these differences we adopted the working hypothesis that many enzymes which operate in intact cells may not do so in the homogenate for reasons such as dilution of cofactors. Indeed many premutagens are only activated by homogenate when additional NADPH is provided. In this study we show that addition of cofactors of further enzymes considerably altered mutagenicity. The alterations differed with different test compounds and the results became more similar to results obtained with intact cells. This was particularly the case with 3-OH-BP, 9,10-diol and with a low dose of BP, which all became very weak mutagens as was observed with intact cells. In contrast, 7,8-diol remained strongly mutagenic in agreement with its activity with whole cells. 9-OH-BP, a potent mutagen with homogenate, but only a weak mutagen with cells, was an exception, since its mutagenicity was reduced only slightly more than that of 7,8-diol. However, in this study we took into account a few of many possible inactivation pathways. Therefore, it remains to be determined whether metabolic factors other than those modulated by the additions performed in this study are crucial for the inactivation of 9-OH-BP in intact hepatocytes, or whether with this compound pharmacokinetic parameters such as permeability barriers are more important for differences in mutagenicity between whole and broken cells.

Use of intact hepatocytes instead of NADPH-fortified homogenate considerably improved the correlation of mutagenicity with whole animal carcinogenicity. At first glance, this is surprising since polycyclic aromatic hydrocarbon carcinogens only rarely cause liver tumors and it is assumed that carcinogens normally are activated close to their target cells. This may indicate that metabolic differences among different intact cells are significantly smaller than differences between target cell and a rudimentary drug metabolizing system consisting of a liver subcellular preparation and NADPH. Intact hepatocytes may well not be the optimal metabolizing system in short-term tests for carcinogenicity and mutagenicity. However, the present study shows that the metabolizing system can very strongly affect the result of a test. Therefore, if inactivation occurs *in vivo* it is reasonable to take the inactivating systems into account also in *in vitro* tests. More complete, less artificial metabolizing systems are certainly an important means for improvement of the predictive value of many short-term tests for carcinogenicity.

ACKNOWLEDGEMENT

This work was supported by The Council for Tobacco Research -- USA, Inc.

REFERENCES

1. Jeffrey, A.M., Weinstein, J.B., Jennette, K.W., Grzeskowiak, K., Nakanishi, K., Harvey, R.G., Autrup, H. and Harris, C. (1977) Nature, 269, 348-350.
2. Phillips, D.H., Grover, P.L. and Sims, P. (1978) Int. J. Cancer, 22, 487-494.
3. Chouroulinkov, I., Gentil, A., Grover, P.L. and Sims, P. (1976) Br. J. Cancer, 34, 523-532.
4. Kapitulnik, J., Levin, W., Yagi, H., Jerina, D.M. and Conney, A.H. (1976) Cancer Res., 36, 3625-3628.
5. Kapitulnik, J., Wislocki, P.G., Levin, W., Yagi, H., Thakker, D.R., Akagi, H., Koreeda, M., Jerina, D.M. and Conney, A.H. (1978) Cancer Res., 38, 2661-2665.
6. Slaga, T.J., Bracken, W.M., Dresner, S., Levin, W., Yagi, H., Jerina, D.M. and Conney, A.H. (1978) Cancer Res., 38, 678-681.
7. Survey of Compounds which have been Tested for Carcinogenic Activity, PHS Publication no. 149, Washington, D.C. (through 1972 - 1973 volume).
8. Wislocki, P.G., Chang, R.L., Wood, A.W., Levin, W., Yagi, H., Hernandez, O., Mah, H.D., Dansette, P.H., Jerina, D.M. and Conney, A.H. (1977) Cancer Res., 37, 2608-2611.
9. King, H., Osborne, M. and Brookes, P. (1977) Int. J. Cancer, 20, 564-571.
10. Pelkonen, O., Boobis, A.R., Yagi, H., Jerina, D.M. and Nebert, D.W. (1978) Mol. Pharmacol., 14, 306-322.
11. Malaveille, C., Bartsch, H., Grover, P.L. and Sims, P. (1975) Biochem. Biophys. Res. Commun., 66, 693-700.
12. McCann, J., Choi, E., Yamasaki, E. and Ames, B.N. (1976) Proc. Natl. Acad. Sci. U.S.A., 72, 5135-5139.
13. Oesch, F. and Glatt, H.R. (1976) in Screening Tests in Chemical Carcinogenesis (Montesano, R., et al. eds.) IARC, Lyon, pp. 255-274.
14. Owens, I.S., Koteen, G.M. and Legraverend, C. (1979) Biochem. Pharmacol., 28, 1615-1622.
15. Wood, A.W., Levin, W., Lu, A.Y.H., Yagi, H., Hernandez, O., Jerina, D.M. and Conney, A.H. (1976) J. Biol. Chem., 251, 4882-4890.
16. Bentley, P., Oesch, F. and Glatt, H.R. (1977) Arch. Toxicol., 39, 75-75.
17. Glatt, H.R., Vogel, K., Bentley, P. and Oesch, F. (1979) Nature, 277, 319-320.
18. Glatt, H.R., Schwind, H., Zajdela, F., Croisy, A., Jacquignon, P.C. and Oesch, F. (1979), Mutation Res., 66, 307-328.
19. Billings, R.E. and Tephly, T.R. (1976) Biochem. Pharmacol., 25, 2351-2356.

© 1980 Elsevier/North-Holland Biomedical Press
Mechanisms of Toxicity and Hazard Evaluation
B. Holmstedt, R. Lauwerys, M. Mercier, M. Roberfroid eds

CELL CULTURE SYSTEMS TO STUDY GLIAL TRANSFORMATION

JOSEPH P. BRESSLER, RUTH COLE AND JEAN DE VELLIS
Laboratory of Nuclear Medicine and Radiation Biology, University of California, Los Angeles, California 90024, USA

INTRODUCTION

A significant number of human cancers are environmentally related[1]. To focus on the identification of these environmental factors and to understand the mechanisms of induction, many researchers have developed models employing fibroblasts[2]. Though these models have answered many interesting questions, fibrosarcomas are not a common human tumor; therefore, it becomes pertinent to employ other cell types.

Gliomas are prevalent among human cancers. Compared to other types of malignancies, very little has been done to understand mechanisms which induce them. One problem in an experimental approach to gliomas has been the heterogeneity of brain tissue. Brain is composed of three main cell types, neurons and two types of glial cells, oligodendrocytes and astrocytes[3]. These cells are intricately dependent on one another for many functions, such as nutrient supply and growth regulation[3]. Therefore, *in vivo* studies cannot define cell specific functions. For example, induction of brain tumors by implanting carcinogen pellets could not determine the cell types metabolizing the carcinogen. Also, with this type of tumor induction, it is difficult to accurately identify the type of tumor, because cells may lose differentiation markers during transformation.

The purpose of the proceeding studies is to define *in vitro* model systems to study the transformation of pure populations of glial cells. This method is based on a technique developed by McCarthy and de Vellis[4], where oligodendrocytes and astrocytes were selected from brain cell cultures of neonatal rat cerebral tissue. We have been able to study the transformation of two different types of glial cells using an *in vivo-in vitro* model and a complete *in vitro* model. Data will be presented to demonstrate that the transformed cells were glial and tumorigenic.

MATERIALS AND METHODS

The preparation of primary brain cell cultures and purification of the glial cell types were done as described[4]. The oligodendroglial cultures were maintained in BME* with 0.6% glucose and 15% FCS (medium A) unless otherwise noted. The astroglial cultures were passed with 2.5% trypsin and maintained in medium A except with 10% FCS. Media, trypsin and FCS were purchased from Irvine Scientific, Irvine, CA, and plasticware was purchased from Falcon, Oxnard, CA. ENU (10 μg/g body weight) dissolved in PBS was administered via the femural vein on the 19th day of gestation. To test for tumorigenicity, 21-day-old rats were irradiated with 400 r and injected with 10^6 cells no later than 24 h after irradiation. The induction and assay of LDH and GPDH were done as described[4], and the CNPase assay was done as described[4].

RESULTS

After 7 d, primary brain cells in culture form a bilayer where the phase-dark, process-bearing oligodendrocytes can be seen growing on top of a bed layer of flat cells composed mostly of astrocytes (f 1a). The spherical oligodendrocytes on top of the flat epithelioid-shaped astrocyte can be seen more clearly with SEM (f 1b). After vigorously shaking the flasks, the oligodendrocytes can be selectively removed and plated. A 99% pure oligodendrocyte culture is prepared (f 1d), and the bed layer of cells is completely devoid of these cells (f 1c).

Pregnant rats were injected with ENU or PBS, and oligodendrocytes were prepared from the 2- to 4-day-old pups. The cells from the PBS-treated group were either grown in media A or in DMEM/F-12 supplemented with 10% FCS and 2% horse serum (media B). Upon confluency, the oligodendrocytes were passed by shaking overnight.

A marked increase in cellular proliferation was observed between 100-150 d in those cultures derived from ENU-treated animals or treated with media B. Four different transformed oligodendrocyte cell lines were obtained, 3, 4, 12 and 13 (t 1) capable of forming tumors. Cells derived from buffer-treated animals and fed with media A did not change their rate of proliferation. These cells were not able to produce tumors, and they have been maintained in culture for at least 18 passages.

In culture all of the cell lines appeared similar to oligodendrocytes. Both the nontransformed (f 1d) and the transformed cells (f 1f) have round cell bodies and long extended, multiple fine processes. The transformed cells can be seen to grow to a much higher density and also tend to aggregate.

*Abbreviations used: BME, Basal Eagles Media; FCS, fetal calf sera; ENU, ethyl-nitrosourea; PBS, phosphate-buffer saline; LDH, lactate dehydrogenase; GPDH, glycerol phosphate dehydrogenase; CNPase, cyclic nucleotide phosphohydrolase; dbcAMP, $N^6,O^{2'}$-dibutyryl cyclic AMP; HC, hydrocortisone

TABLE 1

BIOCHEMICAL CHARACTERIZATION OF TUMORIGENIC CELL LINES

Cell Line	Treatment	CNPase (U/μg protein)	LDH Induction	GPDH Induction
3	Media B	388 ± 17	2.1	Not observed
4	Media B	445 ± 20	1.9	Not observed
12	ENU	365 ± 15	1.8	Not observed
13	ENU	526 ± 62	1.5	Not observed
At	Spontaneous	423 ± 48	1.7	3.2

The cell lines were characterized by various biochemical markers that have been associated with oligodendrocytes. All of the cell lines contained significant levels of CNPase, and all of the cell lines could be induced to increase the levels of LDH after a 24-h exposure to 1 mM dbcAMP (t 1), but induction of GPDH by HC was not observed.

The cells composing the bed layer were passed two times per week for the first 12 passages and then on a weekly basis. At each passage the cells were split at either 1:2 or 1:4 ratio to minimize cell-to-cell contact. After 26 passages, small foci of cells growing on top of each other were observed a few days after the cells reached confluency (f 2a) (At), but 25th passage cells (Ac) formed a confluent monolayer (f 2b). Upon further culture, the foci could be visualized by the naked eye.

Morphologically, the At line was quite distinct from cells in primary culture, transformed oligodendrocytes, or the Ac line (f 1e). In these cells the levels of LDH and GPDH were inducible with dbcAMP and HC respectively (t 1). These cells were capable of growing tumors when injected *in vivo*, in contrast to the Ac cell line.

DISCUSSION

Our results demonstrate that pure populations of glial cells can undergo neoplastic transformation in culture. We found that oligodendrocytes could be induced to transform by special media or by a transplacental injection of ENU, and these cells became tumorigenic after 100-150 d in culture. Other investigators, using a similar *in vivo-in vitro* system, observed mixed glial transformation after 100-200 d in culture[5]. In contrast to our results, these investigators found that control cells did not survive in culture. We do not believe that this difference can be accounted for by our use of pure glial populations,

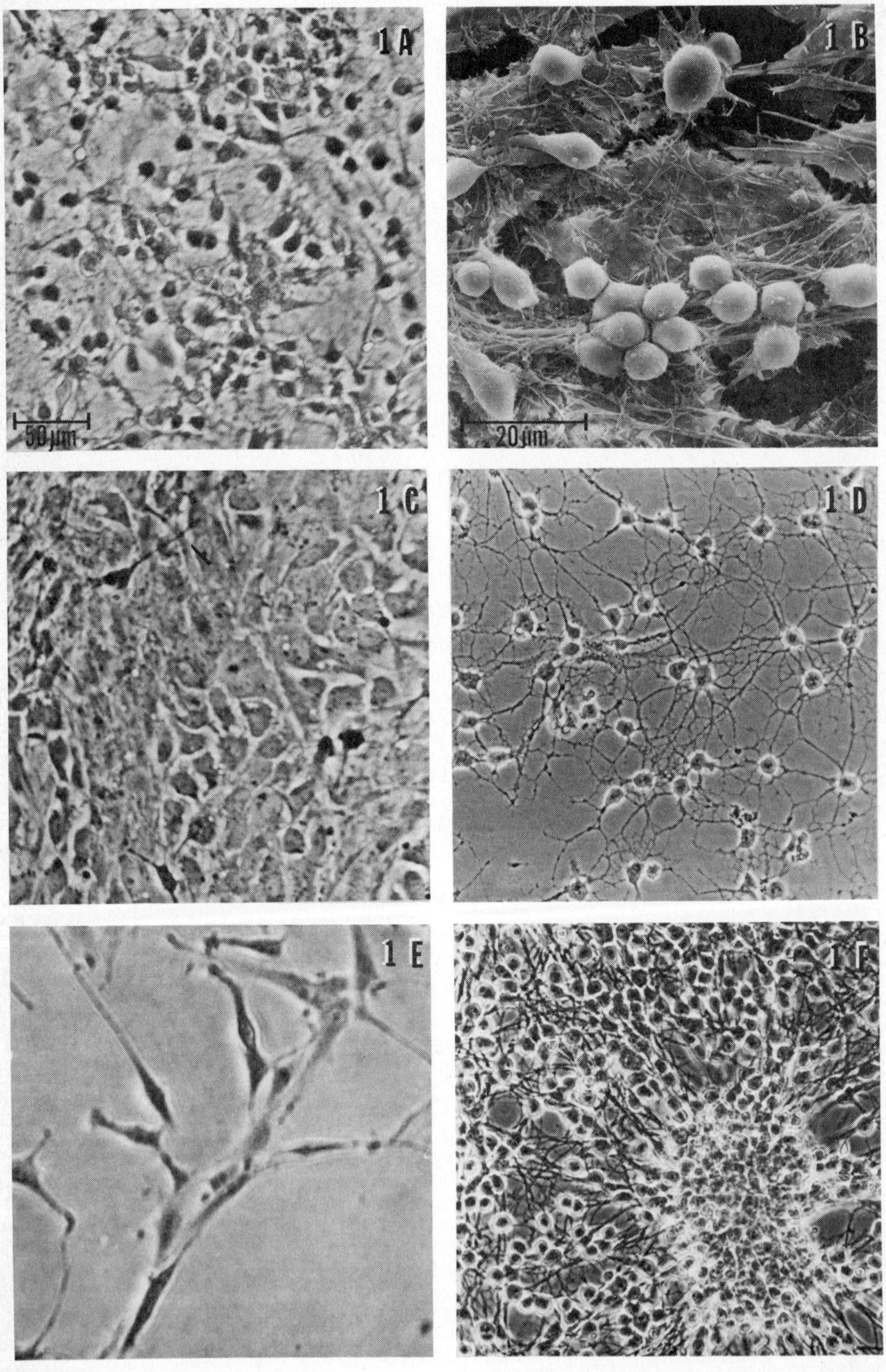
1A
50 µm
1 B
20 µm
1 C
1 D
1 E
1 F

Fig. 1. Phase contrast micrographs of mixed brain cell culture (f 1a), purified oligodendrocytes (f 1d), bed layer without oligodendrocytes (f 1c), At line (f 1e), and the 12 cell line (f 1f). SEM of mixed cell cultures (f 1b).

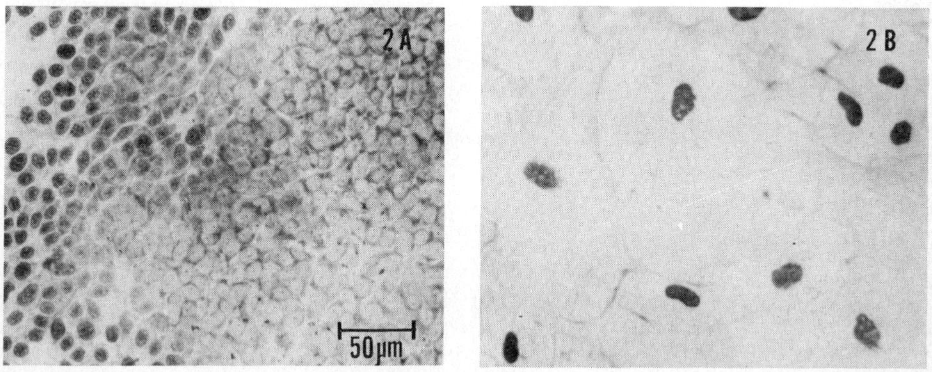

Fig. 2. Giemsa staining of a pile-up colony at 26th passage (f 2a) or cell monolayer at 25th passage (f 2b).

rather we attribute this difference to our culture conditions and use of postnatal pups.

The possibility that our purified oligodendrocyte population was contaminated by other cell type(s) must be ruled out since the transformed cells possessed various oligodendrocyte-specific markers, such as CNPase, inducibility of LDH as well as various morphological criteria. Rajewsky *et al.*[5] characterized various glial cell lines transformed *in vitro*. They were unable to detect glial fibrous acidic protein or myelin basic protein, but did find S-100 protein. Our lines were also positive for S-100 protein (unpublished observations) and negative for both myelin basic protein and GPDH inducibility. The transformation event might have caused these cells to lose these characteristics. An alternative explanation would be that the carcinogen "hit" a glial stem cell that expressed selected glial functions, afterwhich the cell was inhibited from differentiating and eventually transformed.

In three different experiments a population of cells, originating from the bed layer, spontaneously transformed after 26 passages. These cells lost cell-to-cell contact inhibition and formed pile-up colonies. The cells were tumorigenic, as opposed to the cells that grew in a normal monolayer. They possessed certain biochemical oligodendroglial properties, but morphologically they were quite different from the primary cultures or the Ac cell line. Therefore, we believe that these cells represent a population of less mature oligodendrocytes.

Postnatal nonfibroblast cells usually do not survive in culture for extended periods unless they transform[5,6,7]. To our knowledge, only liver cells can proliferate in culture without transforming[8]. In this report we describe two different glial cell types capable of *in vitro* transformation that do not lose proliferative capabilities in the nontransformed state. This allows us now to compare transformed and nontransformed glial cells to determine characteristics that permit tumor growth. Particular attention will be focused on the cells composing the bed layer. The observation that these cells form pile-up colonies after transformation now gives us a method to screen for glial-specific carcinogens in an *in vitro* system.

ACKNOWLEDGEMENTS

These studies were supported in part by the Department of Energy Contract DE-AM03-76-SF00012 and Environmental Protection Agency Contract EPA-IAG-D5-E-681-AQ. J.P. Bressler is the recipient of a National Research Service Award AG-05145 from NIA.

REFERENCES

1. Higginson, V. (1972) Environment and Cancer. 24th Symposium on Fundamental Cancer Research, Williams and Wilkins, Baltimore, p. 62.
2. Heidelberger, C. (1973) Advances in Cancer Research, Academic Press, New York, pp. 317-360.
3. Jacobson, M. (1978) Developmental Neurobiology, Plenum Press, New York, pp. 27-180.
4. McCarthy K. and de Vellis, J. (1980) J. Cell Biol., 85, 890-902.
5. Laerum, O.D. and Rajewsky, M.F. (1975) J. Nat. Cancer Inst., 55, 1177-1188.
6. Colburn, N.H., Bruegge, W.F.V., Bates, J.R., Gray, R.H., Rossen, J.D., Kelsey, W.H. and Shimada, T. (1978) Cancer Res., 38, 624-634.
7. Steele, V.E., Marchok, A.C. and Nettesheim, P. (1977) Int. J. Cancer, 20, 234-238.
8. Williams, G.M., Elliott, J.M. and Weisburger, J.H. (1973) Cancer Res., 33, 606-612.

© 1980 Elsevier/North-Holland Biomedical Press
Mechanisms of Toxicity and Hazard Evaluation
B. Holmstedt, R. Lauwerys, M. Mercier, M. Roberfroid eds

STUDIES ON THE MECHANISM OF THE SYNERGISTIC CARCINOGENIC RESPONSE REPORTED BETWEEN ETHYLENE DIBROMIDE AND DISULFIRAM AND THE IMPLICATIONS FOR SHORT TERM PREDICTIVE SCREENING TESTS.

BM ELLIOTT and J ASHBY
Central Toxicology Laboratory, Imperial Chemical Industries Limited, Alderley Park, Macclesfield, Cheshire, UK.

INTRODUCTION

Ethylene dibromide (EDB) is carcinogenic in the rat and mouse[1]. Disulfiram however is non-carcinogenic in these species[2] and is usually considered an inhibitor of carcinogenesis[3], a property ascribed to its ability to reduce the activity of certain enzymes including the mixed function oxidase system[4]. It was therefore of great interest when rats exposed to low levels of EDB and disulfiram developed a high incidence of tumours compared to animals given either EDB or disulfiram alone[5]. In this study we have examined possible mechanisms for this synergistic carcinogenic response and assessed the implications for *in vitro* predictive screening tests.

METHODS

Animals. Male Alderley Park (Wistar-derived) or Sprague-Dawley (maintained at Alderley Park) rats (180-200g) were dosed daily by gavage with a suspension of disulfiram in 0.5% (w/v) carboxymethylcellulose. Liver subfractions were prepared as described by Tottmar *et al*[6].

Enzyme Assays. Aldehyde dehydrogenase[6] and glutathione-S-transferase[7] activities were measured using acetaldehyde and 1-chloro-2,4-dinitrobenzene (CDNB) respectively as substrates. Cytochrome P450 levels were estimated as described by Omura & Sato[8].

Bacterial Mutation Assay. The plate incorporation reverse mutation assay of Ames was carried out with strains TA 1537, 1538, 98, 1535 and 100 of *Salmonella typhimurium*. At least 4 dose levels (4-2500μg/plate) with 3-5 plates per dose were used.

RESULTS

In Vitro Experiments. EDB consistently increased the number of revertants in a dose-related fashion in *Salmonella typhimurium* strains TA1535 and 100. The response was enhanced in the presence of an S-9 fraction derived from

Aroclor-induced rats (9000g supernatant from a liver homogenate) Fig 1. Disulfiram showed no mutagenic effects in any of the strains used, either in the presence or absence of S-9. When EDB was tested with S-9 in the presence of the highest non-toxic dose of disulfiram (100μg), no significant overall increase in the number of revertants was seen over that observed with EDB alone. Similarly, when EDB was tested in the presence of an S-9 fraction derived from disulfiram-induced rats ($0.4gkg^{-1}$ for 4 days), no difference in the mutagenicity was seen compared to an uninduced or Aroclor-induced fraction (Fig 1).

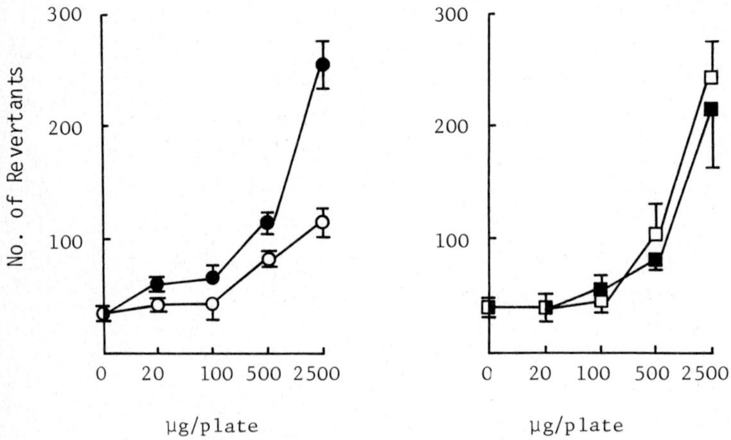

Fig.1. Response of strain TA1535 in the *Salmonella* assay to ethylene dibromide alone ○, and in the presence of (i) an Aroclor-induced S-9 fraction ●, (ii) a disulfiram-induced S-9 fraction ($0.4gkg^{-1}$ daily for four days) □, and (iii) an Aroclor-induced S-9 fraction together with 100μg/plate of disulfiram ■. The bar lines show standard deviations.

Disulfiram was found to inhibit the glutathione-S-transferase activity of rat liver supernatant with a derived K_i value for CDNB as substrate of 28μM. The inhibition was of a 'mixed' or 'non-competitive' nature. A similar inhibition profile was found with an Aroclor-induced rat liver fraction. The high K_m aldehyde dehydrogenase activity of an Aroclor-induced S-9 fraction was also inhibited by disulfiram, but only after a 30 minute preincubation period. The activity of the low K_m enzyme was too small to be measured accurately. Neither of these effects on enzymes observed *in vitro* therefore affected the mutagenicity of EDB in the *Salmonella* assay.

In Vivo Experiments. Liver aldehyde dehydrogenase and glutathione-S-transferase activities were measured in rats dosed daily with $0.4gkg^{-1}$

disulfiram over a period of 8 days. The low K_m mitochondrial aldehyde dehydrogenase activity was reduced by 85% within 24 hours, while the glutathione-S-transferase activity was increased by up to 150% after 6 days (Fig 2). Cytochrome P450 levels were depressed by 30-40% over the period studied. Similar changes in enzyme activities were observed after 9 days dosing of $0.1 gkg^{-1}$ disulfiram. This is approximately the dose which would have been received in the EDB/disulfiram carcinogenicity study.

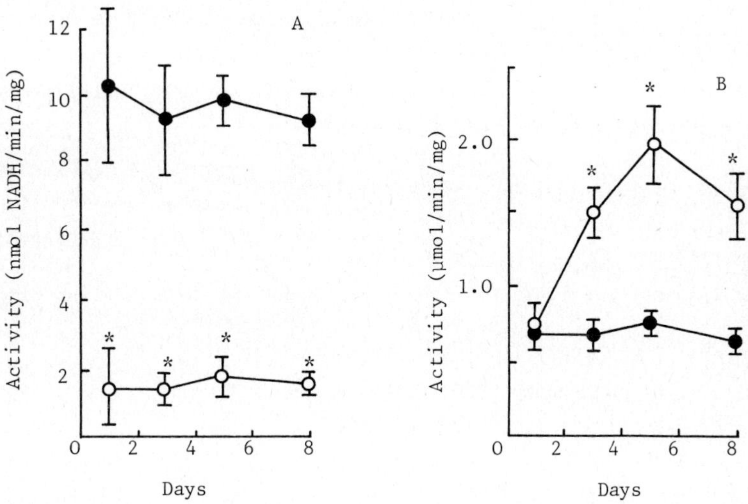

Fig. 2. Changes in activity of the mitochondrial low K_m aldehyde dehydrogenase (A) and supernatant glutathione-S-transferase (B) enzymes in the livers of Alderley Park rats dosed daily with disulfiram, ○ ($0.4 gkg^{-1}$). *p 0.05 c.f. controls, ●. n = 4 ± standard deviations.

DISCUSSION

There is evidence for two distinct pathways in the metabolism of EDB (itself an alkylating agent) each of which may produce metabolites capable of reacting covalently with DNA. The first, conjugation with glutathione via the glutathione-S-transferase enzymes[10] (normally a detoxification pathway) may yield a potentially carcinogenic sulphur half-mustard. The second, an oxidative pathway, yields bromoacetaldehyde[11] which by analogy with chloro-acetaldehyde would be expected to react with DNA[12].

In the rat we have shown disulfiram to increase the activity of the glutathione-S-transferase enzymes and to decrease the activity of certain aldehyde dehydrogenase enzymes (those responsible for the oxidation of acetaldehyde *in vivo*), each of which changes could enhance the reactivity to

DNA of EDB as outlined above. However, the studies *in vitro* showed that disulfiram *inhibits* the activity of the glutathione-S-transferase enzymes and only inhibits the aldehyde dehydrogenase enzymes after a period of pre-incubation with the enzyme. When EDB was tested for mutagenicity in the *Salmonella* assay (widely used as a predictive test for carcinogenicity) in the presence or absence of disulfiram or in the presence of a disulfiram-induced S-9 fraction, no significant change in test response was observed. The marked synergism seen *in vivo* between EDB and disulfiram therefore appears to be specific to the intact animal and incapable of being simulated *in vitro*. It is therefore important to consider that certain protective or synergistic effects which rely upon enzyme induction or another process requiring the whole animal may not be seen in *in vitro* screening tests.

REFERENCES

1. National Cancer Institute Carcinogenesis Technical Report Series (1978) NCI-CG-TR-86.
2. National Cancer Institute Carcinogenesis Technical Report Series (1979) NCI-CG-TR-166.
3. Wattenberg, L.W. (1978) Adv. Cancer Res. 26, 197-226.
4. Zemaitis, M.A. and Greene, F.E. (1976) Biochem. Pharmacol. 25, 1355-1360.
5. Plotnick, H.B. (1978) J.A.M.A. 239, 1609.
6. Tottmar, S.O.C., Petterson, H. and Keissling, K.H. (1973) Biochem. J. 135, 577-586.
7. Habig, W.H., Pabst, M.J. and Jakoby, W.B. (1974) J. Biol. Chem. 249, 7130-7139.
8. Omura, T. and Sato, R. (1964) J. Biol. Chem. 239,2370-2385.
9. Ames, B.N., McCann, J. and Yamasaki, E. (1975) Mut. Res. 31, 347-364.
10. Nachtomi, E. (1970) Biochem. Pharmacol. 19, 2853-2860.
11. Hill, D.L., Shih, T.W., Johnson, T.P. and Struck, R.F. (1978) Cancer Res. 38, 2438-2442.
12. Green, T. and Hathway, D.E. (1978) Chem. Biol. Interact. 22, 211-224.

© 1980 Elsevier/North-Holland Biomedical Press
Mechanisms of Toxicity and Hazard Evaluation
B. Holmstedt, R. Lauwerys, M. Mercier, M. Roberfroid eds

INCREASED SENSITIVITY OF THE SCE-TEST WITH RABBIT LYMPHOCYTES BY AN EXOGENEOUS METABOLIC SYSTEM

D.H. Waalkens, H.F.P. Joosten, T.D. Yih and A. Hoekstra
Drug Safety R&D Labs, Organon International B.V., Oss, The Netherlands

INTRODUCTION

Sister-Chromatid Exchanges (SCEs) were discovered in 1958[1]. Since then, several investigators reported that many physical and chemical agents could increase the frequency of SCEs. The idea was born to use SCEs for the detection of environmental mutagens[2]. However, the autoradiographic method used by Taylor was impractical for large-scale testing of chemicals. Important progress in the development of the SCE test was made when staining techniques became available.

The chromatids of each chromosome can be differentially stained when the thymidine analogue 5-bromodeoxyuridine (BrdUrd) is incorporated into DNA during two successive cell cycles. Differential incorporation of BrdUrd causes differential stainability with the fluorescent dye Hoechst 33258 and Giemsa stain[3] and this practical technique can be applied in mutagenicity testing. The method is quick and simple and can be used in vitro as well as in vivo.

The studies of Carrano et al.[4] indicated a linear relationship between induced SCEs and gene mutations. Furthermore, SCEs are a far more sensitive parameter for chromosome damage than chromosome aberrations[5]. As a result of the many advantages mentioned, the SCE test is now considered to be a practical and useful cytogenetic test for the prediction of mutagenicity and carcinogenicity of chemicals.

A severe limitation of the in vtro SCE test is its lack of response to chemicals that require metabolic activation. Many cultured cell types have a poor drug metabolic activity, but cultured lymphocytes are better than most other types of cells in this respect. For example, the indirect-acting mutagens urethane and benzpyrene cause SCEs in cultured human lymphocytes[6,7]. Rabbit lymphocytes can also activate benzpyrene, but Chinese Hamster Ovary (CHO) cells need exogeneous metabolic activation to produce SCEs with benzpyrene [9]. Cyclophosphamide, another indirect-acting mutagen[10,11], causes SCEs in rabbit, rat and human lymphocytes[12], but is only slightly active or inactive in CHO cells[5,13].

Although cultured lymphocytes possess the drug metabolic machinery to convert indirect-acting mutagens into their mutagenic metabolites, their capacity is too low for their use, without an exogeneous metabolic system, for the detection of indirect-acting mutagens. This problem can be solved by incorporating into the test system a post-mitochondrial (S-9) fraction prepared from rat liver[14] plus an NADPH-generating system, together forming the socalled S-9 mix.

This paper describes the results obtained with cultured rabbit lymphocytes exposed to cyclophosphamide in the absence and in the presence of S-9 mix.

MATERIAL AND METHODS

Lymphocyte culture. Microcultures of peripheral lymphocytes were set up from heparinized blood obtained by ear venipuncture from 3 to 4 adult male Dutch rabbits. Cultures comprised 0.3 ml whole blood and 5 ml medium (pH 7.2). The medium consisted of RPMI (Flow, U.K.), 69 ml; foetal calf serum (Gibco, U.K.), 20 ml; 200 mM L-glutamine (Gibco, U.K.), 1.4 ml; a mixture of penicillin and streptomycin (10.000 units per ml) (Gibco, U.K.), 1.77 ml; 7.5% $NaHCO_3$, 2.7 ml; reconstituted phytohaemagglutinin (PHA) (Wellcome) or 5-bromo-2'-deoxyuridine (Koch-Light, U.K.) (0.1 mg BrdUrd per ml), 5 ml.

The cells were grown in the dark in glass tubes with a metal cap for 53 h at 37°C in a humidified atmosphere of 5% CO_2 in air at pH 7.2. Colchicine (1μg per ml) was added for the final 3 h.

Metabolic activation system. Lymphocyte cultures were exposed to cyclophosphamide (CP) (Asta Werke, Brackwede) (dissolved in HBBS) at several concentrations and a mixture (S-9 mix) of a 9000 g post-mitochondrial supernatant prepared from homogenized Aroclor-induced rat livers (S-9) and cofactors. S-9 was prepared according to Ames et al.[14]. The S-9 mix contained 50% (by volume) S-9 rat liver extract. The cofactor solution was composed as follows : 25 mM $MgSO_4$, 33 mM KCl, 5 mM glucose 6-phosphate, 4 mM NADP and 0.1 M

Na_2HPO_4 - NaH_2PO_4 buffer (pH 7.4). S-9 mix was added to the cultures at a volume of 50 μl per ml medium resulting in a final S-9 content of 2.5%.

Induction of SCEs

(a) exposure for 29 hours without S-9 mix

Lymphocytes were first grown for 24 h with PHA but without BrdUrd, after which the culture tubes were centrifuged and the supernatant discarded. The pelletted cells were then resuspended in medium containing CP at the desired concentration and BrdUrd, but no PHA. Incubation was then continued for 29 h before fixation.

(b) exposure for 3 hours with and without S-9 mix

To lymphocyte cultures incubated for 24 h, CP and S-9 mix were added. The culture tubes were centrifuged after 3 h of exposure and the supernatant discarded. The pelletted cells were washed in phosphate-buffered saline and finally resuspended in culture medium with BrdUrd but no PHA for continued growth for an additional 26 h before fixation.

Preparation of slides and staining. After 53 h, the cells obtained from treatment (a) or (b) were spun down and treated at room temperature with 0.075 M KCl for 5 min, spun down again and fixed in methanol - glacial acetic acid 3 : 1 (3 washes). Fixed cells were spread on to wet, chilled micoscope slides followed by ignition of the fixative in a gas flame. Cell preparations were stained by the Fluorescence Plus Giemsa (FPG) technique[3]. First they were stained with a solution of the fluorescent dye Hoechst 33258 (Riedel-de Haën, Hannover) (50 μg per ml) in 0.067 M Sörensen buffer pH 7.0 for 15 min. The slides were next mounted in 0.16 M phosphate - 0.04 M citrate buffer pH 7.0 and exposed to light from an UV lamp (Philips MPW 125W) at a distance of 30 cm for 2 h. After illumination the slides were kept in 2x SSC (0.3 M NaCl in 0.03 M trisodium citrate, pH 7.2) at $\pm$ 60°C for 20 min. Finally, the slides were rinsed with distilled water and stained for 30 min in 5% Giemsa dye (Merck, Darmstadt) dissolved in 5 mM phosphate buffer (pH 6.8).

Collection of data. The yield of SCEs expressed as the number of SCEs per cell was obtained from scoring 15-20 differentially stained metaphases per culture for each concentration by direct observation of slides under oil immersion (magnification x1000). Mean values were calculated for the parallel cultures from 3 - 4 rabbits. Differences between CP-exposed and control cultures were statistically assessed with the Wilcoxon test.

RESULTS

The frequency of SCEs in control cells was about 5 SCEs per cell. Exposure for 29 h in the absence of S-9 mix caused a significant increase in the number of SCEs per cell at a CP concentration of 10^{-4} M. When the time of exposure in the absence of S-9 mix was reduced to 3 h, an increased frequency of SCEs could still be demonstrated, but the effect was smaller and occurred at higher concentrations of CP, the lowest effective concentration being 10^{-3} M. Under similar conditions of exposure for 3 h, but in the presence of S-9 mix, a significantly increased SCE frequency was observed at much lower concentrations of CP. The lowest effective concentration in the presence of S-9 mix was 10^{-6} M.

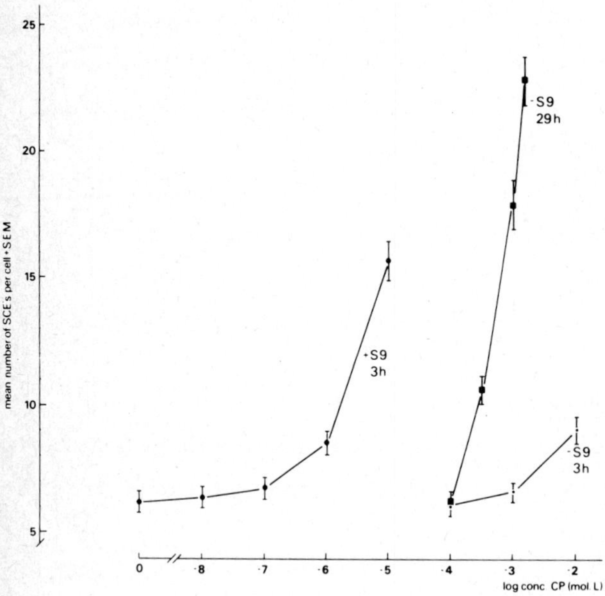

Fig. 1. SCE induction in rabbit lymphocytes with CP. ●——● with S-9 mix for 3h, ▣——▣ without S-9 mix for 3h, ■——■ without S-9 mix for 29 h.

DISCUSSION

As reported previously[12], incubation of rabbit lymphocytes with CP for 29 h beginning at 24 h after starting the culture, caused a significant increase in the SCE frequency at concentrations of 10^{-4} M and higher. This fact indicates that cultured lymphocytes have some drug metabolic activity of their own, as it is known that CP must first be metabolized in order to become effective as a chromosome damaging drug[10] or as a mutagen in bacteria[11]. However, the

capacity to metabolize this indirect-acting mutagen is small in view of the fact that a long exposure time and a relatively high concentration of CP were required to produce the effect. Even when the exposure time was restricted to 3 h, an effect on SCE frequency could be demonstrated, but the effect was small and occurred at a 10 x higher concentration of CP as compared with incubation for 29 h. Under similar conditions of exposure for 3 h, but in the presence of S-9 mix, an increased SCE frequency was established at 10^{-6} M. This concentration of CP is 1000 x lower than the effective concentration in the absence of S-9 mix.
This observation shows that the sensitivity of the test system for CP was very much increased by the addition of S-9 mix. The results further indicate that the duration of exposure of 3 h and the composition of the S-9 mix were adequate, but this does not necessarily mean that they were optimal.

Several combinations of S-9 content, duration and time of exposure and composition of the cofactor solution have been shown to be effective. It is well known that high concentrations of S-9 are toxic to the lymphocytes. An S-9 content of 5% in the culture was too toxic for human lymphocytes, but good results were obtained with 2%[15]. Positive results were reported with lower S-9 contents of 0.5 and 0.2 % in a study with CP in CHO cells[16]. The duration of exposure varies also between laboratories. Periods of 20 min[16], one hour[6] and two hours[15] have been used with success. Large variations between laboratories with respect to NADP and G-6-P concentrations in the incubation mixture can be found in the published reports. These are caused mainly by differences in dilution of the cofactor solution when the S-9 mix is prepared and when the S-9 mix is added to the culture. Another variable is the location in time during the culture period when exposure takes place. Human lymphocytes at 48 h after setting up the cultures responded better to CP with S-9 mix than those exposed immediately at the start of culture[15]. This could be related to the PHA-mediated stimulation of the induction of enzymes in the lymphocytes[8]. A systematic study of the relevance of these variables with the aim to establish the optimal conditions should be undertaken.

The present results show that the sensitivity of the SCE test for an indirect-acting mutagen like CP can be very much increased by incorporating an exogeneous drug metabolic system prepared from rat liver.

The use of the cultured lymphocytes may offer a special advantage in that the cells own drug metabolic machinery is complemented by the exogeneous rat liver drug metabolic system.

ACKNOWLEDGEMENTS

The authors gratefully acknowledge the skillful technical assistance of Mrs W. Benneker and Mr A. v.d. Bergh.

REFERENCES

1. Taylor, J.H. (1958) Genetics, 43, 515-529.
2. Perry, P.E. (1980) in : Chemical Mutagens, Plenum Press, vol. 6., pp.1-39.
3. Perry, P. and Wolff, S. (1974) Nature, 251, 156-158.
4. Carrano, A.V., Thompson, L.H., Lindl , P.A. and Minkler, J.L. (1978) Nature, 271, 551-553.
5. Perry, P. and Evans, H.J., (1975) Nature, 258, 121-125.
6. Csukas, I., Gungl, I., Fedorcsak, I., Vida, G., Antoni, F., Tutoczky, I. and Solymory, F. (1979) Mut. Res., 67, 315-319.
7. Rüdiger, H.W., Kohl, F., Mangels, W., von Wichert, P., Bartram, C.R., Wöhler, W. and Passarge, E. (1976) Nature, 262, 290-292.
8. Takehisa, S. and Wolff, S. (1978) Mut. Res., 58, 321-329.
9. Takehisa, S. and Wolff, S. (1977) Mut. Res., 45, 263-270
10. Foley, G.E., Friedman, O.M. and Drolet, B.P. (1961) Cancer Res., 21, 57.
11. Herbold, B. and Buselmayer, W. (1976) Mut. Res. , 40, 73-84.
12. Waalkens, D.H., Joosten, H.F.P., Taalman, R., Scheres, J.M.J.C., Yih, T.D. and Hoekstra, A. (1980) Mut. Res., 74, 222.
13. De Raat, W.K. (1977) Chem. Biol. Interac., 19, 125-131.
14. Ames, B.N., McCann, J. and Yamasaki, E. (1975) Mut. Res., 31, 347-365.
15. White, A.D. and Hesketh, L.C., (1980) Mut. Res. , 69, 283-291.
16. Stetka, D.G. and Wolff, S. (1976) Mut. Res. , 41, 343-350.

EARLY CHANGES IN CHEMICAL CARCINOGENESIS

Symposium chairmen: W.N. Aldridge and J.E. Gielen

© 1980 Elsevier/North-Holland Biomedical Press
Mechanisms of Toxicity and Hazard Evaluation
B. Holmstedt, R. Lauwerys, M. Mercier, M. Roberfroid eds

ACTIVATION OF CHEMICALS TO PROXIMAL CARCINOGENS

TAKASHI SUGIMURA, KEIJI WAKABAYASHI, MICHIYUKI YAMADA, MINAKO NAGAO and TADAHIKO FUJINO
National Cancer Center Research Institute, 5-1-1, Tsukiji, Chuo-ku, Tokyo 104 (Japan)

I. GENERAL ASPECTS

It is well established that most carcinogens are metabolically activated to ultimate forms through proximate forms[1-3]. The ultimate form, which is called an ultimate carcinogen, readily reacts with cellular macromolecules, such as DNA, RNA and proteins, and also reacts with low-molecular weight cellular constituents, such as glutathione. The change produced in DNA bases by the ultimate carcinogen results in mutation; namely, change in the DNA base sequence through various mechanisms, such as error-prone repair[4]. In this sense, procarcinogens, proximate carcinogens and ultimate carcinogens correspond to promutagens, proximate mutagens and ultimate mutagens, respectively. Some carcinogens, including N-methyl-N'-nitro-N-nitrosoguanidine, methylnitrosourea and β-propiolactone, are directly reactive, *per se*, but most carcinogens, especially those occurring in our environment are procarcinogens, and must be metabolically activated in the body. Many enzymes are involved in this metabolic activation, the most intensively studied of which are drug-metabolizing enzymes located in the microsomal fraction of liver and represented by cytochrome P-450s[1-3].

Most typical carcinogens, such as benzo(a)pyrene, 2-acetylaminofluorene and aflatoxin B_1 are metabolized by microsomal enzymes. Benzo(a)pyrene is converted to various metabolites, the most important ultimate form being 7,8-dihydrodiol-9,10-epoxide[5,6], and cytochrome P-448 is involved in this conversion[7,8]. The ultimate form of 2-acetylaminofluorene is N-sulfonoxy-2-acetylaminofluorene. Its conversion involves N-hydroxylation catalyzed by cytochrome P-448[9], followed by esterification by 3'-phosphoadenosine 5'-phosphosulfate and sulfotransferase[10]. Aflatoxin B_1 is converted to its ultimate form, aflatoxin B_1-2,3-oxide, by cytochrome P-450[11,12]. The pathways of these metabolic activations are illustrated in Fig. 1. P-448 and P-450 of rat liver are induced by intraperitoneal injections of methylcholathrene and phenobarbital, respectively, and both can be induced by injection of polychlorinated biphenyls (PCB)[13,14]. Thus PCB has been most widely used in preparation of microsomes rich in both P-448 and P-450. But use of PCB is actually unsuitable, because PCB is scarcely degraded in the body, and so it is safer to induce both P-448 and P-450 by simultaneous administration of β-naphthoflavone and phenobarbital[15,16]. The ultimate metabolites are mostly electrophiles and can form various adducts with nucleic acid bases, typical examples being N-(guan-2-yl)-7,8,9,10-tetrahydrobenzo(a)pyrene[17], N-(guan-8-yl)-2-acetylaminofluorene[18] and 2-(guan-7-yl)-3-hydroxyaflatoxin B_1[19].

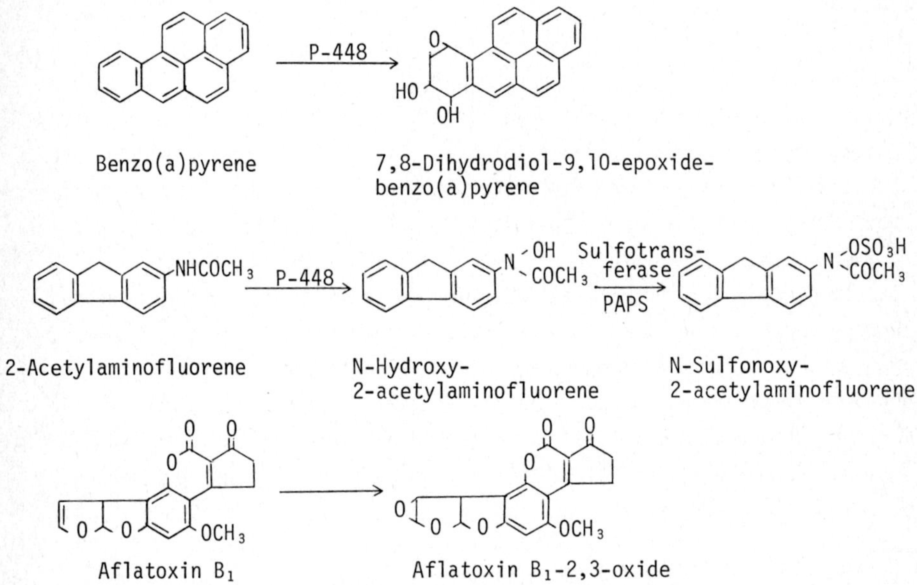

Fig. 1. Metabolic activation of benzo(a)pyrene, 2-acetylaminofluorene and aflatoxin B_1.

II. SPECIFIC FEATURE OF ACTIVATION OF 4-NITROQUINOLINE 1-OXIDE

A little known, but unique, metabolic pathway for activation is that of the potent mutagen and carcinogen, 4-nitroquinoline 1-oxide (4-NQO). This potent mutagen is first reduced to 4-hydroxyaminoquinoline 1-oxide (4-HAQO). In rat liver this reduction is mainly catalyzed by DT-diaphorase[20], but in most living cells, ranging from mammalian fibroblasts to *Escherichia coli*, this reduction was catalyzed by a not well defined oxidoreductase with concomitant oxidation of NADH or NADPH. On further reduction, 4-aminoquinoline is formed, which has far less mutagenicity[21] and carcinogenicity[20].

It is noteworthy that 4-HAQO is a proximate carcinogen, not an ultimate one; the ultimate form of 4-HAQO has not yet been isolated as a stable compound. However Tada and Tada found that ATP, L-serine and the supernatant fraction of rat liver were required for formation of the 4-HAQO-base adduct[22], and it has been postulated that seryl-tRNA synthetase can yield a reactive metabolite in the presence of L-serine and ATP. Seryl-4-HAQO is a putative ultimate form of 4-NQO. Since an oxidoreductase yielding 4-HAQO and seryl-tRNA synthetase is present in most living cells, 4-NQO is mutagenic with a microbial system and carcinogenic with a *in vivo* mammalian system. 4-NQO exerts its mutagenicity without any addition of rat liver microsomal enzymes. 4-NQO is neither a direct mutagen nor a direct carcinogen, but it is activated to its ultimate form by enzyme systems present in both microbes and mammalian cells. This is one reason why 4-NQO has been widely used as a tool in molecular biological studies on mammalian cells cultured *in vitro* as well as on microbial cells. The activation of 4-NQO to an ultimate form is shown schematically in Fig. 2. 4-NQO can produce several adducts with DNA-bases and these are removed by excision repair[23]. UV-Sensitive mutant cells, represented by human xeroderma pigmentosum cells, are abnormally sensitive to 4-NQO, and in these cells the 4-NQO derived base adducts of quinoline in DNA persist for longer than in normal cells[24,25]. The same is true of a UV-sensitive mutant of *Escherichia coli*[23].

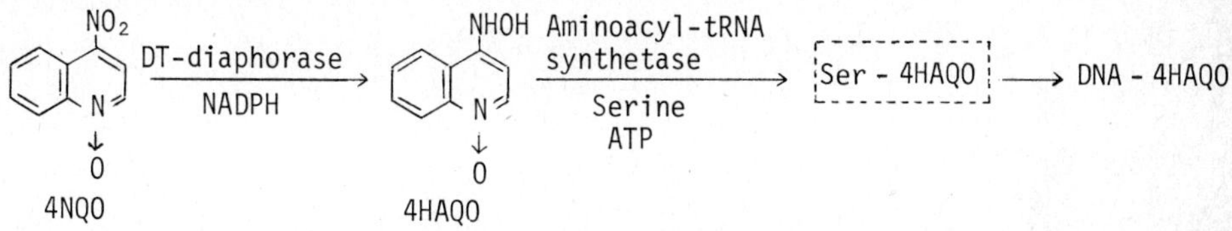

Fig. 2. Metabolic activation of 4-nitroquinoline 1-oxide

Some aromatic amines and azo-dyes have also been suggested to be activated by seryl-tRNA synthetase in a step yielding an ultimate mutagen[26]. However, before this step, these compounds must be metabolized by enzymes located in the microsomal fraction and catalyzing N-hydroxylation or N-demethylation[3,27].

III. METABOLIC ACTIVATION OF HETEROCYCLIC AMINE MUTAGENS FROM PYROLYSATES OF AMINO ACIDS

Our laboratory has been engaged in studies on naturally occurring mutagens and carcinogens for several years. Many new potent mutagens have been isolated from pyrolysates of amino acids and proteins and also from cooked foods, and identified as shown in Table 1. Most of these compounds are heterocyclic aromatic amines, and some of them have higher specific mutagenic activities than

TABLE 1. NEW MUTAGENS FROM PYROLYSATES

Full Name (Abbreviation)	Structure	Source	Spec. Mut. Act. Revertants/μg TA98, +S-9 mix	*In Vitro* Carcino-genicity	*In Vivo* Carcino-genicity	Existing in
3-Amino-1,4-dimethyl-5*H*-pyrido[4,3-*b*]indole (Trp-P-1)	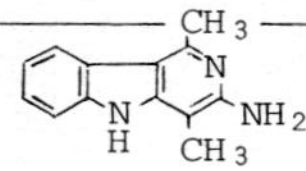	Tryptophan pyrolysate[28]	39,000	+	+	Broiled sardine, pyrolysates of casein, gluten, globulin, albumin, chicken meat, horse mackerel
3-Amino-1-methyl-5*H*-pyrido[4,3-*b*]indole (Trp-P-2)	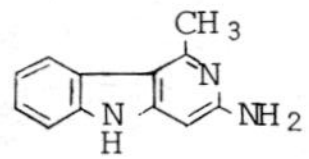	"	104,000	+	+	
2-Amino-6-methyldipyrido-[1,2-*a*:3',2'-*d*]imidazole (Glu-P-1)	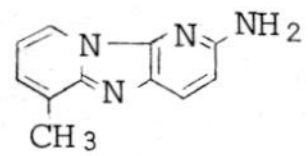	Glutamic acid pyrolysate[29]	49,000	+	a	
2-Amino-dipyrido[1,2-*a*:3',2'-*d*]imidazole (Glu-P-2)	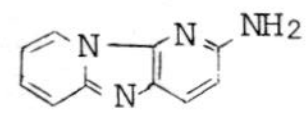	"	1,900	-	a	Broiled dried-squid, pyrolysate of casein
2-Amino-5-phenylpyridine (Phe-P-1)	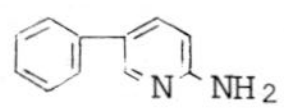	Phenylalanine pyrolysate[28]	41	b	b	
3,4-Cyclopentenopyrido-[3,2-*a*]carbazole (Lys-P-1)	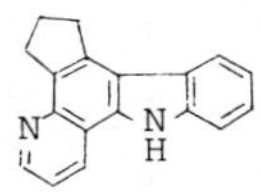	Lysine pyrolysate[30]	86	-	b	
2-Amino-α-carboline (AαC)	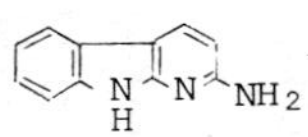	Soybean globulin pyrolysate[31]	300	-	a	Pyrolysates of tryptophan, casein gluten, globluin, albumin, chicken meat, horse mackerel
2-Amino-3-methyl-α-carboline (MeAαC)	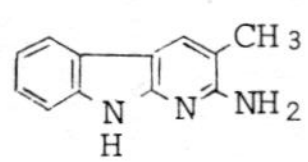	"	200	-	a	
2-Amino-3-methylimidazo-[4,5-*f*]quinoline (IQ)	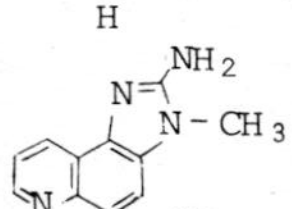	Broiled sardine[32]	433,000	a	a	Heated beef extract
2-Amino-3,4-dimethyl-imidazo[4,5-*f*]quinoline (MeIQ)	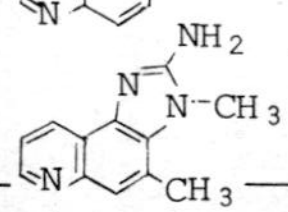	"	661,000	b	a	

[a] On going. [b] Not tested yet.

aflatoxin B_1. *In vitro* and *in vivo* carcinogenesis tests on these compounds are in progress. *In vivo* carcinogenicity tests have already shown that Trp-P-1 and Trp-P-2, isolated from pyrolysates of DL-tryptophan, are hepatocarcinogenic[33]. Trp-P-1 and Trp-P-2 are 3-amino-1,4-dimethyl-5*H*-pyrido[4,3-*b*]indole and 3-amino-1-methyl-5*H*-pyrido[4,3-*b*]indole, respectively[28], and they are more mutagenic *Salmonella typhimurium* TA98 than to TA100[34].

Recently, information was obtained about the metabolism of Trp-P-1. To exert their mutagenicity Trp-P-1 and the other new mutagens must be metabolically activated by S-9 mix of rat liver, or enzymes in human liver. The S-9 fraction from rats injected intraperitoneally with 3-methylcholanthrene has a higher capacity to induce mutagenicity of Trp-P-1 than of phenobarbital[35], indicating that P-448, but not P-450, is mainly involved in the activation. Consistent with this, in experiments using mixtures of purified P-448 or P-450 with NADPH oxidoreductase and a necessary lipid component, the mutagenicity of Trp-P-1 was demonstrated with the system containing P-448, but not P-450[35]. P-448 and P-450 were purified from the livers of rats treated with 3-methylcholanthrene and phenobarbital, respectively[35]. Experiments using genetically defined mice, responsive (Ah^b) and nonresponsive (Ah^d), showed that enzyme activating Trp-P-1, Trp-P-2, Glu-P-1, Glu-P-2, AαC and MeAαC was present in the liver of responsive (Ah^b) mice, but not nonresponsive (Ah^d) mice, after injection of PCB[36]. These data are also consistent with the results described above on systems containing purified P-448 and P-450.

Incubation of Trp-P-2 with microsomes and cofactors yielded several metabolites, which could be separated by thin layer chromatography and high pressure liquid chromatography. One metabolite among several showed mutagenicity toward TA98 without addition of S-9 mix. It may be the hydroxyamino derivative[37]. This compound is probably activated by enzymes present in *Salmonella* cells themselves. When Trp-P-2 was incubated *in vitro* with DNA and S-9 mix, the mutagen was covalently bound to DNA. The structure of the adduct (Fig. 3) indicates that the hydroxyamino derivative of Trp-P-2 reacted with DNA[38]. Since Glu-P-1, Glu-P-2, AαC and MeAαC are structurally related, as shown in Table 1, these compounds may have a common metabolic pathway and reactive form[39].

Recently two potent new mutagens were isolated from broiled sardines, cooked in the way generally used in Japanese homes. These compounds, with the structures 2-amino-3-methylimidazo[4,5-*f*]quinoline (IQ) and 2-amino-3,4-dimethylimidazo[4,5-*f*]quinoline (MeIQ), as shown in Table 1, are probably identical to the mutagens found in broiled hamburger and beef extract after prolonged cooking[40]. These heterocyclic aromatic amines seem to be important in relation to human cancer, because they are found in heated or cooked human foods.

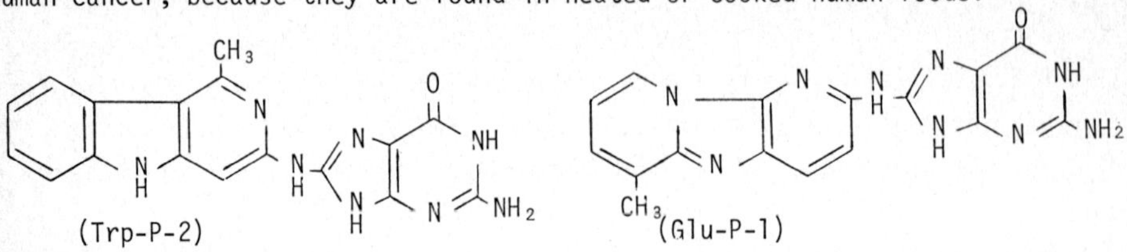

Fig. 3. 3-(C[8]-guanyl)amino-1-methyl-5*H*-pyrido[4,3-*b*]indole   2-(C[8]-guanyl)amino-6-methyl-dypyrido[1,2-*a*:3',2'-*d*]imidazole

An interesting reaction is involved in the metabolism these heterocyclic amines. Peroxidase in the presence of hydrogen peroxide (H_2O_2) was reported to activate aromatic hydrocarbon and to produce N-acetoxy-2-acetylaminofluorene from N-hydroxy-2-acetylaminofluorene[41,42]; in other words, peroxidase causes metabolic activation. Yamada et al. purified myeloperoxidase from human promyelocytic leukemia, HL-60 cells[43]. Incubation of Trp-P-1 with myeloperoxidase and H_2O_2 resulted in loss of the mutagenic activity of Trp-P-1 on *Salmonella typhimurium* TA98. Of course, in the presence of myeloperoxidase and H_2O_2, Trp-P-1 did not induce any revertants of *Salmonella typhimurium* TA98. Similar decreases in mutagenicities of other heterocyclic amines, Trp-P-2, Glu-P-1, and AαC, were observed, as shown in Table 2. At least two metabolites were separated after incubation of ^{14}C-Trp-P-2 with myeloperoxidase and H_2O_2, and none of them was mutagenic toward *Salmonella typhimurium* TA98, indicating that myeloperoxidase catalyzed the reaction in the direction of inactivation of the promutagen and/or proximate mutagen[43]. Thus this reaction is entirely different from the activation reaction of procarcinogenic aromatic hydrocarbons by peroxidase and H_2O_2 [41,43,44]. However, it was observed that the radioactivity of ^{14}C-Trp-P-2 bound with albumin, added during incubation of ^{14}C-Trp-P-2 with myeloperoxidase and H_2O_2; both myeloperoxidase and H_2O_2 were essential for this binding of radioactivity. Inclusion of DNA or RNA instead of protein did not result in any significant incorporation of radioactivity into nucleic acids. These results do not rule out the possiblity that a small amount of binding of Trp-P-2 with DNA is catalyzed by the peroxidase-H_2O_2 system, but they show that the activated form of Trp-P-2 produced with the peroxidase and H_2O_2 system reacts more readily with protein. This binding with protein is much faster than that with nucleic acids. Thus even supposing that the activated metabolite of Trp-P-2 formed with the peroxidase-H_2O_2 system does in fact react with nucleic acids, proteins seem to act as a protective system, removing the reactant before it can react with nucleic acids.

TABLE 2
THE LOSS OF MUTAGENICITIES BY MYELOPEROXIDASE (MPO) AND HYDROGEN PEROXIDE (H_2O_2)

Compound	Additon	Induced revertants (%)
Trp-P-1	None	100
	MPO+H_2O_2	20.0
Trp-P-2	None	100
	MPO+H_2O_2	1.3
Glu-P-1	None	100
	MPO+H_2O_2	23.9
AαC	None	100
	MPO+H_2O_2	26.7

As described above, a metabolic system that acts as an activation step for a certain procarcinogen, acts as an inactivation step for another procarcinogen. Glucuronides have been considered as typical inactive metabolites of many carcinogens. However, Miller and Miller and their associates found that N-hydroxy-2-acetylaminofluorene glucuronide is actually a reactive form that can bind directly with nucleic acids[45]. Thus the metabolic pathways of promutagens to ultimate forms and to inactive forms seems to cris-cross in cells, and the actual metabolic paths may be even more complicated than those known at present.

IV. COMUTAGENIC ACTION OF NORHARMAN-METABOLIC ASPECTS

Norharman is β-carboline produced by pyrolysis of tryptophan[28]. Holmstedt and his colleagues reported the presence of many β-carboline derivatives also in plants[46,47]. Norharman is itself non-mutagenic, but it was found to enhance the mutagenicities of Trp-P-1 and Trp-P-2[48]. This enhancement was observed in the presence of an appropriate amount of S-9[49]. Norharman also enhances the mutagenicity of N-dimethylaminoazobenzene with any amount of S-9[50]. Furthermore, an interesting finding was that although aniline and *o*-toluidine are carcinogenic[51,52], their mutagenicities could not be demonstrated in Ames' test even with a preincubation step, but on adding of norharman and S-9 mix during preincubation these compounds became mutagenic to *Salmonella*, as illustrated in Fig. 4[53]. This mutagenicity was dose-dependent. *m*-Toluidine and *p*-toluidine themselves were not mutagenic, even in the presence of norharman[53]. Incidentally *m*-toluidine and *p*-toluidine are non-carcinogenic. The mutagenicities of chemicals demonstrated in the presence of norharman are closely related to their carcinogenicities. Furthermore the mutagenicity of yellow OB, a known carcinogen[54], was demonstrated in the presence of norharman, as also shown in Fig. 4[49,55].

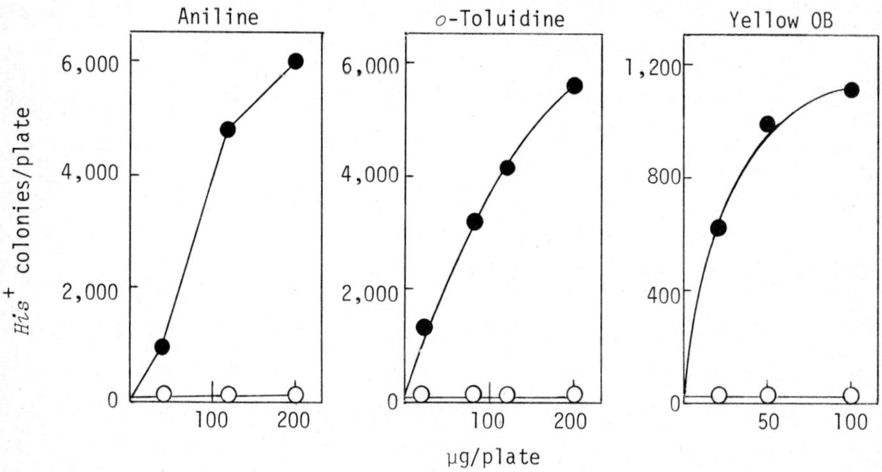

Fig. 4. Comutagenic effect of norharman with aniline, *o*-toluidine and yellow OB. Each test compound was preincubated with 0.1 ml of culture of TA98 and 0.5 ml of S-9 mix with (o——o) or without (o——o) 200 μg of norharman.

Norharman intercalates weakly between DNA base-pairs[56]. This intercalation was confirmed by demonstrating change in the UV spectrum and fluorescence of norharman solution on addition of DNA solution. Agarose gel electrophoresis of phage fd DNA after treatment with DNase and DNA ligase in the presence of norharman indicated unwinding of the double helix of DNA. This intercalation, which was also confirmed by Pezzuto et al.[57], may result in a local structural change in DNA, to a form which is more susceptible to an ultimate carcinogen or which produces conditions favouring error-prone repair.

Norharman also has metabolic effects . Ho et al. found that norharman and related β-carboline derivatives inhibit monoamine oxidase[58], and Fujino et al. found that norharman inhibited the conversion of hydrophobic metablites of benzo(a)pyrene to hydrophilic metabolites[59]. The effects of norharman on cultured mammalian cells have also been studied[60,61].

When a compound is not itself mutagenic, but becomes mutagenic in the presence of norharman, norharman is said to act as a comutagen. Norharman itself is not mutagenic at all. It is interesting that this comutagenic action has been observed only with aromatic amines, aniline, *o*-toluidine and yellow OB, and recently also with 3-aminopyridine[62]. Table 3 shows its comutagenic actions with various aromatic amines and heterocyclic amines.

TABLE 3

COMUTAGENIC ACTIONS OF NORHARMAN ON AROMATIC AND HETEROAROMATIC AMINES

Compound	Comutagenic effect by norharman
Aniline	+
p-Aminophenol	-
Phenylhydroxylamine	+
o-Toluidine	+
m-Toluidine	-
p-Toluidine	-
Yellow OB	+
2-Aminopyridine	-
3-Aminopyridine	+
4-Aminopyridine	-

During studies under the International Program for the Evaluation of Short-term test for Carcinogenicity coordinated by de Serres and Ashby, N,N-diphenylnitrosamine (DPhN) was subjected to mutation-tests using *Salmonella typhimurium*. DPhN has been thought to be noncarcinogenic. When the program was inaugurated in 1976, DPhN was selected as a negative control for N-nitrosomorpholine. However, in 1979, Lijinsky et al. demonstrated the carcinogenicity of DPhN[63] and Nagao and Takahashi demonstrated its mutagenicity in the presence of norharman[64]. Wakabayashi et al. examined its comutagenic effects with various derivatives of DPhN[65]. These data are summarized in Table 4. N-methyl-N-phenylnitrosamine, N-ethyl-N-phenylnitrosamine and N-phenyl-N-benzylnitrosamine were mutagenic in the presence of norharman. These four N-nitrosoaromatic amines are good nitrosating agents[66,67]. Therefore, norharman may exert a comutagenic effect through formation of N-nitrosonorharman. However, the mutagenicity of this compound is not enough to explain the comutagenicity of norharman. More revertants were obtained with N,N-diphenylamine than with DPhN in the presence of norharman and S-9 mix. Therefore, the comutagenic action of norharman with DPhN may be due to a metabolite of N,N-diphenylamine produced from DPhN.

The comutagenic actions so far observed have all been greater on TA98, than on TA100. Several possible mechanisms of the comutagenic activity of norharman have been examined. Norharman is converted to several metabolites by S-9 mix, but these metabolites and phenylhydroxylamine did not induce any revertants without S-9 mix. However, when norharman had been incubated with phenylhydroxylamine and S-9 mix, the acetone soluble fraction of the mixture induced many revertants without S-9 mix. Therefore, production of a mutagenic compound from norharman and phenylhydroxylamine seems to be the most plausible mechanisms of the comutagenic action of norharman. The formation of a mutagen(s) in a mixture of norharman and phenylhydroxylamine is catalyzed by visible light.

TABLE 4
COMUTAGENIC ACTIONS OF NORHARMAN ON N-NITROSOAROMATIC AMINES

Compound	Mutagenicity	
	-Norharman	+Norharman
N,N-Diphenylnitrosamine	-	+
N-Methyl-N-phenylnitrosamine	-	+
N-Ethyl-N-phenylnitrosamine	-	+
N-Phenyl-N-benzylnitrosamine	-	+
N-Phenyl-N-naphthylnitrosamine	-	-
N,N-Dibenzylnitrosamine	-	-

V. CONCLUSIVE COMMENTS

Activation of chemicals to proximate and ultimate carcinogens is one of the most important contribution for the past two decades to understand the mechanisms of carcinogenesis. Furthermore the knowledge is being applied to environmental carcinogen screening and also human cancer prevention.

VI. REFERENCES

1. Miller, J.A. and Miller, E.C. (1969) Prog. Exp. Tumor Res., 11, 273-301.
2. Miller, J.A. (1970) Cancer Res., 30, 559-576.
3. Miller, E.C. (1978) Cancer Res., 38, 1479-1496.
4. Witkin, E.M. (1976) Baceteriol. Rev., 40, 869-907.
5. Jerina, D.M., Yagi, H., Hernandez, O., Dansette, P.M., Wood, A.W., Levin, W., Chang, R.L., Wislocki, P.G. and Conney, A.H. (1976) Carcinogenesis-A Comprehensive Survey Vol 1. Polynuclear Aromatic Hydrocarbons: Chemistry, Metabolism, and Carcinogenesis, Raven Press, New York, pp. 91-113.
6. Yang, S.K., McCourt, D.W., Leutz, J.C. and Gelboin, H.V. (1977) Science, 1199-1200.

7. Wood, A.W., Levin, W., Lu, A.Y.H., Yagi, H., Hernandez, O., Jerina, D.M. and Conney, A.H. (1976) J. Biol. Chem. 251, 4882-4890.

8. Kawajiri, K., Yonekawa, H., Harada, N., Noshiro, M., Omura, T. and Tagashira, Y. (1980) Cancer Res., 40, 1652-1657.

9. Kawajiri, D., Personal communication.

10. DeBaun, J.R., Miller, E.C. and Miller, J.A. (1970) Cancer Res., 30, 577-595.

11. Gurtoo, H.L., Dahms, R.P., Kanter, P.M. and Vaught, J.B. (1978) J. Biol. Chem., 253, 3952-3961.

12. Raina, V., Gurtoo, H.L., Berrigan, M. and Paigen, B. (1980) Biochem. Biophys. Res. Commun., 94, 737-743.

13. Alvares, A. and Kappas, A. (1977) J. Biol. Chem., 252, 6373-6378.

14. Ryan, D.E., Thomas, P.E., Korzeniowski, D. and Levin, W. (1979) J. Biol. Chem., 254, 1365-1374.

15. Haugen, D.A., van der Hoeven, T.A. and Coon, M.J. (1975) J. Biol. Chem., 250, 3567-3570.

16. Matsushima, T., Sawamura, M., Hara, K. and Sugimura, T. (1976) In Vitro Mutagenic Activation in Mutagenesis Testing, Elsevier/North-Holland, Amsterdam, pp. 85-88.

17. Jeffrey, A.M., Jennette, K.W., Blobstein, S.H., Weinstein, I.B., Beland, F.A., Harvey, R.G., Kasai, H., Miura, I. and Nakanishi, K. (1976) J. Am. Chem. Soc., 98, 5714-5715.

18. Westra, J.G., Kriek, E. and Hittenhausen, H. (1976) Chem.-Biol. Interactions,15, 149-164.

19. Essigmann, T.M., Croy, R.G., Nadzan, A.M., Busby, W.F. Jr., Reinhold, V.N., Büchi, G., Wogan, G.N. (1977) Proc. Natl. Acad. Sci. USA, 74, 1870-1874.

20. Matsushima, T. and Sugimura, T. (1971) Recent Results Cancer Res., 34, 53-60.

21. Yahagi, T., Nagao, M., Unpublished data,

22. Tada, Mi., and Tada, Ma. (1975) Nature, 255, 510-512.

23. Ikenaga, M., Ichikawa-Ryo, H., Kondo, S. (1975) J. Mol. Biol., 92, 341-356.

24. Takebe, H., Furuyama, J., Miki, Y. and Kondo, S. (1972) Mutation Res., 15, 98- 100.

25. Ikenaga, M., Takebe, H. and Ishii, Y. (1977) Mutation Res., 43, 415-427.

26. Hashimoto, Y., Degawa, M., Watanabe, H. and Tada, M. (1978) Proc. Jap. Cancer Association, The 37th Annual Meeting, pp. 21

27. Arcos, J.C. and Argus, M.F. (1974) Chemical Induction of Cancer, Vol. IIB, pp. 233-243.

28. Sugimura, T., Kawachi, T., Nagao, M., Yahagi, T., Seino, Y., Okamoto, T., Shudo, K., Kosuge, T., Tsuji, K., Wakabayashi, K., Iitaka, Y. and Itai, A. (1977) Proc. Jpn. Acad., 53, 58-61.

29. Yamamoto, T., Tsuji, K., Kosuge, T., Okamoto, T., Shudo, K., Takeda, K., Iitaka, Y., Yamaguchi, K., Seino, Y., Yahagi, T., Nagao, M. and Sugimura, T. (1978) Proc. Jpn. Acad., 54B, 248-250.

30. Wakabayashi, K., Tsuji, K., Kosuge, T., Takeda, K., Yamaguchi, K., Shudo, K., Iitaka, Y., Okamoto, T., Yahagi, T., Nagao, M. and Sugimura, T. (1978) Proc. Jpn. Acad., 54B, 569-571.

31. Yoshida, D., Matsumoto, T., Yoshimura, R. and Matsuzaki, T. (1978) Biochem. Biophys. Res. Commun., 83, 915-920.

32. Kasai, H., Yamaizumi, Z., Wakabayashi, K., Nagao, M., Sugimura, T., Yokoyama, S., Miyazawa, T., Spingarn, N.E., Weisburger, J.H. and Nishimura, S. (1980) Proc. Jpn. Acad., 56B, 278-283.

33. Unpublished data of our laboratory.

34. Sugimura, T. and Nagao, M. (1979) CRC Critical Reviews in Toxicology, 6, 189-209.

35. Ishii, K., Ando, M., Kamataki, T., Kato, R. and Nagao, M. (1980) Cancer Lett., 9, 271-276.

36. Nebert, D.W., Bigelow, S., Okey, A.B., Yahagi, T., Mori, Y., Nagao, M. and Sugimura, T. (1979) Proc. Natl. Acad. Sci. USA, 76, 5929-5933.

37. Yamazoe, Y., Ishii, K., Kamataki, T., Kato, R. and Sugimura, T. (1980) Chem.-Biol. Interactions, 30, 125-138.

38. Hashimoto, Y., Shudo, K. and Okamoto, T. (1979) Chem. Pharm. Bull., 27, 1058-1060.

39. Hashimoto, Y., Shudo, K. and Okamoto, K. (1980) Biochem. Biophys. Res. Commun., 92, 971-976.

40. Spingarn, N.E., Kasai, H., Vuolo, L.L., Nishimura, S., Yamaizumi, Z., Sugimura, T., Matsushima, T. and Weisburger, J.H. (1980) Cancer Lett., 9, 177-183.

41. Reigh, D.L., Stuart, M. and Floyd, R.A. (1978) Experientia, 34, 107-108.

42. Bartsch, H. and Hecker, E. (1971) Biochim. Biophys. Acta, 237, 567-578.

43. Yamada, M., Tsuda, M., Nagao, M., Mori, M. and Sugimura, T. (1979) Biochem. Biophys. Res. Commun., 90, 769-776.

44. Rogan, E.G., Katomski, P.A., Roth, R.W. and Cavalieri, E.L. (1979) J. Biol. Chem., 254, 7055-7059.

45. Miller, E.C., Lotlikar, P.D., Miller J.A., Butler, B.W., Irving, C.C. and Hill, J.T. (1968) Mol. Pharmacol., 4, 147-154.

46. Holmstedt, B. and Lindgren, J.-E. (1967) In: Ethnopharmacologic Search for Psychoactive Drugs (Efron, D.H., Holmstedt, B. and Kline, N.S., eds.) Public Health Service Publications No. 1645, Washington, pp. 339-373.

47. Agurell, S., Holmstedt, B., Lindgren, J.E., and Schultes, R.E. (1969) Acta Chem. Scand., 23, 903-916.

48. Nagao, M., Yahagi, T., Kawachi, T., Sugimura, T., Kosuge, T., Tsuji, K., Wakabayashi, K., Mizusaki, S. and Matsumoto, T. (1977) Proc. Jpn. Acad., 53, 95-98.

49. Nagao, M., Yahagi, T. and Sugimura, T. (1978) Biochem. Biophys. Res. Commun., 83, 373-378.

50. Nagao, M., Yahagi, T., Honda, M., Seino, Y., Kawachi, T., Sugimura, T., Wakabayashi, K., Tsuji, K. and Kosuge, T. (1977) Cancer Lett., 3, 339-346.

51. U.S. DHEW Publ. No. (NIH) 78-1385 (1978) Public Health Serv., Natl. Inst. Health, Bethesda.

52. Int. Agency Res. Cancer (1978) IARC Monographs on the Evaluation of Carcinogenic Risk of Chemicals to Man, vol. 16, Int. Agency Res. Cancer, Lyon, pp. 349-366.

53. Nagao, M., Yahagi, T., Honda, M., Seino, Y., Matsushima, T. and Sugimura, T. (1977) Proc. Jpn. Acad., 53B, 34-37.

54. Int. Agency Res. Cancer (1975) IARC Monographs on the Evaluation of Carcinogenic Risk of Chemicals to Man, vol. 8, Int. Agency Res. Cancer, Lyon, pp. 287-294.

55. Sugimura, T., Nagao, M., Matsushima, T., Yahagi, T. and Hayashi, K. (1977) Nucl. Acids Res., Spec. Publ. No. 3, 41-44.

56. Hayashi, K., Nagao, M. and Sugimura, T. (1977) Nucl. Acids Res., 4, 3679-3685.

57. Pezzuto, J.M., Lau, P.P., Lau, Y., Moore, P.D., Wogan, G.N. and Hecht, S.M. (1980) Proc. Natl. Acad. Sci. USA, 77, 1427-1431.

58. Ho, B.T. (1972) J. Pharm. Sci. 61, 821-837.

59. Fujino, T., Fujiki, M., Nagao, M., Yahagi, T., Seino, Y. and Sugimura, T. (1978) Mutation Res., 58, 151-158.

60. Levitt, R.C., Legraverend, C., Nebert, D.W. and Pelkonen, O. (1977) Biochem. Biophys. Res. Commun., 79, 1167-1175.

61. Chang, C.C., Castellazzi, M., Glover, T.W. and Trosko, J.E. (1978) Cancer Res., 38, 4527-4533.

62. Komatsu, T., Unpublished data.

63. Cardy, R.H., Lijinsky, W. and Hildebrandt, P.K. (1978) Ecotoxicol. Environ. Safety, 3, 29-35.

64. Nagao, M. and Takahashi, Y. (1980) International Program for the Evaluation of Short-term Tests for Carcinogenicity. Elsevier, Amsterdam, in press.

65. Wakabayashi, K., Nagao, M., Kawachi, T. and Sugimura, T. (1980) Mutation Res., in preparation.

66. Biggs, I.D. and Williams, K.L.H. (1976) J. Chem. Soc., Perkin Trans., 2, 691-695.

67. Challis, B.C. and Osborne, M.R. (1972) J. Chem. Soc., Chem. Commun., 518-519.

© 1980 Elsevier/North-Holland Biomedical Press
Mechanisms of Toxicity and Hazard Evaluation
B. Holmstedt, R. Lauwerys, M. Mercier, M. Roberfroid eds

REACTION WITH DNA AND DNA-REPAIR IN CHEMICAL CARCINOGENESIS

P.F. SWANN and S.A. KYRTOPOULOS, Courtauld Institute, Middlesex Hospital Medical School, London W1P 7PN, United Kingdom.

The early 1960's introduced two closely linked concepts in chemical carcinogenesis: first, that the initiation of cancer is the consequence of a covalent reaction between the carcinogen and a cellular macromolecule; second, that most chemical carcinogens require metabolic activation for this reaction to take place.

The first covalent reactions to be discovered between carcinogens and cellular macromolecules were between azo dyes and protein (1), but after the discovery that a metabolite of dimethylnitrosamine methylates DNA (2) it was shown that metabolites of polycyclic hydrocarbons (3), 2-fluorenylacetamide (4) and other carcinogens bind to nucleic acids. At the same time, there was rapid progress in the understanding of drug metabolism, in particular the importance of the endoplasmic reticulum (5) and of cytochrome P_{450} (6), the conditions necessary for the metabolism of carcinogens in vitro, and the importance of metabolism as a mechanism for the formation of chemically reactive products capable of reacting with nucleic acids.

These discoveries lead in 1970 Miller to suggest that chemical carcinogens share the common property that they form positively charged metabolites which react with DNA (7).

This concept has been adopted widely as a working hypothesis and, among other things, provided the conceptual basis for the Ames Test. The hypothesis demands that we should identify the chemically reactive metabolites of carcinogens; discover which of these metabolites is involved in carcinogenesis; identify the products of the reaction between these and nucleic acids; and define the biological role of each of these reaction products.

These are deceptively simple questions and the difficulty of achieving even the first two of these four objectives can be illustrated by recent work on the polycyclic aromatic hydrocarbons. Recent brilliant work has shown that the tertiary metabolites, the

Bay Region diol-epoxides of Benzo(a)pyrene

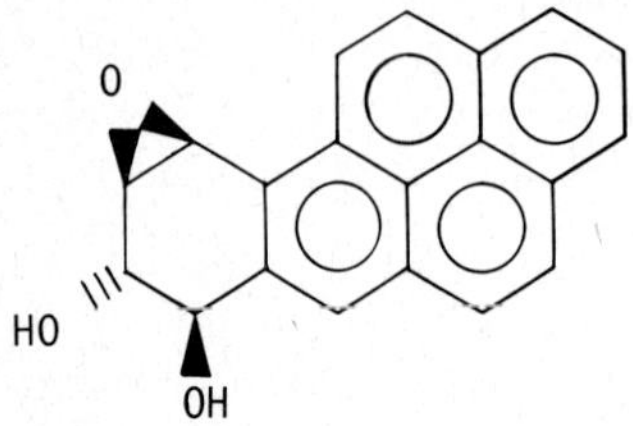

(-) BP-7β,8α-diol-9β,10β-epoxide

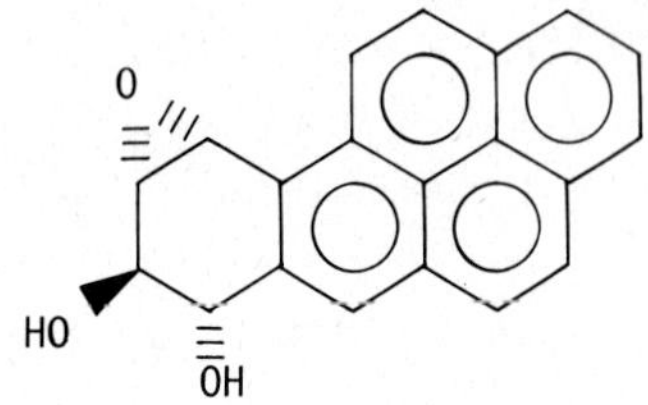

(+) BP-7α,8β-diol-9α,10α-epoxide

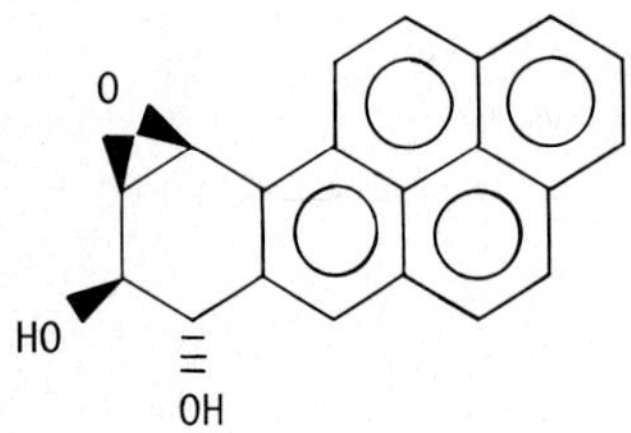

(-) BP-7α,7β-diol-9β,10β-epoxide

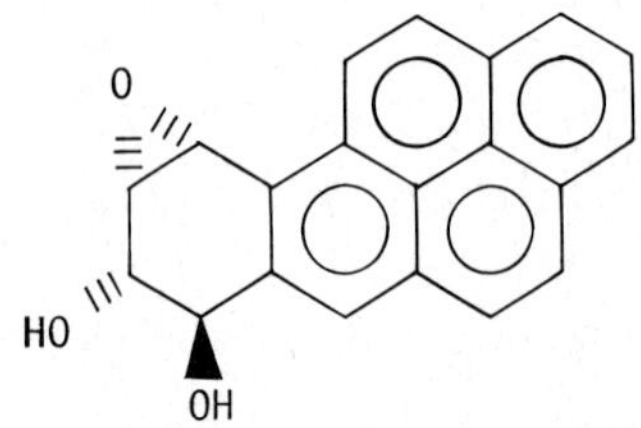

(+) BP-7β,8α-diol-9α,10α-epoxide

'Bay-Region' diol-expoxides (Fig. 1), may be the most (8, 9, 10, 11), although not the only (12), important carcinogenic metabolites of these compounds. They are complex molecules and their metabolism and carcinogenic activity depends upon their absolute stereochemistry as well as their gross chemical structure. For example one of the four enantiomers of benzo(a)pyrene-7,8-diol-9,10-epoxide, the (+)-7β,8α-dihydroxy-9α,10α-epoxy (Fig. 1), is preferentially formed when benzo(a)pyrene is metabolized by rat liver microsomes (13) and has much greater carcinogenic activity than the other enantiomers (14, 15). For benz(a)anthracene also one stereoisomer of the 'Bay-Region' diol is preferentially formed by metabolism (16) and this enantiomer is the most carcinogenic in mice (17).

The most common reaction between the active metabolites of benzo(a)pyrene and DNA is with the N^2-amino group of guanine and the N^6-amino group of adenine (18). The structure and stereochemistry of these adducts has been published (19). Differences

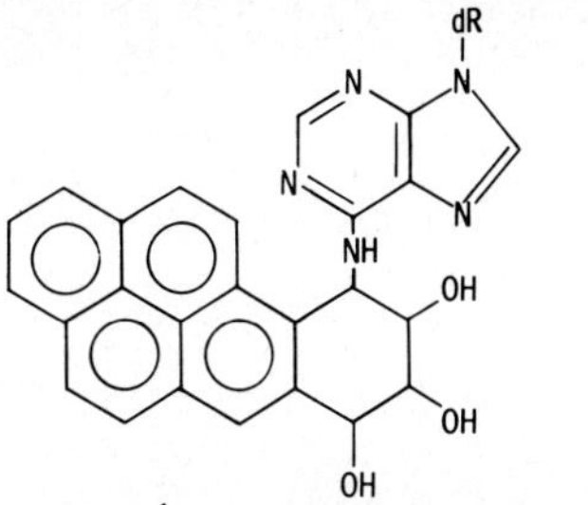

2'-deoxy-N^6-(7,8,9,10-tetrahydro-7β,8α,9α trihydroxybenzo(a)pyrene-10-yl)adenosine

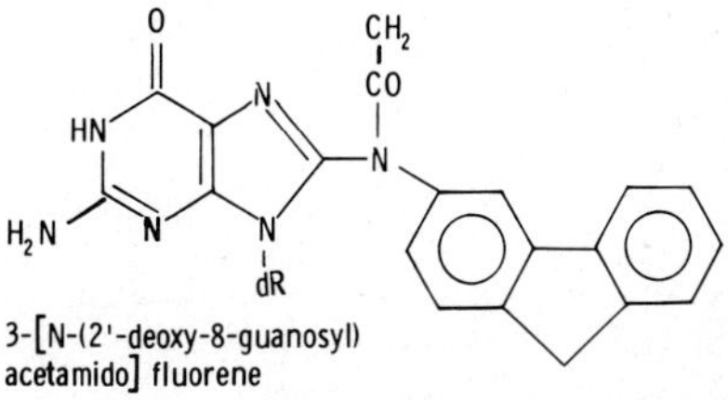

3-[N-(2'-deoxy-8-guanosyl) acetamido] fluorene

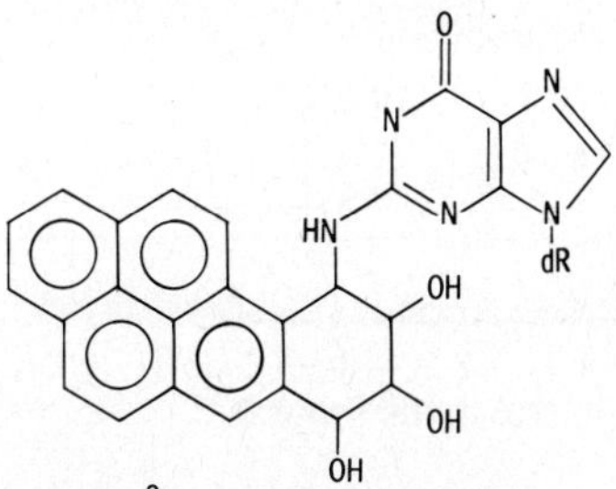

2' deoxy-N^2-(7,8,9,10-tetrahydro-7β,8α,9α trihydroxybenzo(a)pyrene-10-yl) guanosine

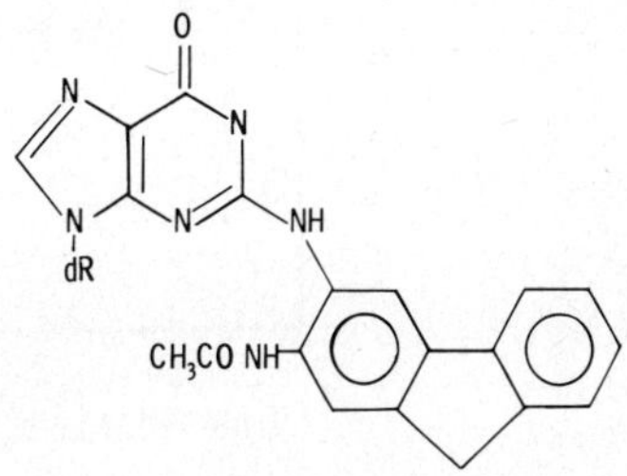

2-acetamido-3-(2'-deoxy-N^2-guanosyl) fluorene

in the biological activity of the isomers may be explained by the recent discovery that only (+)-7β,8α-dihydroxy-9α,10α-epoxy-benzo (a)pyrene binds to guanine residues in double stranded DNA, while both optical isomers bind to guanine in denatured DNA and to adenine in native or denatured DNA (20, 21). The conformation of the DNA also plays an important role in the reaction with AAF. AAF reacts preferentially with single stranded DNA and RNA, attacking only the C-8-position of guanine but in vivo and with native DNA in vitro AAF also reacts with the N^2-position of guanine as well (18). Polycyclic hydrocarbons also react with the N^4-amino group of cytosine, possibly the 7-position of guanine and the phosphate backbone of DNA (18). Probably, other reaction products have yet to be identified. Similarly not all the reactive metabolites of aromatic amines are known yet, and their reaction with DNA is, in most cases, unknown (22).

Under these circumstances, it is impossible to ascribe a specific biological role to any particular reaction product between these carcinogens and DNA. The reaction between the

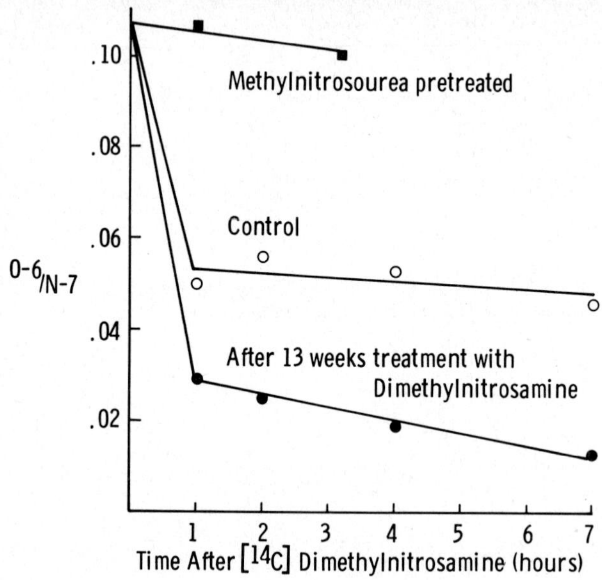

Fig. 3. Disappearance of O^6-[^{14}C]methylguanine from rat liver DNA after 0.7 mg [^{14}C]dimethylnitrosamine/kg. The figure compares the rate in Controls with a) the rate in animals given 8.5 mg dimethylnitrosamine/litre drinking water for 13 weeks, and, b) amount formed and the rate after inhibition of the enzyme by N-methyl-N-nitrosourea pretreatment.

N-nitroso compounds and DNA is also complex but in this case there has been considerable progress towards understanding the biological role of individual reaction products.

When N-nitroso compounds are given to animals they are transformed into alkylating agents which react with DNA. The methylating compounds react with at least 8 positions in DNA (23); the ethylating compounds with 12 positions (24). There is a very strong correlation between the amount of alkylation of one of these positions - the O^6 of guanine - and the incidence of kidney tumours in the rat (23) and thymic lymphomas in the mouse (25). Alkylation of this position has considerable biological significance, for example it is probably responsible for most of nitrosamide-induced mutations in bacteria (26) and eukaryotic cells (27), but the correlation between O^6-alkylation and tumour induction cannot be taken as sufficient evidence of case-and-effect because it is possible that there is an equally good correlation

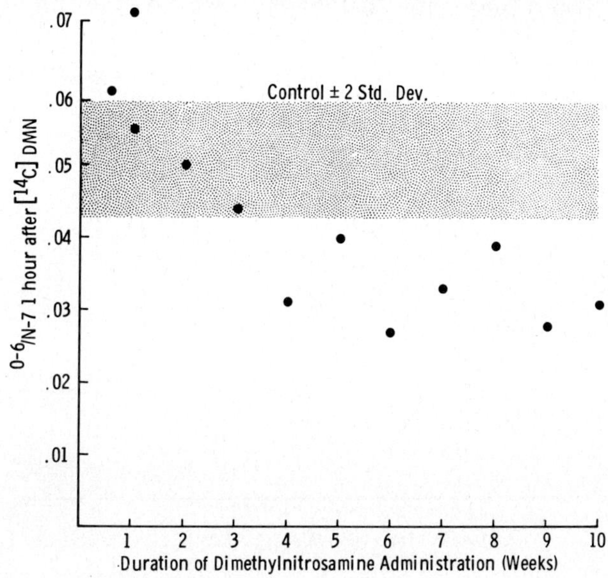

Fig. 4. Changes in the amount of $[^{14}C]O^6$-methylguanine disappearing in the 1st hour after 0.7 mg $[^{14}C]$dimethylnitrosamine/kg in rat liver after prolonged dimethylnitrosamine administration.

between carcinogenic activity and the alkylation of other sites (24) (e.g. the 4-position of thymine - an alkylation which is also promutagenic (28). However, further evidence linking O^6-alkylation and carcinogenesis has come from studies on DNA repair.

Earlier studies had shown that if alkylation induces cancer organs must differ in their susceptibility to it. Brain tumours were induced in the rat, particularly if the rats were treated with ethylnitrosourea in the foetus or shortly after their birth, by a relatively small single dose of nitrosamides; a larger dose also produced tumours in many other organs including kidney; but, even the largest single dose did not induce liver tumours. This range of susceptibility paralleled the ability of these organs to remove O^6-alkylguanine from their DNA: the brain was unable to remove (29) it, the kidney removed it slowly and after some delay (30), and the liver removed it very rapidly (29).

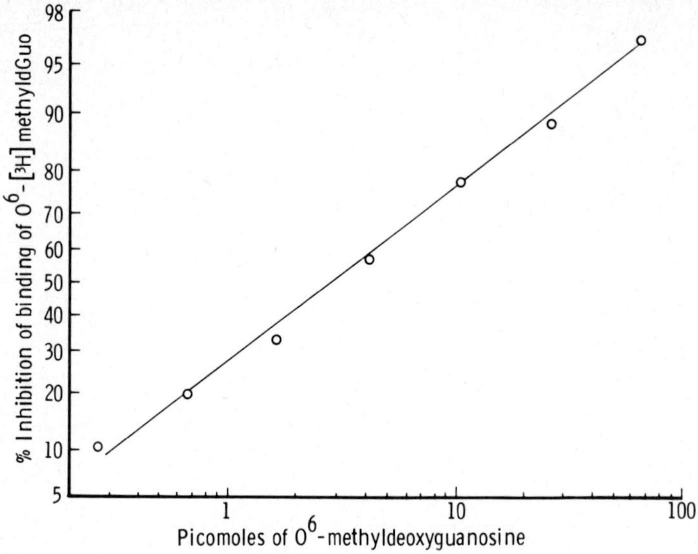

Fig. 5. Radioimmunoassay of O^6-methyldeoxyguanosine. The sensitivity in this case is limited only by the low specific radioactivity of the radioligand (1.4 Ci/mmol).

So far as is known (although there is evidence for differences in the rate of enzymic removal of the O-alkylated pyrimidines (31) their persistence in rat organs has not been measured) this parallel exists only with O^6-alkylguanine, and not with the removal of other alkylated products. Taken with the quantitative relationship between the carcinogenic activity of alkylating agents and their ability to produce O^6-alkylguanine in DNA, this has seemed to indicate a preeminent role for O^6-alkylation in carcinogenesis. Unfortunately, administration of O^6-methyl and ethylguanine to rats derivatives did not result in the incorporation of O^6-alkylguanine into DNA so that a direct test of the biological effect of O^6-alkylation has not been carried out yet (32).

However, these experiments have not explained why dimethylnitrosamine is a potent hepatocarcinogen when given continuously in minute quantity in the diet even though the liver can remove O^6-methylguanine so quickly from DNA (33). After it had been

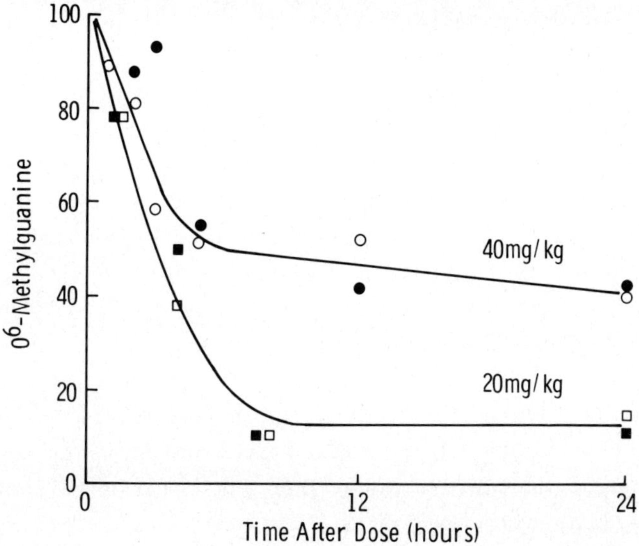

Fig. 6. Loss of O^6-methylguanine from mouse liver main-band ○ □ and satellite DNA ● ■ after dimethylnitrosamine. The numbers have been reduced to percentages to facilitate comparison.

found that one large dose of nitroso compound inhibits the loss of O^6-methylguanine produced in DNA by N-methyl-N-nitrosourea (34) it was thought that prolonged administration of dimethylnitrosamine might exhaust the removal system and allow the O^6-methylguanine to persist as it does in the rat organs which are susceptible to a single dose of methylnitroso compounds. It does not: the rate of loss of O^6-methylguanine is increased by feeding dimethylnitrosamine (35).

Study of the loss of O^6-methylguanine from rat liver DNA after a small dose of dimethylnitrosamine (DMN) has shown most interesting kinetics. The amount of O^6-methylguanine produced can be estimated either by inhibiting the removal by pretreatment of the rat with N-methyl-N-nitrosourea, or by calculation from the known O^6 to N^7-guanine alkylation ratio. A daily dose of 0.7 mg DMN/kg wt/day in the drinking water gives liver tumours in every rat. When this dose is given approximately half the O^6-methylguanine in the DNA is removed in the first hour; the remainder is removed more slowly (Fig. 3). Pretreatment of the rat with 0.7 mg DMN/kg/day does not alter the amount of O^6-methylguanine formed by a single dose but increases the amount lost during the first hour and the remainder is also lost more rapidly (Fig. 3). With this daily dose the increase in rate of loss takes 4 weeks to become established (Fig. 4). The delay may be dose dependent because it occurs faster and to a greater extent if a larger dose of dimethylnitrosamine is given (36).

The nature of the enzyme system carrying out this removal is not yet known but there is some similarity between it and an inducible enzyme system in E. coli which can remove O^6-methylguanine from DNA (37). This system which is error free and is not dependent on the uvr genes has one remarkable characteristic: it is apparently used once only and is effectively titrated by its substrate (38). The enzyme in rat liver appears to have a similar characteristic: as the dose of dimethylnitrosamine is changed between 0.5 mg/kg and 1.8 mg/kg, an almost constant amount of O^6-methylguanine (29 pmoles/g wet wt) is lost in the first hour.

It is difficult to reconcile these findings with the high carcinogenic effectiveness of these low doses of dimethylnitrosamine. The bacterial enzyme appears to be a trans-methylase (40) which repairs the DNA without error (37). It is disputed that the bacterial and mammalian enzyme are similar because the failure of xeroderma cells to remove O^6-methylguanine suggests that the mammalian system is similar to the uv excision system (41), but if the enzyme in bacteria and liver is similar, and, if cancer is the result of the mutagenic properties of O^6-methylguanine, this enzyme should protect against cancer. It is clear that there must be factors we do not understand (for example why a very large and persistent alkylation of the O^6 of guanine has not yet produced tumours in xenopus laevis (39)) or that mutation as the result of O^6-alkylation may not cause cancer.

The studies described above were carried out by radiotracer methods. These methods have limitations which may be overcome by the development of immunological techniques. Recently, radioimmunoassays have been developed for alkylated bases (42-45) and for DNA altered by the carcinogens benzo(a)pyrene (46) and

2-fluorenylacetamide (47). Even at the present state of development immunological techniques are more sensitive than conventional radiotracer techniques for the detection of O^6-methyl and O^6-ethyldeoxyguanosine.

A standard curve for the estimation of O^6-methyl-2'-deoxyguanosine by radioimmunoassay is shown in Fig. 3. We have used radioimmunoassay to study the formation and disappearance of O^6-methylguanine from the 'main band' and satellite DNA of mouse liver after a dose of dimethylnitrosamine (Fig. 6). Mouse DNA can be separated into two fractions of different bouyant density. One of these fractions, the satellite comprising about 10% of the total is a DNA of highly repetitive sequence located in heterochromatin around the centromere (48). The satellite DNA is not transcribed; the main band DNA contains all the active genes. The analysis showed that the alkylation in the satellite DNA is 20-30% less than in the main band DNA (this result was confirmed by radiotracer methods). However, the O^6-methylguanine disappeared at a similar rate from both main band and from satellite DNA (Fig. 6).

The function of this highly repetitive DNA in the mouse is not known (48) but highly repetitive DNA, representing up to 40% of the genome, is found in most eukaryotes (49). Most of it may have no function in shaping the phenotype of the cell (50) but Davidson and Britten (49) have proposed that part of it has a major role in the control of gene expression. Whether this is the case, or not, this experiment has shown that immunological methods may be used to study the interaction of carcinogens, and the repair of damaged DNA in specific fractions of the genome isolated in small quantities. The rate of repair is not the same throughout the genome (e.g. 51) and there is evidence that carcinogens might have a predilection for DNA in specific conformation. As the structure of the genome is unravelled, and the functional units isolated, it will become increasingly necessary to have methods for the analysis of DNA-carcinogen adducts in very small amounts of DNA. It is possible that immunological techniques will be most valuable not only for this but also for the demonstration by immunocytology of the distribution of carcinogen-DNA adducts from cell to cell or even within the chromosome; and, the analysis of human tissue for the presence of carcinogen-DNA adducts. This might allow us to discover whether the numerous drugs which have the potential to be nitrosated in vivo (e.g. 46) react with DNA in vivo.

I am most grateful to Miss Y.C. Chan for typing this manuscript, and the Cancer Research Campaign.

REFERENCES

1. Miller, E.C. and Miller, J.A. (1955) Cancer Res., 7, 468-480.
2. Magee, P.N. and Farber, E. (1962) Biochem. J., 83, 114-124.
3. Brookes, P. and Lawley, P.D. (1964) Nature, 202, 781-784.
4. Marroquin, R.F. and Farber, E. (1965) Cancer Res., 25, 1262-1269.
5. Brodie, B.B. (1955) Science, 121, 603.
6. Estabrook, R.W. (1971) Handbook of Experimental Pharmacology (Brodie, B.B. and Gillette, J.R., ed.) Springer-Verlag, Berlin, pp., 264-284.
7. Miller, J.A. (1970) Cancer Res., 30, 559-576.
8. Sims, P., et al. (1974) Nature, 252, 326-328.
9. Jerina, D.M., et al. (1977) Origins of Human Cancer (Hiatt, H.H., Watson, J.D. and Winsten, J.A., ed.) Book B, Cold Spring Harbor Press, pp., 639-658.
10. Kapitulnik, J., et al. (1978) Cancer Res., 38, 354-358.
11. Bartsch, H., et al. (1979) Chem. Biol. Interact., 26, 185-196.
12. MacNicoll, A.D., et al. (1979) Biochem. Biophys. Res. Commun., 91, 490-497.
13. Yang, S.K., et al. (1976) Proc. Nat. Acad. Sci. (U.S.A.) 73, 2594-2598.
14. Buening, M.K., et al. (1978) Proc. Nat. Acad. Sci. (U.S.A.) 75, 5358-5361.
15. Brookes, P. (1979) Cancer Lett., 6, 285-289.
16. Thakker, D.R., et al. (1979) Chem. Biol. Interact., 27, 145-161.
17. Wislocki, P.G., et al. (1979) J. Nat. Cancer Inst., 63, 201-204.
18. Grunberger, D. and Weinstein, I.B. (1979) Prog. Nucleic Acid Res. Mol. Biol. (Cohen, W.E., ed.) 23, 106-150.
19. Jeffrey, A.M., et al. (1979) Science, 206, 1309-1311.
20. Meehan, T. and Straub, K. (1979) Nature, 277, 410-412.
21. Pulkrabek, P., et al. (1979) Biochemistry, 18, 5128-5134.
22. Miller, E.C. (1978) Cancer Res., 38, 1479-1496.

23. Lawley, P.D. (1976) Screening Tests In Chemical Carcinogenesis (Montesano, R., Bartsch, H. and Tomatis, L., ed.) IARC Scientific Publication No. 12., pp., 181-208.

24. Singer, B. (1979) J. Nat. Cancer Inst., 62, 1329-1339.

25. Lawley, P.D. (1980) Brit. Med. Bull., 36, 19-24.

26. Coulondre, C. and Miller, J.H. (1977) J. Mol. Biol., 117, 577-606.

27. Newbold, R.F., et al. (1980) Nature, 283, 596-599.

28. Singer, B. and Kröger, M. (1979) Prog. Nucleic Acid Res. Mol. Biol. (Cohen, W.E., ed.) 23, 151-194.

29. Goth, R. and Rajewsky, M.F. (1974) Proc. Nat. Acad. Sci. (U.S.A.) 71, 639-643.

30. Nicoll, J.W., et al. (1975) Nature, 254, 261-262.

31. Bodell, W.J., et al. (1979) Nucleic Acids Res., 6, 2819-2829.

32. Pegg, A.E. and Swann, P.F. (1979) Biochim. Biophys. Acta., 565, 241-252.

33. Pegg, A.E. and Hui, G. (1978) Cancer Res., 38, 2011-2017.

34. Kleihues, P. and Margison, G.P. (1976) Nature, 259, 153-155.

35. Montesano, R., et al. (1979) Cancer Res., 39, 1798-1802.

36. Montesano, R., et al. (1980) Cancer Res., 40, 452-458.

37. Samson, L. and Cairns, J. (1977) Nature, 267, 281-282.

38. Robins, P. and Cairns, J. (1979) Nature, 280, 74-76.

39. Hodgson, R., et al. (1980) Europ. J. Cancer, 16, 481-486.

40. Karran, P., et al. (1979) Nature, 280, 76-77.

41. Altamirano-Dimas, M., et al. (1979) Mutation Res., 60, 197-206.

42. Briscoe, W.T., et al. (1978) Biochemistry, 17, 1896-1901.

43. Meredith, R.D. and Erlanger, B.F. (1979) Nucleic Acids Res., 6, 2179-2191.

44. Mueller, R. and Rajewsky, M.F. (1980) Cancer Res., 40, 887-896.

45. Kyrtopoulos, S.K. and Swann, P.F. (1980) J. Cancer Res. Clin. Onkol. (in press).

46. Poirier, M.C., et al. (1980) Cancer Res., 40, 412-416.

47. Poirier, M.C., et al. (1977) Nature, 270, 186-188.

48. John, B. and Miklos, G.L.C. (1979) Intern. Rev. Cytol., 58, 1-114.

49. Davidson, E.H. and Britten, R.J. (1979) Science, 204, 1052-1059.

50. Doolittle, W.F. and Sapienza, C. (1980) Nature, 284, 601-603.

51. Feldman, G., et al. (1980) Biochemistry, 19, 1095-1101.

52. Elder, J.B., et al. (1979) Lancet (i), 1005-1006.

Mechanisms of Toxicity and Hazard Evaluation
B. Holmstedt, R. Lauwerys, M. Mercier, M. Roberfroid eds

MORPHOLOGICAL CORRELATES OF IRREVERSIBLE TUMOUR FORMATION

GORDON C. HARD
Fels Research Institute, Temple University School of Medicine, Phila., PA 19140

In addressing this topic, an attempt will be made to briefly review the morphological responses of tissues and cells which become manifest during the process of chemical carcinogenesis. In keeping with the symposium theme of seeking a stronger foundation for devising short-term predictive tests in chemical carcinogenesis which are quantitatively more acceptable for human risk assessment, the discussion will concern mainly those alterations occurring during the early days or weeks after commencement of carcinogen exposure, that is long before overt tumour development. A model of carcinogenesis which serves to illustrate a number of the events that will be considered in this review utilises a single, high dose of dimethylnitrosamine (DMN), inducing kidney cancer (comprising both mesenchymal and cortical epithelial tumours) in 100% of rats.[1] The renal mesenchymal tumours have been shown to originate from connective tissue elements in the interstitial space of the outer kidney zones,[2] and the epithelial tumours from convoluted tubules of the cortex.[3]

Attributes intrinsic to the morphological approach enable certain problems in chemical carcinogenesis to be confronted. These latter are, on a diminishing scale from whole animal to cellular unit, organ specificity, target cell population specificity and clonal evolution of cancer. Such aspects acknowledge in turn, the variation in susceptibility of animal tissues to the carcinogenic effects of different chemicals, the cellular heterogeneity of all individual organs amongst which (usually) only one cell population or subpopulation will be transformation-sensitive, and the fact that within this susceptible target cell community the cancer process will be restricted to a minutia of cells. Some of these characteristic features pose interpretive problems for various *in vitro* short-term tests, while others hinder efforts to define the critical subcellular mechanisms involved in carcinogenesis. Indeed, the morphological approach will be of paramount importance in identifying and surmounting the technical research problems inherent in the clonal aspect of cancer. The discovery and development of histological techniques such as immunofluorescent markers which can be used to identify the target cells specifically involved in the cancer process will be prerequisite for devising methods of access to those subpopulations for more critical biochemical analysis.

As we consider the chronological sequence of a tissue's response to a chemical carcinogen, one of the most immediate alterations is that of cytotoxicity. The available evidence indicates that all cancer-inducing chemicals adequately studied at suitably carcinogenic doses, elicit visualisable toxic injury in the same target cell populations as are sensitive to the carcinogenic action of those compounds. This is a point of no little consequence for in the very early stages of the process it provides focus on likely tissue candidates for the organotropic effect of a suspect carcinogen. It must be stressed that the cell injury need not be of an irreversible, lethal nature, nor need it to be extensive. The aspect is well illustrated in the DMN-rat kidney tumour model for, although no acute damage was reported in earlier studies using conventional histological technique, microscopic appraisal of perfusion-fixed tissue demonstrated toxic alterations in specifically the target cell populations from which the tumours were derived.[3,4] In the resident interstitial cells of the outer kidney zones, cytotoxic structural alterations were of a reversible nature (lipid droplet accumulation, formation of autophagosomes, dilation of endoplasmic reticulum and nuclear envelopes) and lethal injury was remarkably infrequent. On the other hand, cells of the convoluted cortical tubules showed more extensive involvement, with mainly reversible changes, but also sporadic necrosis.

Although interference with membrane-ribosome associations, visualised as polysome or membrane degranulation, is regarded as a common property of chemical carcinogens[5,6] the ultrastructural lesions induced by carcinogens in target cell populations offer nothing as a specific signal to the later chronic effects.[6] This does not exclude the possibility however, in acknowledgement of the clonal origin of cancer, that specific and early, morphologically-detectable alterations might exist in the small generation of target cells which will become committed to the neoplastic process. Again, with the advent of increasingly sophisticated methods for studying the ultrastructure of informational macromolecules such as DNA, there may, ultimately, be scope for discovering some molecular alteration in target cell populations that has predictive value for carcinogenic action. Isolated electronmicroscopic studies during recent years such as the one illustrating that specific antibodies can be used to map carcinogen binding sites along the DNA molecule *in vitro*,[7] may represent initial steps in this approach.

A second property common to chemical carcinogens, which is detectable by morphological technique including autoradiography, is the early effect on cell proliferation. The tissue response is complex, for carcinogens are known to exert not only a stimulatory effect on DNA synthesis and mitosis in target cell populations, but also to act as inhibitors of cell proliferation.[8] The apparent paradox of these opposite effects can be resolved into some chronological perspective by consideration of both single dose models of carcinogenesis and those involving continuous low-dose exposure. A single administration of DMN at a dose which induces a 100% incidence of tumours in the kidney, causes an immediate inhibition of DNA synthesis and mitosis in all cell populations of that organ for a period of 24 to 72 hours depending on cell type.[9] This blanket effect is followed some days later by increased cell division in specifically those target cell populations from which the mesenchymal and epithelial tumours will arise later. Accordingly, there is enhanced DNA synthesis in resident interstitial cells of the cortex commencing at 3 days, and also in cortical proximal and distal tubules with a peak of response at 10 days after the single dose of DMN.

A similar sequence can be demonstrated in rodent liver during continuous administration of the hepatocarcinogens aflatoxin B_1[10] and 3'-methyl-4-dimethylaminoazobenzene.[11] During the first three weeks of dietary exposure to these carcinogens, there is an inhibition of DNA synthesis and/or mitosis. This is followed by a pronounced stimulation of cell proliferation as measured by these same parameters between the third and sixth week of dosing. Emphasizing the importance of cell proliferation to the cancer induction process, this sequence correlates with the demonstration that a 3-week exposure to either chemical is not hepatocarcinogenic whereas a 6-week schedule is necessary for producing a 100% incidence of liver tumours.[11,12] A review of examples where tissue reaction to chemicals has been adequately examined, suggests that an initial nonspecific inhibition of cell proliferation followed by a selective stimulation of target cell populations may represent a consistent feature of the response to carcinogens.

A morphological aberration which follows as a direct result of the carcinogen's early effects on the cell proliferative cycle is that of conspicuous nuclear enlargement (karyomegaly, megalocytosis). The development of greatly enlarged nuclei, implying progressive polyploidy, has been recorded in response to a number of carcinogens and in a variety of target organs. It has been suggested recently that the correlation between this short-term effect and long-term tumour production in mouse skin is sufficient for application in detecting topical carcinogens, particularly those related to benzo[a]pyrene.[13] At least in epidermis, increase in ploidy level is one of the primary tissue changes of a specific nature that is evoked at an early stage by chemical carcinogens.[8]

The mechanism leading to nuclear enlargement appears to involve a blocking of cells in G_2 of the cell cycle, with a bypassing of mitosis followed by entry to another cell cycle. Repeated cycles thus result in progressive polyploidy.[14] Generally, the morphological alteration takes several weeks to develop in the liver[15] and kidney[8] (karyomegaly is well developed 6 weeks after a single carcinogenic dose of DMN)[3] but only a few days in skin[16] and stomach[17] following administration of the carcinogen. The rapidity with which enlarged nuclei are induced in different organs is likely to be related to the degree of cell turnover intrinsic to the normal tissue, skin and gastric mucosa being continuously renewing cell populations whereas liver and kidney constitute fairly permanent but slowly expanding populations. Discrepancies in correlating gross nuclear enlargement with carcinogenicity do exist. It has not always been recorded as a consistent accompaniment of carcinogen treatment nor is there complete accord with organ specificity. Karyomegaly is a characteristic tissue response of pyrrolizidine alkaloids but the carcinogenicity of some of these compounds has, in the past, been disputed. Increase in nuclear size can result from such physical procedures as partial organ ablation[18] but when compared with the effect of carcinogens, there is a difference in degree of enlargement which may become apparent only when size distribution in a cell population is subject to histogram analysis.[19] Certainly, continued study is warranted to determine the relationship that such nuclear aberrations may have with organ susceptibility to cancer, if any, for they are easily detectable alterations developing well within the desirable time-frame requirement of predictive assay. Gross nuclear enlargement is a common feature of malignant neoplasms induced by a variety of chemicals and of chemically-transformed, neoplastic cell-lines *in vitro*, but there is no evidence to indicate that such cells play any role in the progressive development of cancer from transformed clones.

Histological lesions which occur in target organs during the latent or interim period of carcinogenesis represent a productive area for concerted research. Such pathological entities are commonly termed precursor or preneoplastic lesions but in most cases final proof implicating various examples as inevitable stages in the progression to autonomous growth awaits verification. Different organs respond with differing lesions, a variation which may be dependent on the local environment and primary function(s) of the tissue.

By far the major research effort on interim-stage lesions has been devoted to the liver. Hepatic tissue functions as the main pathway by which foreign chemicals of toxic potential are degraded, and, as emphasized recently, this may be the underlying basis for the generation of a range of controversial early lesions in both rat and mouse liver.[20] Currently a number of hepatocyte populations are believed to be involved in rat liver carcinogenesis. These include clear cell foci, "ground glass" (eosinophilic) foci, foci of resistant hepatocytes, hyperplastic or enzyme-altered foci, early and late hyperplastic nodules (the latter are synonymous with neoplastic nodules), and hyperbasophilic foci. Consensus has yet to be reached on the extent to which various terms relate to the same lesion. Hyperplastic foci and nodules can be readily identified as enzyme-altered lesions by various markers including glycogen storage,[21] γ-glutamyltranspeptidase activity,[22] adenosinetriphosphatase deficiency[23] and resistance to iron storage during dietary overload.[24] However, the foci, as well as the induced liver cancers, display a marked phenotypic heterogeneity[25] which complicates the sequential analysis of lesion progression from early to late stage. Certain studies have demonstrated convincingly the reversibility of some of these lesions[26] while others acknowledge the numerical discrepancy (several thousand-fold) between the high incidence of early foci and the ultimate neoplasms.[27] Although hyperplastic foci are inducible by most if not all hepatocarcinogens, similar lesions are also seen following dietary stress (e.g., choline deficiency)[28] and the administration of certain compounds of doubtful carcinogenicity such as phenobarbitone.[29] Thus early hepatic foci are considered to be obligate precursors, and predictive of hepatocarcinogenesis by some, but within the scope of compensatory hyperplasia in physiological response to cell injury and death by others.[20] Early hyperplastic nodules appear to represent enlargement of the smaller foci[30] but the relationship of neoplastic nodules to carcinoma development is more controversial.[31] In any case, the late appearance of neoplastic nodules precludes their usefulness in the concept of rapid prediction of carcinogenic activity. The induction of hyperbasophilic foci has been recorded mainly as a late phenomenon in hepatocarcinogenesis[32] and such lesions are generally regarded as positively related to cancer development, or even as microcarcinomas.[33] In addition small aggregates of hyperbasophilic cells have been identified amongst normal parenchymal cells at a relatively early stage during aflatoxin carcinogenesis, and these areas are considered also to be likely progenitors of cancer.[34]

Some caution in the interpretation of early liver lesions still seems warranted at this stage, and the induction of nodules by surgical manipulation of the vascular flow, namely portocaval anastomosis[35] supports the adoption of a reserved position. Relevant to the general issue is the recognition that early lesions may represent an adaptation by the liver to generate tissue with a survival advantage in an adverse environment. Enzyme-altered foci not only show enhanced resistance to the acute toxic effects of hepatocarcinogens[36] but they possess a markedly increased content of glutathione which is involved in detoxification mechanisms.[37] However, for the purpose of seeking more extrapolatable phenomena for the early prediction of carcinogenicity by chemicals, using the intact animal, the question concerns not just the fate of the various interim lesions induced, but whether the induction of any particular one characterises the action of a carcinogen. Regardless of issues yet to be resolved concerning the interpretation and significance of interim hepatocellular lesions, it is of interest that the rapid production of early foci of alteration can be achieved in a specialized hepatic system, with a range of carcinogens that are not normally organotropic for liver.[38] Because of the resultant positive correlation with known carcinogenicity in other tissues by these chemicals, this system has been proposed as a possible basis for the short-term testing of carcinogenic potential *in vivo*.

As we turn our consideration from the liver to alternative tissue models of chemical carcinogenesis that have been studied in depth, it becomes apparent that there is a consistent histological aberration common to each of these systems which emerges during the latent period. The feature is that of focal cellular atypia involving specifically, proliferating target cell populations. Thus every organ in which the early stages of carcinogenesis have been examined in detail reveals a chronological sequence which usually involves the induction of a regular form of hyperplasia (or metaplasia), followed by the development of focal hyperplasia (metaplasia, dysplasia) of atypical character. The latter lesions appear to correlate with, and progress to irreversible tumour formation. The particular morphological features which typify the aberrant cell subpopulations vary from tissue to tissue but can include any combination of the alterations listed in Table 1. By way of example, the reaction of the mouse colon to a carcinogenic regime of 1,2-dimethylhydrazine commences during the early weeks as a regular form of hyperplasia in the lower parts of the crypts, followed about 9 weeks after initiation of treatment by development in the upper crypt segments of focal atypical hyperplasia characterised mainly by abnormal cell organization, cellular pleomorphism, basophilia and mitosis. These lesions appear to proceed to colonic cancer.[39] Similar sorts of observations have been convincingly demonstrated with *N*-nitrosobis(2-oxopropyl)amine in the hamster pancreas,[40] 7,12-dimethylbenz[a]anthracene in the rat mammary gland,[41] *N*-nitrosomethylurea and benzo[a]pyrene in the hamster lung[42] and *N*-nitrosomethylurea, dibutylnitrosamine and *N*-[4-(5-nitro-2-furyl)-2-thiazolyl]formamide in the rat bladder.[43] Focal atypical hyperplasia in the latter example was characterised by the novel appearance of surface microvilli.

TABLE 1

MORPHOLOGIC ALTERATIONS ASSOCIATED WITH ATYPICAL HYPERPLASIA

Disorganization of architecture	Nuclear pleomorphism
Disturbance of cell orientation	Nucleolar hypertrophy
Expanded intercellular spaces	Aberrant intercellular junctions
Decreased cell adhesion	Aberrant mitochondria
Cellular pleomorphism	Novel microvilli
Hyperchromatism[a]	Annulate lamellae
Increased nucleus:cytoplasm ratio	

[a]Usually hyperbasophilia.

The phenomenon of cellular atypia occurs during the induction of chemical carcinogenesis in nonepithelial tissues also. For instance hypercellular lesions develop in the interstitial space of the kidney cortex from 3 weeks after a carcinogenic dose of DMN, preceding the development of renal mesenchymal tumours.[2,4] The hypercellular foci consist mainly of mononuclear inflammatory cells, but also in low incidence, hypertrophic fibroblast-like cells which can be identified as aberrant constituents of the intertubular connective tissue by their cytological features. Similar observations have been recorded in subcutaneous mesenchymal carcinogenesis induced by benzo[a]pyrene.[44]

The results of these various detailed studies lead to the conclusion that chemical carcinogens are capable of inducing two morphological types of hyperplasia during the process of carcinogenesis, regular hyperplasia which can result also from a range of non-specific agents causing tissue loss including physical injury, infection and toxic injury; and later, atypical hyperplasia (atypical metaplasia or dysplasia) which appears to be positively correlated with the development of neoplasia. Consideration of precursor lesions in man further supports the idea that cellular atypia is an important stage of cancer development for a consistent correlation seems to be emerging between individuals or populations at high risk to certain cancers, and the presence of such abnormalities in target organs, for example in lung,[45] liver,[46] colon,[47] pancreas[48] and gall-bladder.[49] With the criterion of morphological aberration in mind, further clarification of the rat liver lesions may be provided by recent electronmicroscopic studies which demonstrate no cellular atypia in early hyperplastic foci, but the emergence of aberrant cytological features in some hyperplastic nodules after 10 weeks.[50] In the light of evidence from other organ systems, this result could be interpreted as suggesting that enzyme-altered foci possibly may represent regular, that is compensatory, hyperplasia, whereas early hyperplastic nodules displaying morphological atypia may identify more specifically with the irreversible process of carcinogenesis. In this general area, there is a need to consolidate the distinction between physiological and atypical hyperplasias by defining more clearly the spectrum of cellular aberrations characteristic for each organ system, and then to determine whether such defined lesions can be regarded as pathognomic of later cancer development.

As a directly related extension of the morphological events occurring *in vivo*, the *in vivo-in vitro* system of cell culture appears to offer a basis for morphological correlation with tumour induction in the intact animal. Transformation using this technique has been demonstrated in mesenchymal and epithelial cells of the DMN-exposed rat kidney[51,52] and rat liver,[53] epithelial cells from 7,12-dimethylbenz[a]anthracene-exposed rat trachea,[54] neural cells from the brains of rats exposed *in utero* to ethylnitrosourea,[55] and hamster embryo cells exposed *in utero* to a variety of chemical carcinogens.[56] In this system, cells are isolated into monolayer or organ culture from target tissues shortly after the administration of the inciting carcinogen, usually within hours or days. After a lag period, in the case of the DMN-treated rat kidney approximately 65 days,[57] morphologically transformed cell populations develop which usually conform with the cell type from which the *in vivo* tumours would have been derived. Transformation is manifest by the sudden emergence of an immortal population of rapidly proliferating morphologically altered cells which show a reduced density-dependence or contact inhibition, followed by loss of anchorage-dependence as indicated by formation of colonies in semi-solid media and cellular aggregates (multicellular tumour spheroids) in suspension. The extent to which these various markers of transformation are manifest in particular populations depends on cell lineage. The method offers considerable scope for developing criteria that correlate short-term phenomena with chronic changes in the live animal. Of equal importance is the potential for producing more purified target cell populations to facilitate the study of mechanisms in chemical carcinogenesis. The system is presently hampered to some degree however, by a continuing requirement to define more suitable *in vitro* conditions for culturing epithelial cell populations from a variety of host organs, without attendant fibroblast contamination.

Clearly, the morphological approach in chemical carcinogenesis provides a substantial potential for identifying early markers which presage irreversible tumour formation. Whether any one of the morphological events can be adapted to function as a self-sufficient economic strategy for detecting carcinogens remains to be determined. Certainly there appears to be some scope for developing adjunct assays for *in vivo* corroboration of established *in vitro* short-term tests, which would encompass the concepts of potency, dose-response, species sensitivity and organ and target cell specificity.

ACKNOWLEDGEMENTS

The author acknowledges support from grants CA-24216 and CA-12227, awarded by the National Cancer Institute, DHEW.

REFERENCES

1. Hard, G.C. and Butler, W.H. (1970) Cancer Res., 30, 2796-2805.
2. Hard, G.C. and Butler, W.H. (1970) Cancer Res., 30, 2806-2815.
3. Hard, G.C. and Butler, W.H. (1971) Cancer Res., 31, 1496-1505.
4. Hard, G.C. and Butler, W.H. (1971) Cancer Res., 31, 337-347.
5. Williams, D.J. and Rabin, B.R. (1971) Nature, 232, 102-104.
6. Svoboda, D. and Higginson, J. (1968) Cancer Res., 28, 1703-1733.
7. deMurcia, G., Lang, M-C.E., Freund, A-M. et al. (1979) Proc. Natl. Acad. Sci., 76, 6076-6080.
8. Oehlert, W. (1973) Cell Tissue Kinet., 6, 325-335.
9. Hard, G.C. (1975) Cancer Res., 35, 3762-3773.
10. Godoy, H.M., Judah, D.J., Arora, H.L. et al. (1976) Cancer Res., 36, 2399-2407.
11. Hughes, P.E. (1969/70) Chem.-Biol. Interactions, 1, 301-305.
12. Neal, G.E. and Butler, W.H. (1978) Brit. J. Cancer, 37, 55-60.
13. Ingram, A.J. (1979) Chem.-Biol. Interactions, 26, 103-113.
14. Ingram, A.J. and Grasso, P. (1977) Exp. Path., 14, 233-242.
15. Schoental, R. and Magee, P.N. (1957) J. Path. Bact., 74, 305-319.
16. Pullinger, B.D. (1940) J. Path. Bact., 50, 463-471.
17. Toledo, J.D. (1965) Beitr. Path. Anat., 131, 63-120.
18. James, J., Schopman, M. and Delfgaauw, P. (1966) Exp. Cell Res., 42, 375-379.
19. Grasso, P. (1980) personal communication.
20. Newberne, P.M. and McConnel, R.G. (1980) in Principles and Methods in Modern Toxicology (Eds. Galli, C.L., Murphy, S.D., Paoletti, R.) Elsevier, Amsterdam, in press.
21. Bannasch, P., Mayer, D. and Hacker, H-J. (1980) Biochim. Biophys. Acta, 605, 217-245.
22. Cameron, R., Kellen, J., Kolin, A. et al. (1978) Cancer Res., 38, 823-829.
23. Rabes, H.M., Scholze, P. and Jantsch, B. (1972) Cancer Res., 32, 2577-2586.

24. Williams, G.M. and Yamamoto, R.S. (1972) J. Natl. Cancer Inst., 49, 685-692.

25. Pitot, H.C., Barsness, L., Goldsworthy, T. et al., (1978) Nature, 271, 456-458.

26. Teebor, G.W. and Becker, F.F. (1971) Cancer Res., 31, 1-6.

27. Watanabe, K. and Williams, G.M. (1978) J. Natl. Cancer Inst., 61, 1311-1314.

28. Newberne, P.M., Harrington, D.H. and Wogan, G.N. (1966) Lab. Investig., 15, 962-969.

29. Butler, W.H. (1978) Brit. J. Cancer, 37, 418-423.

30. Williams, G.M. Klaiber, M., Parker, S.E. et al. (1976) J. Natl. Cancer Inst., 57, 157-165.

31. Williams, G.M., Ohmori, T. and Watanabe, K. (1980) Am. J. Path. 99, 1-12.

32. Daoust, R. and Calamai, R. (1971) Cancer Res. 31, 1290-1296.

33. Grundmann, E. and Sieburg, H. (1962) Beitr. Pathol. Anat. Allgem. Pathol., 126, 57-90.

34. Newberne, P.M. (1976) Cancer Res., 36, 2573-2578.

35. Weinbren, K. and Washington, S.L.A. (1976) Nature, 264, 440-442.

36. Farber, E., Parker, S. and Gruenstein, M. (1976) Cancer Res., 36, 3879-3887.

37. Deml, E. and Oesterle, D. (1980) Cancer Res., 40, 490-491.

38. Tsuda, H., Lee, G. and Farber, E. (1980) Cancer Res., 40, 1157-1164.

39. Chang, W.W.L. (1978) J. Natl. Cancer Inst. 60, 1405-1418.

40. Takahashi, M., Pour, P., Althoff, J. et al. (1977) Cancer Res., 37, 4602-4607.

41. Russo, I.H. and Russo, J. (1978) J. Natl. Cancer Inst., 61, 1439-1449.

42. Harris, C.C., Kaufman, D.G., Sporn, M.B. et al. (1973) Cancer Chemother. Rep., 4, 43-54.

43. Hicks, R.M. and Wakefield, J. St. J. (1976) Cancer Res., 36, 2502-2507.

44. Westwood, F.R., Longstaff, E. and Butler, W.H. (1979) Brit. J. Cancer, 39, 761-772.

45. Auerbach, O., Stout, A.P., Hammond, E.C. et al (1962) New Eng. J. Med., 267, 111-125.

46. Anthony, P.P. (1976) Cancer Res., 36, 2579-2583.

47. Lipkin, M. and Deschner, E. (1976) Cancer Res., 36, 2665-2668.

48. Cubilla, A.L. and Fitzgerald, P.J. (1976) Cancer Res., 36, 2690-2698.

49. Albores-Saavedra, J., Alcantra-Vazquez, A., Cruz-Ortiz, H. et al. (1980) Cancer, 45, 919-927.

50. Ogawa, K., Medline, A. and Farber, E. (1979) Brit. J. Cancer, 40, 782-790.

51. Borland, R. and Hard, G.C. (1974) Europ. J. Cancer, 10, 177-184.

52. Hard, G.C., Brown, C. and King, H. (1980) Cancer Letters, in press.

53. Mondal, S. (1975) Brit. J. Cancer, 31, 245-249.

54. Marchok, A.C., Rhoton, J.C. and Nettesheim, P. (1978) Cancer Res., 38, 2030-2037.

55. Laerum, O.D. and Rajewsky, M.F. (1975) J. Natl. Cancer Inst., 55, 1177-1187.

56. Di Paolo, J.A., Nelson, R.L., Donovan, P.J. et al. (1973) Arch. Path., 95, 380-385.

57. Hard, G.C. and Borland, R. (1977) J. Natl. Cancer Inst., 58, 1377-1382.

© 1980 Elsevier/North-Holland Biomedical Press
Mechanisms of Toxicity and Hazard Evaluation
B. Holmstedt, R. Lauwerys, M. Mercier, M. Roberfroid eds

ALKYLATION OF NUCLEIC ACID BASES BY EPOXIDES AND GLYCIDYL ETHERS

KARI HEMMINKI and HARRI VAINIO
Department of Industrial Hygiene and Toxicology, Institute of Occupational Health, Haartmaninkatu 1, SF-00290 Helsinki 29 (Finland)

INTRODUCTION

Simple epoxides such as propylene oxide, glycidol, epichlorohydrin and styrene oxide are widely used in industry[1] because of the epoxide group. However the chemical properties of the epoxides are quite different. The rate of alkylation[2, 3] and the mutagenicity[2] of the epoxides varies extensively depending on their electrophilic properties. Glycidyl ethers, widely used as components of epoxy resins[1], share the epoxide group with the above compounds. Thus it is of interest to compare the alkylation properties and the nucleic acid base adducts formed by the simple epoxides and by several types of glycidyl ethers.

METHODS

The alkylation rates were determined fluorometrically using guanosine and deoxyguanosine as the nucleophile[3]. The fluorometric identification of the guanosine adducts was based on the pH-dependent fluorescence properties of the specific adducts[4]. Nucleoside adducts were also purified chromatographically and UV and NMR spectroscopy was applied in the identification[5].

RESULTS AND DISCUSSION

The rate of guanosine alkylation by four different glycidyl ethers was shown in Fig. 1. Phenyl glycidyl ether was most reactive followed by butyl, allyl and isopropyl glycidyl ether. Three commercial epoxy resins, Epikotes 828, 1001 and 1004, each derivatives of bisphenol A glycidyl ether were tested together with epichlorohydrin (Fig. 2). Epikote 828 (molecular weight 370) had about 50 % of the activity of epichlorohydrin, while Epikote 1001 (m.w. 1000) and Epikote 1004 (m.w. 1300) had, respectively, 20 and 10 % of the activity of epichlorohydrin.

The types of guanosine adducts formed by the glycidyl ethers were assayed fluorometrically[4] as shown in Fig. 3. The reaction mixture of isopropyl glycidyl ether and guanosine exhibited a fluorescence excitation peak at about 290 nm at neutral pH while at alkaline pH very low fluorescence was recorded. This is a typical property of N-7 alkyl derivatives of guanosine[4]. Similar

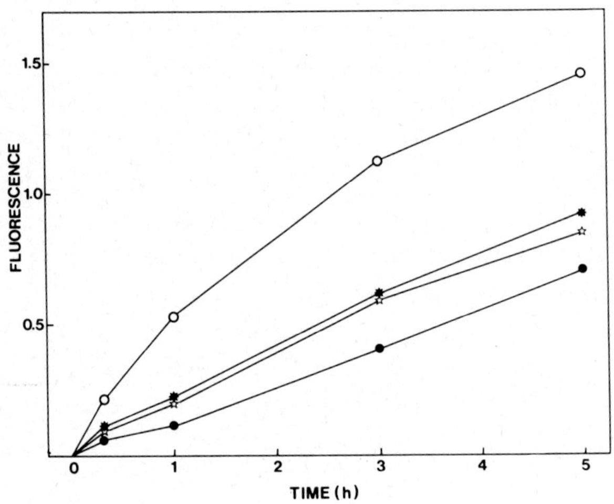

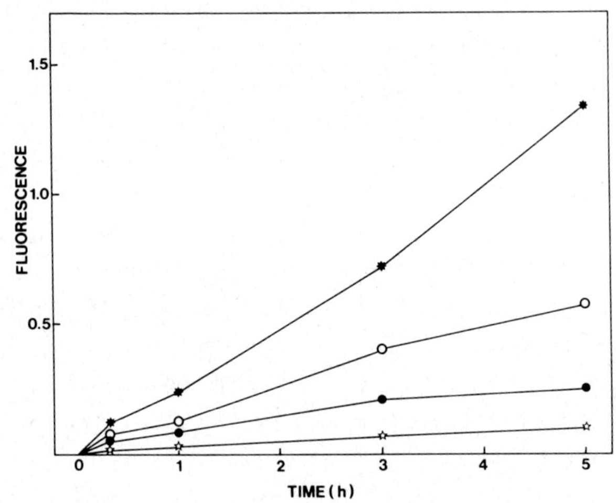

Fig. 1. Alkylation of guanosine by glycidyl ethers (from top): phenyl, butyl, allyl, and isopropyl;

Fig. 2. Alkylation by (from top) epichlorohydrin, Epikotes 828, 1001, and 1004.

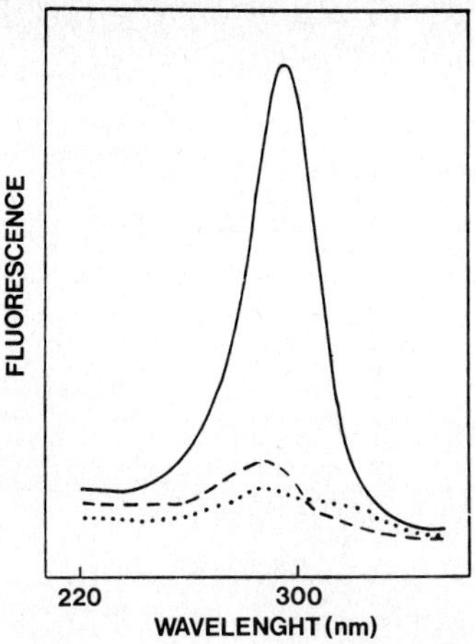

Fig. 3. Fluorescence excitation spectra (emission at 400 nm) of the reaction products of isopropyl glycidyl ether with guanosine at pH 7 (——), in NaOH (---), and at pH 6 after a NaOH treatment (···).

fluorescence properties were also exhibited by the other glycidyl ethers tested indicating alkylation at N 7.

TABLE 1

REACTIONS OF EPOXIDES AND GLYCIDYL ETHERS WITH NUCLEOSIDES

Compound	Guanosine alkylation rate	Alkylation products, with		
		dA	dC	dG, G
Epichlorohydrin	100	N 6	-	N 7
Propylene oxide	40	N 6	-	N 7
Glycidol	60	N 6	N 3	N 7
Styrene oxide	60	-	N 3	N 7
Phenyl g.e.	140	··	··	N 7
Butyl g.e.	70	··	··	N 7
Allyl g.e.	60	··	··	N 7
Isopropyl g.e.	40	··	··	N 7

dA = deoxyadenosine, dC = deoxycytidine, dG = deoxyguanosine, G = guanosine; g.e. = glycidyl ether; - = no adduct, ·· = no results.

Table 1 summarizes the alkylation activities and the base adducts of the epoxides and glycidyl ethers. In so far as information is available, the compounds form same types of adducts. Such results have lead to a suggestion that within a group of structural analogues the biological effects, such as mutagenicity, may be largely determined by the reactivity of the compounds[5].

REFERENCES

1. Fishbein, L. (1979) Potential Industrial Carcinogens and Mutagens, Elsevier, Amsterdam.
2. Hemminki, K. and Falck, K. (1979) Toxicol. Lett., 4, 103.
3. Hemminki, K. (1979) Chem.-Biol. Interactions, 28, 269.
4. Hemminki, K. (1980) Carcinogenesis, 1 (in press).
5. Hemminki, K. et al. (1980) Chem.-Biol. Interactions, 30, 259.

© 1980 Elsevier/North-Holland Biomedical Press
Mechanisms of Toxicity and Hazard Evaluation
B. Holmstedt, R. Lauwerys, M. Mercier, M. Roberfroid eds

MECHANISM OF INHIBITION OF ENZYMATIC DNA METHYLATION BY N-2-ACETYL-AMINOFLUORENE BOUND TO DNA

A. PFOHL-LESZKOWICZ, C. SALAS, R.P.P. FUCHS and G. DIRHEIMER
Institut de Biologie Moléculaire et Cellulaire du CNRS, 15 rue René Descartes, 67084 Strasbourg, and Laboratoire de Toxicologie et de Biologie Moléculaires, Faculté de Pharmacie, Strasbourg (France)

INTRODUCTION

N-acetoxy-N-2-acetylaminofluorene (N-AcO-AAF) a model ultimate metabolite of N-2-acetylaminofluorene (AAF) reacts with DNA giving essentially N-(deoxyguanosin-8-yl)-AAF. This substitution induces a conformational change in the vicinity of the adduct leading to a local denaturation of the double helix (for a review see[1]). In this paper we investigate how the enzymatic methylation of DNA by a DNA-(cytosine-5)methyl transferase is affected by the presence of the covalently bound AAF residues.

MATERIALS AND METHODS

Chicken erythrocytes DNA was a kind gift of Professor Daune. The synthesis of N-AcO-AAF was done as described elsewhere[2]. Reaction of DNA with N-AcO-AAF and subsequent purification of modified DNA was performed as described previously[3,4]. Preparation of purified rat brain DNA-(cytosine-5)methyl transferase was as published[5]. The standard assay mixture contained in 0.2 ml 50 mM Tris-HCl pH 7.8, 0.5 mM dithioerythritol : 40 μg DNA, 0.35 μg pancreatic RNAase, 50 μg partially purified enzyme, 3 μCi S-adenosyl-L-|^{3}H|-methionine (SAM) 50-75 Ci/mmole (New England Nuclear Corp.), 9 nmoles of cold SAM (Boehringer-Mannheim). After incubation at 37°C for various times 20 μl of proteinase K (Merck) (1 mg/ml in 10 mM Tris-HCl pH 7.8, 10 mM EDTA, 10 mM NaCl, 0.5% SDS) was added and the tubes reincubated for 30 min at 60°C. After addition of 1 mg carrier DNA and 0.4 ml of acetic acid 6 N, NaCl 3 M, 2 vol. ethanol were added and the recovered pellet was treated by 0.5 ml 0.5 M NaOH for 10 min at 60°C. The DNA was treated by 2 ml of TCA 15% for 10 min in ice and the precipitate collected on GFC Whatman filters, washed 6 times with 2 ml of 5% TCA, twice with ethanol and counted. With this method the recovery of the DNA was about 85%.

RESULTS

Fig. 1 shows the results obtained when, double or single stranded DNA, AAF substituted or not, was enzymatically methylated. With the AAF substituted DNA samples both the initial velocity of methylation and the overal methylation plateau are decreased as compared to the non-modified DNA samples.

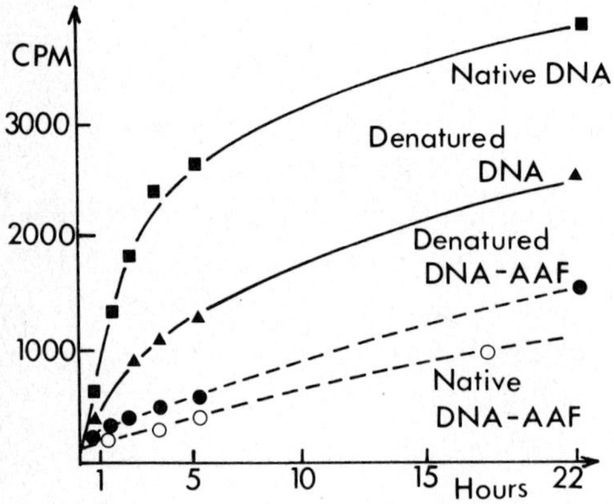

Fig. 1. Methylation of double and single stranded DNAs substituted or not with AAF (4.6% of substituted bases).

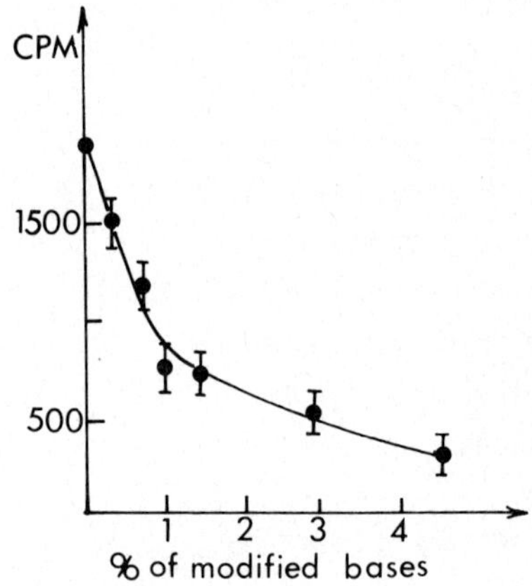

Fig. 2. Methylation of DNA substituted with various amounts of AAF. 45 min of methylation.

Fig. 2 shows that an inverse relation can be established between the degree of DNA modification and its methyl acceptor capacity. Moreover not only the substituted DNA is less methylated but added simultaneously with native DNA it inhibits the methylation of this native DNA (Fig. 3). It appears that about 1 μg of DNA-AAF inhibits to about 50% of the rate of methylation of 20 μg of non-modified DNA.

The initial methylation velocities of variable amounts of non-modified DNA were measured both in the absence and presence of DNA-AAF, modified to variable extent. The plotting of the reciprocals (1/v versus 1/S) shows a mixed type of inhibition (Fig. 4). Km for non-modified DNA expressed in phosphate residue is 250 μM. The Ki can also be calculated from the curves obtained[6] (Fig. 4). It is 37 μM for a DNA with 1.4% of modified bases. Thus the affinity of the enzyme for the substituted DNA is higher than for native DNA.

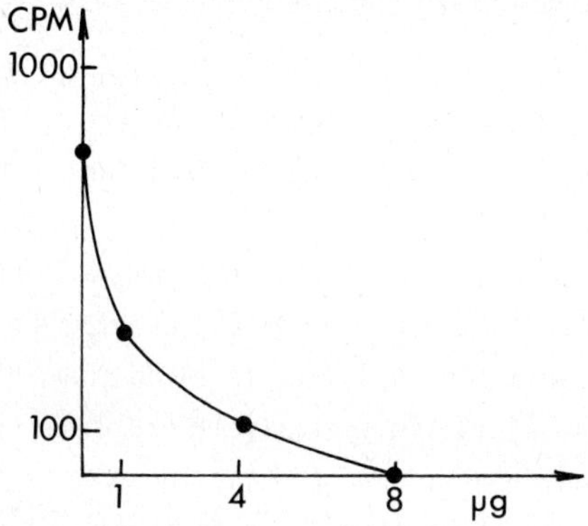

Fig. 3. Inhibition of native DNA (20 µg) methylation by various amounts of DNA-AAF (4.6% of substituted bases). The CPM due to the methylation of DNA-AAF are substracted. 120 min of methylation.

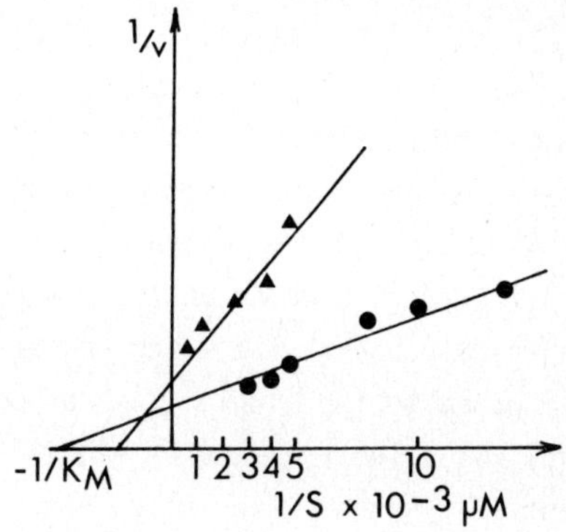

Fig. 4. Lineweaver and Burk plot of inhibition of native DNA methylation by DNA-AAF.

This higher affinity could be due to the AAF induced local denaturation regions in the substituted DNA (insertion-denaturation model[1,4]). We tested therefore the affinity of the enzyme for heat denatured DNA. This was however not the case since the Lineweaver and Burk plot showed that the affinity of the single stranded DNA is 1.6 times lower (400 µM) than that of the native double stranded DNA.

Additional experiments were performed in which instead of mixing simultaneously DNA and DNA-AAF before adding the enzyme, either the DNA or the DNA-AAF was mixed with the enzyme prior to addition of the other substrate. When 4 µg of DNA-AAF (1.8% of modified bases) were incubated with SAM and limited amounts of DNA methyl transferase either for 5 min or 20 min followed by addition of 30 µg of native DNA the methylation does not increase and remains the same that in the control where only DNA-AAF is present. Thus native DNA does not displace the enzyme from DNA-AAF and the binding of the enzyme to DNA-AAF is irreversible.

On the other hand if one preincubates native DNA with the enzyme and adds DNA-AAF afterwards one finds that the inhibition of methylation starts only after a lag time.

DISCUSSION

The lower methylation of AAF substituted DNA can be explained if we consider the model proposed for the methylation reaction[7,8] which assumes that the enzyme "walks" along the DNA strand to methylate several cytosine residues in its way, before being detached from the nucleic acid. We may therefore expect that AAF bound to the guanine residues obstacles the moving of the enzyme along the helix. Once blocked at the AAF substituted site of the DNA the enzyme is irreversibly bound. The lower degree of methylation of double stranded DNA-AAF as compared to the single stranded one (Fig. 1) can be tentatively explained as follows : The presence of AAF in the guanine residues opposing to some potential cytosine methylation sites suppresses the methylation of these cytosines. This last mechanism would only occur in double stranded DNA.

Methylation of cytosine is the only post-replicational modification so far detected in DNA of higher eucaryotes and thus has been made the basis of several proposed mechanisms of gene activity, cellular differentiation and oncogenesis. The hypomethylation of DNA caused by its substitution with AAF could have an importance in these biological mechanisms.

ACKNOWLEDGEMENTS

This work was supported by the Ligue Nationale Française contre le Cancer and the Institut National de la Santé et de la Recherche Médicale (A.T.P. n° 77-79.109 and C.R.L. n° 79-1.154.3).

REFERENCES

1. Daune, M.P. and Fuchs, R.P.P. (1976) Mécanismes d'altération et de réparation du DNA, relations avec la mutagénèse et la cancérogénèse chimique, CNRS edit., pp. 83-102.
2. Lotlikar, P.D., Scribner, J.D., Miller, J.A. and Miller, E.C. (1966) Life Sci., 5, 1263-1269.
3. Miller, E.C., Juhl, U. and Miller, J.A. (1966) Science, 153, 1125-1127.
4. Fuchs, R. and Daune, M. (1972) Biochemistry, 11, 2659-2666.
5. Pfohl-Leszkowicz, A., Salas, C., Fuchs, R.P.P. and Dirheimer, G. (1980) Biochemistry, in press.
6. Segel, I.H. (1975) Enzyme Kinetics, John Wiley Interscience, pp. 183-184.
7. Kalousek, F. and Morris, N.R. (1969) J. Biol. Chem., 244, 1151-1163.
8. Drahowsky, D. and Morris, N.R. (1971) J. Mol. Biol., 57, 475-484 and 61, 343-356.

Mechanisms of Toxicity and Hazard Evaluation
B. Holmstedt, R. Lauwerys, M. Mercier, M. Roberfroid eds

FORMATION OF PRECANCEROUS ISLANDS IN RAT LIVER AND MODIFICATION OF DNA BY ETHYL CARBAMATE: IMPLICATIONS FOR ITS METABOLISM

E. SCHERER, A.P. STEWARD[x] and P. EMMELOT
Division of Chemical Carcinogenesis, Antoni Van Leeuwenhoek-Huis,
The Netherlands Cancer Institute, 121 Plesmanlaan, 1066 CX Amsterdam
(The Netherlands)

INTRODUCTION

Ethyl carbamate is carcinogenic in several species[1,2], and mutagenic[3]. The results concerning its modification of nucleic acids are still controversial[2], and it is not known how ethyl carbamate is activated in vivo. Recently, however, Dahl et al.[4], based on the much higher carcinogenicity and mutagenicity of vinyl carbamate, proposed that oxidation of the ethyl moiety of ethyl carbamate may be the initial step in the activation process. Vinyl carbamate, however, could not be detected in vivo during the metabolism of ethyl carbamate. Nevertheless, since after administration of [ethyl-1-^{14}C; 1,2-^{3}H]ethyl carbamate the ^{3}H/^{14}C ratios of DNA, rRNA and protein adducts were considerably decreased, a metabolism leading to desaturated and/or oxidized ethyl groups remained indicated. Accordingly, one would expect that ethyl carbamate leads to similar and/or identical modifications of macromolecules as does vinyl chloride in vivo, i.e., etheno derivatives of adenosine and cytidine in RNA[5,6], or a 7-alkylguanine in DNA[7,8]. In the present study we dèscribe the formation of precancerous islands in rat liver by ethyl carbamate and its putative metabolites ethyl N-hydroxycarbamate and vinyl carbamate, and the modification of rat and mouse liver DNA in vivo by [1-^{14}C]ethyl carbamate and [carbonyl-^{14}C]ethyl carbamate. The results are consistent with the proposed activation of ethyl carbamate by oxidation of the ethyl moiety.

MATERIALS AND METHODS

Random-bred female Sprague-Dawley rats (Zentralinstitut für Versuchstiere, Hannover, G.F.R.) weighing 220-300 g, and male C3Hf/A mice (our own inbred colony), weighing 30 g, were fed a standard diet (Hope Farms, Woerden, The Netherlands) and given water ad libitum.

---

[x]Present address: Renal Unit, Small Animals Centre, Animal Health Trust, Kennett, Nr. Newmarket, Suffolk, Great Britain.

Induction of precancerous islands was studied in intact and two-third hepatectomized rats (210-240 g)[9]. Ethyl carbamate (300 mg/kg; Merck, Darmstadt, G.F.R.) and ethyl N-hydroxycarbamate (300 mg/kg; Aldrich, Milwaukee, Wis., U.S.A.) and vinyl carbamate (10 mg/kg; a gift from Dr.J.A.Miller) were applied in saline by i.p. injection, 24 h after the operation. 70 Days later the animals were sacrificed, kryostat sections of the livers were stained for Mg^{++}-dependent ATPase and evaluated quantitatively (6 cm^2 of section area per animal) for the number of ATPase-deficient islands per cm^3 of liver[10].

[1-^{14}C]Ethyl carbamate (4.8 mCi/mmole) and [carbonyl-^{14}C]ethyl carbamate (2.21 mCi/mmole) were purchased from NEN (Dreieichenhain, G.F.R.). It was used without further purification, the radiochemical purity being better than 98.5% in both cases as checked by thin-layer chromatography on silica gel G, benzene : methanol (7:3 v/v).

1,N^6 ethenodeoxyadenosine was prepared by alkaline phosphatase treatment of 1,N^6 ethenodAMP (Sigma, St.Louis, Mo., U.S.A.) or reaction overnight, 37° C, of deoxyadenosine (10 mg/ml) with a 2 M solution of chloroacetaldehyde (Fluka, Buchs, Switzerland, used as obtained or freshly distilled), adjusted to about pH 4 with NaOH[11,12]. 3,N^4 ethenodeoxycytidine was prepared in the same way from deoxycytidine. Salmon sperm DNA (Calbiochem., San Diego, Ca., U.S.A.) was modified in vitro with chloroacetaldehyde[13]. 7-2'-hydroxyethylguanine was prepared according to Ehrenberg et al.[14].

DNA from pooled livers of 2 rats or 12 mice was isolated by the SDS-Phenol method of Kirby and Cook (1967). DNA (up to 25 mg, about 5 mg/ml) was hydrolyzed either by (a), neutral heating (0.1 SSC, 100°C for 1 h), (b) acid treatment (0.1 n HCl, 70°C for 1 h), or (c) enzymically[16]. The hydrolysates from (a) and (b) were fractionated by Sephadex G10 column chromatography[17], from (c) by Dowex 50W-X4 column chromatography[16]. Absolute radioactivity of whole fractions was determined by liquid scintillation counting[17]. Due to the low degree of modification of DNA, scintillation counting in some cases was extended to several hours per fraction to get reliable results.

RESULTS AND DISCUSSION

Formation of precancerous islands, which are precursors of liver cancer formation[18], by ethyl carbamate and its putative metabolites ethyl N-hydroxycarbamate and vinyl carbamate in intact and partially hepatectomized rats is given in Table 1. Islands in the different groups were qualitatively similar, and similar to islands induced by DEN[10]. Also the size distribution was the same in all groups (up to 300 μm diameter). Island induction by ethyl carbamate was increased by partial hepatectomy by a factor of about 3, and was similar to

TABLE 1

INDUCTION OF ATPase DEFICIENT ISLANDS IN RAT LIVER

Agent	2/3 Hepatectomy	Dose, mg/kg	Islands/cm^3 $\pm$ S.E.
Ethyl carbamate	-	300	23 $\pm$ 10
Ethyl carbamate	+	300	73 $\pm$ 15
Ethyl *N*-hydroxy-carbamate	+	300	56 $\pm$ 15
Vinyl carbamate	+	10	170 $\pm$ 15

the induction by ethyl *N*-hydroxycarbamate. Administration of vinyl carbamate to partially hepatectomized rats resulted in considerably more islands, and if island induction is expressed on a molar basis, vinyl carbamate was about 60 times more active than the other carbamates. This is consistent with published results concerning the initiation of skin papillomas and lung adenomas in mice[4,19], and supports the hypothesis that oxidation of the ethyl moiety is essential for the carcinogenic potential of ethyl carbamate.

Rat liver DNA modified by [1-^{14}C]ethyl carbamate, whether hydrolyzed by neutral heating or hydrochloric acid, yielded a similar elution pattern on Sephadex G10 chromatography (Figure 1, Table 2). 3 Hours after application of ethyl carbamate (15 mg/kg) little radioactivity was incorporated into parent bases, and 50-60% of all the radioactivity, which was evidently heat labile,

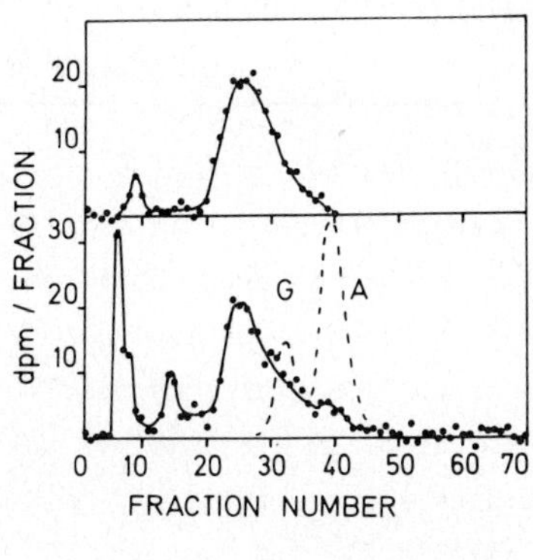

Fig. 1. Sephadex G10 chromatography of (top) the supernatant from neutral heating and (bottom) HCl hydrolysis of DNA isolated from rat liver 3 h after intraperitoneal injection of 15 mg [1-^{14}C]ethyl carbamate/kg.

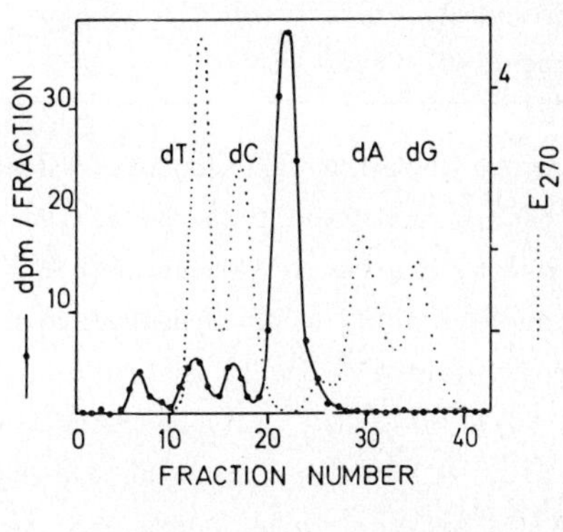

Fig. 2 Dowex 50W-X4 (NH_4^+-form) chromatography of an enzymic hydrolysate of DNA isolated from rat liver 3 h after application of 34 mg [1-^{14}C]-ethyl carbamate/kg.

eluted as a broad peak before guanine. DNA from mouse liver yielded an analogous pattern. 24 Hours after [1-^{14}C]ethyl carbamate (54 mg/kg) the broad peak was still present at about the same extent as at 3 h (Table 2). This indicates that the DNA modification(s) concerned is(are) reactively stable in rat liver. Using [carbonyl-^{14}C]ethyl carbamate and acid hydrolysis of rat liver DNA, all the radioactivity eluted in the fractions containing the apurinic acids and the parent purine bases.

TABLE 2.
BINDING TO LIVER DNA OF ETHYL CARBAMATE IN VIVO
Binding is expressed as µmoles per mole DNA-P, linearily reduced to a dose of 1 mmole/kg. Values in brackets were measured at the limit of detectability.

Position of label	Animals	Dose mg/kg	Time of killing	Hydro-lysis	Apurinic acids	Main peak	Guanine	Adenine
Ethyl-1-C	rats	15	3 h	neutral		1.6		
Ethyl-1-C	mice	1000	10 h	neutral		1.8		
Ethyl-1-C	rats	15	3 h	HCl	0.5	2.3	(0.1)	(0.2)
Ethyl-1-C	rats	38-54	24 h	HCl	5.6	1.6	1.2	1.2
Ethyl-1-C	mice	1000	10 h	HCl	3.6	1.5		(0.1)
Ethyl-1-C	mice	1000	24 h	HCl	5.6	1.3		(0.1)
Ethyl-1-C	rats	34	3 h	enzymic		1.3 ± 0.3	0	0
Ethyl-1-C	mice	28	3.5 h	enzymic		2.7	0	0
Carbonyl-C	rats	70	2.5 h	HCl	(0.1)	0	(0.03)	(0.04)
Carbonyl-C	rats	73	24 h	HCl	1.1	0	0.3	0.6

Since the high carcinogenic, mutagenic and island inductive capacity of vinyl carbamate indicated that the activation of ethyl carbamate could lead finally to epoxyethyl carbamate, which should lead to similar and/or the same modifications of nucleic acids as chloroethylene oxide, the putative reactive metabolite of vinyl chloride[20-24], it was further studied whether DNA modifications described for vinyl chloride could be detected after administration of [1-^{14}C]ethyl carbamate. 1,$\underline{N}^6$-Ethenoadenosine and 3,$\underline{N}^4$-ethenocytidine are modifications of RNA[5,6], and the former adduct has been reported also in DNA[13].

Enzymic hydrolysis and ion exchange chromatography of rat or mouse liver DNA from [1-^{14}C]ethyl carbamate treated animals led to one main radioactive peak (Figure 2) eluting between deoxycytidine and the purine deoxynucleosides (fraction 62, the elution position of deoxyguanosine is set to 100). The etheno compounds, however, added as markers or derived from enzymic hydrolysis of chloroacetaldehyde modified salmon sperm DNA, eluted in different fractions: 3,$\underline{N}^4$-ethenodeoxycytidine fraction 75, 1,$\underline{N}^6$-ethenoadenine fraction 125 and 1,$\underline{N}^6$-ethenodeoxyadenosine fraction 165. This radioactive peak was not present if DNA was heated to 100°C and precipitated again prior to enzymic hydrolysis, indicating that the broad peak on Sephadex and the main peak on Dowex stem from the same modification of DNA. This is substantiated by the quantitative data (Table 2).

Recently, Bolt et al.[8] reported that, in disagreement with earlier studies[13] rat liver DNA modified by vinyl chloride in vivo contained no etheno derivatives of deoxyadenosine or deoxycytidine, but another product which eluted close to deoxyguanosine from an Aminex A6 column. This could have been a modification of N-7 of guanine[7].

Work on the identification of the DNA modification reported here is in progress: it seems that it is identical with the main DNA-adduct resulting from vinyl chloride, since on rechromatography in the Aminex A6 system it eluted with the same volume as the vinylchloride derived modification. Furthermore, reaction of chloroethylene oxide with deoxyguanosine followed by hydrochloric acid hydrolysis yielded a modified product with the UV spectrum characteristic for 7-alkylguanine. This compound eluted from the Dowex 50W as well as the Aminex A6 column with the same volume as the [1-^{14}C] ethyl carbamate derived DNA modification. On reduction by sodium borohydride this marker cochromatographed (silicagel, ethanol-n-butanol-water, 10:80:25) with 7-2'-hydroxyethylguanine. This supports the hypothesis[4] that vinyl chloride and ethyl carbamate are activated by a similar metabolic pathway, and that in both cases 7-2'-oxoethylguanine[7] might be the main modification of DNA.

ACKNOWLEDGEMENT

We are grateful to Dr.J.A.Miller for the gift of vinyl carbamate and Dr.R.J.Laib for the rechromatographies performed in the Aminex A6 system,

REFERENCES

1. Mirvish, S.S. (1968) Adv. Cancer Res., 11, 1-42.
2. IARC (1974) IARC Monographs Vol.7, 111-140.
3. Bateman, A.J. (1976) Mutation Res., 39, 75-96.
4. Dahl, G.A. et al. (1978) Cancer Res., 38, 3793-3804.
5. Laib, R.J. and Bolt, H.M. (1977) Toxicology, 8, 185-195.
6. Laib, R.J. and Bolt, H.M. (1978) Arch. Toxicol., 39, 235-240.

7. Osterman-Golkar, S. et al. (1977) Biochem. Biophys. Res. Commun., 76, 259-266.
8. Bolt, H.M. et al. (1980) Arch. Toxicol. Suppl. 3, 129-142.
9. Higgins, G.M. and Anderson, R.M. (1931) Arch. Pathol., 12, 186-202.
10. Scherer, E. et al. (1974) J. Natl. Cancer Inst., 49, 93-106.
11. Kochetkov, N.K. et al. (1971) Tetrahedron Lett., 22, 1993-1996.
12. Barrio, J.R. et al. (1972) Biochem. Biophys. Res. Commun., 46, 597-604.
13. Green, T. and Hathway, D.E. (1978) Chem.-Biol. Interact., 22, 211-224.
14. Ehrenberg, L. et al. (1974) Mut. Res., 24, 83-103.
15. Kirby, K.S. and Cook, E.A. (1967) Biochem. J., 104, 254-262.
16. Scherer, E. et al. (1980) Cancer Lett., 10, 1-6.
17. Scherer, E. et al. (1977) Chem.-Biol. Interact., 19, 1-11.
18. Emmelot, P. and Scherer, E. (1980) Biochim.Biophys.Acta, 605, 247-304.
19. Berenblum, I. et al. (1959) Biochem. Pharmacol., 2, 168-176.
20. Göthe, R. et al. (1974) Ambio, 3, 234-236.
21. Barbin, A. et al. (1975) Biochem. Biophys. Res. Commun., 67, 596-603.
22. Bonse, G. et al. (1975) Biochem. Pharmacol., 24, 1829-1834.
23. Kappus, H. et al. (1975) Nature, 257, 134-135.
24. Green, T. and Hathway , D.E. (1977) Chem.-Biol. Interact., 17, 137-150.

Mechanisms of Toxicity and Hazard Evaluation
B. Holmstedt, R. Lauwerys, M. Mercier, M. Roberfroid eds

ON THE METABOLISM OF VARIOUS POLYCYCLIC AROMATIC HYDROCARBONS (PAH) BY LIVER MICROSOMES OF VARIOUSLY PRETREATED RATS

ACHIM SCHMOLDT, JÜRGEN JACOB AND GERNOT GRIMMER
Institute of Pharmacology, University of Hamburg, Martinistr. 52, D-2000 Hamburg 20 (W.Germany)(A.S.) and Biochemisches Institut für Umweltcarcinogene, Sieker Landstr.19,D-2070 Ahrensburg (W.Germany)

INTRODUCTION

In comparison to benzo(a)pyrene little is known about the metabolism of other PAH. In respect to carcinogenic risk we are interested in the metabolism of relevant environmental PAH.

Metabolites formed by rat liver microsomes were analyzed by means of GC/MS technique which allows a better separation and detection than HPLC. Moreover, the influence on the microsomal monooxygenase system after pretreating rats with various PAH was studied.

MATERIALS AND METHODS

Animals. Male Wistar rats (180±15 g b.w.) were pretreated with PAH, 5,6-benzoflavone (40 mg/kg daily for 3 days), phenobarbital (80 mg/kg daily for 3 days), polychlorinated biphenyls (PCB) or 3,4,3',4'-Cl_4-biphenyl (200 mg/kg 3 days before sacrifice). Control rats received the same doses of the vehicles (2 ml arachis oil or NaCl-solution/kg).

Incubations. Incubations were carried out in a total volume of 2 ml containing 50 mM tris/HCl (pH 7.4), 0.15 M KCl, 5 mM $MgCl_2$, 0.2 mM NADPH, 1 mg microsomal protein, 20 μg PAH (dissolved in 20 μl acetone), 0.5 mM NADPH, 8 mM isocitrate, and 50 μg isocitrate dehydrogenase. After incubation at 37° C for 30 min the incubations were stopped by addition of acetone.

Analytical procedures. The samples were deluted with water (10 ml), acidified with acetic acid and extracted with ethyl acetate (twice with 20 ml). The residue of the organic phase was dissolved in isopropanol and cleaned up by column chromatography[1]. The fraction containing PAH and metabolites was silylated with trisil (PEARCE) and BSTFA (Pierce).

GC/MS conditions: 25 or 50 m glass capillaries coated with SE 30 splittless injection, injection temperature 100° C, temperature program 40°/min to 200° C, 1^{O} C/min to 250° C, helium as carrier gas, ion source 250° C, 70 eV (Varian MAT 112 S).

RESULTS

A high resolution of the silylated metabolites can be achieved best by capillary GC. Figure 1 shows the separation of a synthetic mixture of benz(a)anthracene phenols and dihydrodiols. Thus it can be assumed that the method will separate metabolites of other PAH as well. Phenols and higher hydroxylated metabolites can be characterized by their mass spectra.

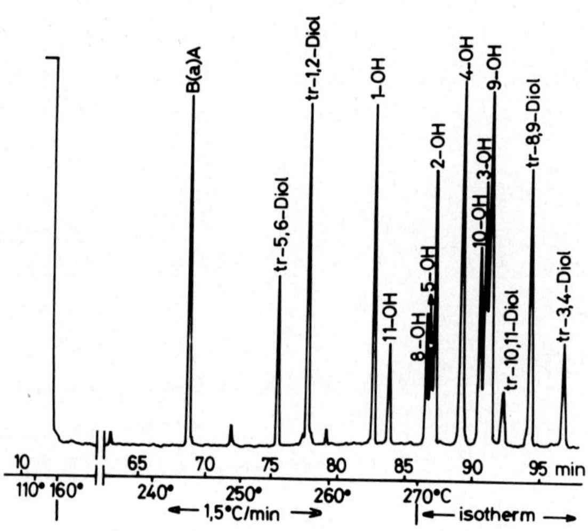

Fig. 1. Gaschromatogram of a synthetic mixture of benz(a)anthracene phenols and dihydrodiols.

The metabolic rates of various PAH with microsomes of normal rats differed significantly (Table 1). Phenanthrene was nearly quantitatively metabolized, only traces of metabolites could be observed in case of crysene, benzo(ghi)perylene and the benzopyrenes. Metabolites of benzo(k)fluoranthene could not be detected.

TABLE 1.

METABOLISM OF PAH BY LIVER MICROSOMES OF NORMAL RATS

Substrate	nmoles/mg x 30 min (number of metabolites)	Substrate	nmoles/mg x 30 min (number of metabol.)
Phenanthrene	111 (2)	B(a)P[a]	1.6 (2)
Fluoranthene	31 (6)	B(e)P[a]	0.8 (2)
Pyrene	32 (6)	B(b)F[a]	5.2 (3)
B(a)A[a]	12 (6)	B(k)F[a]	-
Chrysene	0.7 (2)	I(1,2,3 -cd)P[a]	-
C(cd)P[a]	39 (6)	B(ghi)P[a]	1.6 (2)

[a] B(a)A=benz(a)anthracene, C(cd)P=cyclopenta(cd)pyrene, B(a)P=benzo (a)pyrene, B(e)P=benzo(e)pyrene, B(b)F=benzo(b)fluoranthen, I(1,2,3-cd)P=Indeno(1,2,3-cd)pyrene, B(k)F=benzo(k)fluoranthene, B(ghi)P=benzo(ghi)perylene

TABLE 2

BENZ(a)ANTHRACENE AND BENZO(a)PYRENE METABOLISM BY LIVER MICROSOMES OF PRETREATED RATS

Pretreatment	Induction factor benz(a)-anthracene	Induction factor benzo(a)-pyrene	cyt.P450/448 (λ max)
Controls	1[b]	1[b]	1.0[b] (450.5)
5.6-Benzoflavone	4.4	4.2	1.6 (449)
PCB	6.2	5.2	3.9 (449.5)
3,4,3',4'-Cl_4-biphenyl	5.8	6.2	2.2 (449)
Phenobarbital	7.2	2.4	3.6 (450.5)
B(a)A[a]	6.5	4.2	1.5 (449)
Pyrene	0.4	1.1	1.3 (450.5)
Chrysene	9.1	6.0	1.7 (448)
B(a)P[a]	5.0	11.0	1.7 (448.5)
B(e)P[a]	1.6	1.9	1.1 (449.5)
B(b)F[a]	4.1	8.6	1.9 (447.5)
B(j)F[a]	6.5	5.8	1.5 (448)
B(k)F[a]	3.4	4.7	1.5 (448)

[a] B(j)F=benzo(j)fluoranthene; further abbreviations see table 1.
[b] Control values: Benz(a)anthracene 6.1 nmoles/mg microsomal prot./30 min; benzo(a)pyrene (fluorimetric assay): 1.06±0.12 nmoles/mg/15 min; cyt.P450: 0.75±0.12 nmole/mg microsomal protein.

Table 2 shows the influence of the pretreatment of rats with well known inducers and of PAH on the metabolism of benz(a)anthracene. The PAH studied caused considerable differences in the metabolic rate. Chrysene was more effective than 5,6-benzoflavone or benzo(a)pyrene, whereas pyrene decreased the metabolic rate; benzo (e)pyrene did not show any effect.

Different increases of the metbaolic rate were observed in case of benz(a)anthracene and benzo(a)pyrene. To clarify whether this results only from the detection method (benzo(a)pyrene metabolites were measured fluorimetrically) the metabolic rates of some PAH-substrates were measured after pretreating rats with benzo(k)-fluoranthene. In comparison to controls the following increase factors (metabolism pretreated/unpretreated) were observed: Fluoranthene 2.1, pyrene 2.1, chrysene 31.1, benz(a)anthracene 3.4, benzo(b)fluoranthene 9.5, benzo(j)fluoranthene 7.5, benzo(a)pyrene 23.1, benzo (e)pyrene 57.3, indeno(1,2,3-cd)pyrene 55.0. Besides these remarkable differences benzo(k)fluoranthene has shown to be a potent inducer causing already effects at almost 0.2 mg/kg dose level.

CONCLUSIONS

GC/MS is an effective method for qualitative and quantitative analysis of PAH metabolites. After derivatization even polyhydroxylated metabolites can be detected.

The metabolic rates od various PAH vary considerably and increase to a different extent after pretreatment with carcinogenic or non-carcinogenic PAH. Since generally an exposure occurs to mixtures of various PAH, some of which being potent inducers, an increased conversion of carcinogenic PAH to ultimate carcinogens should be considered. Further investigations will show whether the different increase factors for the metabolism of the series of PAH studied result from the PAH caused induction of different P450-isocytochromes.

ACKNOWLEDGEMENT

The authors are grateful for the supply of benz(a)anthracene metabolites by the National Cancer Institute U.S.A.

REFERENCE

1. Grimmer,G. and Böhnke H. (1972) Z.Anal.Chem. 261, 310-314.

© 1980 Elsevier/North-Holland Biomedical Press
Mechanisms of Toxicity and Hazard Evaluation
B. Holmstedt, R. Lauwerys, M. Mercier, M. Roberfroid eds

SYNERGISTIC EFFECTS OF CIGARETTE SMOKE EXTRACTS, BENZ(A)PYRENE AND NICKEL SULPHATE ON MORPHOLOGICAL TRANSFORMATION OF HAMSTER EMBRYO CELLS

EDGAR RIVEDAL, JAN HEMSTAD AND TORE SANNER
Norsk Hydro's Institute for Cancer Research, The Norwegian Radium Hospital, Oslo (Norway)

INTRODUCTION

The risk for development of lung cancer among cigarette smokers depends on a number of factors. Thus,people working with asbestos as well as nickel refinery workers have a much higher frequency of lung cancer than expected from their smoking habit alone[1-4]. Moreover, the lung cancer frequency is higher in urban than rural areas[5,6]. Air pollution from coal and oil powered plants as well as car emission contain airborne particles covered with polycyclic aromatic hydrocarbons, i.e. benz(a)pyrene[7,8].

The purpose of the present work was to study whether cigarette smoke extract would affect morphological transformation of hamster embryo cells by benz(a)pyrene and nickel sulphate.

MATERIALS AND METHODS

Test chemicals. Benz(a)pyrene (BP) and 12-O-tetra-decanoyl-phorbol-13-acetate (TPA) were purchased from Sigma Chem Co (St. Louis, MO., USA). $NiSO_4 \cdot 6H_2O$(p.a.) was obtained from Merck (Darmstadt, FRG). Smoke extracts were prepared by dimethylsulphoxide (DMSO) extraction of glass fiber filters exposed to cigarette smoke. The chemicals were dissolved in DMSO and diluted with warm complete medium to the desired concentration shortly before use. The final concentration of DMSO was consistently less than 0.2%.

Transformation assay. Primary cultures of Syrian hamster embryos at 14 d of gestation, were prepared according to the method of Pienta et al[9]. The bioassay[9,10] was used with small modifications as previously described[11]. Essentially, 200 target cells were seeded in Petri dishes on a feeder layer consisting of $6x10^4$ X-irradiated (5000R) cells. The test chemicals were added 24 h later and the dishes washed and stained after 7 d incubation. In experiments where the promoting effect of smoke extract and TPA was tested, the dishes were washed twice with phosphate buffered saline 4 d after addition of BP, and new medium was added containing smoke extract or TPA. The colonies were stained 4 d later. Morphological transformation is defined as altered colony morphology consisting of criss crossing and piling up of cells not observed in control dishes. All experiments have been repeated 3 - 5 times with consistent results. One set of data is presented for each experiment.

RESULTS

The frequency of morphological transformation by smoke extract, BP and nickel sulphate given separately and in combination is shown in table 1. In separate experiments (not shown)

TABLE 1

MORPHOLOGICAL TRANSFORMATION BY SMOKE EXTRACT, BENZ(A)PYRENE AND NICKEL SULPHATE GIVEN SEPARATELY AND IN COMBINATION

Additions[a]	Total no.colonies	Cloning eff.(%)	Total no transf. colonies	Transformation frequency[b] (%)
Control	306	26	0	0
Smoke extract	324	27	2	0.6
BP	240	20	3	1.4
$NiSO_4.6H_2O$	300	25	1	0.3
BP+smoke extract	192	16	9	4.7
$NiSO_4.6H_2O$ + smoke extract	312	26	11	3.5

[a]The following concentrations were used: Smoke extract 5 ug/ml; BP 0.01 µg/ml; $NiSO_4.6H_2O$ 5ug/ml.

[b]The transformation frequency is calculated as the number of transformed colonies divided by the total number of surviving colonies multiplied with 100. 6 dishes were used for each concentration.

the transformation frequency was found to increase with increasing concentration of the test substances. It is apparent from the table that with the concentrations used, the combination of BP and smoke extract gave a transformation frequency of 4.7% which is more than twice that expected. Likewise, the combination of nickel sulphate and smoke extract gave 3 - 4 times as many transformations as expected. The results clearly demonstrate that the transformation frequency found in the presence of BP or nickel sulphate are enhanced by addition of smoke extract.

To study the interaction between BP and smoke extract in more details, an experiment was carried out in which the medium on the dishes was changed 4 d after addition of the test chemical. When BP was present during the first period with no additions during the second period, the transformation frequency

TABLE 2

EFFECT OF SMOKE EXTRACT AND TPA ON PROMOTION OF TRANSFORMATIONS INITIATED BY BENZ(A)PYRENE

Additions[a] 1.period (4 d)	2.period (4 d)	Total no. colonies	Cloning eff. (%)	Total no. transf. colonies	Transformation frequency (%)[b]
None	None	612	26	0	0
BP	None	420	18	2	0.5
None	Smoke extr.	636	27	0	0
None	TPA	480	20	2	0.4
BP	Smoke extr.	504	21	19	3.8
BP	TPA	420	18	26	6.2

[a] The following concentrations were used: BP 0.05 µg/ml; smoke extract 5 µg/ml; TPA 0.1 µg/ml.

[b] The transformation frequency is calculated as the number of transformed colonies divided by the total number of surviving colonies multiplied with 100. Twelve dishes were used for each concentration.

was 0.5% (table 2). No transformation was observed when smoke extract was present during the second period with no additions during the first period. Interestingly, when BP was present during the first period and smoke extract during the second period, a transformation frequency of 3.8% was observed, which is more than 7 times higher than expected. This suggests that smoke extract promotes transformations initiated by BP. Further support for this was obtained in experiments where the tumor promotor TPA[12] was present during the second period in stead of smoke extract. Also in this case, the transformation frequency was about 7 times higher than expected from experiments where BP and TPA were tested separately in the two periods.

DISCUSSION

The present results demonstrate a potentiating effect of cigarette smoke extract on morphological transformation of Syrian hamster embryo cells by BP and nickel sulphate. Experiments where the exposure period was divided into two parts and smoke extract or TPA were present during the last part, suggest that smoke extract has a promotion like effect on formation of transformed cells initiated by BP. The results also show that transformation can be induced by cigarette smoke itself. Thus, smoke extract can both initiate and promote morphological transformation of hamster embryo cells.

ACKNOWLEDGMENTS

The excellent technical assistance of Mrs. Astri Nordahl is greatly acknowledged. Thanks are due to Tiedemanns Tobaksfabrik, Oslo, Norway for providing smoke exposed filters. E.R. is Research Fellow of the Norwegian Research Council for Science and Humanities.

REFERENCES

1. Selikoff, I.J. Hammond, E.C. and Churg, J. (1968) J.Am. Med.Assoc., 204, 106-112.
2. Hammond, E.C. and Selikoff, I.J. (1973) Int.Agency Res. Cancer, Scientific Publication No.8, Lyon, France, pp.312-317.

3. McEvan, J.C. (1976) Ann.N.Y.Acad.Sci., 271, 365-369.

4. Kreyberg, L. (1978) Br.J.Ind.Med., 35, 109-116.

5. Burrascano, J.J. (1978) N.Y.State J.Med., 78, 924-934.

6. Smoking and Health, a report of the Surgeon General (1979) Chapter 5. US Dep.of Health, Education and Welfare, Washington, pp.1-74.

7. Natusch, D.F.S. (1978) Envir.Health Perspec., 22, 79-90.

8. Handa, T., Kato, Y., Yamamura T. and Tadahiro, I. (1980) Envir.Sci.Tech., 14, 416-422.

9. Pienta, R.J., Poiley, J.A. and Lebherz, W.B.III (1977) Int.J.Cancer, 19, 642-655.

10. DiPaolo, J.A., Donovan, P. and Nelson, R. (1969) J.Natl. Cancer Inst., 42, 867-876.

11. Rivedal, E. and Sanner, T. (1980) Cancer Letters, 8, 203-208.

12. Van Duuren, B.L., and Orris, L. (1965) Cancer Res., 25, 1871-1875.

Mechanisms of Toxicity and Hazard Evaluation
B. Holmstedt, R. Lauwerys, M. Mercier, M. Roberfroid eds

IRREVERSIBLE MACROMOLECULAR BINDING OF THE FLAME RETARDANT TRIS-(2,3-DIBROMOPROPYL)PHOSPHATE IN VITRO AND IN VIVO

ERIK DYBING, ERIK J. SÖDERLUND AND SIDNEY D. NELSON
Department of Toxicology, National Institute of Public Health, Oslo, Norway and Department of Medicinal Chemistry, University of Washington, Seattle, Washington, USA

INTRODUCTION

The flame retardant tris(2,3-dibromopropyl)phosphate (Tris-BP) can be activated to a potent mutagen in the *S. typhimurium* test[1,2,3] and causes kidney tubular adenomas and carcinomas in long-term feeding experiments with rats and mice[4]. We have studied the role of metabolism for the activation of Tris-BP to covalently (irreversibly) macromolecular bound products in vitro and in vivo.

MATERIALS AND METHODS

Chemicals. ^{3}H-Tris-BP was synthesized by acylation of ^{3}H-2,3-dibromopropanol (^{3}H-2,3-DBP) with phosphoryl chloride. ^{3}H-2,3-DBP was synthesized by reducing 2,3-dibromopropionaldehyde with sodium boro(^{3}H)hydride (Amersham Radiochemical Centre, U.K.). 2,3-Dibromopropionaldehyde was prepared from bromine and acrolein in carbon tetrachloride.

Covalent binding. Washed microsomes were prepared from control or phenobarbital (PB)-, β-naphthoflavone (BNF)-, polychlorinated biphenyl (PCB)- or $CoCl_2$-pretreated Wistar rats. For determination of ^{3}H-Tris-BP covalent protein binding in vitro, microsomes, label and a NADPH-generating system were incubated at 37 °C for 15 min and stopped by addition of trichloroacetic acid (TCA)[5]. In DNA binding experiments in vitro DNA was added to the microsomal incubation and DNA extracted with phenol:chloroform:isopentyl alcohol[6]. For determination of in vivo protein binding, rats were given ^{3}H-Tris-BP 250 mg/kg i.p. and 9 hr later homogenates of liver, kidney and muscle were prepared and precipitated with TCA[7]. DNA binding in liver and kidney were determined according to Viviani and Lutz[8].

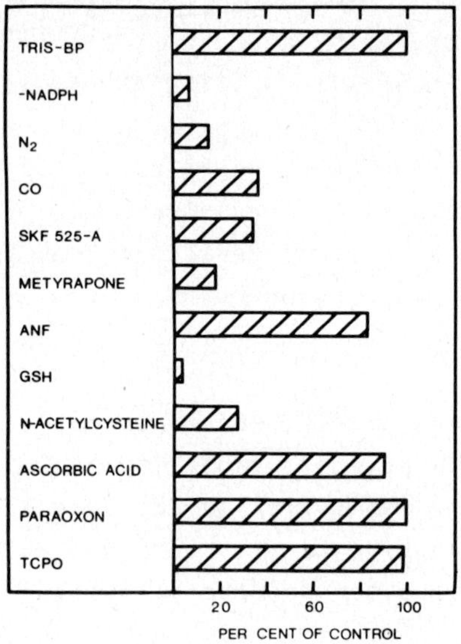

Fig. 1 Conditions for covalent binding of ^{3}H-Tris-BP to rat liver microsomal protein in vitro

RESULTS

^{3}H-Tris-BP was metabolically activated to a product(s) which bound covalently to rat liver microsomal protein in the presence of NADPH and oxygen (Fig. 1). The binding rate was markedly reduced by CO and cytochrome P-450 inhibitors such as SKF 525-A and metyrapone. Addition of the nucleophiles glutathione (GSH) and N-acetylcysteine strongly inhibited ^{3}H-Tris-BP binding, whereas the radical reducing agent ascorbic acid, the esterase inhibitor paraoxon and the epoxide hydratase inhibitor 1,1,1-trichloropropene epoxide (TCPO) were without effects. Pretreatment of rats with PB increased ^{3}H-Tris-BP binding rates 6-fold, but BNF-pretreatment did not induce binding (Fig. 2). $CoCl_2$-pretreament almost abolished ^{3}H-Tris-BP binding. The binding rate with kidney microsomes was only 7 % of the rate with liver microsomes, but it was doubled using PCB-pretreated microsomes. ^{3}H-2,3-DBP, a hydrolysis product of ^{3}H-2,3-Tris-BP[9], also bound covalently to liver microsomal protein; this occurred at 17 % of the rate seen with ^{3}H-Tris-BP.

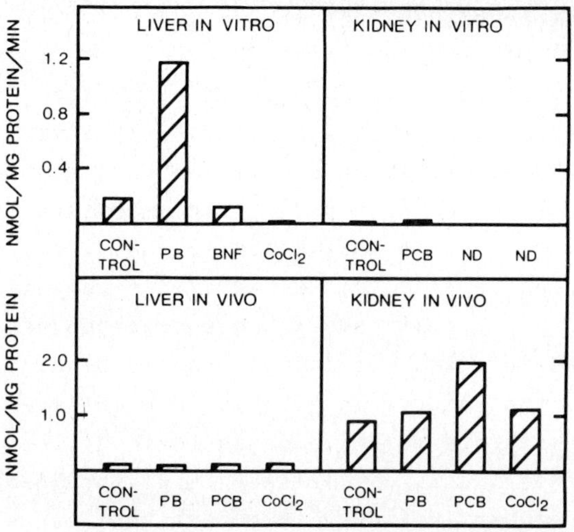

Fig 2. Effect of pretreatments on ^{3}H-Tris-BP covalent binding to liver and kidney microsomal protein in vitro and to liver and kidney protein in vivo. N.D.: Not determined.

Administration of ^{3}H-Tris-BP to rats lead to its covalent binding to proteins in kidney and liver (Fig. 2). Kidney binding levels were 5 times higher than in liver. ^{3}H-Tris-BP binding in vivo was not altered by PB- or $CoCl_2$-pretreatment, however, kidney binding was doubled after PCB-pretreatment. ^{3}H-Tris-BP also bound covalently to DNA, either when DNA was added to liver microsomal incubations or when DNA was extracted from kidney and liver of rats given ^{3}H-Tris-BP in vivo. In vitro DNA binding rates were tripled using PCB-pretreated liver microsomes compared to controls (45.7 vs. 16.0 pmol/mg DNA/20 min). Four times higher binding levels were found in kidney DNA than in liver DNA in vivo (66.3 vs. 15.6 pmol/mg DNA). DNA binding in kidney was increased by 44 % after PCB-pretreatment.

DISCUSSION

From the effects of inducers and inhibitors of cytochrome P-450 on the covalent binding of ^{3}H-Tris-BP it is evident that ^{3}H-Tris-BP is metabolically activated to an electrophile(s) by a cytochrome P-450 dependent oxidation reaction. Tris-BP appears to be a substrate for the PB-inducible form of the cytochrome(s). Because of the lower rate of binding seen with ^{3}H-2,3-DBP compared to ^{3}H-Tris-BP and the lack of effect of the esterase inhibitor paraoxon, it seems unlikely that 2,3-DBP is a proximate reactive metabolite of Tris-BP. Further, since ascorbic acid and TCPO were without effects on ^{3}H-Tris-BP binding, a radical intermediate or an epoxide is probably not involved in the metabolic activation of Tris-BP. We tentatively propose that Tris-BP is oxidatively debrominated yielding either reactive α-bromo ketones or aldehydes.

In contrast to in vitro microsomal protein binding, protein binding in vivo was much higher in kidneys than in liver. This correlates very well with the relative organotoxic potential of Tris-BP in single dose experiments[10]. Tris-BP covalent DNA-binding was also considerably higher in kidney than in liver, corresponding to the organotropy of the carcinogen[4].

ACKNOWLEDGEMENTS

This study was supported by the Royal Norwegian Council for Scientific and Industrial Research.

REFERENCES

1. Prival, M.J., McCoy, E.C., Gutter, B. and Rosenkranz, H.S. (1977) Science, 195, 76-78.
2. Blum, A. and Ames, B.N. (1977) Science, 195, 17-23.
3. Söderlund, E.J., Nelson, S.D. and Dybing, E. (1979) Acta Pharmacol. Toxicol., 45, 112-121.
4. Reznik, G., Ward, J.M., Hardisty, J.F. and Russfield, A. (1979) J. Natl. Cancer Inst., 63, 205-212.
5. Dybing, E., Aune, T. and Nelson, S.D. (1979) Biochem. Pharmacol., 28, 43-50.
6. Neal, G.E., Mattocks, A.R. and Judah, D.J. (1979) Biochim. Biophys. Acta, 585, 134-142.
7. Dybing, E., Aune, T. and Nelson, S.D. (1979) Biochem. Pharmacol., 28, 51-55.
8. Viviani, A. and Lutz, W.K. (1978) Cancer Res., 38, 4640-4644.
9. St. John, Jr., L.E., Eldefrawi, M.E. and Lisk, D.J. (1976) Bull. Environ. Contamin.. Toxicol., 15, 192-197.
10. Söderlund, E., Dybing, E. and Nelson, S.D. Toxicol. Appl. Pharmacol., in press.

© 1980 Elsevier/North-Holland Biomedical Press
Mechanisms of Toxicity and Hazard Evaluation
B. Holmstedt, R. Lauwerys, M. Mercier, M. Roberfroid eds

CARCINOGENIC POTENTIAL OF DICHLOROACETYLENE

D.REICHERT, U.SPENGLER, W.ROMEN and D. HENSCHLER
Institut für Pharmakologie und Toxikologie der Universität, Versbacher Straße 9, D-8700 Würzburg, FRG.

INTRODUCTION

Dichloroacetylene (DCA) occurs as a decomposition product of trichloroethylene, tetrachloroethane and acetylene. Additionally DCA is a by-product of the synthesis of certain chlorinated hydrocarbons. The synthesis of vinylidene chloride, in particular, is accompanied by DCA formation. DCA inhalation experiments with animals substantiate this compound's strong nephrotoxic properties; moreover a carcinogenic potential has been proposed[1]. This assumption is supported by studies of the chemical reactivity of DCA: it is chemically highly reactive. In contact with air DCA decomposes to a series of, for the most part, perchlorinated hydrocarbons[2]. Some of these are established strong mutagens (e.g. trichloroacryloyl chloride[3]) or carcinogens (e.g. hexachlorobutadiene[4]). It is assumed that DCA decomposition in mammalian organisms may occur in a similar manner.

To evaluate the biological risk of DCA exposure we conducted, as a first step, a one year inhalation study with groups of 30 male and 30 female NMRI mice. Preliminary results of this study are reported in this paper.

MATERIALS AND METHODS

Chemicals. DCA was freshly synthesized from trichloroethylene in steady state concentration as described previously[5]. DCA is stable in pure nitrogen. In the exposure mixture with air, DCA is stabilized by admixture of acetylene (1:2, v:v)[2,5].

Animals. Groups of 30 male and 30 female NMRI mice each (Zentralinstitut für Versuchstiere, D-3000 Hannover, FRG) were used for DCA exposed animals and controls. They were kept in an air-conditioned room with an artificial 12 h day/night rhythm. Feed (Altromin®) and tap water were freely available. For the duration of the exposure (8 a.m.- 2 p.m.) animals had no access to food and water. The experimental period was determined by the length of survival of the various animals (6-8 weeks old at start). Animals were checked twice daily for mortality.

Exposure system. During the exposure the bodies of the animals were kept in place in tubular, transparent plexiglass casings on the outside of the actual exposure chamber (300 x 240 x 35 mm). Only the noses were in contact with the exposure mixture which was streamed through the chamber from bottom to top. The duration of the exposure was 6 h/day, 1 day/week, 12 months.

DCA was selectively and quantitatively determined by a Hall electrolytic conductivity detector. A special gas-sampling system allowed continuous control of the concentrations of synthesized DCA vapor[5]. The concentration was adjusted to 9 ppm.

Histological examination. Deceased animals were autopsied, organs were weighed (liver, spleen, kidney, lung, heart), tissue sections were fixed in 10% formalin before they were embedded in Paraplast. Eyes and Harderian glands were fixed in a 1:1 (v:v) mixture of formalin (10%), and glutaraldehyde (2%), and subsequently decalcified in a 1:1:8 (v:v:v) mixture of formalin (40%), formic acid (98%) and water. Hematoxylin-eosin staining was used routinely, but other stains were employed when needed.

RESULTS AND DISCUSSION

Body weight and survival. Body weight gain differed markedly between control and DCA exposed animals after 25 weeks exposure time, indicating an early manifestation of toxicity. Polyuria and glucosuria pointed to a nephrotoxic effect. The survival time for both exposed male and female mice is significantly reduced in comparison with control animals; mean survival times are as follows (controls in parentheses): males 54.8 ± 3.0 weeks (97.2 ± 5.5 weeks) females 70.9 ± 2.6 weeks (88.5 ± 4.6 weeks). The reduced life expectancies of exposed male mice are consistent with the general observation that male mice inhale, due to their substantially higher respiratory rate as compared to female mice, a considerably larger dose.

Histology. The acute toxic lesion is characterized by extensive necrosis of the proximal tubules of the kidneys. The renal damage still persists later on in the form of atypical cells and poorly differentiated tubular epithelia. It is suggested that this damage leads to disturbed reabsorption, subsequently to nephro-

TABLE 1

TUMORS OBSERVED IN MALE AND FEMALE MICE AFTER DCA EXPOSURE

		MALES		FEMALES	
		CONTR.	9 PPM	CONTR.	9 PPM
NO. OF AUTOPSIED ANIMALS		27	30	29	30
ORGAN	TUMOR				
KIDNEY	CYSTADENOMA	8(29.6%)	23(76.7%)	0(0%)	15(50%)
	ADENOCARCINOMA	0(0%)	4(13.3%)	0(0%)	0(0%)
LUNG	ADENOMA	3(11.1%)	2(6.7%)	4(13.8%)	1(3.3%)
	CARCINOMA	0(0%)	0(0%)	1(3.4%)	0(0%)
HARDERIAN GLAND	CYSTADENOMA	5/23[1](21.7%)	5/22[1](22.7%)	2/23[1](8.6%)	8/29[1](27.6%)
SKIN	ADENOMA	0(0%)	0(0%)	0(0%)	1(3.3%)
	CARCINOMA	0(0%)	0(0%)	1(3.4%)	2(6.7%)
STOMACH	ADENOMA	2(7.4%)	0(0%)	1(3.4%)	0(0%)
	CARCINOMA	0(0%)	0(0%)	1(3.4%)	0(0%)
MAMMARY GLAND	ADENOMA	0(0%)	0(0%)	0(0%)	0(0%)
	CARCINOMA	0(0%)	0(0%)	1(3.4%)	0(0%)
THYROID GLAND	ADENOMA	0(0%)	0(0%)	0(0%)	0(0%)
	CARCINOMA	0(0%)	0(0%)	1(3.4%)	1(3.3%)
UTERUS	MYOMA	-	-	0(0%)	1(3.3%)
OVARY	GRAN. CELL TUMOR	-	-	1(3.4%)	0(0%)
TESTICLE	INTERST. CELL TUMOR	1(3.7%)	0(0%)	-	-
HEMOPOIETIC SYSTEM	MALIGNANT LYMPHOMA	13(48.1%)	1(3.3%)	17(58.6%)	2(6.7%)
TUMORS (TOTAL)		32	35	30	31

[1]No. of sectioned glands

hydrosis and cystic degeneration.

Tumor incidence. The results of tumor incidences, which represent the almost completed experiment, are given in Table 1. The most important result is a striking increase in the formation of renal cystadenomas in male and female mice as related to DCA exposure. Four adenocarcinomas were found in male mice.

A considerable incidence of tumors in the Harderian gland was observed in all groups. Not all organs were available for histological investigation, since the detection of this tumor proved to be very difficult, on account of the tiny structure and remote position of this organ; only 73 - 97% of the animals could be taken into the evaluation. From these results (Table 1), no significant differences between exposed and control groups were found.

Both male and female control animals show a high rate of malignant lymphomas formation. The high incidence of this type of tumors in control groups correlates well with their higher life expectancies. As outlined above, the life expectancies of the exposed animals are significantly decreased, paralleling a decrease of the rate of malignant lymphomas.

These preliminary data are indicative of a carcinogenic potential of DCA in mice. Interestingly, the acute and chronic toxic effects as well as the organ specificity of tumor formation are identical (at least in part) for DCA, chloroform and hexachlorobutadiene. We therefore hypothesize a common molecular mechanism for all these compounds; this assumption is particularly supported by our previous finding of the formation of chloroform (with its metabolite phosgene) and hexachlorobutadiene from DCA.

ACKNOWLEDGEMENTS

This work was supported by a grant from BG Chemie, D-6900 Heidelberg. The skilful technical assistance of Ms. C. Fabian and C. Hölterhoff is gratefully acknowledged.

REFERENCES

1. Reichert, D., Henschler, D. and Bannasch, P. (1978) Food Cosmet. Toxicol. 16, 227-235.
2. Reichert, D., Metzler, M. and Henschler, D. (1980) J. Environ. Pathol. Toxicol. in press
3. Reichert, D., Neudecker, T., Spengler, U. and Henschler, D. (1980) in preparation
4. Kociba, R.J., Keyes, D.G., Jersey, G.C., Ballard, J.J., Dittenber, D.A., Quast, J.F., Wade, C.E., Humiston, C.G. and Schwetz, B.A. (1977) Am. Ind. Hyg. Ass. J. 38, 589-602.
5. Reichert, D., Spengler, U. and Henschler, D. (1979) J. Chromatogr. 179, 181-183.

© 1980 Elsevier/North-Holland Biomedical Press
Mechanisms of Toxicity and Hazard Evaluation
B. Holmstedt, R. Lauwerys, M. Mercier, M. Roberfroid eds

CHRONIC TOXICITY AND CARCINOGENICITY OF CYTOSTATIC N-NITROSO-(2-CHLOROETHYL)UREAS AFTER REPEATED INTRAVENOUS APPLICATION TO RATS

GERHARD EISENBRAND and MICHAEL HABS
Institute of Toxicology and Chemotherapy, German Cancer Research Center, Heidelberg, F.R.G.

SUMMARY

Clinically established 2-chloroethylnitrosourea derivatives (CNU-derivatives) and newly developed analogs with high cytostatic activity in experimental animal tumors were given intravenously to rats in dosages simulating clinical application schemes (9.5-150 mg/m^2, every six weeks for up to 10 applications). Among ring-substituted analogs, highest median survival times (MSTs were reached and, consequently, highest median total doses were tolerated by two clinically established drugs, methyl-CCNU and CCNU. The water-soluble ring-substituted analogs morpholino-CNU and chlorozotocin were considerably more toxic, leading to significantly reduced MST. Morpholino-CNU was a stronger carcinogen than CCNU and methyl-CCNU, inducing malignant as well as benign tumors and premalignant alterations predominantly in the lung, but also in the nervous system and forestomach. Among open-chain analogs, the clinically established drug BCNU had the highest toxicity and also was an effective carcinogen, inducing 23% malignant lung tumors at a median total dose of 300 mg/m^2 (4 x 75 mg/m^2) within only 164 days MST. The new analogs hydroxyethyl-CNU and hydroxyethyl-CNU-methanesulfonate were significantly less toxic than BCNU. HECNU, which had been proven to be cytostatically superior to BCNU in experimental animal tumors, was the least toxic of the open-chain analogs, achieving the highest MST. On the other hand, BCNU at the highest dosages induced significantly more malignant tumors than HECNU and HECNU-MS, although the BCNU-treated group had a much shorter MST than the groups treated with the two new analogs.

The results demonstrate that cytostatic acitivity and long-term toxic and carcinogenic effects in animals are not necessarily linked: analogs of clinically similar cytostatic activity like BCNU, CCNU and Methyl-CCNU show strong differences in long-term toxicity and carcinogenicity and experimental drugs like HECNU and HECNU-MS with cytostatic activity superior to BCNU are less toxic and less carcinogenic.

MATERIALS AND METHODS

Compounds:

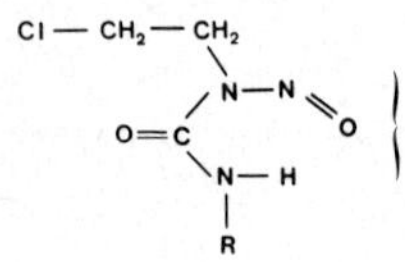

CNU

CNU-Derivatives tested	—R
CCNU	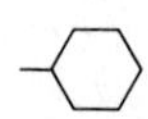
Methyl- CCNU	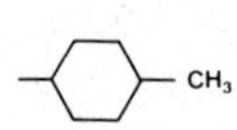
Morpholino-CNU	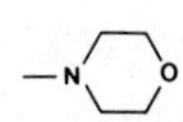
Chlorozotocin	D-Glucopyranose
BCNU	$-CH_2-CH_2Cl$
Hydroxyethyl-CNU	$-CH_2-CH_2OH$
Hydroxyethyl-CNU-methanesulfonate	$-CH_2-CH_2-OSO_2CH_3$

Male Wistar rats (30 animals per group) received every six weeks doses of 9.5-150 mg/m^2 of the nitrosoureas, dissolved in Cremophor EL/ethanol/water (1.5/1.5/20 vol. parts) by intravenous injection. Controls (120 animals) received the same amount of solvent. Treatment was discontinued either when severe lethal toxicity became apparent or after the maximum dose of 10 applications had been given. All animals were observed for life time.

Organs showing abnormalities at autopsy were examined histologically. Statistical calculations were made using the U-test for comparison of individual MSTs and the x^2-test for comparison of tumor incidences in a modification which accounts for differences in survival times (Peto, 1974)

RESULTS AND DISCUSSION

Chronic toxicity (Table 1)

The clinically established ring-substituted analogs CCNU and methyl-CCNU were the least toxic substances, achieving MSTs at individual doses of 9.5-75 mg/m^2 similar to that of the control

TABLE 1: CHRONIC TOXICITY AND CARCINOGENICITY OF N-NITROSO-(2-CHLOROETHYL)UREA DERIVATIVES AFTER REPEATED INTRAVENOUS APPLICATION TO RATS: MAX. NUMBER OF APPLICATIONS, MEDIAN TOTAL DOSES AND MEDIAN SURVIVAL TIMES
INITIAL NUMBER OF ANIMALS (♂ WISTAR RATS): 30 PER EXPERIMENTAL GROUP - 120 IN THE CONTROL

		150 MG/M^2	75 MG/M^2	38 MG/M^2	19 MG/M^2	9.5 MG/M^2
CCNU	MAX. NUMBER OF APPLICATIONS	7	10	10	10	-
	MEDIAN TOTAL DOSE (MG/M^2)	1050	750	380	190	-
	(95% RANGE)	('')	('')	('')	('')	-
	MEDIAN SURVIVAL TIME (DAYS)	369	530	601	661	-
	(95% RANGE)	(327-617)	(487-617)	(504-619)	(597-702)	-
METHYL-CCNU	MAX. NUMBER OF APPLICATIONS	8	10	10	10	-
	MEDIAN TOTAL DOSE (MG/M^2)	1200	750	380	190	-
	(95% RANGE)	(1050-1200)	('')	('')	('')	-
	MEDIAN SURVIVAL TIME (DAYS)	374	599	619	555	-
	(95% RANGE)	(304-395)	(558-624)	(563-657)	(509-664)	-
MORPHO-LINO-CNU	MAX. NUMBER OF APPLICATIONS	4	4	10	10	10
	MEDIAN TOTAL DOSE (MG/M^3)	600	300	380	190	95
	(95% RANGE)	('')	('')	('')	('')	('')
	MEDIAN SURVIVAL TIME (DAYS)	158	251	467	533	499
	(95% RANGE)	(138-168)	(158-462)	(451-476)	(510-632)	(467-523)
CHLOROZO-TOCIN	MAX. NUMBER OF APPLICATIONS	-	-	10	10	10
	MEDIAN TOTAL DOSE (MG/M^2)	-	-	380	190	95
	(95% RANGE)	-	-	('')	('')	('')
	MEDIAN SURVIVAL TIME (DAYS)	-	-	474	590	583
	(95% RANGE)	-	-	(436-513)	(518-613)	(565-638)
BCNU	MAX. NUMBER OF APPLICATIONS	-	4	10	10	10
	MEDIAN TOTAL DOSE (MG/M^2)	-	300	266	152	95
	(95% RANGE)	-	('')	(228-304)	(152-190)	('')
	MEDIAN SURVIVAL TIME (DAYS)	-	164	263	314	568
	(95% RANGE)	-	(157-211)	(230-312)	(295-410)	(514-588)
HYDROXY-ETHYL-CNU	MAX. NUMBER OF APPLICATIONS	-	10	10	10	10
	MEDIAN TOTAL DOSE (MG/M^2)	-	565	380	190	95
	(95% RANGE)	-	(525-600)	('')	('')	('')
	MEDIAN SURVIVAL TIME (DAYS)	-	331	541	572	558
	(95% RANGE)	-	(294-456)	(518-627)	(522-617)	(492-606)
HYDROXY-ETHYL-CNU METHANE-SULFONATE	MAX. NUMBER OF APPLICATIONS	-	4	10	10	10
	MEDIAN TOTAL DOSE (MG/M^2)	-	300	380	190	95
	(95% RANGE)	-	('')	('')	('')	('')
	MEDIAN SURVIVAL TIME (DAYS)	-	262	502	530	530
	(95% RANGE)	-	(194-485)	(477-525)	(490-554)	(461-547)

group. Even at 150 mg/m^2, these compounds could be given 7-8 times, respectively, before late lethal toxicity became apparent. Such late toxic effects were similar for all compounds: there was a considerable loss of body weight and the animals mainly succumbed to infections, e.g. pneumonia, enterocolitis and meningoencephalitis. Almost invariably there was some toxic damage to the liver with fatty degeneration, single cell necroses, fibrosis and bile duct proliferation. CCNU showed some, chlorozotocin a high degree of dose-dependant renal toxicity (necroses, tubular degeneration, glomerulo- and pyelonephritis).

Morpholino-CNU, a new water-soluble ring-substituted analog with high cytostatic activity in rat leukemia L 5222 (Zeller & Eisenbrand, 1980) was much more toxic than CCNU and methyl-CCNU, as evidenced by significantly reduced MST even at low doses (38 mg/m^2: $p < 0,01$; 19 and i.5 mg/m^2: $p < 0.05$ vs. control). Chlorozotocin could not be given at doses exceeding 38 mg/m^2, because 7/30 animals died after one dose of 75 mg/m^2 within 14 days. MST was still significantly reduced at 38 mg/m^2 ($P < 0.01$), but lower dosages gave MSTs similar to that of the control.

BCNU, an open-chain analog which is in clinical use since the early 1960s (Carter, 1980), was the most toxic compound of the whole series: 75 mg/m^2 could only be given 4 times and an MST of only 164 days was reached. At 19 mg/m^2 the MST was still significantly reduced, compared to the control ($p < 0.01$). The water-soluble analog hydroxyethyl-CNU, however, showed strongly reduced toxicity compared to BCNU ($p < 0.01$): at 75 mg/m^2, a median total dose of 565 mg/m^2 was reached which gave an MST of 331 days. Lower dosages were well tolerated and could be fully applied. Hydroxyethyl-methane-sulfonate was slightly more toxic than hydroxyethyl-CNU, but was still significantly less toxic than BCNU (comparison of MSTs at 75 mg/m^2: $p < 0.01$).

Carcinogenicity (Table 2)

Gross inspection of carcinogenicity data indicated a preference of tumorigenic effects in experimental groups for nervous system, lung and forestomach. CCNU and methyl-CCNU again compared favorably and exerted only weak tumorigenic response in the target tissues mentioned. Methyl-CCNU at 19 mg/m^2 gave rise to some

TABLE 2: CARCINOGENIC ACTIVITY OF N-NITROSO-(2-CHLOROETHYL)UREA DERIVATIVES AFTER REPEATED INTRAVENOUS APPLICATION TO RATS [1)]

COMPOUND	MEDIAN TOTAL DOSE (MG/M^2)	MALIGNANT TUMORS (%)	Σ %	NERVOUS SYSTEM MALIGNANT %	NERVOUS SYSTEM Σ [2)] %	LUNG MALIGNANT %	LUNG Σ [2)] %	FORESTOMACH MALIGNANT %	FORESTOMACH Σ [2)] %
CCNU	1050	10	17	-	-	3	7	-	-
	750	7	30	-	-	-	13	-	10
	380	-	10	-	-	-	-	-	7
	190	-	3	-	-	-	-	-	-
METHYL-CCNU	1200	4	19	-	-	4	8	-	8
	750	8	27	-	-	-	-	-	-
	380	18	27	-	-	-	-	-	4
	190	18	23	9	9	-	-	5	5
MORPHOLINO-CNU	600	19	30	4	4	15	19	-	7
	300	7	20	-	4	7	7	-	15
	380	14	21	4	4	7	7	4	8
	190	5	24	-	-	5	9	-	9
	95	-	7	-	-	-	-	-	-
CHLOROZOTOCIN	380	10	15	-	-	5	5	-	5
	190	-	-	-	-	-	-	-	-
	95	8	16	4	4	-	-	4	8
BCNU	300	27	32	5	5	23	23	-	5
	266	-	13	-	-	-	13	-	-
	152	-	3	-	-	-	-	-	3
	95	4	12	4	-	-	8	-	-
HYDROXYETHYL-CNU	565	12	32	4	4	-	8	4	16
	380	9	22	9	9	-	4	-	9
	190	8	8	-	-	-	-	-	-
	95	6	12	6	6	-	-	-	6
HYDROXYETHYL-CNU-METHANESULFONATE	300	7	17	7	7	-	-	-	10
	380	7	14	3	3	-	-	-	7
	190	7	10	-	-	-	3	-	-
	95	-	4	-	-	-	-	-	4
SOLVENT CONTROL	-	8	15	1	1	-	1	-	6

1) PATHOLOGY NOT FULLY COMPLETED YET

2) SUM OF INCIDENCES (%) OF PRENEOPLASTIC ALTERATIONS, BENIGN AND MALIGNANT TUMORS, BASED ON NUMBERS OF EVALUABLE ANIMALS. IF AN ANIMAL HAD MORE THAN ONE TUMOR IN DIFFERENT ORGANS, THESE WERE COUNTED SEPERATELY.

malignant tumors in the nervous system and forestomach, but there was no indication for a dose-response relation. CCNU showed some effect in the lung (adenomas, adenoakanthomas) and in the forestomach (papillomas, basal cell proliferation and atypias). Morpholino-CNU on the other hand, showed quite strong, dose-dependent carcinogenic effects, inducing malignant and benign tumors in the lung. Since in the two highest dosage groups the MSTs were very low (Table 1), it might be concluded that even more tumors would have been seen if longer MSTs would have been reached. Chlorozotocin, which could only be applied in dosages of 9.5-38 mg/m^2, showed some indication for a possible tumorigenic effect to the lung, forestomach and nervous system. The compound had shown considerable local carcinogenicity, however, when given in a comparable median total dose (300 mg/m^2) intraperitoneally to SD-rats (Habs et al., 1979).

BCNU at 75 mg/m^2 showed the strongest carcinogenic effects, inducing malignant tumors, mainly in the lung. The high frequency (23%) of these malignancies is especially remarkable, since the MST in this group was only 164. As with morpholino-CNU, it could be concluded that much more malignant tumors would have been seen if the MST would have been longer.

Hydroxyethyl-CNU shows some tumorigenic effects in the nervous system, forestomach and lung, but is significantly less carcinogenic than BCNU at 75 mg/m^2 ($p < 0.05$). The same is true for hydroxyethyl-CNU-methanesulfonate at the same dose level ($p < 0.05$)

CONCLUSIONS

For the clinically used analogs of the series tested, indications for cytostatic superiority in chemotherapy of human tumors have not been seen, except of a slight superiority of CCNU over BCNU and Methyl-CCNU in treatment of advanced Hodgkins disease (Wasserman et al., 1975). The present study shows however strong differences in long-term toxic and carcinogenic effects to rats within the series of clinically used compounds (CCNU, Methyl-CCNU, BCNU, Chlorozotocin) with BCNU being the most toxic compound and the strongest carcinogen. In the absence of any clear data for clinical superiority of BCNU over the other analogs, and in view of the results reported here, this compound should be replaced by analogs with reduced toxicity and carcinogenicity.

REFERENCES

Carter, S.K. (1980) The clinical evaluation of analogues. IV.Nitrosoureas. In: Recent Results in Cancer Res., New Anticancer Drugs. S.K. Carter, Y. Sakurai, eds., Springer (Berlin-Heidelberg, New York), pp. 119-123

Habs, M., Eisenbrand, G., Schmähl, D. (1979) Carcinogenic activity in Sprague-Dawley rats of 2-[3-(2-chloroethyl) -3-nitrosoureido] -D-glucopyranose (Chlorozotocin). Cancer Letters 8, 133-137

Peto, R., (1974) Guidelines on the analysis of tumor rates and death rates in experimental animals. Br. J. Cancer 29, 101-105

Zeller, W.J., Eisenbrand, G., Fiebig, H.H. (1978) Chemotherapeutic activity of new 2-chloroethylnitrosoureas in rat L 5222 leukemia: comparison of bifunctional and water-soluble derivatives with 1,3-Bis(2-chloroethyl)-1-nitrosourea. J. Natl. Cancer Inst. 60, 345-348

Zeller, W.J., Eisenbrand,G. (1980), Oncology, in press

© 1980 Elsevier/North-Holland Biomedical Press
Mechanisms of Toxicity and Hazard Evaluation
B. Holmstedt, R. Lauwerys, M. Mercier, M. Roberfroid eds

COMPARATIVE STUDY ON THE METABOLISM AND ACTIVATION OF AFLATOXIN B_1 IN NUCLEI, MICROSOMES AND RECONSTITUTED P-450 SYSTEM OF RAT LIVER

YOSHIO UENO, HIROKO YOSHIZAWA AND REIKO UCHIMARU
Department of Toxicology and Microbial Chemistry, Faculty of Pharmaceutical Sciences, Tokyo University of Science, Ichigaya, Tokyo 162 (Japan)

INTRODUCTION

Recent approaches to the molecular mechanism of aflatoxin B_1(AFB_1) toxicity revealed that microsomal monooxygenase mediates the biotransformation of AFB_1 into several metabolites such as AFM_1, AFQ_1 and the activation into 2,3-oxide[1,2]. Recently, the similar biotransformation was observed with the nuclei[3]. In the present paper, we have analysed the metabolism and activation of AFB_1 in the isolated nuclei and microsomes. Furtheremore, by employing the reconstituted P-450 system, we have compared the molecular specificity of cytochrome P-450s in order to evaluate the data observed with the nuclei and microsomes.

MATERIALS AND METHODS

Animals. Male Sprague-Dawley rats were either untreated or injected intraperitoneally with phenobarbital (PB, 25 mg/kg/day for 4 days), 3-methylcholanthrene (MC, 75 mg/kg/day for 4 days) or Kanechlore 400 (PCB, 670 mg/kg for one day). Nuclei and microsomes were prepared from the same liver speciments by sequential centrifugation of 0.25 M sucrose- or 0.8 M sucrose-homogenates.

Cytochromes. Cytochrome PB-450, MC-P-448, PCB-P-450 and PCB-448, purified from the respective microsomes of pretreated rats, were supplied from Dr.Kamataki (Keio Univ., Tokyo), and cytochrome b_5 of rabbit liver was kindly provided by Dr.Imai (Protein Res.Inst., Osaka).

Estimation of aflatoxin B_1 metabolites. Chloroform-soluble fraction of the reaction mixture was analysed by silica gel TLC (chloroform-methanol, 95:5) and the fluorescence intensity was estimated by a Shimadzu dual-wavelength chromatoscanner (Shimadzu Co., Osaka).

Binding of [^{3}H]aflatoxin B_1 to DNA. Nuclei (0.5 mg DNA) were incubated with 0.125 µmole of [^{3}H]AFB_1 for one hour under the condition described in TABLE 1, and DNA was extracted and the radioactivity was counted. In the case of reconstituted system, 150 µg of calf thymus DNA and 0.57 µCi of [^{3}H]AFB_1 were supplemented, and the reaction was proceeded at 37°C for one hour. The reaction was terminated by an addition of SDS and followed by phenol extraction.

RESULTS AND DISCUSSION

Formation of aflatoxin M_1. In the microsomal and nuclear systems, the major metabolites were AFM_1 and AFQ_1, and the formation of AFM_1 was enhanced by PCB and MC. The optimal pH was 8.3 in the both enzyme systems, and the kinetic analysis revealed similar K_m and V_{max} values for AFM_1 formations. In the reconstituted system, the formation of AFM_1 was mediated only by P-448. The pH optimum was 8.0, and its V_{max} was about 4 times higher than that of MC-microsome as shown in Table 1. These findings indicate that the monooxygenase of nuclei is very similar to that of the microsomes, and the metabolic activity of the purified P-448 was much higher than that of the membrane-bound form.

TABLE 1

KINETIC COMPARISON OF AFLATOXIN M_1 FORMATION IN NUCLEI, MICROSOMES AND RECONSTITUTED CYTOCHROME P-450 SYSTEM

System	Inducers	Optimal pH	K_m (M)	V_{max} (AFM_1 nmol/nmol P-450/min)
Nuclei[a]	MC	8.3	9.3×10^{-5}	0.663
Microsomes[a]	MC	8.3	8.6×10^{-5}	0.313
	PB		1.6×10^{-4}	0.043
P-448[b]	PCB	8.0	1.7×10^{-5}	1.333
P-450[b]	PB		(not produced)	

[a]150 µmoles of Tris HCl buffer (pH 8.3), 12.5 µmoles of $MgCl_2$, 0.75 µmole of NADP, 25 µmoles of G-6-P, 0.25 unit of G-6-P dehydrogenase, 25 µmoles of nicotinamide, 32 nmoles of AFB_1 and 1-4 mg protein of nuclei or 0.2-1 mg of microsomes, in total volume of 1.25 ml, were incubated at 37°C for 20 min.

[b]0.75 nmole of fp_T, 15 µg of dilauroyl L-3-phosphatidylcholine suspended in 20% glycerol, 0.1 nmole of cytochrome P-448/450, 50 µg of sodium deoxycholate, 0.05 µmole of EDTA, 25 µmoles of Tris HCl buffer (pH 8.0), 0.25 µmole of NADP, 2.5 µmoles of G-6-P and 0.5 unit of G-6-P dehydrogenase, in total volume of 0.5 ml, were incubated at 37°C for 30 min.

Formation of aflatoxin Q_1. The production of AFQ_1 in the nuclei and microsomes was induced by PCB and PB and was maximum at pH 7.4. In the reconstituted system, MC-P-448 as well as PB-P-450 mediated the formation of AFQ_1 with the maximum at pH 8.0, and the speed (AFQ_1 pmol/nmol cytochrome/min) of P-448 was several times higher than that of P-450. Therefore, it is presumed that the nuclear and microsomal P-450s, induced by PB, could not express their maximum activity for the formation of AFQ_1.

Formation of aflatoxin B_1-diol. In the nuclei and microsmes, a minor amount of AFB_1-diol was detected. However, in the reconstituted system, 150 and 50 pmoles of AFB_1-diol was accumulated in P-448 and P-450 systems, respectively, and these accumulated AFB_1-diol, which was maximum at pH 7.4, was dimished when DNA was supplemented to the reaction system. Therefore, it is highly possible that "AFB_1-2,3-oxide" mediated by P-450 and P-448 is hydrolysed spontaneously to give rise AFB_1-diol in the absence of acceptors such as DNA.

Binding of aflatoxin B_1 to DNA. The nuclei, isolated from PB or PCB-pretreated rat livers, resulted in 4-fold increment of AFB_1 binding to DNA, and its K_m value was estimated to 1.1×10^{-4} M. Since the treatment of nuclei by Triton -X 100 abolished the AFB_1 binding to DNA, loss of drug-metabolizing activity and resulted in a marked decrease of phospholipid content, the nuclear binding of AFB_1 is presumed to be mediated by the monooxygenase system localized in the outer nuclear membrane. In the reconstituted system, both species of P-448 and P-450 mediated the binding of $[^3H]AFB_1$ to DNA with the maximum at pH 8.0, and the binding speed (AFB_1 bound pmole/nmole cytochrome/min) was estimated to 11 and 17, respectively. These results indicate that the activation of AFB_1, estimated by the binding to DNA, is mediated both types of cytochrome P-448 and P-450, and the relative activity of P-448 was about 50 % less than that of P-450. Guengerich[4] also reported that multi species of cytochrome P-450s contribute to the activation of AFB_1.

Effects of cytochrome b_5 on the metabolism and activation of aflatoxin B_1. In the present experiments, we have established some similarity and difference among the nuclei, microsomes and reconstituted systems for the metabolism and activation of AFB_1. Since the reconstituted system composed from the purified cytochrome P-450s and fp_T, the possible contribution of other factors is not ruled out. In this respect, we have investigated the effect of cytochrome b_5 on the metabolism and activation of AFB_1 in the reconstituted cytochrome system. As shown in Table 2, the supplement of cytochrome b_5 enhanced markdely the binding of AFB_1 to DNA in proportional to the amounts added, and the stimulation effect of cytochrome b_5 was more effective in P-450 system than in P-448 system. A slight enhancement of AFQ_1 was also observed in P-450 system.

Experiments with the intact nuclei and microsomes have revealed that PB was effective for the enhancement of AFB_1 binding to DNA. That is, the activation of AFB_1 is predominantly mediated by the cytochrome P-450 type. The present data about the stimulating effect of cytochrome b_5, therefore, demonstrated that the combination of P-450 with cytochrome b_5 gives rise an important role for the activation of AFB_1 into "reactive intermediate".

Summing up the above data and discussion, it is concluded that the the enzymatic characteristics of monooxygenase system of the nuclei and microsomes are quite similar each other in regards to pH dependency, inducer specificity

TABLE 2

EFFECTS OF CYTOCHROME b_5 ON THE ACTIVATION AND METABOLISM OF AFLATOXIN B_1 IN RECONSTITUTED CYTOCHROME SYSTEM

Cytochromes	Cytochrome b_5 (nmole)	DNA Binding (pmole AFB_1 bound /nmole P-450/min)	AFM_1 (pmole/nmole P-450/min)	AFQ_1
PB-P-450[a]	–	22.3 (100)[c]	ND[d]	6.2 (100)
	0.017	29.1 (130)		
	0.058	40.8 (180)	ND	8.0 (130)
	0.116	59.7 (270)		
PCB-P-448[b]	–	12.4 (100)	451	23.8
	0.116	17.7 (140)		

[a]0.054 nmole/assay
[b]0.094 nmole/assay
[c]Percent of the control
[d]Not detected

and kinetic values. The experiments with the reconstituted cytochrome system revealed that AFM_1 is strictly mediated by P-448, and the formation of AFQ_1 and the activation into DNA-binding form are mediated both by P-450 and P-448. Possible contribution of cytochrome b_5 for P-450-dependent binding of AFB_1 was demonstrated.

ACKNOWLEDGEMENTS

This experiment was supported in part by a Cancer Research Grant [53-2] from the Ministry of Health and Welfare. The authors wish to thank Drs. Kamataki (Keio Univ.) and Imai (Protein Res.Inst.) for supply of cytochrome P-450s and cytochrome b_5, respectively.

REFERENCES

1. Croy, R.C., Essigmann, J.M., Reinhold, V.N. and Wogan, G.N.(1978) Proc. Natl.Acad.Sci. U.S.A., 75, 1747-1759.
2. Essigmann, J.M., Croy, R.C., Nadzan, A.M., Busby, W.F.Jr., Reinhold, N.V., Buchi, G. and Wogan, G.N. (1977) Proc. Natl.Acad.Sci. U.S.A., 74, 1870-1874.
3. Vaught, J.B., Klobs, W. and Gurtoo, H.L. (1977) Life Sciences, 21, 1497-1504.
4. Guengerich, F.P. (1977) J.Biol.Chem., 252, 3970-3979.

Mechanisms of Toxicity and Hazard Evaluation
B. Holmstedt, R. Lauwerys, M. Mercier, M. Roberfroid eds

CARCINOGENICITY OF FORMALDEHYDE VAPOR: INTERIM FINDINGS IN A LONG-TERM BIO-ASSAY OF RATS AND MICE

J. SWENBERG, W. KERNS, K. PAVKOV, R. MITCHELL AND E. J. GRALLA
Chemical Industry Institute of Toxicology, Research Triangle Park, North Carolina and Battelle Memorial Laboratories, Columbus, Ohio

INTRODUCTION

Formaldehyde is a widely used chemical with annual production exceeding 9 billion pounds in the United States[1]. Considerable human exposure to formaldehyde vapor occurs at concentrations around 1 ppm[2]. Formaldehyde is known to cause local irritation and skin sensitization; however, little information is available on its chronic toxicity and potential for carcinogenicity. Formaldehyde is weakly mutagenic[3], causes unscheduled DNA repair[4] and protein-DNA crosslinks[5].

The present study was initiated to more thoroughly assess the chronic toxicity and carcinogenicity of formaldehyde vapor in rats and mice. The results are based on data generated during the first 18 months of the study. A more complete presentation of the data will be published elsewhere[6].

MATERIALS AND METHODS

Groups of 120 male and female Fischer-344 rats and B6C3F1 mice were exposed to 2, 6 or 15 ppm formaldehyde vapor for 6 hours/day, 5 days/week in 5 m^3 Hinners-type chambers. The test atmosphere was generated by heating solid paraformaldehyde to 130-180°F and metering this vapor into filtered incoming air. Chamber concentrations were monitored every 30 minutes by infrared spectrophotometry and calibrated by the chromotropic-acid method.

Animals were observed twice daily and examined more closely during weekly and later biweekly weighings. Interim sacrifices were performed on 10 randomly selected rats and mice of each sex per exposure group at 6 and 12 months and on 20 per group at 18 months. Complete necropsies were performed on these and on all animals found dead or moribund during the course of the study. Histopathology was conducted on all tissues of control and 15 ppm animals and on four sections of nasal turbinates from all exposure concentrations.

RESULTS

Exposure to formaldehyde vapor caused dose-related decreases in body weight in rats and mice of both sexes. Male mice of all groups experienced considerable mortality during the first year due to fighting, while female mice and all rats exhibited minimal mortality. However, a sharp increase in mortality occurred in rats exposed to 15 ppm during the subsequent six months (Fig. 1). This increase was primarily due to the development of squamous cell carcinomas of the nasal cavity (Fig. 2). Large osteolytic tumors frequently penetrated into the subcutis, forming external masses (Fig. 3), while early lesions were usually located on or lateral to the nasal- or maxillo-turbinate (Fig. 4). No such tumors have been detected in mice simultaneously exposed to formaldehyde vapor.

Fig. 1 Cumulative mortality of rats exposed to formaldehyde vapor.

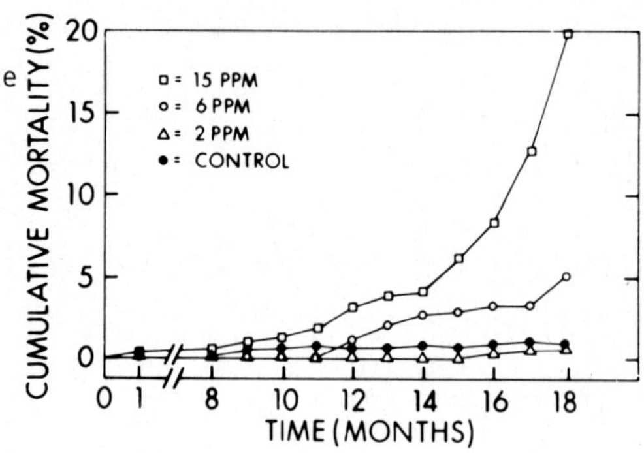

Fig. 2 Cumulative number of nasal carcinomas in 200 Fischer-344 rats exposed to 15 ppm formaldehyde vapor.

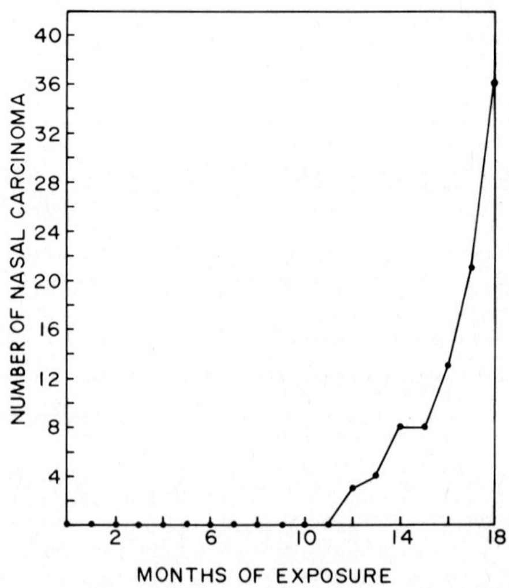

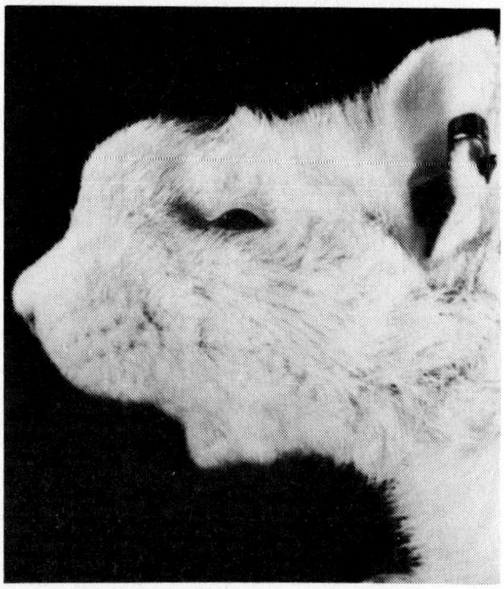

Fig. 3 Appearance of a 15 ppm formaldehyde exposed rat bearing a large squamous cell carcinoma of the nasal cavity which extends into the subcutis over the premaxilla.

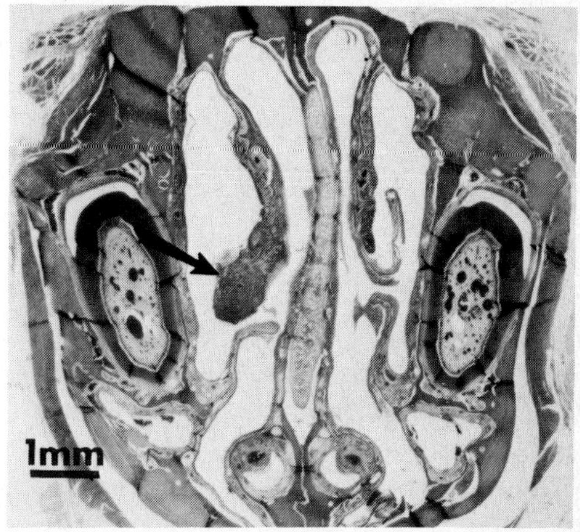

Fig. 4 Low-power view of an early squamous cell carcinoma arising in the nasoturbinate (arrow) of a rat exposed to 15 ppm formaldehyde vapor. H&E.*

Compound related changes were not evident in tissues other than the upper respiratory tract. An outbreak of sialodacryoadenitis occurred near the end of the first year of exposure which resulted in characteristic lesions in the lacrymal and salivary glands and upper respiratory tract in rats sacrificed at 12 months. Sequential sacrifices after 6, 12 and 18 months of exposure demonstrated that rats exposed to 2, 6 and 15 ppm of formaldehyde vapor developed rhinitis, epithelial dysplasia and squamous metaplasia that was dose-related in severity and extent. Progressive lesions including squamous papillary hyperplasia, cellular atypia and squamous cell carcinoma were evident in the nasal cavities of randomly selected rats exposed to 15 ppm for 18 months (Table 1). In contrast, rhinitis, epithelial dysplasia and squamous metaplasia were present in mice exposed to 15 ppm for 18 months, but not in those exposed to 2 or 6 ppm formaldehyde vapor. No progression to carcinoma was evident in mice.

---

*Figs. 1-4 are reproduced with the permission of Cancer Research.[6]

TABLE 1
SUMMARY OF HISTOPATHOLOGY IN THE NASAL TURBINATES OF RATS EXPOSED TO FORMALDEHYDE FOR 18 MONTHS

Diagnosis	Exposure level	0 ppm	2 ppm	6 ppm	15 ppm
	No. rats examined	40	40	40	40
Rhinitis, acute suppurative or seropurulent		0	2	7	39
Focal turbinate atrophy		0	0	0	2
Epithelial dysplasia		0	35	37	13
Squamous metaplasia		0	24	35	39
Squamous or epithelial hyperplasia		0	0	0	15
Squamous papillary hyperplasia		0	0	0	4
Squamous metaplasia with cellular atypia		0	0	0	7
Adenomatous polyp		0	1	1	1
Squamous cell carcinoma		0	0	0	8

DISCUSSION

Squamous cell carcinomas were clearly induced in the nasal cavities of rats exposed to 15 ppm formaldehyde vapor, but have not occurred in rats exposed to 2 or 6 ppm nor in mice exposed to all three levels. This sharp dose and species difference requires careful interpretation for accurate risk assessment. This will be best accomplished after the 24-month study is completed. By allowing time for further expression and regression of lesions, a better understanding of the pathogenesis of formaldehyde-induced disease will be achieved.

REFERENCES

1. 1979 Directory of Chemical Producers: United States of America. SRI International, Menlo Park. pp 637-638.
2. Formaldehyde - An assessment of its health effects. (1980). Nat. Acad. Sci., Washington, DC.
3. Auerbach, C., et al (1977). Mutation Res. 39:317-62.
4. Martin, C. N. et. al. (1978). Cancer Res. 38:2621-2627.
5. Wilkins, R. J. and H. D. MacLeod. (1976). Mutation Res. 36:11-16.
6. Swenberg, J. A. et. al. (1980). Cancer Res. (In press).

Mechanisms of Toxicity and Hazard Evaluation
B. Holmstedt, R. Lauwerys, M. Mercier, M. Roberfroid eds

DETECTION OF MUTAGENS IN VARIOUS ALCOHOLIC BEVERAGES, PARTICULARLY IN APPLE BRANDY, A PRODUCT OF WESTERN FRANCE

C. LOQUET[1)], G. TOUSSAINT[2)] and J.Y. LeTALAER[3)]
[1)]Gesellschaft für Strahlen- und Umweltforschung, Abteilung für Toxikologie, Ingolstädter Landstrasse 1, 8042 Neuherberg, (West Germany), [2)]International Agency for Research on Cancer, Unit of Environmental Carcinogens, 150 cours Albert Thomas, 69008 Lyon (France), [3)] Centre Francois Baclesse, route de Lion s/mer, 14000 Caen, (France)

INTRODUCTION

Epidemiological studies have indicated a good correlation between the high mortality rate from oesophageal cancer and the mortality rate from alcoholism of males in the west of France[1]. The risk of oesophageal cancer is increased with the consumption of strong beverages. In these areas the spririt most often consumed is apple brandy, which has an alcohol content of 40° or more. The mutagenic activity of homemade and commercial apple brandies produced in Normandy was examined and compared to that of other spirits (whiskys, rums, armagnacs, cognacs) using the Salmonella/microsome assay[2] in the presence or absence of liver homogenate fraction S-9.

MATERIALS AND METHODS

Samples. Thirty homemade apple brandies were collected from farms in different areas of Normandy. 18 commercial apple brandies and 28 other commercial spirits i.e., 8 whiskeys, 8 cognacs, 4 armagnacs and 8 rums of various brands, were purchased.

Fractionation Procedure. 50 ml of each of the 76 samples were distilled at 78^oC under atmospheric pressure to separate the alcoholic fraction. The non-volatile fraction was obtained from the aqueous fraction by evaporation to dryness under vacuum at 45^oC. The non-volatile fraction was dissolved in 3 ml DMSO (spectrograde) so that 200 ul were equivalent to 3 ml of the initial volume.

From one homemade apple brandy, fifteen sub-fractions were obtained from the original aqueous fraction by spinning band distillation. Six sub-fractions were obtained by HPLC from the non-volatile fraction[3].

Mutagenicity test. Mutagenicity was performed by plate incorporation assays[2] using *Salmonella typhimurium* strains TA 98 and TA 100. The liver homogenate fraction S-9 was obtained from Wistar rats (200-230 g) or BD-VI rats (120-130 g) treated with either 0.1% phenobarbital in drinking water for one week or with a single injection of 500 mg/kg Aroclor 1254 i.p. 5 days before the animals were sacrificed. Plating was also carried out after pre-incubation of the whole mixture 20 min at 25^{0}C. To accommodate the changing volume of the aqueous test fractions the concentrations of the top agar were adjusted in the following manner: To test 500 ul of the samples we used 1.6 ml of modified top agar (0.75 g NaCl and 0.75 g agar)/100 ml. For 1000 ul of the sample we added 1.1 ml of modified top agar (1.1 g NaCl and 1.1 g agar) /100 ml.

RESULTS

A mutagenic response was found in some or all three of the fractions (alcoholic, aqueous, non-volatile) using 200 ul per assay with or without metabolic activation, particularly in the homemade apple brandies (Table 1).

TABLE 1

MUTAGENICITY OF ALCOHOLIC BEVERAGES IN SALMONELLA TYPHIMURIUM TA 98 AND TA 100

BEVERAGE	FRACTIONS ALCOHOLIC	AQUEOUS	NON-VOLATILE
Homemade apple brandies	5/30[a]	7/30	2/30
Industrial apple brandies	0/18	2/18	0/18
Other alcoholic beverages - rum, whisky cognac, armagnac	5/28	0/28	0/28

[a]Number of beverage samples found mutagenic over number tested.

Introducing 200 ul to 1000 ul of the aqueous fraction of one homemade apple brandy/plate in the presence of liver S-9, we obtained a dose-response curve in TA 98 (Fig. 1). This aqueous fraction was divided by a spinning band column distillation into 15 ml fractions. Each one was tested alone and in pairs of adjacent fractions. Using 400 ul of pairs of adjacent sub-fractions, mutagenicity occured in TA 98 in three groups, one at the beginning of the distillation (after the alcoholic fraction) with S-9, one in the middle without S-9, and one at the end with S-9.

The non-volatile fraction of 100 ml of the same homemade apple brandy was dissolved in 1 ml DMSO and the resulting dilutions were tested. A dose-response curve was obtained in TA 98 and S-9 (Fig. 2). This non-volatile fraction was then chromatographed by HPLC and 6 sub-fractions were collected and tested. Two out of the 6 subfractions were found to be mutagenic with TA 98 and S-9 (not shown).

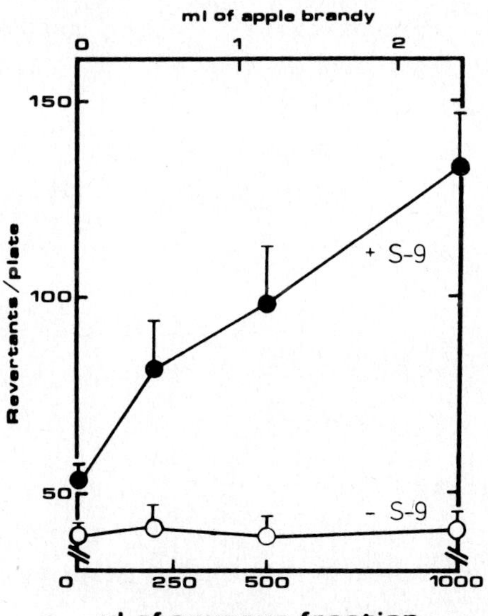

Fig. 1. Mutagenicity was determined in plate assays using liver S-9 (150 ul/plate) from Aroclor or phenobarbital-treated BD-VI rats (●). In control assays S-9 was omitted.

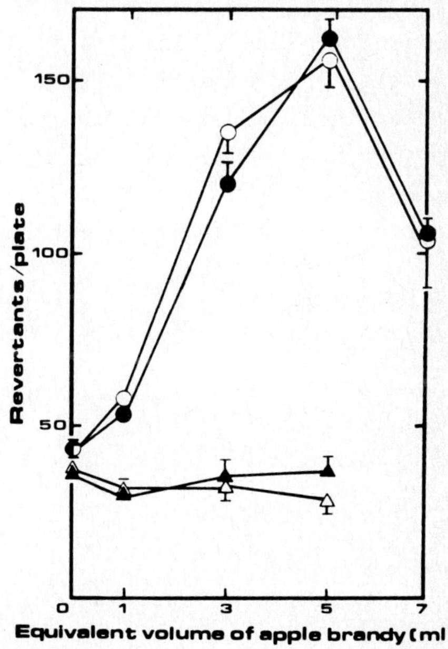

Fig. 2. Plate incorporation assay with S-9 (●), without S-9 (○). Plating after a preincubation step of 20 min at 37°C with (▲) or without (△) S-9.

DISCUSSION

Homemade apple brandies produced in the west of France exhibited a higher mutagenic response (37%, 11/30) than commercial brandies (11%, 2/18) or other types of spirits, such as whiskeys, cognacs, rums and armagnacs (17%, 5/28). Homemade apple brandies were the only samples giving a mutagenic response in all three fractions (alcoholic 5/30, aqueous 7/30, and non-volatile 2/30), this response also being at a higher level than in other types.

Various types of mutagenic compound(s) were found: directly acting compounds and compounds requiring metabolic activation. As TA 100 reacts specifically with base-pair substitution mutagens and TA 98 with frameshift mutagens, the response obtained in one or the other strain may be due to different chemical mutagenic compounds. Moreover, the distribution of the active compounds in the three fractions during the distillation indicates their various chemical natures. The mutagenic activity demonstrated in fractions of spirits cannot be related to the presence of a single compound.

When the chemical structure and action of those mutagens can be determined, their role in the etiology of oesophageal cancer could be defined. Although the mutagenicity found in homemade apple brandy was weak, people exposed to these mutagens over a long period of time may have a greater risk of developing oesophageal cancer.

REFERENCES

1. Tuyns, A.D. (1979) Int. J. Cancer, 5, 152-156.

2. Ames, B.N., McCann, J. and Yamasak, E. (1975) Mutation Res., 31, 347-361.

3. Loquet, C., Toussaint, G. and LeTalaer, J.Y. (1980) Mutation Res., in press.

LONG-TERM EXPOSURE TO OCCUPATIONAL INTOXICANTS

Symposium chairmen: M. Ikeda and A. Heyndrickx

© 1980 Elsevier/North-Holland Biomedical Press
Mechanisms of Toxicity and Hazard Evaluation
B. Holmstedt, R. Lauwerys, M. Mercier, M. Roberfroid eds

EPIDEMIOLOGIC APPROACH TO SUBCLINICAL EFFECTS OF METALS IN LONG-TERM OCCUPATIONAL EXPOSURE

HARUHIKO SAKURAI, M. D.
Department of Preventive Medicine and Public Health, Keio University School of Medicine, 35 Shinanomachi, Shinjuku-ku, Tokyo (Japan)

INTRODUCTION

In toxicological sciences, the importance of experiments using animals or biological systems in vitro is self-evident. However, they cannot substitute observations or experiments made on humans in several aspects.

First of all, they cannot provide information on exposure-effect or exposure-response relationship in man which is necessary for setting environmental standards for preventive purposes. These quantitative relationships between exposure and effects also give clues for diagnosis of poisoning. In the practice of occupational health, for example, differential diagnosis of ill health of workers is often impossible without knowing the extent of exposure and considering its implication by reference to the knowledge of exposure-effect relationship. Most of the individual signs and symptoms of intoxication are non-specific and, if exposure data are not available, it is only after the intoxication has reached a severely disabling stage that the diagnosis can be made on the basis of chracteristic combinations of signs.

Second, it may be difficult to predict, from animal experiments, the sequence of diverse effects occurring in exposed men. Even critical organs, the organs where adverse effects appear at the earliest stage of intoxication, may not be readily identified by animal experiments without very intensive morphological and functional observations being performed. Moreover, there is naturally the difference of species which may alter the sequence of toxicological events. In fact, majority of known health hazards due to environmental pollutants have been discovered by clinical observation. This is intelligible because the exposed population has been far greater in actual human life than in laboratory experiments, the effort to detect unknown health effects have generally been more vigorously made in clinical case finding, and medical data including subjective symptoms can be more easily obtained from humans than from laboratory animals. It should be noted that most of the methods of collecting health information have been developed for clinical purposes.

And third, chronic effects due to long-term occupational or environmental exposure are hard to reproduce in laboratory animals.

For these reasons, it is clear that clinical and epidemiologic observation is indispensable for human toxicology, and particularly in chronic toxicity studies.

When epidemiologic study and clinical case study are compared, epidemiology may be more efficient in finding hitherto unknown health effects, especially at lower exposure levels, and it is definitely needed for establishing exposure-response relationship in humans.[1] However, in making an epidemiologic approach, we must have access to a group of workers with considerable population size. The lower the levels of exposure become, the larger will be the required size of population for obtaining statistically significant results. In actual industrial setting, larger factories have generally achieved considerable improvement of workplaces, accompanied by reduction of exposed population due to automatic control systems. In smaller factories, where unfavorable working condition is still prevalent, the number of workers exposed to a toxic substance is often too small for epidemiologic study. Moreover, negative attitude of the management may sometimes discourage investigative approach to the health of workers and publishing of results. Therefore, it is logical that relatively few epidemiologic studies have been published on metals even though toxicological information about them is of fundamental importance.

The purpose of the present paper is to make a brief overview of known chronic effects of metals in prolonged occupational exposure, and then to show the types of information obtained and methodological problems inherent in epidemiologic approach to long-term low level exposure.

TYPES OF EFFECTS OBSERVED IN LONG-TERM EXPOSURE TO METALS.

Among 67 metal elements, excluding 19 nonmetals(H, He, Ne, Ar, Kr, Xe, Rn, F, Cl, Br, I, At, B, C, N, O, Si, P, S) and 6 radioactive metals(Po, Ra, Ac, Th, Pa, U) from 92 naturally occurring elemetns, only limited number of metals have come to be recognized as established chronic intoxicants for man. In a recently published handbook on metal toxicology[2], 14 metals(Al, Sb, As, Be, Cd, Cr, Co, Fe, Pb, Mn, Hg, Ni, Tl, V) are considered to have caused cases of chronic intoxication in man, while for 13 other metals(Ba, Bi, Cu, Ge, In, Mo, Se, Ag, Te, Sn, Ti, W, Zn), reported chronic effects, if any, are not regarded as confirmed adverse effects or simply there is no description other than for acute effects.

Of 14 recognized chronic intoxicants for humans, 11 are known to have caused chronic respiratory effects as shown in Tab. 1. This is the largest category of effect appearing after long-term exposure to metals. The second largest group is skin involvement seen in antimony, arsenic, beryllium, chromium, cobalt, nickel, thallium and vanadium. On the other hand, chronic effects on the central nervous system have been established only for lead, manganese, and

TABLE 1

METALS KNOWN TO CAUSE CHRONIC RESPIRATORY EFFECTS IN MAN

Al	Pneumoconiosis
Sb	Obstructive lung changes, Pneumoconiosis(?)
As	Nasal perforation, Bronchial carcinoma
Be	Granulomatosis, Bronchial carcinoma
Cd	Emphysema, Obstructive lung changes
Cr	Nasal perforation, Bronchial carcinoma, Asthma, Pneumoconiosis(?)
Co	Pneumoconiosis, Asthma(?)
Fe	Functional lung changes, Pneumoconiosis(?)
Mn	Pneumonia (acute ?)
Ni	Nasal and bronchial carcinoma, Asthma, Pneumoconiosis(?)
Pt[a]	Asthma
V	Asthma, Pneunomia (acute ?)

[a] Added to the list of metals contained in "Handbook on the Toxicology of Metals" (1979)

mercury. Chronic peripheral neuropathy has been described only for arsenic, lead, mercury, and thallium. Liver and kidney involvement in chronic form was found only in arsenic, cadmium, lead, and possibly in mercury. This sort of summary might be by no means indisputable. However, considering the multiplicity of metal elements and abundance of experimental data, the scarcity of established chronic effects in man is remarkable. It surely reflects the lack of information rather than the real situation.

CHRONIC RESPIRATORY EFFECTS

Because the respiratory system is the common route of absorption in occupational exposure, it is logical that the involvement of this organ turns out to be the most common category. However, types of effects are diversified as shown in Table 1, Inflammatory changes of nasal and bronchial mucosa, bronchial asthma, emphysema, interstitial fibrosis, carcinoma, and morphologically undefined functional impairments are of the chief findings.

An approach which appears promising for finding subclinical respiratory effects is pulmonary function test. Recent development of technique has made the test of lung function a sensitive and manageable tool applicable even for epidemiologic survey.

Various indices of lung function have been measured in cadmium workers since Friberg[3] first reported in 1950 that this element impaired pulmonary as well as renal function of chronically exposed subjects. Shortness of breath was complained by many of 43 workers exposed for more than 9 years to cadmium oxide dust in an alkaline battery factory. In about one-third of the subject with long-term exposure, the residual volume—total lung capacity ratio was increased suggesting that emphysema was present. In 1953, Bonnell[4] also found emphysema in 10 workers among 100 men employed at two factories where an alloy of copper and cadmium was manufactured. The diagnosis of emphysema was made by clinical examination supported by radiological finding and lung function test. When the results of lung function tests were compared between 42 exposed and 44 control subjects, it was found that the mean time constant estimated from the expiratory fast vital capacity curve of the exposed group was significantly larger than that of the control group. Bonnell and others[5] made a follow-up study of the same 100 men in 1957, four years after the original study. It was found that the mean values for 1957 were lower than the corresponding values for 1953 for vital capacity, maximum ventilatory capacity, swept fraction, and higher for time constnat. When individual values for time constant for 1957 were plotted aginst the respective values for 1953, the majority of values for time constant were higher in 1957, suggesting a deterioration of respiratory function. After the effect of aging was taken into account, it was concluded that the deterioration in lung function of those men with emphysema in the original survey took place despite the fact that the majority of the men with chronic cadmium poisoning were not further exposed to cadmium after 1953. Although some of the indices of lung function measured by Bonnell and others[4 5] are not in common use nowadays, the effects found in their subjects can be interpreted as obstructive lung changes caused by cadmium exposure. This is an example of cohort study applied to disclose intra-individual changes of function due to chronic exposure. Although cautious attitude is required to maintain comparability of data determined on different points in time, this is one of efficient epidemiologic approaches to working population. Similar cohort studies were used by us to reveal a hypertensive effect of carbon disulfide in viscose rayon workers[6] and slight effect of work load on peripheral blood in lead workers[7]. A cohort of about 300 battery workers were followed for 4 and a half years to detect possible anemic effect of lead. Working condition was drastically improved during the observation period and mean δ-aminolevulinic acid concentration in urine decreased from 8.4mg/l in the spring of 1972 to 2.9mg/l in the autumn of 1975. Specific gravity of blood was determined as an index of anemia because reproducibility of blood specific gravity measurement is remarkably higher than that of other hematological indices such as hemoglobin concentration and red blood cell count. Moreover specific gravity usually holds a very high correlation coefficient of more than 0.9 with other more direct indices of anemia. It was found that the mean specific gravity showed a significant semiannual fluctuation, viz. higher in spring and lower in autumn. The mean length of overtime work showed just the opposite changes, viz. less in spring and more in autumn, corresponding to the annual fluctuation of demand for car batteries. Multiple regression and partial correlation analyses clearly indicated that the work load was one of the significant causal factors of this change whereas lead exposure as estimated from blood lead and urinary δ-aminolevulinic acid was not causally related. This is one of the proofs that the blood lead concentration in the range of up to 80 μg/100ml, as found in this cohort, is not likely to cause anemic effect.

Coming back to subclinical pulmonary effect of cadmium, more recent studies revealed that other indices of pulmonary function such as forced vital capacity[8 9 10], forced expiratory volume in one second[8 9 11], peak expiratory flow rate[8 9], and closing capacity[12] were significantly worsened in cadmium workers with extended exposure than in control workers with comparable age and smoking habit. However, clinically apparent emphysema, as described by the earlier reports, has not been found in most recent studies. Reported deterioration of pulmonary function are mostly subclinical and several recent studies[12 13 14] even failed to find significant results. Thus, in a recent review on this subject[15], Lauwerys concluded that in the absence of acute episodes of overexposure, the changes induced by cadmium in the lung are usually mild and emphysema may not be induced by low level exposure even when it is prolonged.

Similar approaches using pulmonary function tests have been made on subclinical effects of welding. Since welding fumes contain various gases and particles of metals and oxides, this is a field where experimental approach is impracticable. In a recent study[16] made in Sweden, measurements of spirometric parameters, forced expiratory flow volume curve, and closing volume tests were performed on 119 welders and 90 controls. It is now recognized that conventional spirometry and measurements of breathing mechanics are insensitive methods for detection of obstruction located in peripheral small airways. This is mainly because the resistance is very low in the peripheral part of the bronchial tree, constituting only about one-fifth to one-tenth of the total airways resistance. Recently, the amount of airway closure, i.e., the closing volume and flow rates measured at various low lung volume during forced expiration have been claimed to be more sensitive to peripheral airway function than conventional spirometry. The results of the study made on 119 welders and 90 controls, matched with respect to age, height, and smoking habit, indicated that closing volume and closing capacity were significantly higher and total lung capacity was significantly lower in welders. The effect of smoking and of welding on ventilatory lung function appeared to be of compable magnitude.

The problem often encountered in this sort of lung function study is the effect of smoking. Because the deteriorating effects of smoking is usually very clearly detected by most of the ventilatory lung function tests, it tends to mask the effect of other pollutants in low level exposure. Such was also the case in cadmium studies, while in this study made on welders, the effect of welding fume may have been large enough to be significantly revealed.

Another point which is common to epidemiologic studies is the problem of biased selection. In an epidemiologic study with the cross-sectional design, groups of exposed and control workers are observed at a specified point in time. This favours the selection of healthier workers who have successfully tolerated the hazardous environment, while affected workers may have quitted the job. The result of this selection is to understimated the influence of exposure. However, it is assumed that subclinical effects may be detected even when more evident health hazards might have been concealed by autonomous selection. Interestingly, it is pointed out in the study on welders that, with increasing duration of exposure, there appeared to be decreasing differences in ventilatory function between the welders and their matched controls. This was considered to be an effect of selection among the welders.

Third problem is the reproducibility of lung function testing. Since many of the lung ventilatory function tests are dependent on effort and skill of examined persons, intra-individual variation has been found to be considerably large[17]. It might even be influenced by mental attitude of subjects. Therefore, special caution should be excercised in performing lung function tests and in interpreting data, especially concerning intra-individual sequential change in function due to prolonged exposure.

In spite of all those drawbacks, pulmonary function test surely is a useful tool for detecting subclinical effects of inhaled pollutants in humans as evidenced by air pollution studies. Because most metals have irritating capacity to the mucous membrane of respiratory tract when inhaled in high concentration, it seems to me that their effects in long-term low grade exposure need to be reevaluated by modern techniques.

An interesting approach to the upper respitatory effect of a metal has been reported recently[18]. Nasal smears, sputum cells, and biopsies were taken from nasal mucosa of 63 male workers exposed to vanadium dust and the same number of matched control workers exposed to inert dust only. The groups compared were of similar ages and had similar smoking habits. The amount of neutrophils in the nasal smears showed a significant increase. The biopsies from the vanadium workers also showed a significant increase in the number of plasma and round cells, and the histological picture was found to be almost characteristic. There were no signs indicative of allergic inflammation. The earlier level of vanadium exposure was estimated at 0.2 - 0.5 mg/m^3 and the average work period was 11 years. Thus, the finding may represent a subclinical effect of long-term vanadium exposure. A similar study of nasal effect was reported on workers exposes to copper salt dust[19] suggesting that this type of morphological method can be of use for studying effects on the upper respiratory tract.

SUBCLINICAL EFFECTS OF CADMIUM ON KIDNEY, LIVER AND BLOOD

Since chronic pulmonary effect appears to be unique in long-term occupational exposure, cadmium-induced lung impairment was touched upon briefly. However, critical organ in chronic cadmium exposure is generally considered to be the kidney[20]. While exposure to a considerably high concentration of cadmium fume or dust seems to be required to induce pulmonary impairment[15], far lower level of exposure either from respiratory or from alimentary tract is known to cause renal effects when exposure is prolonged[21]. This is because cadmium accumulates in the renal cortex and the liver as expressed by its extraordinarily long biological half-time[21]. Of course, accumulation of an exogenous substance in an organ does not necessarily mean that the organ is affected prior to other organs. However, the organ to which such substance is amply bound either with inert cellular components or by detoxifying mechanisms appears to run a certain level of risk. Are the inert components or detoxifying mechanisms so stable as to warrant a complete protection? As to cadmium, its concentration in renal cortex does not generally have a graded dose-effect relationship with renal functions, but it seems to have a threshold phenomenon. Animal experiments and a few post-mortem examination of cadmium affected workers suggest that the renal damage may occur when a critical level of cadmium concentration has been reached[21].

The characteristic feature of cadmium nephropathy is the impairment of reabsorption function of the proximal tubules. It was first observed as clinical proteinuria by Friberg in 1948[22]. It soon became evident that the proteinuria was mainly of low molecular weight proteins, known as tubular proteinuria. These proteins with lower molecular weight are normal constituents of the plasma. Owing to their smaller molecular size, they are filtered through glomerular membrane, and are usually reabsorbed at proximal tubules. Among several identified low molecular weight proteins, β_2-microglobulin has come to be utilized as a good indicator of the earliest proximal tubular dysfunction.

In a cross-sectional study on 240 workers exposed to cadmium in an alkaline battery factory, Kjellström et al. measured β_2-microglobulin concentration in urine and attempted to correlate the biological results to past airborne concentration. A control group of 87 workers also was examined. Cases in which the β_2-microglobulin level in urine exceeded 290 μg/l were classified as tubular proteinuria. The proportion of workers with urinary β_2-microglobulin exceeding this level was found to increase with duration of exposure. The prevalence rate of abnormal level of urinary β_2-microglobulin exceeded significantly that found in the control group(3.4%) after 6-12 years of employment(19%). The exposure level was about 50 $\mu g/m^3$ for the last 10-15 years.

In a cadmium alloy manufacturing factory, we have recently made a detailed cross-sectional study of renal function and other clinical chemistry determinations on 27 workers[24]. The alloy was mainly hard solder containing copper, zinc, and silver in addition to cadmium. Cadmium levels in blood and urine and length of exposure are summarized in Table 2. Cadmium concentrations in blood and urine were considerably elevated in exposed workers, and the both were positively correlated. Because these indicators of exposure were distributed fairly widely, we relied on regression analyses rather than on dichotomous comparison between exposed and control workers. Observed effects included renal clearances for creatinine, urea, β_2-microglobulin, uric acid, inorganic phosphate, calcium, copper, and zinc, and other routine clinical chemistry measurements. It was found that uric acid/creatinine clearance ratio and phosphate/creatinine clearance ratio showed significant positive linear relationships with blood cadmium concentration, indicating that tubular reabsorption function had been impaired by cadmium. Serum concentrations of uric acid and inorganic phosphate also showed significant changes. However, the decrease in phosphate was not so obvious as in uric acid, probably owing to its hormonal regulation. Creatinine and urea clearances decreased and their concentrations in serum increased significantly, suggesting that glomerular function had also been impaired . Serum β_2-microglobulin concentration was eleveted in spite of the fact that its urinary excretion increased remarkably, suggesting also that glomerular filtration rate had been depressed by cadmium exposure. Hemoglobin, hematocrit, red blood cell count and blood specific gravity showed significant negative linear relationship with blood cadmium, indicating that a slight anemia had been induced. Blood pressure had no association with the indices of exposure. These findings are generally in agreement with earlier clinical observation reported by Friberg[3,22] and Adams et al.[11]. More recent reports[25,26] showed that not only small molecular weight proteins but also larger ones appeared in urine at earlier stage of cadmium poisoning in man. Similar findings have been reported in animals by Nomiyama et al.[30 31]. In our data, urinary β_2-microglobulin concentration of most workers exposed to past high level of cadmium increased to about one hundred times as much as that of workers with normal blood and urine cadmium. However several highly exposed workers showed normal level of urinary β_2-microglobulin. On the other hand, urinary protein showed more consistent increase in highly exposed workers although the extent of increase was about tenfold. It is considered that quantitative determination of total protein in urine might be an equally useful indicator of earlier renal effect of cadmium as β_2-microglobulin in urine, although the problem of differential diagnosis may remain. Other findings in our alloy making workers were slight aminoaciduria, glycosuria, and hyper-calciuria, all of which showed weaker but statistically significant associations with blood cadmium. Another finding of interest was an increased urinary excretion of copper as indicated both by copper clearance and urinary concentration of copper even in workers whose exposure to cadmium, copper and other metals had long been terminated. Usual indicators of liver injury such as GOT, GPT, and γ-GTP values showed no association with cadmium exposure.

Those results of our study of cadmium workers in alloy making factory are mostly in agreement with previous reports although such a sweeping observation on renal and other effects in reference to indices of exposure has not been reported so far.

Recently, we had another opportunity to perform a cross-sectional study on less exposed groups of cadmium workers by exactly the same design as that for alloy makers. The subjects of this study were 119 workers in several factories manufacturing alkaline batteries, of whom 61 were females and 58 were males. Female workers mainly consisted of assembly workers in two small scale factories where exhaust ventilation and other protective devices had been almost absent. On the other hand, male workers were mainly negative active material and platemaking workers in a larger factory with reasonable ventilating facilities. They had been wearing authorized protective masks too. Hence, the level

TABLE 2

LIST OF r INDICATING SIGNIFICANT LINEAR RELATIONSHIPS BETWEEN BLOOD CADMIUM AND EFFECTS FOUND IN CADMIUM WORKERS WITH DIFFERENT EXPOSURE LEVELS

		Workers in alloy factory	Female workers in battery factory	Male workers in battery factory
No. of total subjects		27	61	58
Subjects apparently exposed to cadmium				
No.		14	35	27
Blood cadmium (µg/100ml)	Mean	2.34	1.81	0.73
	Median	2.31	1.50	0.80
	Range	0.47-4.35	0.19-6.30	0.20-1.33
Urine cadmium (µg/l)	Mean	27.7	11.3	4.9
	Median	27.0	5.8	2.8
	Range	0.4-76.4	1.6-86.0	0.1-33.6
Subjects whose lengths of cadmium exposure are known				
No.		14	32	16
Length of exposure (year)	Mean	9.4	5.2	8.2
	Median	8.6	5.6	7.4
	Range	1.0-20.6	1.0-10.8	1.0-15.9
Hemoglobin		-0.559 ** a	NS	NS
Serum				
Creatinine		0.766 ***	NS	NS
Urea		0.393 *	NS	NS
Uric acid		-0.767 ***	NS	NS
Phosphate		-0.521 **	NS	NS
β_2-Microglobulin		0.700 ***	0.343 **	0.320 * c
GPT		NS	NS	0.352 ** a
Urine				
Cadmium		0.817 ***	0.781 ***	0.550 ***
Total protein		0.707 ***	0.256 *	NS
β_2-Microglobulin		0.543 **	NS	NS
Amino acid		0.389 *	NS	NS
Glucose		0.486 *	NS	NS
Calcium		0.480 *	NS	NS
Copper		0.747 ***	0.381 **	NS
Clearance				
Creatinine		-0.771 *** b	NS	NS
Urea		-0.467 * b	NS	NS
Clearance ratio to creatinine clearance				
Uric acid		0.849 ***	NS	NS
Phosphate		0.425 *	NS	NS
Calcium		0.655 **	NS	NS
Copper		0.614 ***	NS	NS

* $p < 0.05$ ** $P < 0.01$ *** $p < 0.001$ NS $p > 0.05$

a. r value calculated for relationship with urine cadmium.

b. n = 23

c. n = 57

of exposure was higher in female than male workers. Durations of cadmium exposure of battery makers were shorter than that of alloy makers, but blood and urine cadmium concentrations of female workers were almost comparable to those of alloy makers as shown in Table 2. Highly significant associations were observed between blood and urine cadmium concentrations in both, male and female groups. However, few effects showed statistically significant linear relationships with blood cadmium levels. In female battery workers, the increases in β_2-microglobulin concentration in serum and total protein and copper concentrations in urine were the only significant findings. The increase in serum β_2-microglobulin concentration was found in male battery makers, too. The only significant finding except the increase of β_2-microglobulin in serum in male battery makers was a slight rise of serum GPT level (Table 2). Since all those changes observed in battery workers were of marginal statistical significance, further study will be needed to confirm them. However, the increase in β_2-microglobulin level was consistently found both in female and male workers without accompanied by changes in glomerular and tubular functions. The increase could not be explained by the age. Tsuchiya et al.[27 28] reported similar findings in a different group of alloy makers although the contribution of reduced glomerular filtration could not be completely excluded. They discussed that the rise of serum β_2-microglobulin may be attributed, at least in part, to the increase in production of this protein due to cadmium exposure. Our finding supports their view and suggests that it may be one of the earliest effects of long-term cadmium exposure. The increase in the urinary excretion of copper, which was found not only in alloy makers but also in female battery makers, is another point of interest. Considering the importance of metallothionein[29] both in cadmium and copper metabolism, the mechanism of this phenomenon surely deserves further study. A very slight proteinuria observed in exposed female workers is worthy of note, because urinary excretion of β_2-microglobulin in this group did not show any change. The positive linear relationship between cadmium in blood and total urinary protein was detected because a few persons in the more exposed group showed scattered increases whereas most others showed no changes at all. Although this finding was of only marginal statistical significance, it may also support the views of Lauwerys et al.[25 26] and Nomiyama et al.[31 32] who stressed the early appearance of higher molecular weight proteins in urine. A positive association between indices of cadmium exposure and serum GPT level was found only in male battery makers and not in more severely exposed groups. It is interesting to note that, even though signs of liver injury have been repeatedly observed in animal experiment[21 30], they have not generally been found in humans.[21] However, our finding supports a possibility of liver injury being induced by cadmium and recovered later in spite of a continued exposure to cadmium. Survey of subjective symptoms did not reveal any indication suggestive of pulmonary or bone changes in all of our exposed groups. Further studies are in progress in which the concentration and particle size distribution of cadmium dusts in workplaces and effects on respiratory tract and bone are to be observed. Moreover, a long-term follow-up of those cohorts, especially the female battery workers, may give us more precise information on earlier effects of chronic cadmium exposure.

CONCLUSION

The types of information obtained by epidemiologic approaches have been shown by several examples performed on workers with prolonged metal exposure. Although animal experiments cannot completely substitute human observation in several aspects, our epidemiologic findings on cadmium workers indicated a good agreement rather than disagreement with animal experimental data. When both approaches are made with reasonable cautiousness, the probability of agreement between them appears to arrive at a satisfactory level even in chronic toxicity studies. In view of the difficulty of finding opportunity to observe groups of workers with sufficient population size, the importance of animal experiment cannot be overemphasized. And the best approach is probably a combination of those different methods whenever practicable.

REFERENCES

1. Sakurai, H. and Tsuchiya, K. (1975) Symposium Proceedings, International Conference on Heavy Metals in the Environment, Vol.III, pp.1-17.
2. Friberg, L., Nordberg, G. F. and Vouk, V. B.,(ed.) (1979) Handbook on the Toxicology of Metals, Elsevier/North-Holland, Amsterdam, pp.1-709.
3. Friberg, L. (1950) Acta Med. Scand. 138, Suppl. 240.
4. Bonnell, J. A. (1955) Br. J. Ind. Med. 12, 181-195.
5. Bonnell, J. A., Kazantzis, G. and King, E. (1959) Br. J. Ind. Med. 16, 135-147.
6. Sakurai, H. and Seki, Y. (1977) Keio J. Med. 26, 223-233.
7. Sakurai, H., Omae, K., Sugita, M, Kusumoto, M., Toyama, T., Adachi, S., Okubo, T. and Tsuchiya, K. (1980) Jap. J. Hyg. 35, 267.
8. Lauwerys,R., Buchet, J.P., Roels, H. A., Brouwers, J. and Stanescu, D.(1974) Arch. Environ. Health 28, 145-148.
9. Materne, D., Lauwerys, R., Buchet, J. P., Roels, H., Brouwers, J. and Stanescu, D. (1975) Cah. Méd. Travail, 12, 1-76.
10. Smith, T. J., Petty, T. L., Reading, J. C. and Lakshminarayan, A. (1976) Am. Rev. Resp. Dis. 114, 161-169.

11. Adams, R. G., Harrison, J. F., and Scott, P. (1969) Q. J. Med. 38,425-442.

12. Stanescu, D., Veriter, C., Frans, A., Goncette, L., Roels, H., Lauwerys, R. and Brasseur, L. (1978) Scand. J. Resp. Dis. 68, 289-303.

13. Teculescu, D. B., and Stanescu, D. C. (1970) Arch. Arbeits. Med. 26,335-345.

14. Gill, P. F. (1978) Proceedings, First International Cadmium Conference, Metal Bulletin Limited, London, pp. 207-210.

15. Lauwerys, R. (1979) in "The Chemistry, Biochemistry,and Biology of Cadmium" Elsevier/North Holland, Amsterdam, pp. 433-455.

16. Oxhoj, J., Bake, B., Wedel, H. and Wilhelmsen, L. (1979) Arch. Environ.Hlth. 34, 211-217.

17. Love, R. G., Attfield, M. D. and Isles, K. D. (1980) Br. J. Ind. Med. 37, 63-69.

18. Kiviluoto, M., Räsänen, O., Rinne, A. and Rissanen, M. (1979) Scand. J. Work, Environ. & Health 5, 50-58.

19. Askergren, A. and Mellgren, M. (1975) Scand. J. Work, Environ. & Health 1, 45-49.

20. Nordberg, G. F. (ed.) (1976) Effects and Dose-Response Relationships of Toxic Metals, Elsevier, Amsterdam, pp. 64-72.

21. Friberg, L., Piscator, M., Nordberg, G. F. and Kjellström, T. (1974) Cadmium in the Environment, 2nd ed., CRC Press, Cleveland.

22. Friberg, L. (1948) J. Ind. Hyg. Toxicol. 30, 32-36.

23. Kjellström, T., Evrin, P. E. and Rahnster, B. (1977) Environ. Res. 13, 303-317.

24. Sakurai, H., Onodera, M., Ohmae, K., and Hosoda, K. (1980) Read at 53th Conference of Japan Industrial Health Association.

25. Bernard, A., Buchet, J. P. Roels, H., Masson, P. and Lauwerys, R. (1979) Eur. J. Clin. Invest. 9, 11-22.

26. Lauwerys, R., Roels, H., Buchet, J. P., Bernard, A. and Stanescu, D. (1979) Environ. Health Perspect. 28, 137-145.

27. Tsuchiya, K., Iwao, S., Sugita, M. and Sakurai, H. (1979) Environ. Health Perspect. 28, 147-153.

28. Iwao, S., Tsuchiya, K., and Sakurai, H. (1980) J. Occup. Med. 22, 399-402.

29. Webb, M.(ed.) (1979) The Chemistry, Biochemistry and Biology of Cadmium, Elsevier/North-Holland, pp. 195-283, 423-431.

30. Nomiyama, K., Nomiyama, H., Nomura, Y., Taguchi, T., Matsui, K., Yotoriyama, M., Akahori, F., Iwao, S, Koizumi, N., Masaoka, T., Kitamura, S., Tsuchiya, K., Suzuki, T. and Kobayashi, K. (1979) Environ. Health Perspect. 28, 223-243.

31. Nomiyama, K., Nomiyama, H., Yotoriyama, M., Okubo, T., Nozaki, R., Akahori, F. and Masaoka, T. (1980) Kankyo Hoken Report, 45, in press.

Mechanisms of Toxicity and Hazard Evaluation
B. Holmstedt, R. Lauwerys, M. Mercier, M. Roberfroid eds

NEUROTOXIC EFFECTS OF LONG-TERM EXPOSURE TO ORGANIC HYDROCARBON SOLVENTS. EPIDEMIOLOGIC ASPECTS

SVEN HERNBERG, Institute of Occupational Health, Helsinki, Finland

Industrial hydrocarbon solvents cover a broad range of different chemical compounds, whose common property is their lipid solubility. Because of this property they have a high affinity to the nervous system and hence solvent poisoning is mainly characterized by impairment of central (CNS) and peripheral (PNS) nervous system function.

The non-specific character of these toxic effects complicates their study. The CNS effects can broadly be referred to as neurasthenia, a syndrome which also occurs in connection with many other conditions, and in severe cases as a psycho-organic syndrome, which also is non-specific. The PNS effects manifest themselves in severe cases as polyneuropathy, but in milder cases the symptoms are less well defined. Because of the non-specificity of the nervous effects, individual etiological clinical diagnosis is difficult, even impossible in mild cases. Cause-effect inferences between exposure to hydrocarbon solvents and morbidity can therefore best be made at the group level, utilizing epidemiologic methods. An epidemiologic study seldom aims at individual diagnosis. Instead, it compares frequencies of isolated neurotoxic symptoms and signs. An prerequisite for inferences from such studies is that they are methodologically valid, in other words, that errors of selection, information and comparison have been avoided. The sensitivity of the study to detect differences between the groups also increases if subjects with a history of conditions which are known to cause neurological manifestations are excluded from both groups. Provided these conditions are met, possible group differences in nervous system dysfunctions between the exposed and the referents can be ascribed to solvent exposure. An epidemiologic study can of course not differentiate between those individuals whose symptoms and signs are due to hydrocarbon solvent exposure and those who have other etiologies. It can only indicate that a given exposure intensity increases the frequency of nervous function impairment.

During recent years several epidemiologic studies using such an approach have been published. Together with clinical studies of manifest cases of poisoning they indicate that long-standing exposure to hydrocarbon solvents indeed causes an excess of various symptoms and signs indicative of nervous function impairment. In the following I shall shortly review some typical studies.

Subjective symptoms

Subjective symptoms in workers exposed to hydrocarbon solvents are either acute and transient, or chronic. Acute symptoms occur during the workday and disappear during weekends and holidays. For example, Swedish workers exposed to jet fuel reported an excess of dizziness, headache, nausea, palpitations and pressure on the chest as compared to a reference group[1]. An excess of the same symptoms also occurred among another group of workers exposed to jet fuel in another plant[2]. Jet fuels contain a large variety of components, of them over 85% saturated hydrocarbons and about 12% aromatic hydrocarbons. Blume and coworkers[3] also found an excess of the same acute symptoms among Swedish house painters, who complained of headache, feeling of drunkenness, dizziness, and anorexia. In a study of 102 Finnish car painters and 102 matched controls, the painters exhibited more nausea, attacks of vomiting, spells of dizziness, feeling of drunkenness, shortness of breath and absentmindedness than pair-matched unexposed controls[4]. A study of 80 Swedish car painters revealed an excess of dizziness, feeling of drunkenness, headache, shortness of breath and slurred speach as compared to two separate reference groups[5]. Also reinforced plastics workers exposed to styrene have reported excess nausea, dizziness and feeling of drunkenness as compared to controls[6]. Altogether these studies show that exposure to solvents causes several acute symptoms.

Chronic symptoms were also inquired about in all the studies mentioned. Exceptional tiredness, concentration difficulties, impaired memory, sleeping disturbances, dysphoria, irritability and nightmares were the symptoms that most clearly differed between exposed and reference subjects [1-6]. All these studies have been fairly consistent in their findings. The symptoms are compatible with what has been referred to as the neurasthenic syndrome. It should be stressed that all studies were well designed and, e.g., alcohol intake did not occur more frequently in the exposed groups than among the referents.

Psychological functions

Earlier studies on patients with severe poisoning caused by high solvent concentrations have revealed severe disturbances of CNS functions [7,8]. More recently, refined techniques such as psychological tests have been applied to detect early impairment. Hane and coworkers[9] compared 52 Swedish house painters with other industrial workers of similar age. They found an excess of disturbances of visual intelligence, dexterity and slowed reaction time among the painters. The primary level of the painters was comparable to that of the reference group, as judged by tests made during military service. Knave and coworkers[2] found differences between workers exposed for several years to jet fuel and unexposed reference persons in tests which made high demands on attention and sensory motor speed, although no differences occurred in tests measuring memory and manual dexterity function.

Psychological tests were also applied in the two surveys on car painters referred to earlier. Hänninen and coworkers[10] found impairments in psychological performances as well as personality changes among the car painters. Impairment in visual intelligence and verbal memory, and reduction of the emotional reactivity were the central features, but the behavioral disturbances also involved several other functions, including performance on a verbal intelligence test. The possible role of differences in the initial intelligence levels was controlled with a separate comparison of the test results of 33 pairs of exposed and non-exposed subjects who were matched for age, and whose intelligence level had been measured during the military service. It was concluded that the primary level was similar in both groups. Elofsson and coworkers[5] also found slowing of the reaction time and impaired performance in tests measuring dexterity, short term memory and perceptual speed. On the other hand, no differences were found with respect to performance in verbal, spatial and reasoning tests.

Härkönen and coworkers[11] studied 98 male workers exposed to styrene in reinforced polyester plastic production. Visuomotor inaccuracy and lowered psychomotor performance were related to a high mean concentration of mandelic acid in urine. Reversals in the Symmetry Drawing tests, form level of straight lines in the Mira test, and errors and omitted reactions in the Bourdon Wiersma Vigilance test were the variables which showed a statistically significant relationship to the mean mandelic acid concentration. However, intellectual functions were not influenced by styrene exposure. Preexposure intelligence levels were evaluated from test results obtained from the files of the Finnish army.

Studies on clinically intoxicated patients confirm these epidemiologic findings[12,13,14]. However, these studies will not be discussed here because of their clinical character.

Electro-encephalographic findings

Several investigations have shown that workers exposed to solvents for long periods exhibit significantly more abnormal EEG's as compared to reference groups, or alternatively, they have shown differences within the normal area[2,15,16,17]. According to Seppäläinen and Härkönen[16], the frequence of theta-activity was increased among workers exposed to styrene. Knave and coworkers[2], on the other hand, observed a less rhythmic and lower amplitude alpha activity among workers exposed to jet fuel as compared to unexposed controls. Elofsson and coworkers[5] also found more alfa activity among 80 car painters as compared with two reference groups of 80 unexposed subjects each. Seppäläinen and coworkers[18], on the other hand, could not demonstrate any differences between 102 car painters and 102 referents, perhaps because the frequency of abnormal EEG's was as high as 29% in the reference group, a finding which the authors could not explain.

Other CNS findings

Two clinical studies have suggested that slight brain atrophy may occur among heavily exposed patients with solvent poisoning [19,20]. These studies had no reference group, however. Elofsson and coworkers[5] also examined their car painters by means of computerized tomography. Some slight changes existed between the groups. The referents had on an average slightly wider cortical fissures and lateral ventricles than the exposed. The authors speculated that slight brain edema among the exposed could have explained this finding.

Neuro-psychiatric disorders as causes for disability retirement

Two case-control studies and one cohort study have investigated the role of solvent exposure as a cause of disability pension due to neuro-psychiatric disorders. Axelson and coworkers [21], using a case-control approach, studied persons on a disability pension because of non-specific neuro-psychiatric disorders (psychoses and oligofrenia were excluded). Occupations where solvent exposure was common such as painters, varnishers and carpet layers, were significantly overrepresented. The rate ratio was 1.8. Moreover, an exposure-response relationship seemed to exist between exposure in terms of occupational years and neuro-psychiatric condititions. Olsen and Sabroe [22] conducted a case-referent study in order to estimate the association between neuro-psychiatric diseases leading to early retirement and exposure to organic solvents in the Danish wood industry. The case group comprised 141 disability pensioners and 28 early old age pensioners, who were matched on the basis of type of pension and age, and whose reasons for being retired were other than neuro-psychiatric conditions. Exposure to organic solvents was studied by means of a questionnaire, and at least 4000 hours of work with organic solvents was the criterion used to define highly exposed subjects. The results showed a statistically significant relationships between neuro-psychiatric disorders and solvent exposure, and an exposure-response pattern was also discernible.

Mikkelsen [23], in a follow-up study of 2601 male Danish painters, found a 3.5-fold rate ratio for disability pensions due to a state of cryptogenic presenile dementia as compared to Copenhagen men and an ad hoc reference group of 1790 male bricklayers. When indications of alcohol abuse, cerebral concussions or other etiologic factors were present, the rate ratio was approximately 2. No excess risk was found for neuro-psychiatric diseases other than presenile dementia.

These studies all indicate that solvent exposure accelerates the aging of the CNS and that the etiology of many non-specific CNS-disorders may, in fact, be solvent exposure.

Peripheral nervous system

The solvents most notorious for causing PNS effects are methylbutylketone and N-hexane. The common denominator for these effects is probably the metabolite 2,5-hexanedione. Billmaier and coworkers[24] have described an outbreak of clinical peripheral neuropathy in a plant that manufactured coated fabrics. The workers were exposed to a mixture of methylbutylketone and methylethylketone. After having seen six severe cases, they examined all 1157 workers in the plant by means of EMG and nerve conduction studies. Of them, 68 had definite and 28 suspect signs, symptoms and electrodiagnostic findings of peripheral neuropathy, mostly in the distal parts of the limbs. Complete paralysis was rarely seen. Achilles tendon and finger reflexes were absent. Some patients had sensory loss. The exposure levels for MBK ranged from a few ppm to about 150 ppm and for MEK from 40 to 760 ppm.

Mallow[25] examined 26 spray painters who had been exposed to methylbutylketone. Of them three had motor impairment, slight impairment of sensory functions (pain and touch) and an elevated threshold for vibration.

Toxic polyneuropathy has also occurred frequently among Italian shoe-industry workers exposed to a mixture of solvents whose most significant component was n-hexane. Cianchetti and coworkers[26] observed a group of 122 workers whose polyneuropathy was characterized by a symmetrical predominantly distal motor deficit, with occasional marked weakness of pelvic girdle muscles, and frequently by only subjective sensory symptoms. Nonspecific disturbances usually preceded neurological signs. Subclinical cases of minimal chronic neuropathy, characterized by alterations of a neurogenic type in the EMG without a reduction of motor nerve conduction velocity, were also observed. Worsening of the clinical picture, with further lowering of nerve conduction velocity, was noted in some cases up to four months after removal from the toxic environment. In the most severe cases clinical recovery took up to three years.

Similar outbreaks of polyneuropathy have occurred in Japan from exposure to glues containing n-hexane[27].

PNS function has also been studied in workers exposed to other hydrocarbon solvents and their mixtures. Unfortunately, however, only very few of these studies have included a clinical neurological examination. Elofsson and coworkers[5] in their study of 80 spray painters found significant group differences as compared to the referents for many neurophysiological parameters measuring peripheral nerve function, most pronouncedly in the long sensory fibres. Also the maximum conduction velocity of the median nerve was lowered among the painters. The exposed group had a significantly higher vibration threshold, especially in the lower extremities.

In the Finnish group of 102 spray painters, significant differences were found for a decrease in the sense of light touch and pain, as well as for an increase in the vibration threshold, which were more frequent among the car painters than among the referents. The vibration sense was affected in the lower extremities of 65 of the car painters but only in 25 of the referents[28]. Abnormally slow motor conduction velocities or sensory conduction velocities and/or prolonged motor distal latencies were found in 12 of the 59 car painters who underwent a complete neurophysiological examination as compared to none of the 53 referents examined in a similar way[18]. There were only few pathological findings and no statistically significant differences between the groups with respect to the cerebellar and extrapyramidal system, the cranial nerves, and peripheral motor and sensorimotor functions[28].

Examinations of workers exposed to styrene have given conflicting results. Rosén and coworkers[17] found an excess of sensory nerve response with low amplitude and long duration, somewhat low sensory conduction velocities, but close to normal motor neurographic findings among 33 workers as compared to 6 unexposed controls, while Seppäläinen and Härkönen [16] did not find any differences in the average maximal motor conduction velocity of the median, ulnar, deep peroneal and posterior tibial nerves, the conduction velocity of the slower motor fibres of the ulnar and deep peroneal nerves and the sensory conduction velocity of the median and ulnar nerves of 40 styrene-exposed workers as compared to unexposed controls.

Exposure-response considerations

Because of insufficient exposure data, very few epidemiologic studies on solvents have provided useful data for exposure-response considerations. The Finnish study on styrene-exposed reinforced plastics workers is an exception, however[11]. In this study the urinary mandelic acid concentrations were used as a measure of current exposure. The urine samples were collected at the end of the workday from every subject once a week, on consequtive weekdays, for five weeks prior to the clinical examination. The arithmetic mean of the five determinations was used for the estimation of the intensity of the individual exposure. This mean varied from 7 to 4715 mg/l (median 808 mg/l).

Abnormal EEG findings and psychological tests measuring visuomotor accuracy and psychomotor performance showed a correlation with the concentration of mandelic acid in urine. For the EEG findings, a notable change in the proportions of normal and abnormal EEG's occurred as the mandelic acid concentration exceeded 700 mg/l. This value corresponds to an estimated TWA styrene concentration of 31 mg/m^3 of air. Those who excreeted less than 700 mg/l had only about 10% abnormal EEG's, which corresponded with the prevalence in the reference group and with usually reported normal frequencies, whereas those with a mandelic acid excretion in excess of 700 mg/l had a prevalence of 30%. With regard to psychological functions, the first change in visuomotor accuracy became discernible when the urinary mandelic acid concentration exceeded 800 mg/l. A more pronounced decrement appeared in both visuomotor accuracy and in psychomotor performance when the mandelic acid concentration exceeded 1200 mg/l, with corresponds to an 8-h TWA exposure of 5 ppm.

Although no such exposure-response data are obtained from the car painter studies reviewed here[4,5,10,18,28], it should be noted that the average exposure had been about 30% of the ACGIH TLV recommendation in the Finnish study and 12-30% of the Swedish TLV's in the Swedish study. The Swedish TLV's are usually the same as or lower than the ACGIH recommendations. In the Finnish study past exposure was assessed by means of interviews and a history-taking of technical improvements, which were compared with the results of current measurements. In the Swedish study a reconstruction of an old painting box was made and the concentrations measured, in addition to similar assessments as in the Finnish study. In the Swedish studies on personnel exposed to jet fuel many measurements were made during the survey[1,2]. Most mean values ranged between 150 and 500 mg/m^3. The highest value was 974 mg/m^3 during 55 min. Peaks of more than 3200 mg/m^3 were recorded. However, exposure conditions in the past may have been considerably worse.

Self-selection of workers

Most of the studies reviewed in this context have used cross-sectional data on neurotoxic effects. However, since solvents cause subjective symptoms, it seems prudent to postulate that affected workers selectively tend to seek new employment. Husman[4] has tried to assess the effect of selection by means of approaching also car painters who during the five years preceding the investigation (January 1969 to December 1973) had changed their employment. He found altogether 124 car painters who had left a car painting job in the 27 car repair garages involved in the study. A total of 101 painters answered the questionnaire. Of them, 39 had chosen a new job without exposure to solvents and of them 26 mentioned health reasons as the main cause. The symptom frequencies of the 39 expainters were of a slightly higher level than those of the current car painters in spite of that the exposure had ceased. Therefore it indeed seems that job turnover had diminished rather than added to the symptom frequency of the car painters who still were active. Unfortunately, no objective examinations could be performed on the expainters for practical reasons.

Conclusions

The studies reviewed here show that long-standing exposure to hydrocarbon solvents causes a variety of symptoms and signs indicating both CNS and PNS impairment. Cross-sectional studies are diluted by selective turnover and hence yield an underestimate of the true effect. The significance of these findings increases in the light of the experience that disability retirement due to neuro-psychiatric disorders is more common than expected among occupations with solvent exposure. Although it is probable that causative exposure levels have been considerably in excess of current permissible exposure limits, there are indications that fairly moderate levels also may increase morbidity. The wide variation in sensity of the CNS to neurotoxic agents is of importance in this context.

REFERENCES

1. Knave, B. et al. (1976) Scand.j.work environ. & health 3, 152-164.
2. Knave, B. et al. (1978) Scand.j.work environ. & health 4, 19-45.
3. Blume, J. et al. (1975) Läkartidningen 72, 702-706.
4. Husman, K. (1980) Scand.j.work environ. & health 6, 19-32.
5. Elofsson, S-A. et al. (1979) Läkartidningen 76, 4127-4148.
6. Härkönen, H. (1977) Int.arch.occup.environ.health 40, 231-239.
7. Grandjean, E. et al. (1955) Br.j.ind.med. 12, 131-142.
8. Münchinger, R. (1963) Proceedings of the 14th international congress on occupational health, Madrid , pp. 687-689.
9. Hane, M. et al. (1977) Scand.j.work environ. & health 3, 91-99.

10. Hänninen, H. et al. (1976) Scand.j.work environ. & health 4, 240-255.

11. Härkönen, H. et al. (1978) Scand.j.work environ. & health 4, 53-59.

12. Lindström, K. (1973) Work environ.-health 10, 151-155.

13. Arlien-Søborg, P. et al. (1979) Acta neurol.Scandinav. 60, 149-156.

14. Juntunen, J. et al. (1980) Int.arch.occup.environ.health (in press).

15. Giuliano, G. et al. (1975) Lav.um. 26, 33-42.

16. Seppäläinen, A.M. and Härkönen, H. (1976) Scand.j.work environ. & health 3, 140-146.

17. Rosén, I. et al. (1978) Scand.j.work environ. & health 4, suppl. 2, 184-194.

18. Seppäläinen, A.M. et al. (1978) Scand.j.work environ. & health 4, 304-314.

19. Gregersen, P. et al. (1978) Ugeskr.laeg. 140, 1638-1644.

20. Juntunen, J. et al. (1980) European neurol. (in press).

21. Axelson, O. et al. (1976) Scand.j.work environ. & health 2, 14-20.

22. Olsen, J. and Sabroe, S. (1980) Scand.j.soc.med. suppl. 16, 44-49.

23. Mikkelsen, S. (1980) Scand.j.soc.med. suppl. 16, 34-43.

24. Billmaier, D. et al. (1974) J.occup.med. 16, 665-671.

25. Mallow, J.S. (1976) J.am.med.ass. 235, 1455-1457.

26. Cianchetti, G. et al. (1976) 39, 1151-1161.

27. Yamamura, Y. (1969) Folia psychiatr.neurol.Jpn. 23, 45-57.

28. Husman, K. and Karli, P. (1980) Scand.j.work environ. & health 6, 33-39.

© 1980 Elsevier/North-Holland Biomedical Press
Mechanisms of Toxicity and Hazard Evaluation
B. Holmstedt, R. Lauwerys, M. Mercier, M. Roberfroid eds

IDENTIFICATION OF HUMAN TOXICITY AND CARCINOGENICITY BY ETHYLENE DERIVATIVES

CARLO H. TAMBURRO and RICHARD A. GREENBERG
Liver Research Center, Departments of Medicine, Community Health and Cancer Center, University of Louisville School of Medicine, Louisville, Kentucky 40202, U.S.A.*

INTRODUCTION

Ethylene derivatives such as vinyl chloride and vinyl bromide are chemicals to which humans have had long term exposure in the occupational environment. These indispensable industrial chemicals have provided untold benefits to our societies. Many, however, have been found to be toxic, carcinogenic or both in man as well as in animals and increasing numbers are becoming suspect.

Most of our current human knowledge of the toxicity and carcinogenicity of ethylene derivatives is derived from medical reports of either intentional, suicidal or accidental ingestion or environmental exposure. Periodically, retrospective epidemiological studies are conducted because of case occurrences in various occupations or industries. Although this type of information gathering eventually provides an outline of the pathogenic process in man, it provides little human data concerning the intermediate stages of the disease process. These gaps are usually filled in by animal data where there is an appropriate animal model available for study.

Our present day knowledge about the early latent injuries that occur during long term but low grade exposure to occupational intoxicants is limited. Less is known about how to identify these processes early. Carbon tetrachloride and vinyl chloride are among the few exceptions in which there has accumulated considerable knowledge concerning latent effects on humans. In order to illustrate the correlation between the clinical methods of detection of ethylene derivative toxicity and carcinogenicity and the human pathogenic process related to chemical injury, vinyl chloride will be used as the model.

Among the ethylene derivatives, vinyl chloride is the best chemical model because its chemical structure is relatively simple and it induces both acute and chronic injury to multiple body systems. In the human, there is direct evidence of toxicity to the liver, spleen, bone and blood system and strong evidence suggesting involvement of the lung and the cardiovascular system. Vinyl chloride has induced multiple cellular types of cancer in animals and at

---

*Portions of this work were supported by the NCI Contract number 1-CN-55212

least one and possibly up to five different cellular types of malignancy in man. These include hepatic angiosarcoma, large clear cell lung carcinoma, glioblastoma of the brain, lymphoma and possible primary hepatocellular carcinoma. In addition, good animal models are available because vinyl chloride induces the same type of toxicity and carcinogenicity in animals as in man. Finally, the use of vinyl chloride and similar agents in industrial environments provide actual human epidemiological settings for determining, if there is any association with human cancer. Four excellent broad literature surveys of ethylene derivatives and their effects on humans have been conducted by Posner and Falk[1], Van Durren[2], Key _et al_[3] and, Nicholson and Moore[4].

METABOLISM OF ETHYLENE DERIVATIVES

Over the past few decades at least one common scenario for the toxicity and carcinogenicity of ethylene derivatives has become increasingly apparent and can be typified by vinyl chloride. Entry into the human body by these chemical agents, although mainly via the lung, can occur to a significant degree by skin absorption and through the gastrointestinal tract. Repeated laboratory studies have established that most chemicals are, in their native state, non-toxic, having to be metabolically activated to become cytotoxic, mutagenic, or carcinogenic[5,6,7]. The primary enzyme system involved in the activation and detoxification of these chemicals is known as mixed function oxidase (microsome hydroxylase, microsome drug metabolizing enzymes, or monoxygenases). This enzyme system oxidizes a variety of both endogenous and exogenous compounds to more polar derivatives which most often undergo secondary enzymatic reactions generally yielding products that are less harmful than the parent compound.

The steady-state level of chemicals and their intermediates appears to be a key determinate in the biological activity of these agents and the ultimate effect they produce at the cellular and organ level. The ethylene derivatives form a group about whom a steadily increasing knowledge is evolving concerning their oxidation and detoxification pathways as related to long term, low grade toxicity, mutagenicity or carcinogenicity.

In the case of vinyl chloride, monoxygenases evidently played a crucial role in the activation of the ultimate carcinogen, and probably function as the common metabolic pathway for ethylene derivatives. Vinyl chloride is believed to form an epoxide as well as an aldehyde. The formation of these intermediate metabolites appears to depend on the dose[8] as well as the presence of other agents or co-factors[9].

At dose levels of less than 50 ppm, vinyl chloride metabolism appears to involve the alcohol dehydrogenase enzyme system. Further oxidization ultimately forms monochloroacetic acid. With chronic progressive exposure, metabolism occurs by epoxidation or peroxidation without significant changes in the proportion of the urinary metabolites excreted when the dose is varied. This data would indicate that the metabolism of vinyl chloride is a saturable process[10]. Covalent binding of vinyl chloride and other ethylene derivatives to hepatic micromolecules and nucleic acids has also been shown[11]. In addition, the decrease in the hepatic glutathione content when exposure exceeds 100 ppm, suggests that vinyl chloride carcinogenicity may be related to a decreased ability to detoxify its active metabolites.[8] However, all of this metabolic data fails to take into account the fact that malignant transformation with vinyl chloride exposure occurs in the mesenchymal cells and not the primary liver cell[12]. Recent studies have shown a 250-500 fold difference in the oxidation and detoxification capability of hepatic vs sinusoidal lining cells[13], suggesting that different carcinogenic susceptibilities may be related to individual cell differences in oxidative or detoxifying ability, or both.

Application of this data to the actual clinical problem in the industrial environment has helped in the development of occupational surveillance systems.

EPIDEMIOLOGICAL IDENTIFICATION OF THE CARCINOGENICITY OF ETHYLENE DERIVATIVES

At present, determination of the real or presumptive toxic or carcinogenic risk to man of chemicals and other agents has been mainly through chemical structural analysis, bacteriological mutagenic assays, and assessment of tumor occurrence in experimental animals. Epidemiological studies have included isolated prospective or retrospective studies initiated because of experimental findings or casual episodic observations.

The effectiveness and ability of epidemiological studies to identify occupational intoxicants in the development of human disease has been well documented. Although many attempts have been made to devise surveillance systems to meet individual industrial needs, there had not been a uniform health surveillance system designed for industry-wide application which was shown to be effective as well as economically practical.

Obviously such a task is not an easy one. Experiments with animals and other biological systems, although able to yield good presumptive evidences of toxicity including carcinogenicity, are limited by expense, time and other biological factors which may not allow test results to be necessarily applicable to man. These problems, monumental as they may seem, are dwarfed by the fact that humans are never, in the work place or otherwise, exposed to just one chemical or agent at a time but usually to complex combinations.

Three major elements are needed in the formation of an occupational monitoring system: (1) uniform methods for maintaining medical surveillance of the incidence and prevalence of occupational disease, (2) a system of monitoring all aspects of the work environment that may contribute to occupational disease, and (3) reliable methods, screening or epidemiological, by which potential relationships between occupational disease and work environments can be established.

Vinyl chloride's induction of a rare but specific liver cancer provided the setting for implementation of such a prospective prototype occupational health surveillance system. Six years of experience in the application of this system in an actual industrial environment, utilizing a wide variety of ethylene derivatives, has evolved a comprehensive surveillance system applicable for industry-wide use.

Since not all industries would require all aspects of such an extensive surveillance system, various components were developed, implemented and assessed as separate entities within the comprehensive program, divided into three major levels composed of a total of 9 components.

INDUSTRIAL/OCCUPATIONAL ENVIRONMENT CLASSIFICATIONS

Each industry or occupational environment can be classified into three categories based on their toxic or carcinogenic environmental potential.

Category A - Possibly toxic/carcinogenic occupational environment: These include all occupations or industries in which the industrial material(s) have not yet been studied for toxicity or carcinogenicity.

Category B - Probably toxic/carcinogenic industrial environment: These include all occupations and/or industries which utilize materials suspected to be toxic or carcinogenic via animal or human data.

Category C - Actual toxins/carcinogens being used within the industrial environment: These include those occupations or industries actively utilizing known toxic or carcinogenic related industrial materials.

Although this system was originally designed for cancer control, it can and should be utilized for the control of the medical illnesses or diseases found within the occupational or industrial environments.

HEALTH SURVEILLANCE SYSTEM: LEVEL I

This level is designed as the core or basic foundation for the comprehensive health surveillance system. It is applicable to any occupation or industry, whether small or large. It does not require an employee medical examination and may be implemented at a minimum cost which is economically practical. This first level includes the following components: (1) a standardized job classification code, (2) an employee work history record, (3) a chemical exposure rating system, and (4) a medical illness and disease data base.

As an example of the effectiveness of this system, a vinyl chloride polymerizing plant, which had been in existence for 35 years, standardized all of its 350 job classifications. Employee work histories were derived from employment and pay records, both retrospectively and prospectively (retrospectively for 35 years and prospectively for 6 years).

A rating system was developed for chemical exposure based on a rank order. This approach was used because most occupational environments do not have specific knowledge as to the potential hazard of all agents that they use. Even those agents which are known to be hazardous are not always monitorable and monitoring of one agent does not adequately take into account interactions between various agents and chemicals. It also took into account the necessity to have an immediately implementable system of relatively low cost which could, at the least, identify developing areas of potential hazard.

A six point rank order scale was developed and applied to 22 chemicals selected from two separate manufacturing processes, one for synthetic rubber and the other, for plastics, based on their potential for hepatic toxicity and carcinogenicity. The six point rating basis used was:

0 - NO EXPOSURE
1 - MINIMUM POSSIBLE EXPOSURE
2 - MINIMAL EXPOSURE TO LOW LEVELS
3 - MODERATE EXPOSURE
4 - WORKS IN AREA SUBJECT TO OCCASIONAL HIGH EXCURSIONS
5 - WORKS IN AREAS WHERE LEVEL IS HIGH
6 - INTIMATE CONTACT - SKIN OR HIGH INHALATION

The selected chemicals rated for exposure indices are listed on the next page.

Finally, a systematic recording of all medical illnesses* and diseases of each individual employee was determined from medical records and verified from histories of the individual employees. For purposes of this analysis and illustration, only liver disease and cancer were considered. The international classification of disease code (ICD) system was used in the classification process.[14,15]

Identification of Ethylene Derivative Carcinogenicity

In order to facilitate its evaluation, this system was applied retrospectively to determine its ability to identify chemical exposure relationships to

*Even industries without medical records can develop a system of annual self-update, by individual employees, of their illnesses or diseases.

LIST OF SELECTED CHEMICALS FOR EXPOSURE INDICES

CODE	CHEMICAL	CODE	CHEMICAL
01	ACRYLIC ACID	12	MECURIC CHLORIDE
02	ACRYLAMIDES - ACRYLAMIDE, METHYL, N-OCTYL, nMA	13	METHANOL
03	ACRYLONITRILE	14	PHENOL
04	ACETYLENE	15	TOLUENE
05	ACRYLATES--ETHYL, METHYL, METHYL-METH, 2 ETHYL HEXYL, N-BUTYL	16	VINYL CHLORIDE
06	BISPHENOL A	17	VINYLIDENE CHLORIDE
07	BUTADIENE	18	VINYL ACETATE
08	CAPRYLYL CHLORIDE	19	PVC DUST
09	CHLORINATED SOLVENTS--CARBON TETRACHLORIDE, CHLOROFORM, TRICHLOROETHYLENE, EDC	20	CATALYSTS
10	CHLORO ETHYL VINYL ETHER	21	STYRENE
11	DIETHYL MALEATE	22	HEXANE

cancer development. The analysis program utilized the vinyl chloride exposure and hepatic angiosarcoma as its prototype example.

Liver Cancer

There were four cases of angiosarcoma in a vinyl chloride polymerization plant from 1974 through 1978. Each of these four cases were matched by age (year of birth), sex, race, year of initial employment and years of continuing employment at the plant through 1974. Each of the angiosarcoma cases were compared with their corresponding matched controls on their Cumulative Exposure Rank Months, separately calculated for each calendar year (Table 1). CERMs for a chemical were determined by the months worked at a job with an exposure ranking for a specific chemical. For example, Table 1 shows that an employee worked at job 576 in building 000 for 6 months. This job had an estimated exposure rank for vinyl chloride of 2, giving the employee 12 cumulative exposure rank months for vinyl chloride during 1944. During 1945, he had a CERM to vinyl chloride of 5 months at Level 2 or 10 CERMs for a total of 45 CERMs for 1945. In this analysis, these were then ranked within each calendar year and the ranks summed over the calendar years. If the work histories and the ordered ranking exposures were no better than random assignment, one would expect the uniform distribution of ranks within each year and independence from year to year. Figure 1 demonstrates a very clear pattern of high exposure to chemical #16, vinyl chloride. This is to be expected apriori if the work history data

TABLE I

DETAILED WORK AND EXPOSURE HISTORY

	1A			1B				
	WORK HISTORY			EXPOSURE RANK FOR EACH CHEMICAL				
YEAR	A BUILDING	D JOB	NO. MONTHS	VINYL CHLORIDE	2*	3*	. . . .	22*
1944	000	576	6	2	1	1	. . . .	4
1945	000	576	5	2	1	1	. . . .	4
1945	111	194	7	5	4	1	. . . .	1
1946	111	194	12	6	4	1	. . . .	1
1947	111	194	12	6	4	3	. . . .	1
1948	111	194	8	5	4	3	. . . .	1
1948	121	192	4	4	3	1	. . . .	1
1949	121	192	4	4	3	1	. . . .	1
1949	112	253	8	2	6	3	. . . .	2
.	.	.	.					
.	.	.	.					
.	.	.	.					
1957	121	235	12	4	3	1	. . . .	1
.	.	.	.					
.	.	.	.					
.	.	.	.					
1972	117	573	5	1	2	1	. . . .	1
1972	000	574	7	2	1	1	. . . .	4
1973	000	574	12	2	1	1	. . . .	4
1974	000	574	8	2	1	1	. . . .	4
1974	TERMINATED							

*OTHER CHEMICAL

and the exposure rank data were valid. The analysis clearly demonstrates the ability to create a valid exposure ranking. A second significant finding was the identification in all four angiosarcoma victims of a significantly high exposure to chemicals #20, #22, and #11. Chemical #20 was a catalysis group used only for vinyl chloride polymerization. Chemical #22, hexane, was used as a solvent for the catalysis group #20 and, chemical #11, diethylmaleate, a specialized catalyst was used only for the specialized vinyl chloride product. None of the chemicals used in the synthetic rubber or in polyvinyl chloride (PVC) areas were significant in this employee group.

In addition, a clear pattern of exposure is apparent for the angiosarcoma victims. All four showed excess exposure to five chemicals. By chance, this would be expected to occur for only 1.25 chemicals. All four angiosarcoma victims also had less than expected exposure to five additional chemicals. This expectation again is only 1.25. When the binomial distribution is looked at, this distribution of numbers of successes in four trials with the probability of success at each end at each trial one half, the results are statistically significant ($P<0.1$). Again, the null hypothesis of random assignment of exposure is rejected validating the use of the rank ordered exposure work history to identify the increased occurrence of malignancies in an occupational environment.

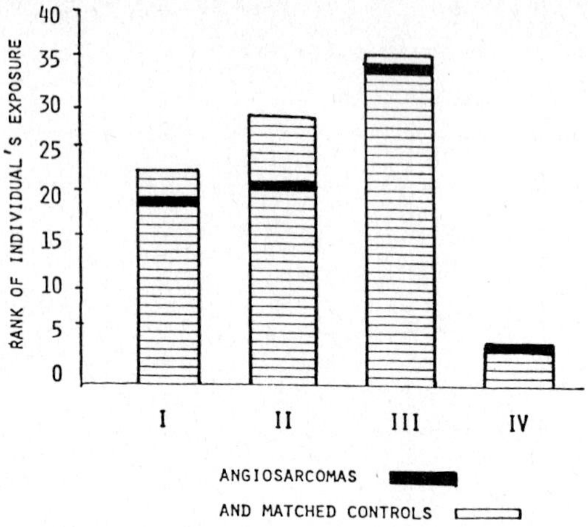

Figure 1 Vinyl chloride exposure rank of individuals with angiosarcoma

LEVEL II - OCCUPATIONAL HEALTH SURVEILLANCE SYSTEM

At this level, medical screening components are added to the basic LEVEL I system. Component five is a medical examination, both a medical history and a physical examination. This is preferably performed by a single group in order to provide uniformity throughout the medical history and examination. This provides for better reproducibility and a continued high degree of voluntary compliance.

The sixth component is laboratory screening studies. Medical screening provides specifically designed or selected studies based on the body system involved, the metabolism of the potentially toxic agent or the type of injury caused by the agent(s).

The selection of proper laboratory screening studies requires special attention. Few of the commonly available medical tests have been adequately evaluated for their sensitivity and specificity in correctly identifying latent disease in an asymptomatic healthy cohort of industrial workers. Most screening studies presently in use have only been previously evaluated in ill or symptomatic populations. This prior medical experience therefore, does not reflect accurately the sensitivity and specificity of these tests for use as screening tools.

Secondly, the screening tests evaluations are performed on ill populations which involves individuals with more advanced or extensive disease in comparison to their industrial counterparts.

Thirdly, the relatively low incidence of most toxic injury and cancer development, related to chronic exposure, requires both careful prospective evaulations with proper controls and adequate time for validation before they are made required screening standards or utilized as effective screening tools. This is illustrated in the following evaluation of government required screening tests to identify hepatic injury which had been selected on the basis of clinical medical experience in ill populations.[16]

The Detection of Chemical Liver Injury From Ethylene Derivatives

Commonly used liver biochemical "function" studies have all demonstrated high degrees of sensitivity in identifying individuals with hepatic disease in general medical practice. Sensitivity alone, however, is insufficient to determine the effectiveness of screening tests. Specificity and sensitivity are both required not only for the identification of all workers with disease but for accurately excluding those without disease.

Figure 2 illustrates the sensitivity, specificity and sum of sensitivity and specificity of common clinical tests in identifying occupational liver disease. The decreased ability to identify liver injury from biochemical enzyme studies occurs because in hepatic cellular injury, increased enzyme release occurs only with major degrees of injury and only during the active phase of the injury. Therefore, enzymatic studies do not adequately detect low grade or chronic injury nor effectively demonstrate the additive effect or progression of intermittent injury. In contrast, indocyanine green (ICG), an anionic dye specific for testing the overall functional capability of the liver to extract anions, can identify early acute injury and can, when used sequentially, identify progressive changes in total liver capability. In actual clinical trial, therefore, the ICG clearance test proved to have the highest sensitivity and specificity for identifying general liver injury.

In order to further document the specificity of these tests, liver biopsies, performed for medical reasons on 100 workers, were histologically classified double blindly as (a) having no hepatic disease, (b) liver injury of non-chemical origin, and (c) liver injury of chemical origin as identified by the critera of Popper, *et al*[17] and Tamburro, *et al*[18]. In addition, the extent of exposure to vinyl chloride among these individuals with liver biopsies was also identified in these three groups. As illustrated in Figure 3, increased exposure ranking was found more frequently among those with chemical liver injury than in those with liver disease without chemical injury or with normal histology.

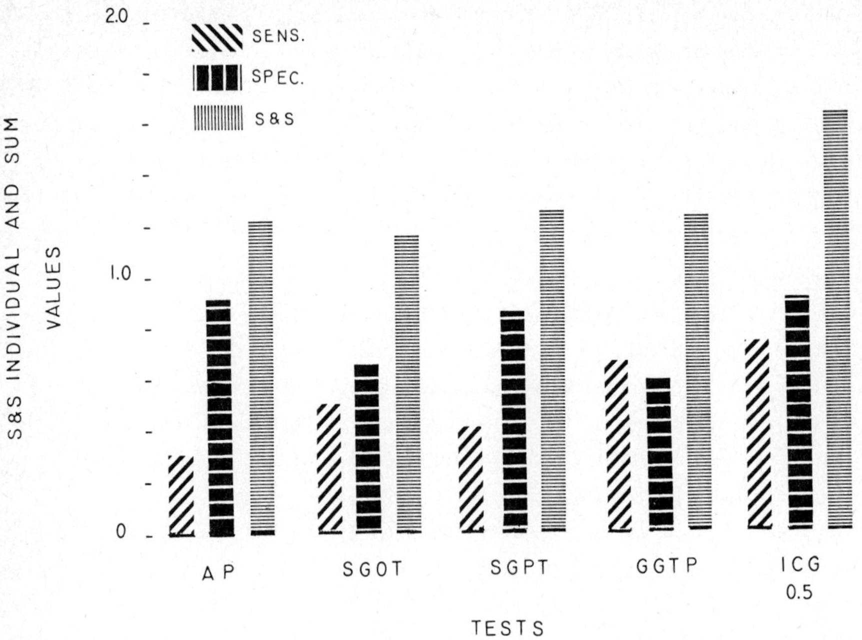

Figure 2. Sensitivity, specificity and sum values of biochemical screening tests in vinyl chloride workers with biopsy documented liver status. SGPT: Serum glutamic pyruvic transaminase; GGT: Gamma glutamyl transpeptidase; ALK PHOS: Alkaline phosphatase; SGOT: Serum glutamic oxaloacetic transaminase; ICD: Isocitric dehydrogenase; ICG: Indocyanine green clearance-0.5 mg and 5.0 mg/Kg.

LEVEL III - OCCUPATIONAL HEALTH SURVEILLANCE SYSTEMS

This LEVEL builds upon the six components of LEVELS I and II and is utilized in areas where occupational toxicity and carcinogenicity has already been identified. At this level, screening studies often will require evaluation for both their potential risk and benefit as well as their effectiveness.

The seventh component adds the use of specified organ studies such as sputum cytology, endoscopic examination, non-invasive cardiovascular function studies, etc.. The eighth component involves radiological or radioisotopic screening studies such as liver, spleen, lung or brain scans. Here the risk of the screening tests is or may be potentially significant and must be weighed against the benefit.

This is illustrated by a study of the value of radioisotopic screening in the detection of injury due to ethylene derivatives and the identification of early tumor development. The effectiveness of radioisotopic scanning vs biochemical screening vs ultrasonographic examination for (a) chemical liver injury, (b) tumors of the liver, and (c) splenomegaly was evaluated. Table 3 illustrates the capability of the liver scan to identify correctly developing anatomical lesions (i.e. cirrhosis, masses, tumor, etc.) before the occurrence of symptoms and at a time when biochemical abnormalities may be minor or first developing. Initial comparison studies, in terms of relative sensitivity and specificity, of radioisotopic scans vs ultrasonography vs biochemical studies to identify (a) hepatocellular injury and (b) tumor masses do not support the usefulness of ultrasound as a screening tool for heaptic disease.[19] The

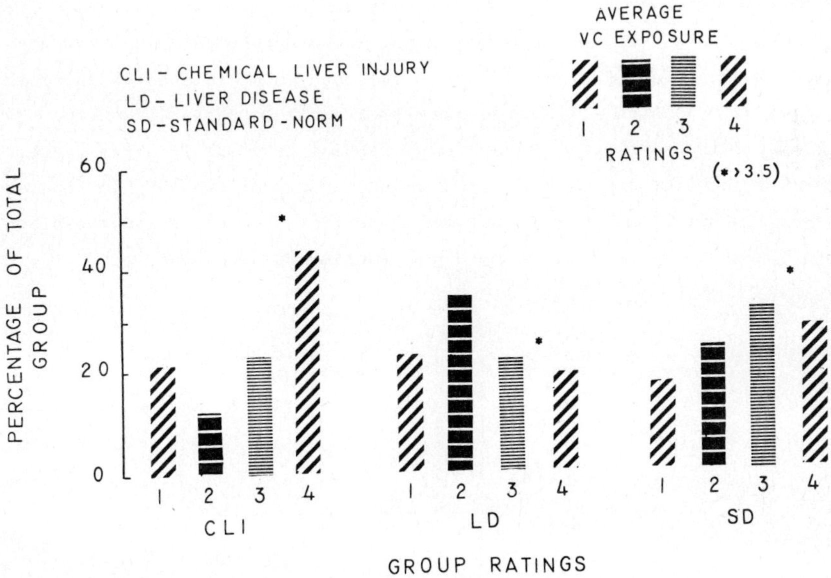

Figure 3. Liver injury-exposure correlation in three groups of vinyl chloride workers with known histological liver status.

TABLE 2

^{99m}Tc SULFUR COLLOID LIVER-SPLEEN SCAN RESULTS RELATED TO BEST MEDICAL DIAGNOSIS

Best Medical Diagnosis	Liver-Spleen Scan Abnormal	Normal	Total
Abnormal	16	3	19
Normal	32	925	957
Total	48	928	976

Sensitivity - 16/ (16+3) = 84%

Specificity - 925/ (32+925) = 97%

possibility of substituting ultrasonography for radioisotopic scanning, however, requires further study as the techniques for ultrasonography become more refined.

It is interesting to note that the clinical tests selected for detecting liver injury are almost totally directed to the hepatocyte, yet vinyl chloride induces its major injury to the non-hepatocytic cells, the endothelial cells, of the hepatic sinusoids and possibly to all vascular endothelial cells in the body, as exemplified by the development of both acro-osteolysis and splenomegaly in vinyl chloride workers. The effects of vinyl chloride on the non-hepatocytic cells is illustrated in Figure 4, where the radioisotopic clearance of 99 Tc sulfur colloid demonstrates two distinct patterns among those ethylene derivative workers with and without splenomegaly. These uptake patterns show changes in reticuloendothelial (RE) cell function believed to be related to chemical stimulation of RE system. Although these preliminary studies illustrate the potential usefulness of specific screening studies to identify organ systems in occupational chemical exposure the cost effectiveness of such highly sophisticated radioisotopic studies and the benefit vs risk from potential radiation exposure, needs to be studied before their routine use is advocated.

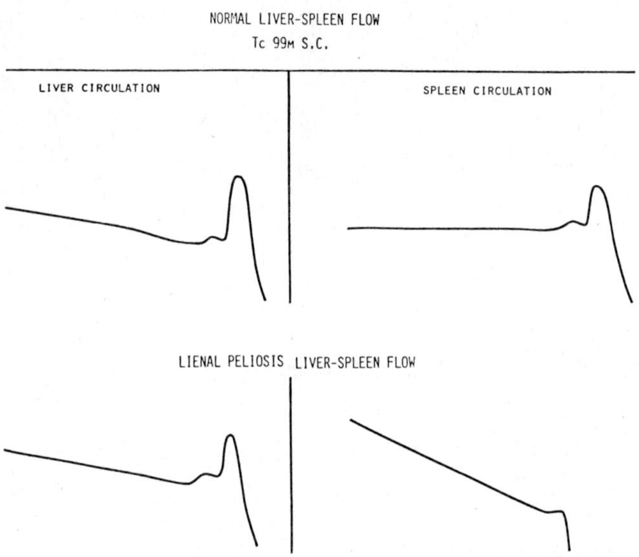

Figure 4. Reticuloendothelial cell uptake in chemical workers: Top patterns in workers with normal angiographic and blood flow studies. Lower patterns in workers with angiographic lienal peliosis and abnormal blood flow.

COST-BENEFIT

In terms of cost, the LEVEL I occupational health surveillance system is easily within the economic practicability of all industries. Initial cost for establishing a program, both retrospectively and prospectively, averaged $20.00 to $30.00/employee and is $4.00-$6.00/employee/year to maintain. LEVEL II costs depend greatly on the care used in the selection and documentation of the medical screening test(s) used. The average cost for single yearly screening is $68.00-$69.00/employee and $138.00/employee requiring multiple screening.

At the present time, it is unlikely that cost-benefit effectiveness can be shown for a LEVEL III health surveillance system for Category C environments. The enormous number of chemicals in use, the complexity of multiple interactions between various agents and chemicals, our limited knowledge in man about the actual mechanism by which certain chemicals with low grade toxicity induce cancer and other co-factors such as obesity, smoking, alcohol intake, medical drugs, and non-occupational medical illnesses all place the cost-benefit of LEVEL III system more in the category of developmental, pilot costs rather than as continuous costs. Average costs for LEVEL III system in Category C environment was $200.00-$450.00/employee/year.

The usefulness of LEVEL I system to industries using ethylene derivatives can be illustrated by the world-wide occurrence of angiosarcoma related to vinyl chloride exposure (Figure 5). The total number of reported cases of angiosarcoma in vinyl chloride workers reached its peak in 1975. Since then, the number of cases have been slowly and progressively falling. Vinyl chloride associated angiosarcoma was first identified in 1973 in animals and 1974 in humans. Major environmental efforts to reduce exposure occurred after 1974. Epidemiological data has demonstrated that there is a latency period of 10 to 30 years (from the initial exposure to the development of the tumor). However, there has been a progressive decrease over the succeeding 6 years in the reported occurrence of angiosarcoma among vinyl chloride workers. It is therefore, unlikely that this decrease was solely due to the changes made in the exposure environments since 1974. Changes in vinyl chloride levels in the industrial environment have occurred in previous years and these reductions could account for this decreased incidence and would support the concept of a biological threshold if not an actual one.

Further studies are required to determine whether this decreased occurrence of vinyl chloride associated angiosarcoma is due to (a) an actual biological threshold, (b) simply a prolonging of the latency period by a reduced exposure level, or (c) that the present exposure levels are within the ability of the biological systems to handle during normal life expectency (i.e. a practical threshold).

A LEVEL I prospective occupational health surveillance system in place in

1955 could have both identified the problem earlier and documented the clinical response to intervention procedures.

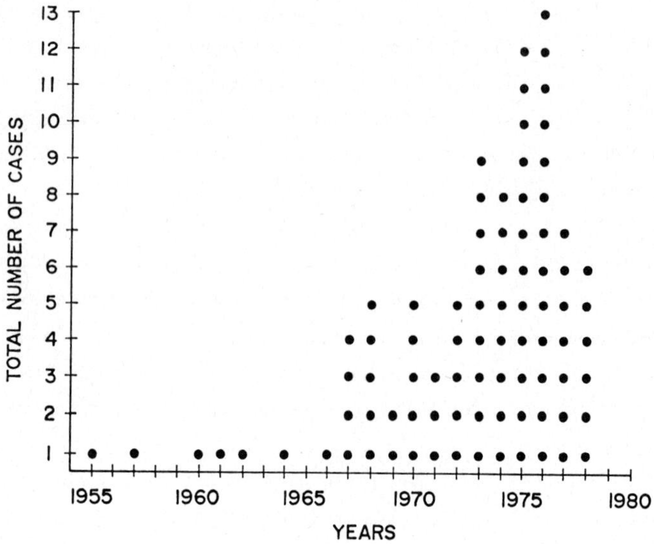

Figure 5. World wide vinyl chloride associated angiosarcoma cases/year.

CONCLUSION

The human toxicity, mutagenicity and carcinogenicity from ethylene derivatives, as well as other chemical agents, require a prospective epidemiological system because of the uniqueness of human species and complexity of human environment. Actual field experience has showed that such a system can work as an early warning, provide verification of environmental safety and document the effectiveness of preventive intervention against cancer and work related problems.

REFERENCES

1. Posner, H.S. and Falk, H.L., (1977). Environ. Health Perspec. 21, 293-326.
2. VanDuuren, B.L. (1980) Oncology Review-PB 80-922904 ICRDB Program Office, 8300 Colesville Road, Silver Springs, Md. 20901, U.S.A.
3. Key, M.N., Henshel, A.F., Bulter, J. etal. (1977) Occupational Diseases: A Guide to their Recognition, DHEW (NIOSH) Public. No. 77-181. Superintendent of Documents, U.S. Government Printing Office, Wash. D.C. 20402.
4. Nicholson, W.J. and Moore, J.A., (1979) Ann. N.Y. Acad. Sci. 320, 1-730.

5. Reynolds, E.S. and Moslen, M.T. (1980) in Toxic Injury of the Liver, Part B, ed. Farber, E. and Fisher, M.M., Marcel Dekker, Inc., New York, pp. 542-587.

6. VanDuuren, B.L. (1980) Oncology Review PB 80-922904, ICRDB Program Office, NCI, Silver Springs, Md., U.S.A. pp. 23-32.

7. Selkirk, J.K. (1980) in Carcinogenesis, Vol. 5, Modifiers of Chemical Carcinogensis, ed. Slaga, T.J., Raven Press, New York, p. 1-31.

8. Watanabe, P.G. and Gehring, P.J. (1977) Environ. Health Perspec. 17, 145-52.

9. Radike, M.J., Stemmer, K.L., Brown, P.G., etal (1977) Environ. Health Perspec. 21, 153-155.

10. Watanabe, P.G., McGowan, G.R., Madrid, E.O., etal (1976) Toxicol. Appl. Pharmacol 36(2), 339-352 and 37(1), 49-59.

11. Watanabe, P.G., Zenpel, J.A., Pegg, D.G., etal (1978) Toxicol. Appl. Pharmacol. 44(3), 571-579.

12. Fortwengler, H.P., Jones D., Espinosa, E., etal (1979) Fed. Proc. 38-(3),999.

13. Du, J.T., Eades, D.S., Tamburro, C.H. (1980) Fed. Proc. 39 (in press).

14. Greenberg, R.A., Tamburro, C.H., Kupchella, C.E. (1978) in Prevention and Detection of Cancer, New York; Part 2, Vol. 2, ed., Nieburgs, H., Marcel Dekker, Inc., pp. 1921-1928.

15. Tamburro, C.H., Davidson, C.S., Fisher, M.M. etal (1979) in Guidelines for Detection of Toxicity Due to Drugs and Chemicals, ed. Davidson, C.S., Leevy, C.M., Chamberlain, E.C., HEW-NIH Pb. No. 79-313, pp. 60-80.

16. Tamburro, C.H., Greenberg, R.A. (1980) Environ. Health Perspec. (in press).

17. Popper, H. and Thomas, L.B. (1975) Ann. N.Y. Acad. Sci. 246, 172-194.

18. Tamburro, C.H., Makk, L., Popper, H. (1979) Gastroenterology 77, A43.

19. Greenberg, R.A., Whelan, J.Jr., Tamburro, C.H., etal (1980) unpublished data.

Mechanisms of Toxicity and Hazard Evaluation
B. Holmstedt, R. Lauwerys, M. Mercier, M. Roberfroid eds

BIOLOGICAL MONITORING OF EXPOSURE TO CHEMICAL POLLUTANTS; EXPOSURE TESTS, BIOLOGICAL LIMITS AND METHODS OF ANALYSIS: A REVIEW

ZDENĚK BARDODĚJ
Department of Medical Chemistry, Charles University, Šrobárova 48, 100 42 Praha 10 (Czechoslovakia)

INTRODUCTION

In the terminology of the International Workshop on the use of biological specimens for the assessment of human exposure to environmental pollutants[1], the term biological monitoring is defined as a systematic collection of human or other biological specimens for which the analysis of pollutants concentrations, metabolites and biotransformation products, is of immediate application; analysis and evaluation will generally be performed within a period of weeks after collection. Unless qualified, "biological monitoring" will refer to human specimens.

In industrial toxicology biological monitoring started to develop about seventy years ago (carbon monoxide 1912[2], lead 1943[3], mercury 1938[4], trichloroethylene 1946[5], benzene 1948[6], cholinesterase inhibitors 1953[7], 5-aminolevulinic acid 1960[8], mutagens 1977[9]). Here, in view of possible immediate health hazards, not only the monitoring itself, but very soon also the indicators of tolerable exposure levels became of primary interest. Biological monitoring and chemical risks evaluation in industry became termed "exposure tests" and "biological limits" became the analogy of TLVs in biological material. Exposure tests have been discussed in numerous monographs[10-21] and reviews[22-32].

GENERAL ASPECTS OF BIOLOGICAL MONITORING AND EXPOSURE TESTS

Prior to the development of an exposure test ten aspects should be considered: (a) fate of pollutant in organism, (b) compound to be determined, (c) material to be analyzed, (d) time of sampling and time interval if collecting urine, (e) storage and preservation of specimens, (f) method of analysis, (g) units to be used to express results, (h) results adjusting and interpretation, (i) frequency of examinations, (j) application of results for setting or re-setting biological limits.

In exposure to toxic elements and their compounds, usually the element is determined, but sometimes also other indicators are used. Most organic pollutants are, however, metabolized in the body and their metabolic products are then estimated.

The retention of aerosols in the respiratory tract depends on size, shape, specific gravity and solubility of particles, the uptake of inhaled vapors and gases is about 60 % (acetone 60, benzene 49, biphenyl 60, ethyl benzene 60, mercury 66; α-methyl styrene 60, phenol 70, pyridine 70, styrene 61, 1,1,1-trichloroethane - uptake decreases, trichloroethylene 60, p-xylene 64 %) [33,34].

The biotransformation starts very often with oxidation, but also reduction and synthetic and other reactions may participate in these processes. Similar compounds are usually metabolized in a similar way (toluene and xylenes, ethyl benzene and styrene, trichloroethylene and vinyl chloride, benzene and biphenyl).

The excretion follows a curve which is a superposition of two or more exponential curves; the main half-life of elimination usually increases at low-level concentrations (half-lives h in urine: benzene - phenol 4.5, ethyl benzene - mandelic acid 5, mercury 720, styrene - mandelic acid 7, trichloroethylene - trichloroacetic acid more than one half-life)[21,34].

The most commonly analyzed biological material is urine. The reason for it lies not only in the fact that many substances are excreted in the urine, but also because its sampling and analysis is relatively easy. Blood and exhaled air analyses are performed if the urine analysis is not adequate, i.e. when no suitable compound is excreted via the kidney. Unfortunately, some substances are metabolized to carbon dioxide and water, or other products of normal metabolism. Determination of enzymes activities and of hemoglobin-related derivatives is also performed in blood.

The time of sampling is not too decisive, if the compound to be determined is excreted very slowly, but its role becomes far more important if the elimination rate is high. Usually, the urine collected at the end of exposure is analyzed. Recently, also samples taken next morning before next exposure have been recommended for the determination of tetrachloroethylene, 1,1,1-

trichloroethane and toluene in blood[35] and of styrene metabolites in urine[36]. It has been also suggested to perform the iodine-azide test for urinary carbon disulfide metabolites before and after working shift to reduce the effect of interfering sulfur compounds from the diet[37]. For the estimation of fluorides the use of urine samples collected after two days without exposure is now also recommended[35].

The specification of time intervals during which the urine is to be collected is quite necessary; the interval lenght may be 2, 3, 4, 8 (working shift) or 24 hours. Longer intervals are sometimes of advantage because the fluctuations in exposure and urine volume have not such an impact on the result, but the result may be influenced by the presence of personel supervising the sample collection, because the working habits and exposure of workers may become voluntarily or involuntarily changed.

Biological material should be stored[38] in a refrigerator at 4 °C, where most substances remain stable for at least 14 days. Urine samples for the determination of coproporphyrin should be stored at -20 °C. Urines for the determination of 5-aminolevulinic acid and of hippuric acid should be acidified to pH = 4; coproporphyrin is more stable in alkalinized urines containing Na_2EDTA. For the preservation of urines that contain mercury potassium persulfate is to be used. Blood for the determination of volatile compounds, as e.g. organic solvents and carbon monoxide, should be stored in entirely filled glass-stoppered tubes.

The method of analysis should be accurate and precise, but also simple, selective, sensitive and fast enough so that the analysis could be performed as often as desirable.

The result of chemical analysis can be expressed in concentration units (μmol/l, mg/l) or as amount excreted per unit of time. Usually the first expression is used, although the last one may be of some advantage in some cases. As the intake of fluids and the excretion of urine fluctuate, the concentration of the compound eliminated depends not only on the dose of pollutant but also on the volumen of eliminated urine. Therefore, the adjustment of results to standard specific gravity of urine or to endogenous creatinine is recommended.

Biological limits should guarantee no health damage to exposed persons. This is possible for most pollutants, but not in carcinogens and mutagens, where the absolutely safe no-effect level can hardly be set and where we have to accept some level of risk - or to prohibit the use of such compounds. Biological limits should be based on long-term observations in industry, where the health status of workers is regularly examined and the exposure monitored by analysing biological material. Where the threshold limit values in air are well documented and the absorption balance, biotransformation pathways and elimination kinetics of pollutant and its metabolic products are known, then the biological limit can be derived from the experimentaly established relationship between pollutant concentrations in air and in biological material.

The frequency of repeatedly conducted analyses of biological material depends as a rule on the severity of the pollutant effect and on the extent of its hazard. The determination should be repeated more often if the substance is highly dangerous, producing irreversible changes in the body, and/or is highly volatile, or if the level of exposure is high, but also at each change in the production technology.

There is no doubt that biological monitoring is one of the best way how to provide reliable data for setting biological limits, or how to justify them. Examples of biological limits are in Table 1.

No big changes have been made in biological limits over the last years; this may be ascribed to exactness of the older data, but also to the difficulties in proving their correctness. Also the number of substances with recommended biological limits has not increased significantly. In spite of it the progress is remarkable, mainly in the methodology of chemical analysis. Some examples may be given here.

EVALUATING EXPOSURE TO CHEMICAL POLLUTANTS

Inorganic pollutants. For screening dangerous exposures of lead, determinations of 5-aminolevulinic acid and coproporphyrin in urine are newly complemented by Zn-protoporphyrin determination[39]. Packed columns with ion exchangers (Biorad) for 5-aminolevulinic acid isolation, Elwalux lamp for fluorimetric coproporphyrin estimation[40] and ESA Hematofluorometer for the determination of Zn-protoporphyrin in one drop blood are now commercially available. The influence of urine volume on exposure test for lead has been investigated[41].

Inorganic mercury as well as methyl mercury are now determined mostly after reduction to metal and subsequent volatilization, using the method of atomic absorption. The half-life of mercury in urine after mercury vapor inhalation was 30 days; if the mercury concentration drops below 0.2 mg/l = 1 μmol/l, the half-life begins to increase[42]. Adjustment of urinary mercury to creatinine led to a reduction in concentrations fluctuations[42]. The respective methyl mercury concentrations in blood, red blood cells and hair were 1 : 2 : 300[43].

Antimony, arsenic, bismuth, germanium, lead, selenium, tellurium and tin can be isolated after reduction with sodium borohydride as volatile hydrides and determined by atomic absorption (Perkin-Elmer, Varian). Methods for the determination of mercury [44], lead[45], 5-aminolevulinic acid[46] and for manganese[45] have become automated. Methods for the determination of cadmium[47], lead [47,48], mercury[47] and 5-aminolevulinic acid[49,50] have been evaluated on an international basis. Mercury[1] and lead[51] can be monitored in single hairs. Exposure tests for chromium[52-54] and nickel[55] have been suggested and also aluminium[56], cadmium[57], cobalt[58], manganese[59] and tungsten[60] have been determined in biological material from exposed workers. Biological limits of some metals in mg/l urine correspond roughly to MACs in mg/m^3 air (As, Be, Cd, Cr, Hg, Ni, Pb, Se, V).

Carbon monoxide can be determined in alveolar air successfully[61]; three methods for the determination of carboxyhemoglobin have been recommended by WHO[62].

Organic pollutants. The fate of halogenated hydrocarbons in the body has been also extensively studied[63,64] and mathematical models of their pharmacokinetics have been developed[65]. Described is also an automated method for the determination of trichloroethylene metabolites in urine[66]. Thiodiglycolic acid has been determined in urine of vinyl chloride workers[67].

Also the determination of phenol in the urine of benzene workers is now successfully automated[68]. GC methods for the determination of benzoic[69], hippuric[70,71], methylhippuric[71,72], mandelic[71,73], phenylglyoxylic[71,73] and 2-furoic acids[74] and of methanol[75] for the evaluation of exposure to toluene, xylenes, ethyl benzene, styrene, fural and methanol have been described. For the production of diazomethane a very simple, but ingenious apparatus has been constructed[70,73]. High pressure liquid chromatography[76] and isotachophoresis[77] is now applied for the determination of phenol, hippuric, methylhippuric, mandelic and phenylglyoxylic acids. The urinary backround of diet-related hippuric acid in persons not exposed to toluene has been studied[78]. Different ways how to express data from chemical analysis have been investigated in balance experiments with xylene[79] and furfural[80] and also in field studies[42]. A Symposium was held on occupational and toxicological aspects of styrene, where also the evaluation of exposure to styrene was discussed[81-83]. Various chlorophenols have been determined in urine by gas chromatography[84,85] and pentachlorophenol by photometry[86].

In humans exposed to biphenyl, 4-hydroxybiphenyl detected in urine has been used for exposure test purposes. Extensive attention has been paid to chlorinated biphenyls, their levels and fate in environment, animals and humans[1]. In organic phosphorus pesticides alkylphosphoric acids are now determined in urine[87]. Kits for the determination of cholinesterase activity are based on the hydrolysis of thiocholine esters and on the determination of thiocholine with 5,5'-dithio-bis(2-nitrobenzoic) acid (Behringer, Merck); the procedure is also automated[88].

Biological limits have been established for 17 cyanogenic aromatic nitro and amino compounds[89].

Experience with quality control of analytical methods in occupational-toxicological laboratory has been published[90]. Some analytical methods have been standardized[91].

Attention has been also focused on alkylating agents and compounds which may be their precursors. It is well known that alkylating agents are a highly dangerous class of substances, that are listed among the most important causes of cancer. Alkylating agents as electrophilic compounds realize their action by reacting with nucleophilic atoms of nucleic DNA bases. Methods for their detection in urine are based on Salmonella typhimurium/microsome tests[1,92,93,94]. Also glutathion is alkylated and after partial degradation and acetylation of cysteine derivative, mercapturic or premercapturic acids occur in urine[95,96]. The presence of mercapturic acids is, however, characteristic also for carcinogenic and mutagenic compounds which themselves are not alkylating agents, but are their precursors, which is quite an important point when screening exposures to unknown carcinogens. The problem is that the splitting of mercapturic acids to thiols, which are determined by reaction with 5,5'-dithio-bis(2-nitrobenzoic) acid, is not quantitative in all substances, and that the backround level of compounds similarly reacting in the urine of non-exposed persons is not negligible. Current methods used to determine mercapturic acids in the urine of persons exposed to styrene vapor appear to be insufficiently sensitive for monitoring styrene exposure in individuals. Some S-cysteine derivatives may undergo further biotransformation as can be demonstrated on two examples: carboxymethylcystein, which is a metabolite of vinyl chloride, undergoes oxidative deamination to thiodiglycolic acid; methylsulfones were detected as metabolites of polychlorinated biphenyls[97].

Development of methods for the determination of mercapturic acids is a very interesting and important field for further research.

Also cytogenetic analysis of human peripheral lymphocytes was used for detecting exposures to alkylating agents in persons at risk[98].

CLOSING REMARK

About twenty five years ago, Goldblatt stated that the words maximum allowable concentrations have been avoided, because at I.C.I. we hold that no concentration is allowable. Some are worse than others, but all are bad[99]. Later wrote H.E. Ayer: "Undoubtedly any method of monitoring dust could be associated with reduction in dust diseases as long as dust exposures are actually reduced"[100]. Exposure tests, biological monitoring and biological limits are only imperfect but valuable means for controlling chemical hazards. Bad though they are, they are better than nothing.

TABLE 1.
LIMITS IN URINE AND IN BLOOD: CS PROPOSAL 1979

Substance	Indicator[a]	Limits in Urine Adjusted to SG 1.024	Creatinine	Limit in Blood
		μmol/l	μmol/mmol	mol/mol
Aniline	p-Aminophenol	350	25	
	Hemiglobin			0.02
Benzene	Phenol	850	60	
Carbon disulfide	-SH and =CS groups	mmol creatinine/l x log T s > 57.5		
Carbon monoxide	Carboxyhemoglobin			0.05
Cholinesterase inhibitors	Cholinesterase inhibition			0.2
Ethyl benzene	Mandelate	6500	500	
Fluoride	Fluoride	150	10	
Lead	5-Aminolevulinate	150	10	
	Coproporphyrin	0.9	0.06	
Mercury	Mercury	0.5	0.035	
Methyl mercury	Mercury μmol/l			0.25
Nitrobenzene	Hemiglobin			0.02
Pentachlorophenol	Pentachlorophenol	7.5	0.5	
Phenol	Phenol	750	55	
Styrene	Mandelate	2000	150	
Toluene	Hippurate	14000	1000	
Trichloroethylene	Trichloroacetate	600	45	
	Trichloroethanol	1300	100	

[a] Methods of determination standardized[91].

REFERENCES

1. The Use of Biological Specimens for the Assessment of Human Exposure to Environmental Pollutants, A. Berlin et al., Eds. (1977) Martinus Nijhoff, Amsterdam, pp. 1-368.
2. Douglas, C.G. et al. (1912) J. Physiol., 44, 275.
3. Teisinger, J. (1934) Čas. lék. čes., 73, 430-434.
4. Stock, A. (1938) Svensk Kemist, 50, 242-250.
5. Forssman, S. and Ahlmark, A. (1946) Nord. Med., 30, 1033.
6. Timár, M. (1948) Iparegészségügyi Kezlemények, 2, 36.
7. Haeger-Aronsen, B. (1959) Scand. J. Clin. Lab. Invest., 12,

Suppl. 47.

8. Sumerford, W.T. et al. (1953) Arch. Ind. Hyg., 8, 383-398.

9. Yamasaki, E. and Ames, B.N. (1977) Proc. Natl. Acad. Sci., 74, 3555-3559.

10. Elkins, H.B. (1950, 1959) The Chemistry of Industrial Toxicology Wiley, pp. 1-406.

11. Teisinger, J. et al. (1956) Chemické metody k vyšetřování biologického materiálu v průmyslové toxikologii. Státní zdravotnické nakladatelství, Praha, pp. 1-128.

12. Teisinger, J. et al. (1959) Khimicheskie metody issledovania biologicheskikh materialov v promyshlennoy toksikologii. Medgiz, Moscow, pp. 1-187.

13. Gage, J. (1960) Gases, Vapors, Mists and Dusts, In: Toxicology. Mechanisms and Analytical Methods, C.P. Stollmann and A. Steward, Eds., Vol. II, Acad. Press, New York, pp. 17-54.

14. Teisinger, J. (1963) Biologische Expositionsteste in der Gewerbetoxikologie. In: Handbuch der gesamten Arbeitsmedizin. E. Baader, Ed. Bd. IV/2, Urban and Schwarzenberg, Berlin, München, Wien, pp. 312-351.

15. Dutkiewicz, T. et al. (1964) Chemiczne badania materialu biologicznego v toksykologii przemyslowej. Panstw. zaklad wydawnictw lekarskich, Warszawa, pp. 1-248.

16. Gadaskina, I.D. and Filov, V.A. (1971) Prevraschenia i opredelenie promyshlennych organicheskikh yadov v organizme, Medicina, Leningrad, pp. 1-221.

17. Linch, A.L. (1974) Biological Monitoring for Industrial Chemical Control. CRC Press, Cleveland, pp. 1-188.

18. Gadaskina, I.D. et al. (1975) Opredelenie promyshlennykh neorganicheskikh yadov v organizme, Medicina, Leningrad, pp. 1-286.

19. Henschler, D. (1976) Analysen in biologischen Material. Analytische Methoden zur Prüfung gesundheitsschädlicher Arbeitstoffe, Bd. 2. Verlag Chemie, Weinheim.

20. Piotrowski, J. (1977) Exposure Tests for Organic Compounds in Industrial Toxicology. US Department of Health, Education and Welfare, Cincinnatti, pp. 1-138.

21. Teisinger, J. et al. (1980) Exposiční testy v průmyslové toxikologii. Avicenum, Praha, pp. 1-368.

22. Elkins, H.B. (1954) Arch. Ind. Hyg. Occup. Med., 9, 212-222.

23. Stockinger, H.W. (1955) Publ. Health Rep., 70, 1-11.

24. Vigliani, E. (1959) Med. Lavoro, 50, 323-327.

25. Gerarde, H.W. (1960) Fed. Proc., 19, 22-25.

26. Bardoděj, Z. (1970) Čs. Hyg., 15, 292-300.

27. Piotrowski, J. (1970) Expozitsionnye testy i sistema predelnodopustimykh koncentraciy v vozdushnoi srede promyshlennykh predpriatiy toxicheskikh veshtshestv. In: Principy i metody ustanovleniya predelno dopustimykh koncentraciy vrednykh

veshchestv v vozdukhe proizvodstvennykh pomeshcheniy. Medicina, Moscow, pp. 5-16.

28. Bardoděj, Z. (1971) Čs. Hyg., 16, 56-61.
29. Zielhuis, R.L. and Verberk, M.M. (1974) Int. Arch. Arbeitsmed., 32, 167-190.
30. Bardoděj, Z. (1975) J. Hyg. Epid. Microb. Immun.,19, 148-162.
31. Lauwerys, D. (1975) Scand. J. Work, Environ. Health, 1, 139-172.
32. Ikeda, M. (1978) Applicability of Urinanalysis as an Exposure Index in Industrial Medicine. In: Industrial and Environmental Xenobiotics. In Vitro Versus in Vivo Biotransformation and Toxicity. Excerpta Medica, Amsterdam, Oxford, pp. 147-155.
33. Bardoděj, Z. (1963) Čs. Hyg., 8, 157-164.
34. Bardoděj, Z. (1964) Acta Univ. Carol. Med. Suppl., 19, 47-54.
35. Hernberg, S. (personal communication).
36. Guillemin, M.P. et al. (1978) Scand. J. Work, Environ. Health, 4, Suppl., 2, 14-21.
37. Grabecki, J. (personal communication).
38. Bardoděj, Z. and Rothe, R. (1978) Workshop CMEA, Moscow.
39. Knecht, U. and Schiele, R. (1978) Verh. Deutsch. Ges. Arbeitsmed., 19. Jahrestagung, 173-178.
40. Hoschek, R. and Fritz, W. (1973) Taschenbuch für den medizinischen Arbeitsschutz und die werksärztliche Praxis, Enke, Stuttgart, pp. 1-225.
41. Araki, S. (1980) Brit. J. Ind. Med., 37, 50-54.
42. Bardoděj, Z. et al. (1975) Čs. Hyg., 20, 146-149.
43. Methylmercury in fish. Report from an Expert Group. (1971) Nord. Hygienisk Tidsk., Suppl., 4, pp. 1-364.
44. Skare, I. (1972) Analyst, 97, 148-155.
45. Ikeda, M. et al. (1978) Amer. Ind. Hyg. Assoc. J., 39,226-232.
46. Lauwerys, R. et al. (1972) Clin. Chim. Acta, 40, 443-447.
47. Lauwerys, R. et al. (1975) Clin. Chem., 21, 551-557.
48. Hoschek, R. and Schittke, H.J. (1973) Vergleichsbestimmungen für Blei im Blut sowie für Blei und Kadmium im Urin. Bundesanstalt für Arbeitschutz und Unfallforschung, Dortmund, pp. 1-188.
49. Roels, H.E. et al. (1974) Clin. Chem., 20, 753-760.
50. Berlin, A. et al. (1974) Clin. Chem., 20, 749-752.
51. Grandjean, P. (1978) Ind. Arch. Occup. Environ. Health, 42, 69-81.
52. Gylseth, B. et al. (1977) Scand. J. Work Environ. Health, 3, 28-31.
53. Mutti, A. et al. (1979) Ind. Arch. Occup. Environ. Health, 43, 123-133.

54. Tola, S. et al. (1977) Scand. J. Work Environ. Health, 3, 192-202.

55. Hogettweit, A.Ch. (1978) Ann. Occup. Hyg., 21, 113-120.

56. Valentin, H. et al. (1976) Ind. Arch. Occup. Environ. Health, 38, 1-17.

57. Friberg, L. et al. (1971) Cadmium in the Environment, CRC Press, Cleveland, pp. 1-248.

58. Barbořík, M. (1972) Pracov. lék., 24, 249-252.

59. Barbořík, M. (1973) Pracov. lék., 25, 82-86.

60. Barbořík, M. (1972) Pracov. lék., 24, 292-297.

61. Baretta, E.D. et al. (1978) Amer. Ind. Hyg. Assoc. J., 39, 202-209.

62. WHO (1976) Selected Methods of Measuring Air Pollutants, Geneva, pp. 49-65.

63. Droz, P.O. and Fernández, J.G. (1978) Brit. J. Industr. Med., 35, 55-60.

64. Monster, A.C. (1970) Kinetics of Chlorinated Hydrocarbon Solvents. Studies in Volunteers Exposed to Trichloroethylene, 1,1,1-Trichloroethane and Tetrachloroethylene, Thesis, Universiteil van Amsterdam, pp. 1-96.

65. Fernández, J.G. et al. (1977) Brit. J. Ind. Med., 34, 43-55.

66. Kaneko, M. et al. (1975) Ind. Arch. Occup. Environ. Health, 34, 165-172.

67. Müller, G. et al. (1978) Ind. Arch. Occup. Environ. Health, 41, 199-205.

68. Heilstand, R.N. and Todd, A.S. (1972) Amer. Ind. Hyg. Assoc. J., 33, 378-381.

69. Flek, J. and Šedivec, V. (1971) Coll. Czechoslov. Chem. Commun., 36, 3108-3114.

70. Šedivec, V. and Flek, J. (1970) Coll. Czechoslov. Chem. Commun., 35, 3265-3273.

71. Roosmalen, P.B. van and Drummond, I. (1978) Brit. J. Ind. Med., 35, 56-60.

72. Flek, J. and Šedivec, V. (1973) Coll. Czechoslov. Chem. Commun., 38, 1754-1959.

73. Flek, J. and Šedivec, V. (1980) Int. Arch. Occup. Environ. Health, 45, 181-188.

74. Flek, J. and Šedivec, V. (1976) Coll. Czechoslov. Chem. Commun., 41, 732-737.

75. Mráz, M. and Šedivec, V. (1980) Pracov. Lék., 32, 18-23.

76. Gossler, K. et al. (1979) Arbeitsmed. Sozialmed. Präventivmed., 14, 236-240.

77. Sollenberg, J. and Baldenstein, A. (1977) J. Chromat., 132, 469-476.

78. Szadkowski, D. et al. (1980) Int. Arch. Occup. Environ.

Health, 45, 141-152.

79. Šedivec, V. and Flek, J. (1976) Int. Arch. Occup. Environ. Health, 37, 219-232.

80. Šedivec, V. and Flek, J. (1978) Int. Arch. Occup. Environ. Health, 42, 41-49.

81. Bardoděj, Z. (1978) Scand. J. Work Environ. Health, 4, Suppl., 2, 95-103.

82. Härkönen, H. (1978) Scand. J. Work Environ. Health, 4, Suppl., 2, 104-113.

83. Wolff, M.S. et al. (1978) Scand. J. Work Environ. Health, 4, Suppl., 2, 114-118.

84. Ahlborg, U.G. et al. (1974) Arch. Toxicol., 32, 271-278.

85. Roosmalen, P.B. et al. (1980) Arch. Occup. Environ. Health, 45, 57-62.

86. Bardoděj, Z. (1978) Čs. Hyg., 23, 116-119.

87. Shaffik, N.T. and Bradway, D.E. (1976) Residue Rev., 62,59-77.

88. Pilz, W. (1974) Cholinesterases. In: Methods of Enzymatic Analysis, U.H. Bergmayer, Ed., Chemie Weinheim, Academic Press, New York, San Francisco, London, pp. 840-855.

89. Linch, A.L. (1974) Amer. Ind. Hyg. Assoc. J., 35, 426-432.

90. Angerer, J. and Schaller, K.H. (1976) Arbeitsmed. Sozialmed. Präventivmed., 11, 311-312 and 12, 33-35.

91. Bardoděj, Z. (1979) Čs. Hyg., 24, 155-164.

92. Durston, W.E. and Ames, B.N. (1974) Proc. Natl. Acad. Sci., USA, 71, 737-741.

93. Legator, M.S. et al. (1975) Ann. New York Acad. Sci., 269, 16-20.

94. Mc Cann, J. and Ames, B.N. (1975) Ann. New York Acad. Sci., 269, 21-25.

95. Seutter-Berlage, F. et al. (1977) Ind. Arch. Occup. Environ. Health, 39, 45-51.

96. Doorn, R. van et al. (1979) Arch. Occup. Environ. Health, 43, 159-166.

97. Yoshida, S. and Nekamuro, A. (1978) J. Food Hyg. Soc. Jap., 19, 185-189.

98. Šrám, R.J. and Kuleshov, N.P. (1980) Arch. Tox. Suppl., 4, 11-18.

99. Goldblatt, M.W. (1955) Brit. J. Ind. Med., 12, 1-20.

100. Ayer, H.E. (1969) Amer. Ind. Hyg. Assoc. J., 30, 117-125.

Mechanisms of Toxicity and Hazard Evaluation
B. Holmstedt, R. Lauwerys, M. Mercier, M. Roberfroid eds

CYTOGENETIC AND CYTOKINETIC INVESTIGATIONS ON LYMPHOCYTES FROM WORKERS OCCUPATIONALLY EXPOSED TO TETRACHLOROETHYLENE

MASAYUKI IKEDA, AKIO KOIZUMI
Department of Environmental Health, Tohoku University School of Medicine, Sendai 980 (Japan)
TOSHIAKI WATANABE, AKIRA ENDO
Department of Hygiene and Preventive Medicine, Yamagata University School of Medicine, Yamagata 990-23 (Japan)
and KUNIHIKO SATO
Kyoto Industrial Health Association, Kyoto 604 (Japan)

INTRODUCTION

Tetrachloroethylene (perchloroethylene, $CCl_2 = CCl_2$; to be abbreviated as TETRA), the most extensively chlorinated ethylene, has been widely employed in industries as a moderate degreasing agent. In addition, its use in dry-cleaning stations has been increasing. Rather recently, National Cancer Institute in the United States reported that TETRA of technical grade produces hepatocellular carcinoma in mice, but not in rats, when given orally over a long period[1]. This study was initiated to examine whether or not occupational exposure to the vapor of this solvent induces any cytogenetic effect on the peripheral lymphocytes of factory workers. Cytokinetic studies were carried out concurrently.

MATERIALS AND METHODS

Ten factory workers with occupational exposure to TETRA were studied. They were devided into two groups depending on the exposure intensity (details will be given in RESULTS) in relation to their workshops. Group 1 consisted of 5 males and 1 female (aged from 20 to 66) in the degreasing department with intensive exposure to TETRA. Those in the support department, 2 males and 2 females (aged from 17 to 31), formed Group 2. They were exposed to the vapor only indirectly.

TETRA of technical grade was the only solvent used in the workshops, and accordingly, Kitagawa detection tubes[2] were considered appropriate for workroom air analysis. Blood samples were taken from the cubital vein, and lymphocytes were cultured for 72 hours in phytohemagglutinin-M (15 μg/ml) containing RPMI

---

*This work was supported in part by a grant-in aid to one of the authors (A.K.) from the Ministry of Education, Science and Culture of the Government of Japan.

1640 supplemented with 20% fetal calf serum and bromodeoxyuridine (5 μg/ml). Chromosomal preparations were prepared by air-drying, and differential staining by FPG[3]. Other examination items were as listed in Table 1.

TABLE 1

EXAMINATION ITEMS

Items	Notes
Exposure intensity measurement	
Vapor concentration	by Kitagawa detection tubes[2]
Urinary metabolites[a]	total trichloro-compound determination[4]
Physical examination	
Subjective symptoms	scored by the interviewer
Hematology[b]	Hb, Ht, RBC & WBC
Hepatic function[b]	GOT, GPT, LDH, ALP, TTT, & ZTT
Peripheral lymphocyte culture[c]	Chromosome aberration, SCEs, proportion of metaphases, mitotic index

[a] Urine samples were collected at 14:00-15:00 on Thursday.
[b] By conventional methods. [c] For details, see text.

RESULTS

Exposure intensity assessments

The people in Group 1 were employed for 10 to 18 years and TETRA concentrations in their workshops ranged from 30 to 220 ppms (25 determinations) with a geometric mean (GM) of 92 ppm. Those in Group 2 had employment records of one quarter to 3 years, and TETRA in workroom air was 10 to 40 ppm with peak exposures up to 80 ppm on rare occasions. In accordance with the vapor concentrations[5], urinary total trichloro-compound level was higher in Group 1 with a GM of 50.7 mg/L (SD range; 41.1-62.6 mg/L), while the GM in Group 2 was 19.0 mg/L with a SD range of 14.8-24.4 mg/L.

Physical examinations

Results from physical examinations well agreed with those from exposure measurements. All workers in Group 1 had one or more subjective symptoms such as dizziness, sore throat, shoulder stiffness or chilly sensation in extremities, while one subject in Group 2 complained such. There was none among the controls. Hepatic function tests were essentially negative and no abnormality was found in hematology.

Cytogenetics and cytokinetics

Despite of the findings in exposure measurements and physical examinations, no dose-related abnormalities were observed in the frequency of chromosome aberrations or SCEs (Table 2). Both the frequencies ($p > 0.05$ by X^2-test) and the percentages ($p > 0.05$ by the Monte Carlo Method[6]) of numerical or structural chromosome aberrations among the exposed workers did not differ significantly from the corresponding values in the controls, except for one case (marked with an asterisk in Table 2) in which the increase in the percentage was barely significant ($p = 0.036$). Structural aberrations observed were mostly gaps and/or breaks, and no more severe anomalies were observed. SCEs were also essentially constant among the groups. As the majority in the exposed group was male, the results from male workers were selected for the comparison with male control results (the bottom two lines in Table 2). No significant difference ($p > 0.05$) was observed in chromosome aberrations or SCEs.

TABLE 2

CHROMOSOME ABERRATIONS, SCEs, AND CELL CYCLE KINETICS

Groups	n[a]	Chromosome aberrations		SCEs	metaphase proportion[a]	Mitotic index[b]
		Numerical	Structural			
Workers	511/10	13(2.5%*)	10(2.0%)	8.6±0.9	77± 7	15±6
Group 1	302/6	6(2.0%)	4(1.3%)	8.9±1.0	78± 4	14±6
Group 2	209/4	7(3.4%)	6(2.9%)	8.2±0.7	77±12	17±5
Controls	550/11	9(1.6%)	11(2.0%)	8.2±1.1	78± 7	19±8
Male workers	359/7	9(2.5%)	9(2.5%)	8.7±1.0	79± 6	16±6
Male controls	300/6	5(1.7%)	5(1.7%)	8.0±1.1	78± 7	16±7

[a] M_2 metaphases analyzed / subjects examined [b] M_2+M_3, x 100 [c] x 1,000

Cell cycle kinetics study (Table 2) also could not detect any dose-related difference among the groups. Both the metaphase proportion and the mitotic index were uniform independent of exposure. Differences between male workers and male controls were insignificant ($p > 0.05$).

The possible difference in susceptibility to mitomycin C was examined at the concentration of 10^{-8} M (Table 3). Lymphocytes from the workers did not show any elevated frequency in chromosome aberrations, while those from the controls revealed some increase in structural anomalies. SCEs increase due to mitomycin C was essentially uniform among the groups.

TABLE 3

EFFECTS OF MITOMYCIN C[a]

Groups	n[b]	Chromosome aberrations		SCEs
		Numerical	Structural	increase
Workers	442/10	7(1.6%)	10(2.3%)	8.8±1.2
Group 1	244/6	3(1.2%)	6(2.5%)	9.2±1.1
Group 2	198/4	4(2.0%)	4(2.0%)	8.3±1.1
Controls	543/11	9(1.7%)	25(4.6%)	9.0±1.5
Male workers	294/7	3(1.0%)	6(2.0%)	9.2±1.0
Male controls	293/6	5(1.7%)	15(5.1%)	9.3±1.5

[a] Mitomycin C at 10^{-8} M
[b] M_2 metaphases analyzed / subjects examined

COMMENTS

Cytogenetics and cytokinetics of peripheral lymphocytes from two exposed groups (one at around 100 ppm of TETRA and another at less than 50 ppm) did not show significant dose-related difference from what was observed in non-exposed controls, while the observation in physical examinations and biological monitoring well corresponded to the results from workroom air analyses. It was discussed[7] that the carcinogenic capacity of industrial trichloroethylene might be attributable to inhibitors rather than trichloroethylene itself. Although this may also be the case of TETRA, no information was available of the formulation of technical grade TETRA under the study.

REFERENCES

1 National Cancer Institute (1977) Bioassay of Tetrachloroethylene for Possible Carcinogenicity, Carcinogenesis Technical Report Series No. 13.

2 Kitagawa, T. (1960) Proc. 13th Int. Congr. Occup. Health, New York, pp. 566-572.

3 Watanabe, T., Endo, A., Kato, Y., Shima, S., Watanabe, T., and Ikeda, M. (1980) Int. Arch. Occup. Environ. Health, 46, 31-41.

4 Tanaka, S. and Ikeda, M. (1968) Br. J. Ind. Med., 25, 214-219.

5 Ikeda, M., Ohtsuji, H., Imamura, T. and Komoike, Y. (1972) Br. J. Ind. Med., 29, 328-333.

6 Tsuda, T. (1977) Monte Carlo Method and Computer Simulation (in Japanese), Baifu Kan, Tokyo.

7 Henschler, D., Eder, E., Neudecker, T. and Metzler, M. (1977) Arch. Toxicol. 37, 233-236.

© 1980 Elsevier/North-Holland Biomedical Press
Mechanisms of Toxicity and Hazard Evaluation
B. Holmstedt, R. Lauwerys, M. Mercier, M. Roberfroid eds

HEALTH EFFECTS OF LONG-TERM OCCUPATIONAL EXPOSURE TO POLYCHLORINATED BIPHENYLS

MARCO MARONI, ANTONIO COLOMBI, CARLA ANTONINI and VITO FOA'
Clinica del Lavoro "L. Devoto", University of Milan, via San Barnaba 8,
20I22 Milan (Italy)

INTRODUCTION

The toxicity of polychlorinated biphenyls (PCBs) has been investigated in several animal species and acute toxic damage in humans was reported after an outbreak of oral poisoning in Japan (Yusho disease)[1]. Few data are available on chronic low-dose effects in humans, such as might occur in occupational and environmental exposure.

In this investigation two groups of workers in the electrical industry were studied in order to evaluate PCB exposure and ascertain health effects.

MATERIALS AND METHODS

Subjects and plants

Eighty workers (40 females and 40 males) were studied, of whom 67 were exposed to Pyralene 3010 (a PCB mixture with a 42% chlorine content) in a plant manufacturing electric capacitors (plant A) and 13 exposed to Apirolio (a PCB mixture containing 42% chlorine) in a plant testing electric capacitors (plant B).

In plant A exposure to PCBs occurs in three departments where respectively high-power, low-power and small capacitors (so called "filters") are manufactured. The most important process is the filling of the capacitors with PCBs which is done in autoclaves.

Plant B is an experimental center, where high-power capacitors are short-circuit tested. PCB exposure occurs during handling of the capacitors contaminated with Apirolio dispersed from explosions sometimes caused by stress in testing. The subjects under study were all employed on capacitor testing.

The mean age (± SD) and length of employment of the 80 workers under study was respectively 37 ± 8 and 12 ± 6 years.

Evaluation of PCB exposure and internal load in workers

PCB exposure was evaluated by means of LGC determination of PCBs on samples collected from the air of the working environment, from workroom surfaces and from the palms of the hands of the workers. The internal load was assessed by determining PCBs in whole blood.

The results were expressed as trichlorobiphenyl (TRI-CB) and pentachlorobiphenyl (PENTA-CB) concentration according to whether the LGC pattern of measured PCB was characteristic respectively of a mixture with 42% or 54% chlorine. Details of the analytical methods have been reported elsewhere[2].

Clinical Methods. The workers underwent routine medical examination and a detailed clinical history was obtained; subjects with suspected skin complaints were also examined by a dermatologist. The following laboratory tests were performed on blood and serum samples from the cubital vein of fasting subjects: red cell and leukocyte count; determination of hemoglobin and volume of packed red blood cells; serum bilirubin (total and indirect); serum protein electrophoretic fractions; serum alkaline phosphatase, serum pseudocholinesterase, serum glutamic-oxalacetic transaminase (SGOT), serum glutamic-piruvic transaminase (SGPT), serum γ - glutamil transpeptidase (γGT) and serum ornithincarbamyl transferase (SOCT) activities.

Complete routine analysis was performed on morning urine samples.

RESULTS

The environmental exposure measurements gave PCB air concentrations of 48-275 $\mu g/m^3$, while considerable amounts of PCBs (0,2-159 $\mu g/cm^2$) were detected on all tested surfaces of the workrooms, thus indicating that this source of exposure should be the most serious due to PCB absorption through the skin. The existence of a percutaneous absorption risk was also confirmed by the determinations performed on the palms of the hands of the workers, where 2 to 27 μg of PCBs per cm^2 of skin were detected.

As regards the body load in the workers, blood PCB concentrations of 41-1319 ppb were measured, and the mean ($\pm$ SD) for current and past exposed workers in plant A was respectively 337 $\pm$ 258 and 292 $\pm$ 161 ppb of total PCBs. Considering TRI-CB and PENTA-CB blood concentrations separately in plant A workers, a significant difference between current and past exposed workers could be seen for TRI-CB values (current 128 $\pm$ 85 ppb versus past 86 $\pm$ 50 ppb), whereas no significant difference was observed for PENTA-CB blood values (240 $\pm$ 190 ppb versus 206 $\pm$ 123).

By dividing plant A workers according to department and job and considering the relationship between duration of exposure and blood PCB concentration, rather good correlations were in general obtained. As an example figure 1 shows such a relationship for filter department workers.

The health survey revealed several abnormal findings involving mainly the skin and liver. In the 80 workers studied, 4 cases of chloracne, 6 cases of folliculitis and 5 cases of irritative or allergic dermatitis were found. Three cases of chloracne showed the simultaneous presence of active skin lesions (comedones, suppurative folliculitis and superficial cysts) and repair processes (vermicular scars) involving face, neck, abdomen, thighs or arms, while there were no active lesions in the other case. Two cases of folliculitis were not diagnosed with certainty, because of the concomitant presence of typical and atypical diagnostic features of chloracne.

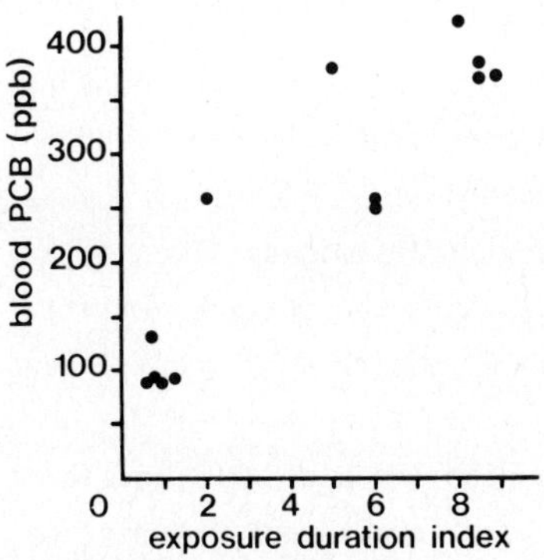

Fig. 1. Blood PCB levels in filter department workers in relation to exposure duration indices. See footnote in Table 1.

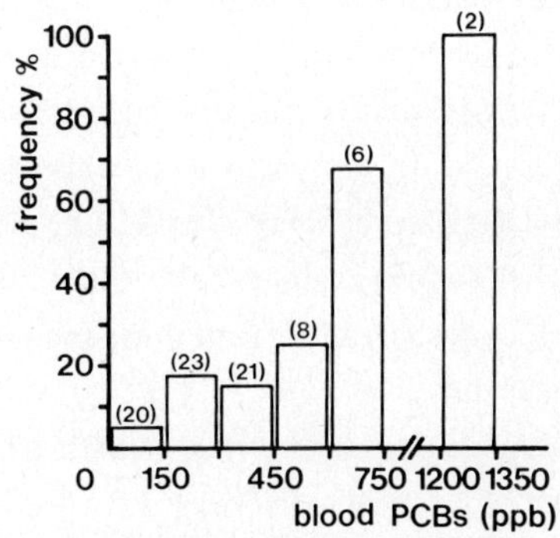

Fig. 2. Frequency of workers with abnormal liver findings for increasing levels of blood PCB concentrations. Number of workers in brackets. χ^2 trend = P< 0.001.

TABLE 1

BLOOD PCB LEVELS IN WORKERS WITH AND WITHOUT ABNORMAL LIVER FINDINGS

Workers	Age (yrs) mean ± SD	Exposure duration index[a] mean ± SD	Blood PCB (ppb) mean ± SD
Hepatic (no. 16)	38 ± 11	4.4 ± 4.0	524 ± 349
Non-hepatic (no. 64)	37 ± 8	3.2 ± 3.0	296 ± 160
Significance	n.s.	n.s.	< 0.001

[a] The exposure duration index was calculated as follows: E.D.I. = YE x 100 x hrs PCB/hrs tot, where YE is the length of employment in years, and hrs PCB and hrs tot are respectively the annual working hours with exposure to PCBs and the total annual working hours.

The workers with chloracne were all males, who had been working for many years on capacitor impregnation with PCBs and had developed chloracne 3 to 27 years ago. None of them had any liver complaints. At the time of the study their blood PCB levels were rather high (mean 450 ppb, range 310-574 ppb).

As deduced from symptoms, clinical examination of the liver, and laboratory tests, sixteen male workers (9 in plant A and 7 in plant B) were observed with more or less marked hepatic involvement. Eight workers complained of symptoms related to digestive difficulties such as post-prandial epigastric distress, epigastric pain with or without burning, post-prandial headache, intolerance to fatty foods, and bad taste in the mouth first thing in the morning. At physical examination, all but two asymptomatic workers showed various degrees of hepatomegalia, in several cases with increased consistency of the liver on palpation and in one case also with facial spider angiomas. The most frequently altered tests were serum gammaGT activity (8 cases), transaminase (7 cases) and OCT (6 cases). Blood cell count, bilirubin, alkaline phosphatase activity, serum electrophoretic fractions and urine analysis were within the normal range in all workers.

In Table 1 the mean age, lenght of exposure to PCBs and blood PCB levels are reported for the workers with and without hepatic involvement. Statistical analysis indicated a significant difference for blood PCB levels, but no significant difference was found for age and length of exposure. Figure 2 reports the frequencies of workers with liver involvement for increasing blood PCB levels: a significant positive association between prevalence of liver disorders and blood PCB levels was found.

Besides dermatological and hepatic abnormalities, two cases of bleeding hemangioma and one case of leukaemia were observed. The first case of hemangioma was in a 29 years old worker who also had hepatomegalia but not chloracne, and had a blood PCB concentration of 1259 ppb. The second case of hemangioma was in a 47 years old worker who also had leukaemia but no skin complaint. This man had been employed on high-power capacitor manufacture in plant A since the age of 30 and for 16 years after had always been well. Shortly before this study, he complained of bleeding from the tongue and was admitted to hospital, where a cavernous hemangioma of the tongue was found and surgically treated. Laboratory tests made during hospitalisation revealed a chronic myelocytic leukaemia and since then the patient has been undergoing antiblastic therapy. After six months, our examination revealed no hepatomegalia but marked alterations of serum enzymes and hematuria; the blood PCB level was 396 ppb.

DISCUSSION AND CONCLUSIONS

In the plants under study, absorption of PCBs occurred mainly through the skin, so the commonly used method to asses industrial exposure by determination of PCB concentration in work place air alone is not sufficient to give exhaustive information on the exposure level of the workers. Furthermore, guidelines for prevention in industry should also consider the protection of the workers against skin absorption of these compounds.

The determination of PCBs in whole blood has been shown to be a useful test to evaluate the internal load in monitoring workers. The blood PCB concentration measured with reference to the length of exposure can be utilized to compare different levels of occupational and environmental exposure.

All the four cases of chloracne observed arose several years ago in workers with long service and in three cases, despite the decrease in intensity of exposure achieved after the onset of chloracne, skin lesions were found that were still active, thus indicating the slowly developing nature of this disease.

As regards the liver, the majority of the workers showed hepatomegalia and moderate increase in serum gammaGT activity. These findings, which are similar to those observed in animals given PCBs experimentally, should probably be interpreted as clinical appearance of microsomal enzymatic activity induction as is also suggested by the results of urinary porphyrin excretion, which will be reported elsewhere. The data reported in Table 1 and Figure 2, coupled to the absence of a history of excessive consumption of alcohol or drugs in the patients, suggest that the liver involvement can probably be connected with PCB exposure.

The carcinogenicity of PCBs has been proved in several animal species and in the opinion of the I.A.R.C., PCBs have to be considered, for practical purposes, as carcinogenic for humans[3]. The discovery of two fast developing cavernous hemangiomas and one chronic myelocytic leukaemia stresses the need for extensive epidemiological studies on cancer incidence among PCB workers.

REFERENCES

1. World Health Organization (1976) Polychlorinated Biphenyls and Terphenyls, Environmental Health Criteria 2, W.H.O., Geneva.
2. Maroni, M. et al. (1980) Occupational Exposure to Polychlorinated Biphenyls in Electrical Workers. I. Environmental and Blood PCB Levels, Brit. J. industr. Med., in press.
3. International Agency for Research on Cancer (1978) Polychlorinated biphenyls and polybrominated biphenyls, I.A.R.C. Monographs on the evaluation of the carcinogenic risk of chemicals to humans, vol. 18, Lyon.

Mechanisms of Toxicity and Hazard Evaluation
B. Holmstedt, R. Lauwerys, M. Mercier, M. Roberfroid eds

BEHAVIOUR OF INDICATORS OF DOSE AND EFFECT AFTER CESSATION OF OCCUPATIONAL EXPOSURE TO LEAD

LORENZO ALESSIO, MARIA ROSA CASTOLDI, PIETRO ODONE, I. FRANCHINI
Clinica del Lavoro, University of Milan. Via S.Barnaba 8 -20122 Milano Italy

INTRODUCTION

Over the years, in working environments where inorganic lead is used, measures have usually been taken to reduce the atmospheric concentrations of the metal. As a result of this, many workers who were exposed to high lead concentrations in the past, are presently exposed to concentrations below the TLV.

Moreover, in working environments where hygienic conditions are not satisfactory, it is common pratice to remove, for varying periods of time, those subjects with biological indicators exceeding the "permissible" values. In spite of interruption of exposure, it is likely that high deposits of lead remain in the organism of such workers and it should be necessary to determine the amount of such deposits accurately before deciding whether they may resume a lead-exposing job.

In consideration of the above, it appeared important to assess whether subjects who in the past had an "abnormal" exposure to lead may show alterations due to the presence of tissue deposits of lead. At the present time the only means which enables evaluation of active deposits of lead is the determination of chelatable lead [1,2]; this test is indicative even when some time has elapsed between termination of exposure and the investigation.

In male subjects who had ceased lead-exposing work for a least one year, we studied the relationships exsisting between chelatable lead and blood lead, between chelatable lead and indicators of effect and, moreover, for comparison, the relationships between blood lead and indicators of effect. The data thus obtained were compared with those relative to subjects currently occupationally exposed to lead.

The criteria followed in selecting subjects and the methods used for the determination of biological tests are indicated in previous papers [3,4].

RESULTS AND DISCUSSION

Blood lead (PbB). In 48 subjects with current lead exposure, the chelatable lead (PbU-EDTA) levels were closely correlated with the PbB levels (r= 0.85;

p < 0.001); in 45 subjects with past exposure, however, the correlation between the two tests was lower (r= 0.54), even though statistically significant (p<0.001). From fig.1 it can be seen that, for an identical variation in PbU-EDTA, the variations in PbB are higher in currently exposed subjects.

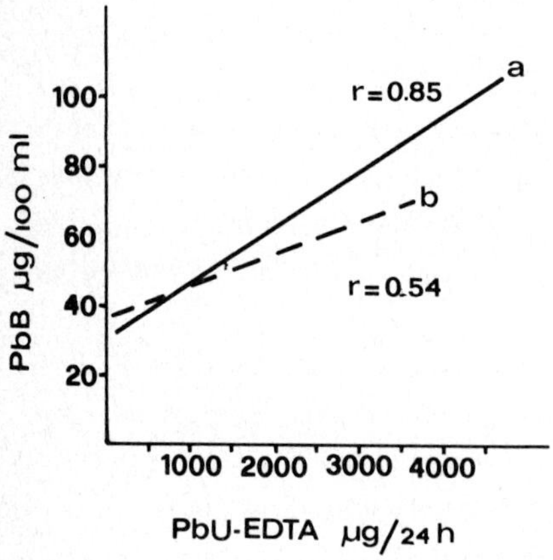

Fig. 1 . Relationships between PbU-EDTA and PbB in currently (a) and past (b) exposed workers. Linear type regression functions.

Statistical analysis showed that the trend of the two lines was significantly different (t= 3.63; p < 0.001).

These data indicate that PbB in subjects who have ceased working with lead cannot be reliably used to indirectly evaluate the active deposit of lead.

Erythrocyte protoporphyrin (EP). In 64 subjects who had ceased work a year before, the correlation coefficient between PbB and EP was decidedly lower (r= 0.45) even still statistically significant (p < 0.001), compared to the findings in 108 currently exposed subjects (r= 0.85; p < 0.001). The comparison made to test any difference in trend of the regression lines between PbB and EP (fig. 2) showed that the slope of the two lines is statistically different (t= 2.28; 0.02 < p < 0.05).

On the contrary a study of the relationship between EP and chelatable lead showed that the two variables were well correlated both in 48 subjects still at work (r= 0.88; p < 0.001) and in 56 subjects no longer exposed (r= 0.72; p < 0.001). The slopes of the regression lines between PbU-EDTA and EP (fig. 3) do not differ (t= 0.93; p n.s.); the latter two lines are also coincident (t= 0.56; p n.s.).

These data confirm that both chelatable lead and EP remain high for a long time after cessation of exposure and suggest that EP stays at high levels possibly due to a direct inhibition of heme synthesis by the lead which is released from the deposits [4].

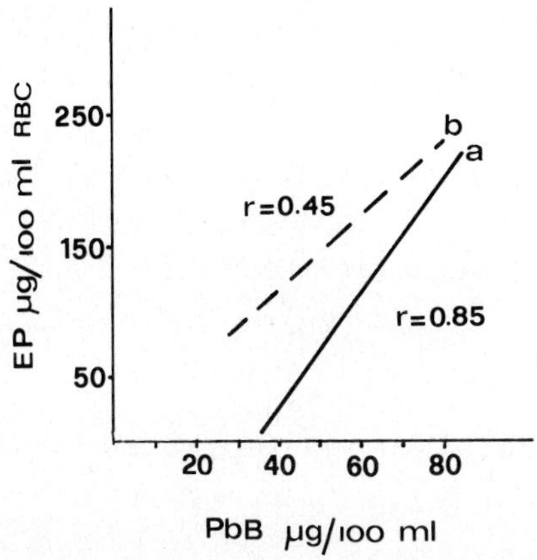

Fig. 2. Relationships between PbB and EP in currently (a) and past (b) exposed workers.
Linear type regression functions.

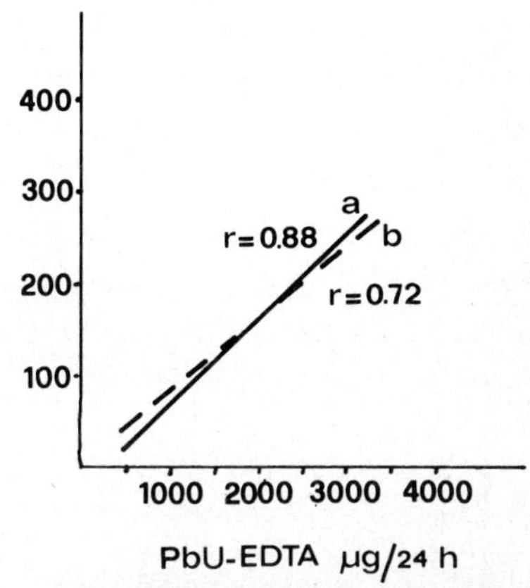

Fig. 3. Relationship between PbU-EDTA and EP in currently (a) and past (b) exposed workers.
Linear type regression functions.

δ-amino-laevulinic acid dehydratase activity of erythrocytes (ALAD)
In 32 currently exposed subjects we found that ALAD was closely correlated with PbB ($r= 0.76$; $p<0.001$); while in 23 subjects who had ceased work with lead, ALAD and PbB were not significantly correlated ($r= 0.22$).

In both groups ALAD was closely correlated with chelatable lead ($r= 0.70$; $p<0.001$ and $r= 0.46$; $p<0.05$ respectively). Comparison of the two lines showed that the functional relationships between PbU-EDTA and ALAD in the currently exposed subjects do not differ; the slope of the curves was the same ($t= 0.77$; p n.s.) and from a statistical point of view the curves themselves were coincidental ($t= 1.89$; p n.s.).

The results obtained should be interpreted with considerable caution in view of the fact that the groups of subjects under study were not large in number. However these data appear to indicate that measurement of ALAD may be used to reveal a severe past exposure to lead when it is necessary, for example, to establish whether a chronic symptomatology is due to past exposure.

Urinary δ-amino laevulinic acid (ALAU). In 48 subjects currently exposed and in 42 past exposed we found a good correlation between PbB and ALAU ($r= 0.68$; $p<0.001$ and $r= 0.61$; $p<0.001$ respectively).
Comparison of the regression curves showed that variations in ALAU with respect to PbB do not differ in the two groups (Fig.4); the slope was the same ($t= 0.48$

p n.s.) and the curves were coincidental (t= 1.40; p n.s.).

The correlation between PbU-EDTA and ALAU was significant in the two groups, even though it was less close in those exposed in the past ($r= 0.84$; $p<0.001$ and $r= 0.48$; $p<0.001$ respectively). Comparison between the lines showed that, in the past exposed subjects the ALAU values were decidedly lower than those found in the currently exposed subjects (fig. 5). Statistical analysis confirmed that the slopes of the two curves were different ($t= 3.2$; $p<0.01$).

These results confirm that ALAU cannot be used after cessation of exposure to establish the amount of active deposit in the organism [5].

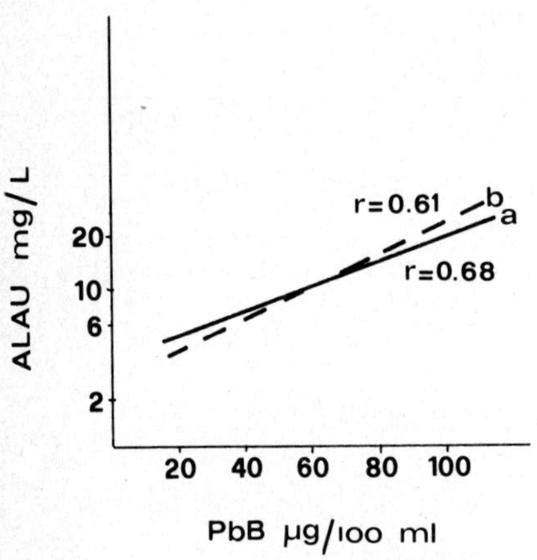

Fig. 4. Relationships between PbB and ALAU in currently (a) and past (b) exposed workers. Exponential type regression functions. Logarithmic scale on ordinate.

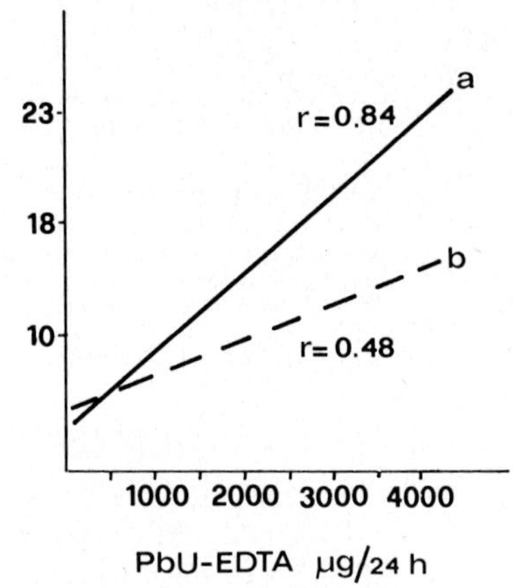

Fig. 5. Relationship between PbU-EDTA and ALAU in currently (a) and past (b) exposed workers. Linear type regression functions.

From the above it is clear that not all the tests that are commonly used for biological monitoring of subjects currently exposed to lead can also be used for the surveillance of subjects who have ceased lead-exposing work. Particularly, PbB is of very limited value in establishing the persistence and degree of an active lead deposit. As far as the indicators of effect are concerned, determination of EP and ALAD permits detection of alterations in heme synthesis, caused probably by the lead that is released from deposit organs even many years after cessation of work. ALAU, however, is of no use for this purpose.

The confirmation that subjects who have stopped working with lead can have high metabolically active deposits of lead, leads us to believe that the problem raised in introduction may be real: that is, subjects working at present exposed to "low" lead concentrations but who have been exposed to higher concentrations in the past could have active deposits of the metal so as to cause more marked effects than would be expected on the basis of an evaluation of the subsequent exposure.

REFERENCES

1. Teisinger, J., Prerovska, I., Sedicev, V., Flek, J., Roth, Z., (1969) Int. Arch. Gewerpath. Gewerhyg., 25, 240-255.
2. Nordberg, G.F., (1976) Effects and dose-response relationship of toxic metals. 7-96 Elsevier Scientific Publishing Company, Amsterdam.
3. Alessio, L., Bertazzi, P.A., Monelli, O., FOA', V. (1976) Int. Arch. Occup. Environ. Hlth. 37, 89-105.
4. Alessio, L., Bertazzi, P.A., Monelli, O., Toffoletto, F. (1976). Int. Arch. Occup. Environ. Hlth 38, 77-86.
5. Prerovska, I., Teisinger, J. (1970). Brit. J. of Ind. Med., 27, 352-355.

© 1980 Elsevier/North-Holland Biomedical Press
Mechanisms of Toxicity and Hazard Evaluation
B. Holmstedt, R. Lauwerys, M. Mercier, M. Roberfroid eds

RENAL FUNCTION IMPAIRMENT IN LEAD-EXPOSED WORKERS: CORRELATIONS WITH ZINC PROTOPORPHYRIN AND BLOOD LEAD LEVELS

RUTH LILIS, ALF FISCHBEIN, JOSE VALCIUKAS, WILLIAM E. BLUMBERG* AND IRVING J. SELIKOFF

Environmental Sciences Laboratory, Mount Sinai School of Medicine, 1 Gustave Levy Place, New York, N.Y., 10029 and *Bell Laboratories, Murray Hill, N.J.

INTRODUCTION

Chronic lead nephropathy associated with severe occupational lead poisoning has been often reported in the past, when lead exposure was considerably higher, and has been documented in experimental models, establishing the transition from acute tubular histological changes to diffuse interstitial fibrosis and renal failure[1]. Exposure to lesser but still significant concentrations of lead has continued and chronic lead nephropathy from occupational exposure in the recent past has been a subject of controversy. Cramer[2] and Wedeen[3] have documented renal function impairment in lead exposed workers, and ultrastructural changes--interstitial fibrosis, glomerular sclerosis and arteriolar damage--underlying the reduction in glomerular filtration rate. An excess mortality from chronic renal disease was found in lead exposed smelter workers and lead battery plant employees.[4]

The investigation of renal function in lead-exposed occupational groups working under conditions currently prevailing in industry was the purpose of this study. It was thought that comparison between occupational groups with different levels of lead exposure and lead absorption would be useful in defining levels at which permanent renal function impairment could result if exposure continues for long periods of time.

POPULATIONS AND METHODS

Two clinical field surveys of <u>secondary lead smelter workers</u> were conducted in two different locations: Group I consisted of 158 males, Group II of 111 males[5,6]. Blood lead (PbB) determination by atomic absorption spectrophotometry (Perkin-Elmer Model 303 combined with a Varian-Techtron carbon rod atomizer, Model 63), serum creatinine and blood urea nitrogen (BUN), as part of SMA-12, urinalysis, and zinc protoporphyrin (ZPP) in blood, determined with a hematofluorometer[7,8] as previously described were part of the study protocol.

Three occupational groups with lower lead exposure were also examined: these consisted of 45 cable manufacturers, 90 cable splicers, and 45 firearm instructors. Lead exposure in splicing telephone cables results from the installation and maintenance of lead sleeves over cable joints, by using a lead containing solder. This type of lead exposure has not generated clinically overt lead poisoning. The lead exposure of cable manufacturers results from handling of lead containing stabilizers added to the polyvinyl chloride coating of electrical wires. The potential hazard of occupational lead exposure in indoor firing ranges has only recently been recognized[9]; mildly symptomatic cases of lead poisoning have been reported, and hazardous levels of airborne lead documented.

Pearson's correlation coefficients were computed between BUN and creatinine levels, as indicators of renal function, and the following characteristics of the lead exposed groups: age, duration of lead exposure, PbB and ZPP levels. Since glomerular filtration rate (GFR) decreases with age, the age dependency of BUN and creatinine were ascertained in two non-lead exposed reference populations. The correlations between age and duration of lead exposure and indicators of renal function were then computed in the lead-exposed groups after controlling for the age-dependent effect by the method of partial correlations.

RESULTS

The distribution by age and duration of lead exposure of the various groups is presented in Tables 1 and 2. Distributions of PbB and ZPP levels are presented in Figure 1. Other important characteristics of secondary smelter workers--Group I were the frequent (59%) occurrence of elevated PbB ($> 80\ \mu g/100ml$) in the past, a history of lead colic (25%), and the frequency (45%) with which chelation therapy had been used. The main distinctive feature of Group II was long duration of exposure, in 38% exceeding 10 years (Table 2). High PbB had been detected in the past in 56% of cases, but such notification had been used for lower PbB levels in recent years. Chelation therapy in this group had been used in only 19% of cases.

In Group I elevated BUN levels (> 21 mg/100ml) were found in 29 of those examined (18%): the prevalence was higher with longer duration of exposure, 13% in those with less than 10 years exposure versus 55% of those exposed for more than 10 years. The correlation between BUN and duration of lead exposure was found to be highly significant ($r = 0.370$, $p < 0.001$). BUN levels were also significantly correlated with age ($r = 0.350$, $p < 0.001$). This was not unexpected, since duration of lead exposure is closely related to age.

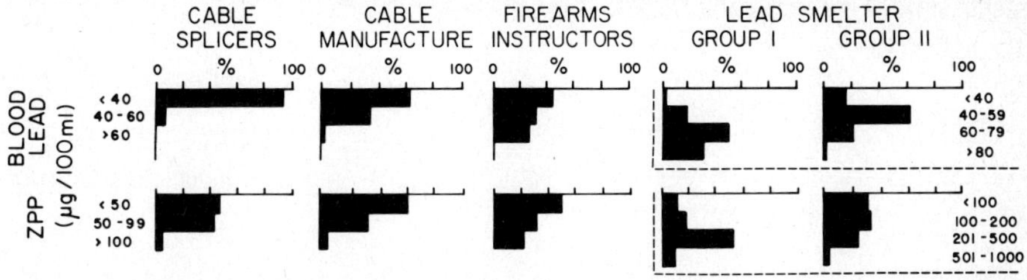

Fig. 1 Frequency distribution of blood lead and zinc protoporphyrin in lead exposed occupational groups.

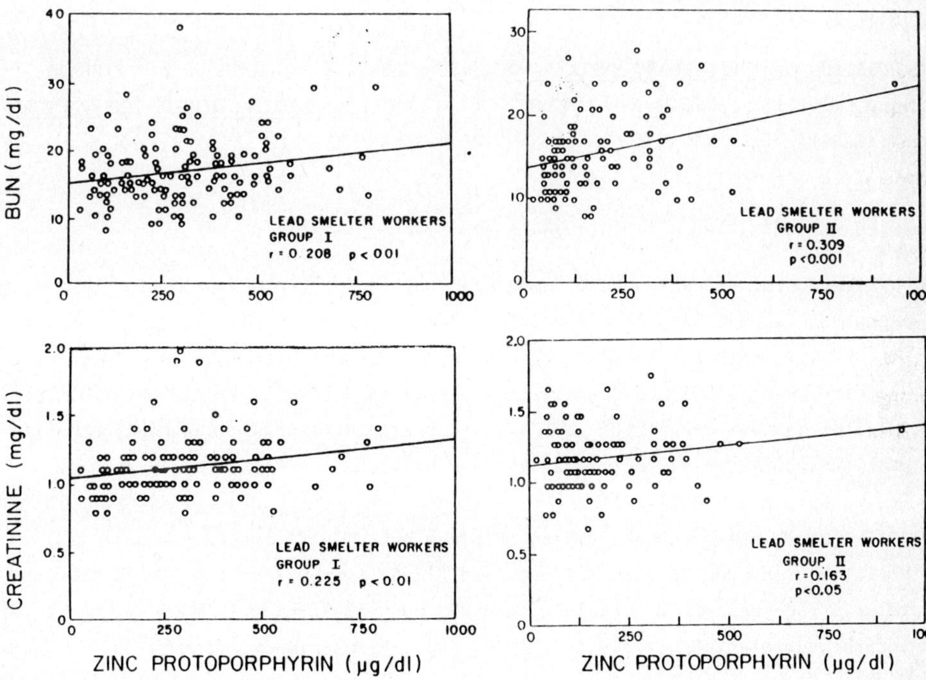

Fig. 2 BUN and creatinine plotted against zinc protoporphyrin and fitted with the least square regression lines.

TABLE 1
AGE DISTRIBUTION

AGE (YEARS)	SECONDARY SMELTER WORKERS				CABLE SPLICERS		CABLE MANUFACTURERS		FIREARM INSTRUCTORS	
	GROUP I		GROUP II							
	N	%	N	%	N	%	N	%	N	%
< 30	70	44	26	24	47	52	10	22	6	13
31 - 50	63	40	52	48	42	47	23	51	34	76
> 50	25	16	31	28	1	1	12	27	5	11

TABLE 2
DURATION OF LEAD EXPOSURE

DURATION OF LEAD EXPOSURE (YEARS)	SECONDARY SMELTER WORKERS				CABLE SPLICERS		CABLE MANUFACTURERS		FIREARM INSTRUCTORS	
	GROUP I		GROUP II							
	N	%	N	%	N	%	N	%	N	%
< 10	138	87	68	62	71	79	33	73	36	80
> 10	20	13	42	38	19	21	12	27	8	18

Similar relationships were found with regard to serum creatinine. Levels in excess of 1.2 mg/100ml were found in 18% and a more marked elevation of creatinine (> 1.4 mg/100ml) in 8% of cases. Of 20 workers with more than 10 years of exposure, nine (45%) had creatinine levels higher than 1.4 mg/100ml. The correlation between creatinine levels and duration of exposure was higly significant ($r = 0.341$, $p < 0.001$), as was that between creatinine levels and age ($r = 0.363$, $p < 0.001$).

The correlation between BUN and PbB was not significant ($r = 0.05$, n.s.) while that between BUN and ZPP was significant ($r = 0.208$, $p < 0.01$). The correlation between serum creatinine and PbB was significant ($r = 0.184$, $p < 0.05$), but the correlation between creatinine and ZPP was higher, ($r = 0.225$, $p < 0.01$) (Figure 2).

For <u>Group II</u>, definitely elevated BUN values (> 25 mg/100ml) were found in 3% of cases, and in 8% the BUN levels were in the range of 22-25 mg/100ml. Correlations between BUN and duration of lead exposure and between BUN and age were found to be high, $r = 0.393$, $p < 0.001$ and $r = 0.428$, $p < 0.001$. Serum creatinine levels were higher than 1.4 mg/100ml in 14 (13%) of cases, while in 30 subjects (28%) they were in the 1.3-1.4 mg/100ml range. Serum creatinine was significantly correlated with duration of lead exposure ($r = 0.335$, $p < 0.001$) and with age ($r = 0.19$, $p < 0.05$). The correlation between BUN and PbB was non-significant ($r = 0.043$, n.s.), but a significant correlation was found between BUN and ZPP levels ($r = 0.309$, $p < 0.001$). There was no correlation between serum creatinine and PbB ($r = 0.029$, n.s.); the correlation with ZPP was again significant ($r = 0.163$, $p < 0.05$).

It was considered that the investigation of age dependency of BUN and creatinine in control, non-lead-exposed populations was necessary in order to establish with a high degree of certainty the lead induced effect. In two reference groups (without lead exposure), 160 male industrial employees and 167 male residents of Michigan state, the correlations of BUN with age were $r = 0.166$, $p < 0.02$ and $r = 0.20$, $p < 0.02$, considerably lower than in the secondary lead smelter workers. Serum creatinine levels showed no significant correlation with age in the two reference populations ($r = 0.062$ n.s. and $r = 0.155$, $p > 0.05$).

Correlations of age and duration of lead exposure with BUN and creatinine for Group I and Group II secondary lead smelter workers were then established, after controlling for the age-related effect found in the non-lead exposed reference population by the method of partial correlations. The results of this analysis are presented in Figure 3 and 4. Thus, significant correlations between duration of lead exposure, characteristic for these two secondary lead smelters and renal function as reflected in BUN and serum creatinine levels, were documented, after appropriate correction for an age dependent effect, as established in two reference populations.

In the three occupational groups with lower lead exposure, a similar analysis indicated the absence of significant correlations between BUN and creatinine, as indicators of renal function, and age, duration of lead exposure, PbB or ZPP levels (Table 3).

TABLE 3

CORRELATION OF BUN WITH AGE, DURATION OF LEAD EXPOSURE, PbB and ZPP IN THREE OCCUPATIONAL GROUPS WITH RELATIVELY LOW LEAD EXPOSURE

	CABLE SPLICERS (N = 90)	CABLE MANUFACTURERS (N = 45)	FIREARM INSTRUCTORS (N = 45)
AGE	-0.104 n.s.	0.271 n.s.	0.330 p = .049
DURATION	-0.067 n.s.	0.152 n.s.	0.103 n.s.
BLOOD LEAD	-0.095 n.s.	0.037 n.s.	0.014 n.s.
ZINC PROTOPORPHYRIN	-0.050 n.s.	0.178 n.s.	0.042 n.s.

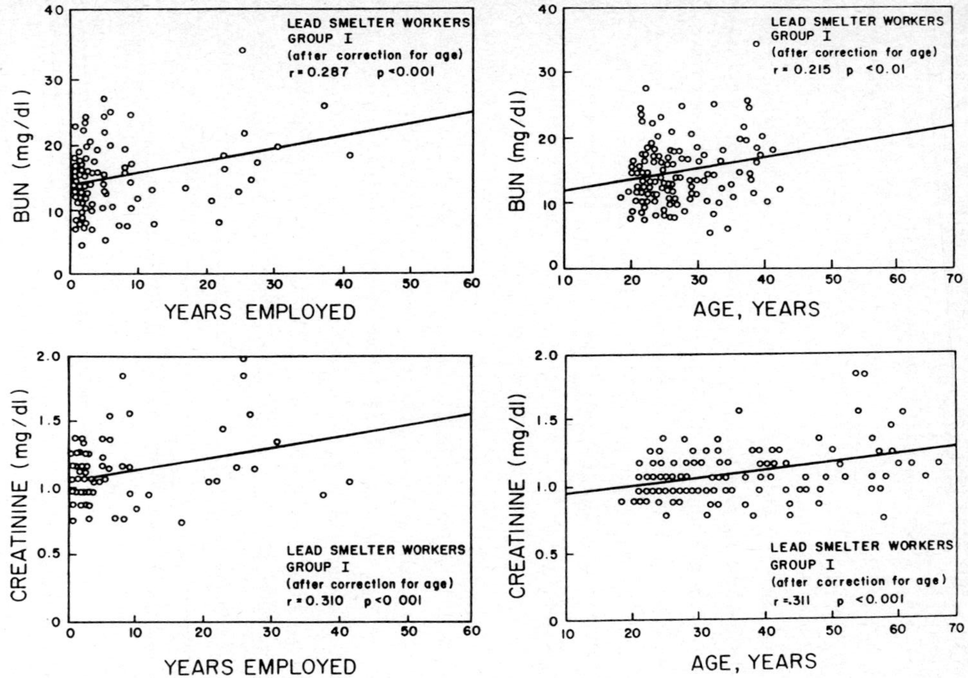

Fig. 3 Group I: BUN and creatinine plotted against duration of employment and age, after correcting for age-effect through partial correlation, and fitted with the least-square linear regression lines.

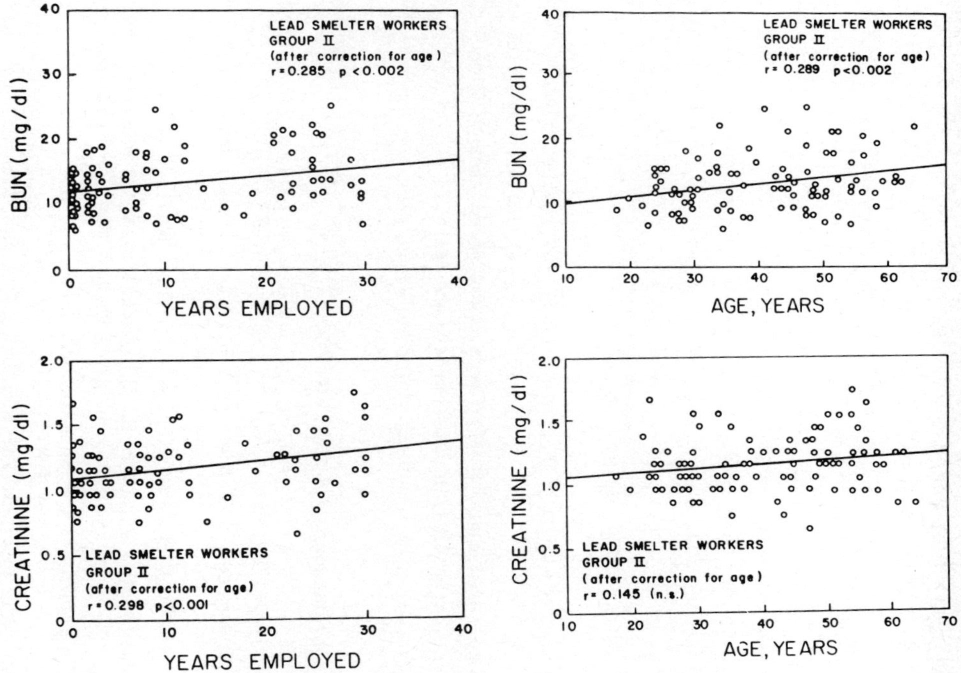

Fig. 4 Group II: BUN and creatinine plotted against duration of employment and age, after correcting for age-effect through partial correlation, and fitted with the least-square linear regression lines.

When comparing the two groups of secondary lead smelter workers with the three occupational groups with lower lead exposure, no major differences in distribution by age and/or length of lead exposure were noted (Table 1 and 2). The major differences consisted in much higher proportions of elevated PbB (> 60 μg/100 ml), ZPP levels (> 100 μg/100 ml) in secondary lead smelter workers: for elevated ZPP levels the proportions were 90% and 67%, as compared to 5%, 6% and 22% in the three groups with lesser lead exposure. These findings are interpreted to indicate that the risk of renal function impairment increases with higher lead exposure and absorption.

CONCLUSIONS

Occupational groups with a high prevalence of PbB levels in excess of 60 μg/100ml and ZPP in excess of 100 μg/100ml are at definite risk for renal function impairment with long-term exposure. The prevalence of kidney function impairment (reduction in GFR) in lead exposed subjects is definitely higher than that of elevated serum creatinine or BUN levels[3].

REFERENCES

1. Goyer, R.A. (1971) Curr. Top. Pathol. 55, 147-176.
2. Cramer, K., Goyer, R.A., Jagenburg, R. and Wilson, M.H. (1974) Brit. J. Ind. Med. 31, 113-127.
3. Wedeen, R.P., Maesaka, J.K., Weinter, B., Lipat, G.A., Lyons, M.M., Vitale, L.F. and Joselow, M.M. (1975) Am. J. Med. 59, 630-641.
4. Cooper, W.C. and Gaffey, W.R. (1975) J. Occup. Med. 17, 100-107.
5. Lilis, R., Fischbein, A., Diamond, S., Anderson, H.A., Blumberg, W.E., Eisinger, J. and Selikoff, I.J. (1977) Environ. Res. 14, 255-285
6. Lilis, R., Valciukas, J., Fischbein, A., Andrews, G. and Selikoff, I.J. (1979) J. Environ. Path. & Toxicol. 2: 1447-1474.
7. Fischbein, A., Eisinger, J. and Blumberg, W.E. Mt. Sinai J. Med. N.Y. (1976) 43, 294-299.
8. Blumberg, W.E., Eisinger, J., Lamola, A.A., and Zuckerman, D.M. (1977) Clinc. Chem. 23, 270-274.
9. Landrigan, P.J., McKinney, A.S., Hopkins, L.C. et al. (1975) JAMA 234, 394.

Mechanisms of Toxicity and Hazard Evaluation
B. Holmstedt, R. Lauwerys, M. Mercier, M. Roberfroid eds

EVALUATION OF OCCUPATIONAL EXPOSURE TO METALLIC MERCURY AND OF ITS EARLY RENAL EFFECTS

M. BERODE, M.P. GUILLEMIN, B. MARTIN[a], L. BALANT[b], R. FAWER, P.O. DROZ, P. MADELAINE, M. LOB
Institut universitaire de médecine du travail et d'hygiène industrielle, Lausanne, Switzerland
[a] Institut universitaire de médecine sociale et préventive, Lausanne
[b] Policlinique universitaire de médecine, Genève, Switzerland

INTRODUCTION

This study was undertaken to investigate the usefulness of a few urinary enzymes analyses in order to detect early renal effects of occupational exposure to metallic mercury. Other aspects, such as early detection of central nervous system effects will be published elsewhere[1].

Based on results of Ansermet[2] and other authors[3,4,5], the following enzymes were selected: lactate deshydrogenase (LDH) (E.C.1.1.1.27) leucine aminopeptidase (LAP) (E.C.3.4.11.1.), alkaline phosphatase (AP) (E.C.3.1.3.1.) and β-glucuronidase (BG) (E.C.3.2.1.31).

To complete the investigation of the renal function, proteins and creatinine clearance were also measured as well as β-glucuronidase in serum.

To define the current state of exposure to metallic mercury, we performed analysis of this metal in air, blood and urine.

METHODS

This study covered 52 male workers from three types of industries: glass blowers in 7 fluorescent tubes factories (FT), workers in a chloralkali plant (CA) and chemical industry-acetaldehyde production-workers (CI). Out of these 52 persons, 26 were exposed to mercury, the other ones are control. The size distribution of population in different factories was the same for both groups, each exposed worker being matched with one control person of comparable age working in the same factory.

Personal air sampling was carried out at 0,05 l/min drawing air through tubes filled with golden coated asbestos according to the method of Aubort et al[6]. After thermal desorption, Hg vapor was analysed by fluorescence spectrometry[7].

Night urine was collected three times consecutively, under precise timing. For the exposed workers one sample was also taken at the end of shift.

Mercury analysis in urine was performed by flameless AAS[8]; creatinine by an automatic Jaffe method[9] and total proteins by a modified Biuret method[10].

For LDH, LAP and AP, the procedure recommended by the German Society of clinical Chemistry (Monotest Boehringer) was applied for urine after dialysis. For BG, the Fishman's method[11] modified for time and temperature of incubation was selected for urine and serum samples.

Mercury in whole blood was measured by fluorescence spectrometry after digestion in HNO_3 at 150 ^{o}C.

Classical methods of clinical chemistry were used for serum creatinine, hematocrite and hemoblogin measurements.

RESULTS AND DISCUSSION

Occupational survey and biological monitoring. The mean exposure level for the exposed group is 26 μg Hg/m³ with a range from 6 to 65.

In Table 1 the workers have been subdivided into three classes according to their exposure level. The mean biological monitoring results for each type of industry and for controls are also given.

TABLE 1

SIZE DISTRIBUTION OF WORKERS AND BIOLOGICAL MERCURY INDEXES ACCORDING TO EXPOSURE LEVEL

Exposure level	Size distribution				Urinary Hg level		Blood Hg level
					End of shift	Next morning	
μg Hg/m³	Number of people				μmole/mole creat. (mean±SE)		nmole/l (mean±SE)
	FT	CA	CI	Total			
< 10	4	4	0	8	6,6 ± 1,2	6,3 ± 1,2	34,9 ± 1,7
10 to 45	2	5	6	13	13,3 ± 1,9	14,3 ± 1,8	38,3 ± 3,1
> 45	1	3	1	5	12,4 ± 2,9	11,4 ± 2,0	59,4 ± 14,4
Exposed	7	12	7	26	11,0 ± 1,3	11,3 ± 1,2	41,3 ± 3,5
Control	7	12	7	26	not determ.	3,4 ± 0,7	16,6 ± 1,6

It is interesting to note the distribution of urinary concentration which is decreased in the upper level contrary to the blood concentration. Is it due to a non representative exposure level or to a physiological difference in mercury excretion? This remains open until more information will be available.

On an individual basis, significant correlation appears between biological and air mercury measurements if urine mercury concentration is corrected for creatinine:
- blood and air ($r = 0{,}39$ $P < 0{,}05$)
- urine "end of shift" and air ($r = 0{,}39$ $P < 0{,}05$
- urine "next morning" and air ($r = 0{,}38$ $P < 0{,}05$)

On a group basis (each group corresponding to a factory), the correlation between urine and air ($r = 0{,}83$ $P < 0{,}01$ for 8 points) became better than these between blood and air ($r = 0{,}34$ not sig. for 8 points).

Possible renal effects. The results of the enzymes analysis used to detect an early renal effect gave values within the normal range. The same was true for proteins excepted for two workers.

The results obtained for these biological indexes are shown in Figure 1 using the subdivision of population according to exposure level defined in Table 1.

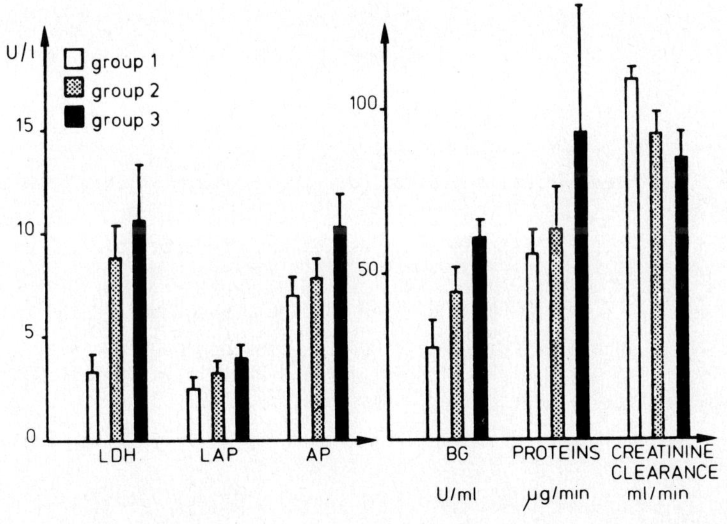

Fig.1 Group 1: exposure level ⩽ 10 µg Hg/m^3
Group 2: exposure level between 10 and 45 µg Hg/m^3
Group 3: exposure level ⩾ 45 µg Hg/m^3

For LDH, BG and creatinine clearance, the differences between groups are significant ($P < 0{,}05$ for Student t test). For the other parameters the difference is not significant but the trend does exist.

As shown in Figure 1, the variation of these tests seems to be in relation with exposure level contrary to the variation of urinary mercury parameter.

CONCLUSIONS

On a small group of workers exposed to relatively weak metallic mercury level, some variations of activity of urinary enzymes, of proteins concentration and of creatinine clearance have been displayed in relation with the level of exposure.

Although the values are in the normal range the trend in the above mentionned parameters sign an early damage of the nephron. It should be stressed that this damage is presumably reversible.

These results have to be confirmed on a larger scale.

ACKNOWLEDGEMENTS

We wish to sincerely thank all the employers and workers who actively participated in the completion of this study.

The technical assistance of Ms M. Dobler and Mrs P. Oswald was highly appreciated.

REFERENCES

1. Fawer, R. et al. To be published
2. Ansermet, F., Miéville, C. and Diezi, J. (1980) Arch. Toxicol. Suppl. 4 pp. 201-207.
3. Mattenheimer, H. (1977) Annals of Clin. and Lab. Science Vol 7, 5 pp. 422-431.
4. Raab, W. (1971) Z. klin. Chem. u. klin. Biochem. 9 Jg, pp. 143-154.
5. Plummer, D.T., Ngaha, E.O., Wright, P.J., Leathwood, P.D. and Blake, M.E. (1979) Diagnostic Significance of Enzymes and Proteins in Urine. Dubach, U.C. and Schmidt, U., Hans Huber Publishers, pp. 71-87, Bern.
6. Aubort, J.D., Rollier, H. and Ramuz A. (1977) Trav. Chim. Alim. Hyg. 68, 155.
7. Thompson, K.C. and Reynolds G.D. (1971) Analyst 96, pp. 771-775.
8. Hatch, W.R. and Ott, W.L. (1968) Analyt. Chem. 40, pp. 2085-2087.
9. Zender, R. and Falbriand, A. (1965) Clin. Chim. Acta 12, pp. 183-190.
10. Savory, J., Pu, P.H. and Sunderman, F.W. (1968) Clin. Chem. 14, 1160.
11. Fishman, W.H., Kato, K., Anstiss, C.L. and Green, S. (1967) Clin. Chim. Acta 15, p. 435.

CLINICAL TOXICOLOGY

Symposium chairmen: L.F. Prescott, E. Fournier and M. Lesne

© 1980 Elsevier/North-Holland Biomedical Press
Mechanisms of Toxicity and Hazard Evaluation
B. Holmstedt, R. Lauwerys, M. Mercier, M. Roberfroid eds

BIOLOGICAL EVALUATION OF HEMOPERFUSION IN ACUTE POISONING.

C. BISMUTH, P.E. FOURNIER
Hôpital Fernand WIDAL. UNIVERSITE PARIS VII. FRANCE

Hemoperfusion with cartridges of coated activated charcoal or resins in acute intoxications has several theoretical indications that are established by previous studies (1, 2, 3, 4, 5) : intoxication must be massive ; the extra-cellular distribution of the drug must be high ; the intoxicants must be measurable ; and epuration should take place when the plasma level is maximum. For the physician working in intensive care units, complications do not appear as an additive indication : respiratory depression, cardiac failure or convulsions, require immediate aggressive supportive treatment.

EVALUTION OF EFFICIENCY

The real problem raised by hemoperfusion is in fact the evalution of its efficiency in removal of intoxicants.

In vitro, this efficiency is excellent in what concerns clearances of substances as well as the disappearance from the plasma of marked molecules (6).

In vivo, it is still debatable.

Our experience is based upon 75 hemoperfusions with charcoal in acute intoxications, five patients having undergone 2 procedures (table 1).

HEMOPERFUSION CASES (1976 - 1979) 75 PATIENTS

Intoxicant	Cases	Deaths	Causes
Bismuth (chronic)	1	1	Septicemia
Selenium	1	0	
Poly pesticides	1	1	Aspiration pneumonia
Meprobamate	14	1	Cardio-respiratory arrest before epuration
Barbiturates			
- slow-acting	8	0	
- medium	14	0	
- short-acting	10	0	
Digitoxine - Digoxine	7	2	Cardiac failure
Paraquat	8	5	Pulmonary fibrosis
Chlorinated and aromatic solvants	3	0	
Tricyclic anti-depressants	3	0	
Colchicine	3	1	Schock
Paracetamol	2	1	Hepatic failure

Clinical appraisal

To toxicologists with pharmacological formation and daily clinical training, it appears that the efficiency of hemoperfusion cannot be appreciated clinically as :
a) amelioration (recovery from coma, apnea, hypotension, disappearance of convulsions or cardiac arythmias) is generally usual often within some hours with only supportive treatment in acute intoxication. (during the last ten years a spontaneous and significant shortening of the duration of acute signs has even been noted in intoxication by short-acting barbiturates (7) which represent more than 50 % of our recrutment of intoxications by hypnotics.)
b) an acute intoxication can exhibit no clinical improvment during hemoperfusion while however a significant removal of drug has occured, for exemple, if the therapy is performed during the period of intestinal absorption (table 2).

PHENOBARBITAL INTOXICATION (15 g)

Deepening of clinical and E.E.G. coma during efficient hemoperfusion (HP)

	Clinical assessment	E.E.G.	Serum barbiturate		Hemoperfusion barbiturate removal
			mg/l	µmol/l	grammes
Two hours before	grade 3	15 s black out and bursts	170	735	
2nd hour during HP	grade 4	No cerebral activity	172	740	1
End of HP	grade 4	No cerebral activity	190	820	1,25
					total : 2,25

Biological estimation

The estimation of hemoperfusion efficiency is then essentially biological: which is the amount of removed drug ?

A - The usual methods in anecdotal reports must be criticized.

I - Repeated measures of serum levels during the procedure appear inadequate as :

1) the fall of blood levels is often indistinguishable from the spontaneous kinetics

in vivo of the drug as it has been shown concerning digoxin (8).
as :
2) the blood level is often a poor reflect of the total body burden of intoxicants. (We shall stress this point later with regard to clearance data).
as :
3) are uncertain the level of digestive absorption of drugs which varies in man from 2 % to 90 %, and the rate of hepatic metabolism (always underestimated).

The treatment by hemoperfusion lasts 4 hours. The variation in serum levels during this interval of time depends partly or mostly on the moment it has been performed compared with the time of oral absorption (table 3). Performed in period (a) the serum level can be higher at the end of epuration, with however a good removal of drugs.

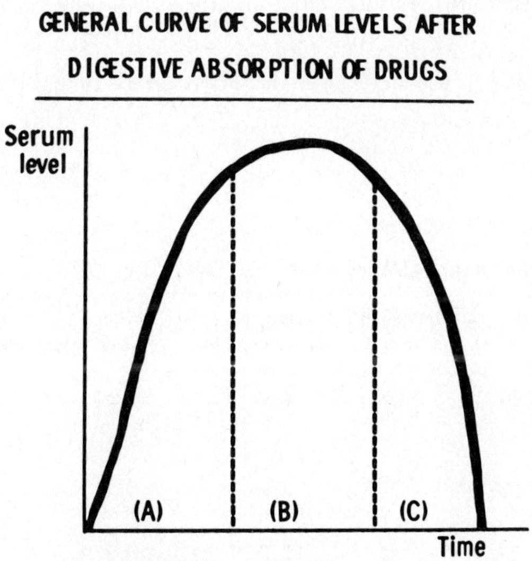

(A) absorption
(B) absorption concomitant with metabolic degradation and elimination
(C) concomitant metabolic degradation and elimination

Performed in period (b) the serum level can remain constant during the procedure: it proves or a good equilibrium between extra and intracellular spaces or a persistent digestive absorption and not inefficiency of hemoperfusion (table 4).

MEPROBAMATE INTOXICATION (45 g)

Hemodialysis + charcoal cartridge

Time hours	Serum meprobamate at arterial inlet (A)		Serum meprobamate at venous outlet (V)		Clearance $\frac{A-V}{A}Q^{+}$	Meprobamate removed
	mg/l	µmol/l	mg/l	µmol/l	ml/mn	mg/h
12.00-13.00	250	1150	200	920	57	600
13.00-14.00	235	1080	200	920	44	420
14.00-15.00	265	1215	170	780	95	1140
15.00-16.00	195	895	175	800	32	240
16.00-17.00	245	1125	165	755	82	960
19.00	290	1330				total: 3350mg

+ Blood flow (ml/mn)
(Lobo & al. Clinical Nephrology, 7, 1977, 73)

Performed in period (c) the decrease in serum level is not only related to HP but is a complex phenomena including urinary elimination and metabolic degradation.

Ex : in 4 cases of meprobamate intoxication (table 5)

PART OF HEPATIC METABOLISM IN MEPROBAMATE REMOVAL

TREATMENT	Plasma level (mg/l)° Day 1	Day 2	Hepatic °° metabolism (g/d)	Urinary excretion (g/d)	Extra-renal method (g/d)
Supportive (unknown intoxication : coma-cardiogenic shock)	200	125	4.8	0.6	
Osmotic diuresis + peritoneal dialysis	250	115	6.1	1	1
Osmotic diuresis + hemodialysis	260	90	5.15	1.7	3.35
Osmotic diuresis + hemoperfusion	250	80	4.5	1.5	3

° Sensitivity = 5 mg/l
°° Derived value obtained by using 75 % of body weight as the distribution space for the drug and by excluding the contribution of diuresis and hemoperfusion
(MADDOCK R. K. & al. : J. Am. Asso., 201, 1967, 999)

II - The evaluation of hemoperfusion should be biological, not according to the differences of plasma level between the beginning and the end of the procedure, but neither according on the *clearances* : here is a very usual method of appraisal of efficiency of dialysis. It is justified in nephrological explorations when methods of extra-renal dialysis are compared with normal renal performances upon usual constituants of the body, as are creatinine, urea, electrolytes, vitamines, hormons.

In toxicology, its introduction is misleading.

The problem there is extraction of foreign substances, with :

1) variable distribution in the body,
2) possible protein and lipid binding,
3) other ways than renal elimination.

a) A high clearance rate for a given substance means only that a large number of plasma-contained molecules are dialyzed. If the quantity of drug contained in the plasma is low besides the absorbed amount, the plasma can be cleared up at the end of epuration with a poor total elimination (table 6).

HEMOPERFUSION IN PARAQUAT INTOXICATION (50 mg/k)

Identical clearances and various removal

Time hours	Serum paraquat at arterial inlet (A)		Serum paraquat at venous out let (V)		Clearance $\frac{A-V}{A}Q^{+}$	Paraquat removed
	µg/l	µmol/l	µg/l	µmol/l	ml/mn	mg/h
12 - 13	800	3,5	120	0,45	170	9,6
13 - 14	540	2,1	140	0,55	150	4,8
14 - 15	340	1,3	120	0,45	130	2,7
15 - 16	200	0,7	50	0,2	150	1,8
19 th	380	1,5	versus 2d hemoperfusion			total : 19 mg

$^{+}$ Q = blood flow (ml/mn)

b) As a corollary, the same high clearances can represent very different excretions beetween the beginning and the end of one performance (table 6). The poor result of the last hour is probably related to the saturation of the cartridge but the disappointing amount removed in spite of good clearances in the 2d and 3d hour is related with progressive drug-free plasma.

B - A better approach to evaluation consists in calculating the total drug removed by determining hourly measurements of arterial-venous levels of drug multiplied by blood flow across the column.

The best method is to determine the elution of the column (it must be remembered that we are working only upon samples of the device : if the distribution in the cartridge is not homogeneous, the total drug content will be approximate).

If the ingested dose is precisely stated, the percent removed by hemoperfusion may be reasonably extrapolated for further case application.

The table 7 gives the expectable results of hemoperfusion in usual intoxications experienced in our Center.

EXPECTABLE RESULTS OF HEMOPERFUSION

Toxin	Number of cases	% of ingested dose	
		Maximum	Minimum
Slow-acting barbiturates	8	15	6
Medium barbiturates	14	12	6
Short-acting barbiturates	10	10	4
Paraquat	8	2	0.2
Digitoxine	3	2.5	0.1
Colchicine	3	4	< 1
Imipramine	3	2.2	< 1
Paracetamol	2	2	0.2
Meprobamate	14	17	7

- Barbiturate excretion is very close the already published cases ; the extraction of short-acting barbiturates is significantly higher than with hemodialysis.

- Digitoxine is very poorly removed with charcoal hemoperfusion. Amberlite hemoperfusion appears more promising (9).

- Paraquat is poorly removed with hemoperfusion (probably more poorly than with hemodialysis). But as intestinal absorption is only a small part of ingested dose, this little paraquat removed may be useful. In our experience, it has no effect upon mortality, but OKONEK published 2 cases with intermediate plasma levels who survived after continuous hemoperfusion (10).

- Meprobamate appears well extracted by hemoperfusion (between 7 and 17 % of ingested dose).

- The failure of Amitryptiline removal is because of discrepancy between weak extracellular and large intracellular distribution, as it is for Colchicine.

- The poor result with Paracetamol depends on the short half-life of the drug : 4 hours.

According to these data, and in a practical purpose, if the initial blood level of the drug is readily available after the patient is hospitalized, the optimum efficiency of hemoperfusion can be estimated beforehand

so that the decision to carry out hemoperfusion can be maintained, post poned or abandoned. We conducted this estimation about 3 clinically severe poisonings, applying the best conditions of activity, that means : complete disappearance of the drug between arterial inlet (A) and venous outlet (V = 0), plasma level of drug in A constant during the procedure, high blood flow (300 ml/mn) and not saturated cartridge in 4 hours. In these optimum approximations, the presumed removal of drug was so low, that we abandoned the indication of HP, estimating that the outcome would not be modified by this invasive treatment. (Table 8)

PREDICTABLE RESULTS OF HEMOPERFUSION
(calculated beforehand)

Intoxicant	Ingest amount	Plasma level (/ l)	Optimum removal of drug (mg)
Arsenic trioxyde	3 g	1.16 mg	85
Imipramine	3 g	2 mg	144
Colchicine	60 mg	60 µg	4.3

Supposing : 1) A (arterial inlet) - V (venous outlet) = A (V = 0)
2) A = constant during the procedure
3) High blood flow = 300 ml/min.
4) Not saturated cartridge in 4 hours.

In conclusion, the indication of this method of therapy which appears costly and not free from specific complications (6) should be reserved :

a) to medical teams quite aware of specific metabolism of the concerned intoxication supported by full toxicological data.

b) to threatening-life intoxications, due to cytoplasmic poisons, in the early clinical course, before the distribution in tissues occurs.

c) to "functional" intoxications having no mortality if hospitalized before respiration and circulatory complications, in the purpose to reduce the socio-economic costs of self-poisoning. We gave our results concerning hypnotic drugs. Whether these results can be judged satisfactory, live-saving or insignificant is largely a matter of personal standards.

SUMMARY

The efficiency of Hemoperfusion in acute poisoning cannot be clinically estimated, because :

a) concomittant intestinal absorption, hepatic metabolism and urinary excretion must be taken into account.

b) with supportive treatment alone, spontaneous recovery usually occurs in 98 % of the intoxications in Intensive Care Units.

The efficiency of hemoperfusion can only be estimated biologically.

Measuring the blood level at the beginning and the end of hemoperfusion as well as measuring the clearances of the drug is misleading. A better method is to measure the amount of extracted drug, either indirectly by calculation (from hourly differences of arterio-venous measures of drug concentration multiplied by the blood flow) or directly by elution of the cartridge.

In a practical way, if the blood level of drug is readily available after the patient is hospitalized, the optimum efficiency of hemoperfusion can be estimated beforehand, so that the decision to carry out the hemoperfusion can be maintened, postponed or abandoned.

For the most part, the experience of toxicologists has shown hemoperfusion to be ineffective for drugs with weak extra-cellular distribution (such as Digitoxine, Tricyclic drugs, Heavy Metals, Colchicine). Its effectiveness for certains drugs, with poor in vitro dialysance (such as Paracetamol) or with small percentage of intestinal absorption (such as Paraquat) is still debatable. In the case of intoxications by hypnotic drugs, one hemoperfusion allows an average of 4 - 12 % of the ingested medium and short barbiturates, 7 - 17 % of the ingested Meprobamate.

Whether these results can be judged satisfactory, life-saving or insignificant is largely a matter of personal standards.

REFERENCES

1. GOULDING, R. (1976) Experience with hemoperfusion in drug abuse. Kidney International, 10 : 338

2. MATIN, A.M. et al (1975) Charcoal hemoperfusion in the managment of severe poisoning. Brit. Med. J. 1. 392.

3. VALE, J.A. et al (1975) The use of charcoal hemoperfusion in the management of severely poisoned patients. Brit. Med. J. 1. 5

4. YATZIDIS, H. (1971) The use of ion exchange resins and charcoal in acute barbiturate poisoning, in "Acute Barbiturate Poisoning", edited by Matthew H. Amesterdam, Excerpta Medica.

5. WINCHESTER, J.F. et al (1977) Dialysis and hemoperfusion of poisons and drug - Update. Trans. Am. Soc. Artif. Intern. Organs, 23, 762.

6. BISMUTH, C. and SCHERRMANN, J.M. (1980) Hémoperfusion sur charbon activé enrobé. Appréciation de son efficacité à propos de 75 intoxications. Méd. Lég. et Toxicol. 1, 23

7. GAULTIER, M et al (1978) Decrease in duration of short actiong barbiturate intoxications. 8th meeting of the European meeting of the international association of Forensic Toxicologists. 21, 51.

8. SLATTERY, J.T. and KOUP, J.R. (1979) Haemoperfusion in the Managment of Digoxin Toxicity : Is it warrented ? Clin. Pharmacok. 4, 395.

9. MATHIEU , D. (1979) Intoxication digitalique massive. Traitement par hémoperfusion (Amberlite X AD 4). Thèse Lille - France.

10. OKONEK, S. et al (1979) Two survivors of severe Paraquat intoxication by "continuous hemoperfusion". Klin. Wochenschr. 57, 957.

© 1980 Elsevier/North-Holland Biomedical Press
Mechanisms of Toxicity and Hazard Evaluation
B. Holmstedt, R. Lauwerys, M. Mercier, M. Roberfroid eds

A TOXICOLOGICAL EVALUATION OF HEMOPERFUSION USING PHARMACOKINETIC PRINCIPLES

G.DE GROOT[1], R.A.A.MAES, Centre for Human Toxicology, State University, Utrecht and A.N.P.VAN HEIJST, Department of Reanimation and Clinical Toxicology, State University Hospital, Utrecht and National Poison Control Centre, National Institute of Public Health, Bilthoven, The Netherlands

INTRODUCTION

Over the last 4 years there has been an even growing interest in the application of hemoperfusion in clinical toxicology using either activated charcoal or Amberlite XAD-4, a polymeric resin, as an adsorbent. Since 1976 we have considered the use of hemoperfusion in the treatment of severe intoxications, primarily involving barbiturates but also including non-barbiturate hypnotics, tranquillisers, anti-depressives, analgesics, metals and pesticides. In the course of the investigations a total of 60 patients were treated with hemoperfusion involving 100 perfusions concerning 30 drugs, metabolites or other poisons.

In the evaluation of hemoperfusion several different parameters are considered. In the first place, hemoperfusion has been judged by its effect on the patient's clinical condition. For example, when a comatose patient awakes during or subsequent to treatment with hemoperfusion, the procedure is assumed to be effective. However, clinical improvement, or the failure of it, may be related to many factors, only one of which is the elimination of ingested poisons or their metabolites. Therefore, consideration of a change in the clinical condition is a final check of the efficiency rather than a judgemental criterion.

Secondly, the amount of drug that has been removed is frequently considered. Usually this parameter is calculated from data including plasma concentrations of the respective drugs at the inlet and outlet of the perfusion column. However, as concentrations in erythrocytes may be considerably lower than in plasma[1,2], calculation of the eliminated amount using plasma data, may lead to an overestimation. Another objection is that for the assessment of the value of the hemoperfusion therapy, a comparison has to be made with the total amount of drug in the body at the start of the perfusion. However, the exact amount of drug that has been ingested and subsequently absorbed is usually unknown as is

---

[1]Present address: Department of Pharmaceutical Toxicology, National Institute of Public Health, Bilthoven, The Netherlands

the part that has already been excreted at the time the perfusion starts. A better, more objective evaluation may be obtained when two pharmacokinetic parameters, the plasma clearance and the elimination half-life, are considered, together providing a useful tool in the evaluation of hemoperfusion.

When, some time after ingestion, an equilibrium between absorption, distribution and elimination of a drug has been attained (pseudo-distribution equilibrium), the relation between its elimination half-life ($t\frac{1}{2}$) and plasma clearance (Cl) is:

$$t\tfrac{1}{2} = 0.693 \frac{V_d}{Cl}$$

in which V_d is the apparent volume of distribution of the drug. For most drugs the plasma clearance can be described as the sum of the renal clearance and the metabolic clearance and in case of extracorporal elimination, it includes the respective extracorporal clearance as well. Thus, when hemoperfusion is performed the plasma clearance is enhanced and as a result the half-life will be shortened. The parameters in this equation can be used for the evaluation of hemoperfusion in relation to normal body elimination as well as other elimination techniques. Besides, when information on these parameters is available for a certain drug, the contribution of hemoperfusion in the total drug elimination can be predicted.

By presenting some cases of poisoning in which hemoperfusion has been applied in this paper it will be demonstrated how the contribution of hemoperfusion in the total drug elimination can be predicted and evaluated. In addition, the principles outlined may equally be applied to intoxications with other poisons.

HEMOPERFUSION IN MAPROTILINE POISONING

Maprotiline is a tetracyclic antidepressive drug, which shows a very large distribution volume (13.4 l/kg), meaning that only a very small fraction of the total amount of drug in the body is present in plasma. The normal plasma clearance of this drug is 240 ml/min, a high value, but due to its large distribution volume a long half-life (58 hours) is shown[3]. In Figure 1 the plasma concentrations are shown in a case of maprotiline intoxication, in which hemoperfusion with a Haemocol (Smith & Nephew Pharmaceuticals Ltd, Harlow, U.K.) column was applied. The average clearance value found was 79 ml/min. As could be expected from the above-mentioned pharmacokinetic parameters, especially from the high normal plasma clearance, only a minor effect of hemoperfusion was demonstrated. During perfusion the plasma level decreased but, probably due to a redistribution rebound, it returned to about the same level as before perfusion, although a residual absorption may not be completely excluded.

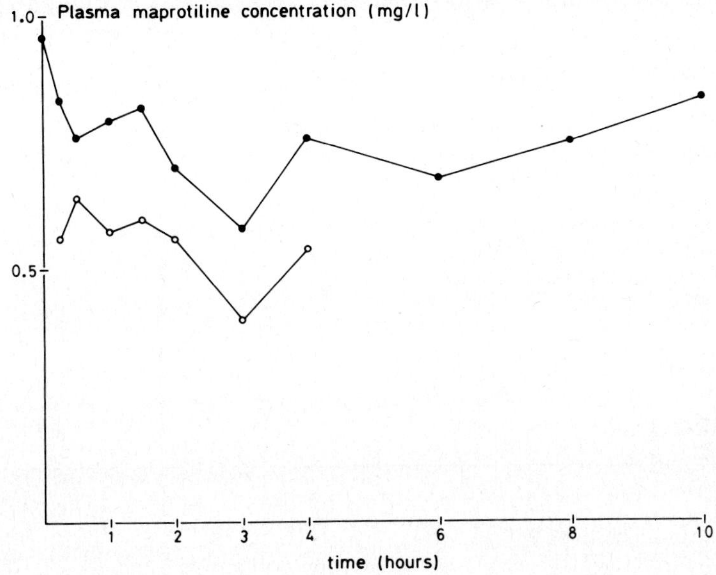

Fig. 1. Plasma concentrations of maprotiline at the inlet (closed dots) and outlet (open dots) of the perfusion column in a case of maprotiline intoxication in which hemoperfusion with the Haemocol was applied.

Other examples of drugs which show large distribution volumes in combination with relatively high normal plasma clearances are the tricyclic antidepressive drugs and their demethylated metabolites and digoxin. For these drugs only a minor contribution of hemoperfusion in the total body elimination may be expected.

HEMOPERFUSION IN MEPROBAMATE POISONING

Meprobamate is a sedative with anti-anxiety properties. It shows a relatively small distribution volume of 0.65 l/kg, which means that a considerable fraction of the drug is present in plasma. The normal plasma clearance of the drug is 50 ml/min and its mean half-life is 11 hours[4].

Table 1 shows clearance and half-life data in 5 cases of meprobamate poisoning in which hemoperfusion was applied, in 3 cases with the Haemocol, in the 2 other cases using the Adsorba 300 C (Gambro Dialysatoren GmbH, Hechingen, GFR). Compared with the half-life values after perfusion the respective values during perfusion were considerably reduced. This could be expected when the clearance values that were achieved with the respective hemoperfusions (between 89 and 300 ml/min) are compared with the normal plasma clearance of 50 ml/min.

HEMOPERFUSION COLUMN	AVERAGE CLEARANCE (ML/MIN)	ELIMINATION HALF LIFE (HOURS)	
		DURING PERFUSION	AFTER PERFUSION
HAEMOCOL	156	2.3	31.2
HAEMOCOL	89	3.2	6.2
HAEMOCOL	157	4.2	15.5
ADSORBA 300 C	118	4.2	11.7
ADSORBA 300 C	300	4.2	8.7

Table 1. Average hemoperfusion clearance and elimination half-life values during and after perfusion, respectively, obtained from 5 cases of meprobamate intoxication.

Consequently, it may be concluded that, unlike with compounds such as maprotiline, hemoperfusion therapy is very effective in meprobamate poisoning.

HEMOPERFUSION IN BARBITURATE POISONING

An important field of application of hemoperfusion is in barbiturate poisoning. In about 50% of the cases in which hemoperfusion has been applied in our hospital at least one barbiturate has been involved. Table 2 shows the relevant pharmacokinetic parameters of some of these drugs. A parameter of primary importance is the normal plasma clearance. From the data presented it can be seen that short-acting barbiturates (barbiturates with short half-lifes) have high normal plasma clearances. Application of hemoperfusion would result here only in a minor contribution to the total body clearance. When the half-life value increases, a decreasing normal plasma clearance is noted and the contribution of hemoperfusion to the total body clearance will be of increasing importance.

COMPOUND	DISTRIBUTION VOLUME (L/KG)	PLASMA CLEARANCE (ML/MIN)	HALF LIFE (HOURS)
METHOHEXITAL	1.13	829	1.6
HEXOBARBITAL	1.10	259	4.4
HEPTABARBITAL	1.30	138	7.7
CYCLOBARBITAL	0.51	35	12.0
VINYLBITAL	0.84	29	23.7
SECOBARBITAL	1.52	53	25.0
BUTOBARBITAL	0.78	18	37.5
PHENOBARBITAL	0.70	5	113

Table 2. Apparent distribution volume, normal plasma clearance and elimination half-life values of some barbiturates. All data refer to the therapeutic concentration range (most of these data originate from ref. 5).

Intoxications caused by barbital overdose

Barbital is a long-acting barbiturate with a long half-life and a low normal plasma clearance. Figure 2 shows 2 cases of poisoning, treated with hemoperfusion, each with a different activated charcoal column. Because of the very high plasma levels in these barbital intoxications the effect of an increasing saturation of the columns on the course of the respective clearances might be observed. Indeed, in both cases clearance values did not remain at a constant level, but declined exponentially, suggesting the occurrence of a progressive saturation. For the Haemocol the initial clearance of 130 ml/min decreased to its half in 147 min. For the Adsorba 300 C half the initial clearance of 293 ml/min was reached after 170 min. At the end of 4 hours of perfusion the clearance effected by the Adsorba 300 C was higher than the initial clearance achieved with the Haemocol.

Intoxications caused by Vesparax^R overdose

Vesparax^R is a hypnotic marketed in the Benelux, containing both secobarbital and brallobarbital. Figure 3 shows the plasma levels of the respective barbiturates in a case of Vesparax^R intoxication in which hemoperfusion was applied using the DX-60 column (Extracorporeal Medical Specialties Inc., King of

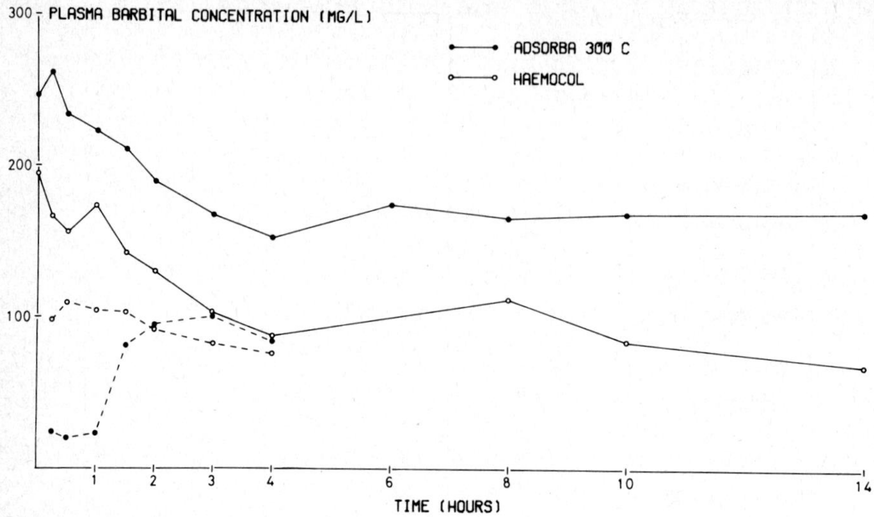

Fig. 2. Plasma concentrations of barbital at the inlet (solid lines) and outlet (broken lines), respectively, of the respective perfusion columns in 2 cases of barbital intoxication in which hemoperfusion was applied.

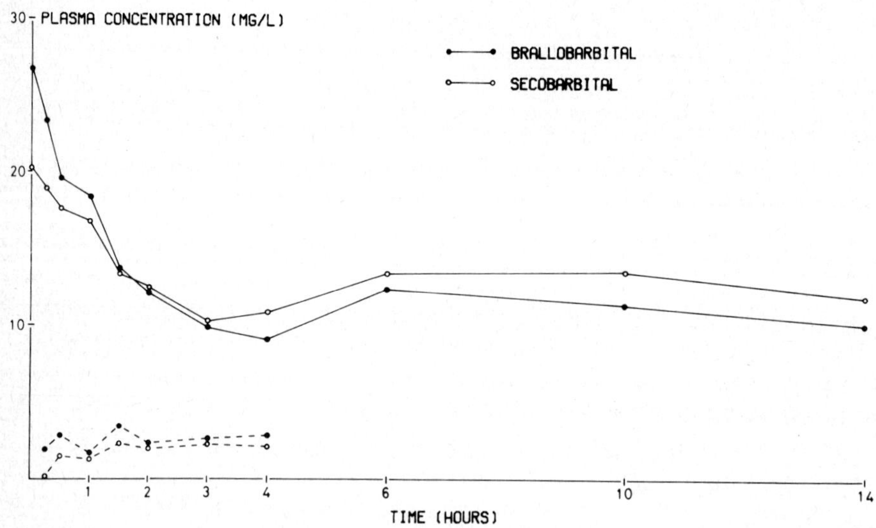

Fig. 3. Plasma concentrations of brallobarbital and secobarbital, respectively, at the inlet (solid lines) and outlet (broken lines) of the perfusion column in a case of Vesparax[R] overdose in which hemoperfusion with the DX-60 was applied.

Prussia, Pa, USA), which contains Amberlite XAD-4 resin as an adsorbent. For barbiturates this column is very efficient, resulting in average clearance values of 240 ml/min for brallobarbital and of 255 ml/min for secobarbital.

The influence of the difference in pharmacokinetic parameters of the two drugs is demonstrated in this figure. The distribution volume of secobarbital is about 3 times that of brallobarbital, meaning that a considerably larger fraction of brallobarbital is present in plasma. Besides, the normal plasma clearance of brallobarbital is smaller[6]. When the concentration curves of the respective drugs are compared, it can be seen that the effect of hemoperfusion is more pronounced with the drug having the lower normal plasma clearance and the smaller distribution volume; the brallobarbital concentration decreases faster. During perfusion the secobarbital concentration decreased with a half-life of 4.0 hours and that of brallobarbital with a half-life of only 2.6 hours.

In this picture another phenomenon that must be considered in evaluating the use of hemoperfusion is shown. As for these two barbiturates, many other drugs are distributed not only over the central plasma compartment but also over the tissue compartment. If extracorporal elimination is very fast, as is demonstrated in this case, hemoperfusion removes drugs faster from the plasma compartment than it can be replaced from the tissue compartment. A result of this multicompartment distribution kinetics is that after hemoperfusion a redistribution rebound of the plasma drug concentration can be expected. However, the occurrence of such an effect does not automatically implicate that the patient's clinical condition will deteriorate after perfusion, for the demonstrated increase in plasma level means that the drug concentration in the tissue compartment is simultaneously decreasing and possibly at the sites of action as well. Nevertheless, this possible rebound should also be taken into account, otherwise consideration of the half-lifes during perfusion may lead to an overestimation of the efficiency of hemoperfusion.

Intoxications caused by vinylbital overdose

Vinylbital is a hypnotic barbiturate with a relatively small distribution volume but, as its normal plasma clearance is low, its half-life is about 24 hours (see Table 2). Table 3 shows clearance and half-life data in 4 cases of vinylbital overdose in which hemoperfusion was applied, in one case with the Haemocol, in the 3 other cases using the DX-60. From the calculated half-life data during and after perfusion, respectively, the efficiency of hemoperfusion is clearly demonstrated. These results could be expected when it is considered

HEMOPERFUSION COLUMN	AVERAGE CLEARANCE (ML/MIN)	ELIMINATION HALF LIFE (HOURS)	
		DURING PERFUSION	AFTER PERFUSION
HAEMOCOL	121	8.5	20.8
DX - 60	289	2.2	20.0
DX - 60	270	1.5	36.3
DX - 60	299	3.0	9.0

Table 3. Average hemoperfusion clearance and elimination half-life values during and after perfusion, respectively, obtained from 4 cases of vinylbital intoxication.

that a considerable fraction of the total amount of vinylbital in the body is present in plasma. Comparison of the achieved hemoperfusion clearances with the normal plasma clearance shows that in the Haemocol case a 5-fold and in the DX-60 cases even a more than 10-fold elimination was achieved. Thus it can be concluded that hemoperfusion may be extremely effective when applied in this type of poisoning.

CONCLUSIONS

In the toxicological evaluation of the efficiency of hemoperfusion the plasma clearance and the elimination half-life together provide a useful tool. When information on these pharmacokinetic parameters is available the contribution of hemoperfusion in the total drug elimination can be predicted.

It has been demonstrated that hemoperfusion therapy is most effective when the drug involved shows a small distribution volume, which means that a considerable fraction of the total amount of drug in the body is present in plasma. Examples of these drugs are intermediate- and long-acting barbiturates and meprobamate. The extent to which the normal elimination half-life is reduced is determined by the hemoperfusion clearance achieved in relation to the normal plasma clearance of the drug involved. Only a minor contribution of hemoperfusion therapy to the total body elimination may be expected involving drugs showing large distribution volumes in combination with high normal plasma clearance values.

Examples of these drugs are tricyclic and tetracyclic antidepressive drugs and digoxin.

In barbiturate intoxications, especially when long-acting barbiturates are involved, drug removal by hemoperfusion is far superior to elimination by the body. At a blood flow rate of 300 ml/min the highest clearance values were found using the DX-60 column which contains Amberlite XAD-4 as an adsorbent (between 240 and 300 ml/min). The columns filled with activated charcoal showed clearances between 150 and 200 ml/min for the Adsorba 300 C and between 80 and 120 ml/min for the Haemocol. Practically, however, in deciding which perfusion column should be used not only the expected efficiency of a particular column, but also clinical considerations should be taken into account.

REFERENCES

1. Ehrnebo, M. and Odar-Cederlöf, I. (1975) Eur. J. Clin. Pharmacol., 8, 445.
2. Kurata, D. and Wilkinson, G.R. (1974) Clin. Pharmacol. Ther., 16, 355.
3. Alkalay, D., Wagner Jr., W.E., Carlsen, S., Khemani, L., Volk, J., Bartlett, F. and Le Sher, A. (1980) Clin. Pharmacol. Ther., 27, 697.
4. Maddock, R.K. and Bloomer H.A. (1967) J. Am. Med. Assoc., 201, 999.
5. Breimer, D.D. (1977) Clin. Pharmacokin., 2, 93.
6. Groot, G.de, Maes, R.A.A. and Heijst, A.N.P.van, unpublished results.

© 1980 Elsevier/North-Holland Biomedical Press
Mechanisms of Toxicity and Hazard Evaluation
B. Holmstedt, R. Lauwerys, M. Mercier, M. Roberfroid eds

LIAISON WITH INDUSTRY IN THE PROVISION OF ESSENTIAL INFORMATION FOR THE MANAGEMENT OF POISONING II

DR. R. GOULDING, B.Sc., M.D., F.R.C.P., F.R.C. Path.
Poisons Unit, Guy's Hospital, London, U.K.

My co-author, Dr. Spooner, has introduced this very critical topic of industry liaison to further the enlightened clinical management of poisoning first by referring to some of the general problems and then by enlarging, very significantly for this purpose, on the saga of paracetamol toxicity. He could not have chosen a better example. It was not until we were forcibly confronted in our hospital wards with cases of liver damage on this account that both sides, industry and clinical medicine, mobilised their by no means feeble resources to tackle this problem and, gratifyingly, to arrive at a satisfactory solution. But, as our trade union friends are increasingly reminding us in the field of occupational toxicology, they do not want the principal parameters of our investigation to be dead human bodies and gravestones! But the story of paracetamol has been repeated, in principle, all too often. Thalidomide, it is needless to state, stands out as the conspicuous example. Still we can go further than that to the adverse reactions of aspirin, to the otoxicity of neomycin, to the peculiar potency of succinycholine in certain subjects, to the peripheral neuropathy of isoniazid, to the S.L.E. syndrome with hydrallazine, to the renal damage caused by phenacetin, to the hepatic effects of halothane and then, more recently, to the odd behaviour of practolol. This list is obviously by no means exhaustive. So how can this deplorable catalogue avoid being repeated in the future?

The major response has been to multiply the premarketing toxicological investigations with even more experiments on vastly more animals, on more species and by more intricate procedures. Toxicological laboratories have proliferated and toxicologists to man them are at a premium, despite the frenzied efforts of the universities and other institutions to train them. Where, we might ask, is all this enormous energy and expense getting us? Woefully, as became all too evident at the previous International Congress on Toxicology, held in Toronto this science has displayed a dubious track record of being a reliable predictive science, despite the overall theme on that occasion.

Let us labour no more on futile recriminations and see how better this task might be approached. First of all I should remind those present - in all probability unnecessarily - that the physician must be concerned with toxicity in its widest sense, not only that from drugs, but also that from industrial chemicals, agricultural pesticides, household products and even cosmetics and veterinary medicines. He must cater also for delayed as well as for acute effects, for cumulation and for strange disadvantageous and novel manifestations. Properly to encompass all these possibilities, is a daunting exercise, so principally, - like my co-author - I will for the moment concentrate upon acute poisoning from drugs, for that is our main preoccupation in Poisons Centres at the present time.

I cannot speak with any authority about what obtains in other countries, but I can explain how we proceed in Britain. Principally, through the individual firms and to some extent through the Association of the British Pharmaceutical Industry, we maintain a close, ongoing relationship. By contrast, we have no direct contact in these matters with the official licensing authority, the government Committee on Safety of Medicines. Their interchange with industry is by a formal, confidential and legal procedure in which we do not, and cannot, intrude. Not that we suffer for this reason. It is our experience - and always has been - that the various firms and, notably, their medical directors, are most forthcoming and we have no indication that they ever withold any vital information from us.

Of course, by the time a licence to market is granted, no cases of acute overdosage have been reported, so in anticipation we must extrapolate from the animal data. This comes to us just as it is submitted to the licensing authority, embracing a wide range of LD_{50}'s for a series of animal species. Taking the cautious attitude we arrive tentatively at an acute fatal dose for man by simple arithmatic from the most sensitive species on a kilogram body weight formula. It will be no surprise to you that we are frequently incorrect in our prognostications, but at least we are usually on the safe side.

When we ask for observational details of the mode of death as a clue to the mechanism, sadly this proves all-too-often of little informative value, for all we gain is a story of restlessness or depressed activity, convulsions or respiratory depression. What more essentially we require here is the precise pathology and that still exists as a somewhat unexplored area into which, on both sides, we are venturing only slowly. Understandably non-medical toxicologists wrestling with the calculation of a set of precise, statistical LD_{50}'s, with the legions of animals so involved, are not attuned to the comprehension of dynamic pathology.

At the same time we can, however, derive some guide as to the likely presentation of acute overdosage if we can accept that it will be an intensification of the pharmaco-dynamic behaviour of the agent in question. Yet, to glance back quickly to paracetamol, this is not universally so.

Assuming that this stage has been reached, then there is the need to know what happens to the drug in the body; in other words its pharmacokinetics and its metabolism in man, of course, and not in some other animal that may be far from analogous in this respect. Increasingly the licensing authority is placing greater emphasis on this aspect and, correspondingly, pharmaceutical firms are better able to advise us about this. Working along these lines we can form some impression of whether excretion is likely to be rapid or delayed, whether sequestration is likely to occur (and where) and whether from the parallel pharmacodynamics the changes wrought are likely to be reversible. All of these data, by painful and diligent appraisal, can afford us some prediction of the probable clinical picture of acute overdose and the manner in which it might be managed. You will not be astonished to learn that events sometimes prove us, in our forecasting, to be wrong. At least we are not entirely destitute of understanding.

Ideally, I suppose, we might search around for a particular animal species which, pharmacodynamically and pharmacokinetically behaved in an identical manner to man and then deliberately to carry out overdose experiments and their management in such a creature. So far, I regret to admit, we have scarcely embarked in this manner. Less still have we probed into the molecular biology to devise antidotes in advance.

So, you see, despite the information which industry readily furnishes to us and despite our assiduous handling of it, we await our first cases with just about as much confidence as you can rely on the meteorologists to tell you the sort of weather to expect when you are booking the tour to the Ardennes organised by this congress. In short, when a new drug is released we are far from being assured that we are equipped to handle any overdose emergencies.

That is where immediate post-marketing monitoring has an almost literally vital part to plan. My colleague, Dr. Volans, and I have written about this in a recent publication (Inman, 1980). Once we are notified by the manufacturers (not by the licensing authority, be it noted) our system is alerted to any enquiries about it in overdose. Simultaneously doctors are encouraged to get in touch with us about any incident, regardless of its lack of severity. Follow-up is enacted, full case details are assembled and the firm concerned is apprised. Thus from the very first we begin building up a picture. Each new case equips us better to deal with the next. Publication may soon follow and the firm can expand its data sheet accordingly. This, we think, is liaison going full circle and we regret not having established this arrangement a decade or more ago.

Inman, W.H.W., Ed. (1980) "Monitoring for Drug Safety". pp. 367-377. London: MTP Press.

© 1980 Elsevier/North-Holland Biomedical Press
Mechanisms of Toxicity and Hazard Evaluation
B. Holmstedt, R. Lauwerys, M. Mercier, M. Roberfroid eds

RESULTS AND PERSPECTIVES OF ELECTROENCEPHALOGRAPHY IN TOXICOLOGY.

F. MELLERIO
INSERM, Unité de Recherche de Toxicologie Expérimentale U. 26, Hôpital Fernand Widal, 200 rue du Fg St Denis, 75475 Paris Cedex 10, (France).

Cerebral electrogenesis modifications due to toxicological effects are still insufficiently explained,some areas and mechanisms of action remain badly understood. The EEG is objective by worthwhile for detecting pattern changes due to intoxications, in spite of its unspecific and empiric nature. This complementary addition to clinical practice is far too seldom used in toxicology ; hence its practical and theoretical interest need to be brought forward.

MATERIAL AND METHODS

Personal research conclusions from 4500 observations and including about 7500 recordings are herewith reported. The majority of these cases are voluntary or accidental acute poisoning (medicinal or industrial) ; cases of chronic professional intoxication are rarer.
20 electrodes were used for the EEG recordings, according to the bipolar method. Eventually simultaneous inscription of EKG, respiration, eye movement and global myograms were carried out. Auditive and nociceptive stimulations (opening the eyes when possible) were done to determine reactivity.

RESULTS

Acute drug intoxications.

1. Barbiturate and various non barbiturate hypnotics (such as gluthetimide, methylprylone, mecloqualone, methaqualone...) and tranquillizers.

Their absorption induces spectacular EEG disturbances which correspond to vigil comae, diffuse rapid rythms between 18 and 30 c/s, with or without an anterior maximum. Reactivity is paradoxically slow or absent.

During moderate coma (grade II or grades II and III depending upon the different classifications) an EEG usually shows a mixture of diffuse rapid rythms and slow high waves characterized by stiff front and varying quantities. If reactivity persists it is translated by a slowing down and amplification of activity with decreasing polymorphism.

During carus coma , a slow-high activity with shorter frequencies is possible. Barbiturates often induce a very unusual pattern : alternation of repeating short electrical silences and recordable discharges. Regardless of this paroxysmal aspect, we have never seen seizures related to this pattern and reversibility is quite common.

Long acting barbiturates must be classified separately because for moderate and deep coma they usually induce quite a different patterns : delta with added frequencies, between 8 and 12 c/s.

Some peculiarities to be noted are :

That with deep short acting barbiturates coma , diphasic slow waves can be observed spreading with anterior predominance, such as in porto-cava-encephalopathy (but without hepatic failure).

That during acute methaqualone poisoning, EEG paroxysms are possible without convulsive manifestations and previous epilepsy.

2. Neuroleptics (phenothiazine, butyrophenones). Even for deep coma , occasionaly with a hypothermia of about 30°, recordings show only a moderate slowing down and wideninh spread of activity.

3. Tricyclic anti-depressants (Imipramine, amitriptyline and derivatives). Despite severe neurological and cardio-vascular symptoms induced by their absorption, only moderate disturbances are seen in the majority of cases. Paroxysmal abnormalities are seldom encountered even when clonus and seizure occur. With amitriptyline, it is possible to observe sharp and high waves which seem be in transition between a sleep pattern and a paroxysmal one.

4. Isoniazide is an infrequently encountered INH poisoning which leads to a convulsive state with a peculiar EEG : a slowing down and widening spread with generalized synchrone output of very slow high waves.

5. Cardiotropes : when various intoxications such as Quinine, Nivaquine, and Ajmaline were studied, EEG's did not modify, except after cardiac arrest. In this particular case EEG alterations must

be related to hypoxia. When alterations are few the prognosis is favorable , when they are significant it is necessary to repeat the recording a few hours later in order to gain further informations. With digitaline poisoning, abnormal slowing down can appear and continue for several days in cases of metabolic disturbances,disorientation and sometimes atropine confusion.

Various

Antalgics : usually no modification.

Amphetamines, anorexigens, increased vigilance, rapide rythm and low voltage.

Atropinics : state of delirium in contrast with the EEG sleep pattern.

Acute non drug poisonings.

1. Carbon monoxyde : EEG is often of great interest in prognosis: organised activity so although slow, furnishes a relatively sound prognosis. However for some observations, it is necessary to monitor the evolution over several weeks for removing become apparent. Nevertheless in serious poisoning it is possible for the EEG return to normal after several months despite sequellae. Hyperbaric oxygenotherapy gives very good clinical results although improvements in EEG often come later than clinical ones (as opposed to visible EEG improvements prior to the clinical emergency when oxygen caisson was not used). A post-interval syndrom can be noticed with secondary worsening after an apparent transitory removal and a slower EEG.

2. Hypoxia, anoxia (CNH, H_2S...)induce slower waves as for CO.

3. Solvents :

Trichlorethylen : EEG disturbances vary according to the means of absorption - by the respiratory pathway, EEG modifications are generally slight : sleepiness, or sharp pointed alpha. Occasionally after acute massive intoxication an hypoxic pattern appears.

- per os, after massive voluntary absorption, at first the EEG is rapid with reactivity translated by very slow high waves ; as the coma deepens the EEG changes, recording slower activity and monomorphism. This accentuation of abnormalities can results in a slowing of activity over short periods (this kind of EEG evolution is never encountered with other toxics aside from incidents of complication). Accidental poisoning is usually moderate.

CCl_4 : no modification at first, followed by a slowing down of activity related to hepato-renal failure.

4. Ethylen glycol : acute oral intoxication induce renal disorders and,convulsions are possible. Slowing EEG and paroxysms are sometime detected.

5. Halogenate carbohydrates : Br CH_3 a very potent nervous system toxic gives convulsive state which can last days or week despite treatment. Recordings are quite disturbed and various with paxysmal features and slight therapeutic modifications.

6. Herbicides : Paraquat : serious pulmonary disease without significant EEG disturbances.

7. Insecticides : - organo chlorinated have a convulsive action, EEG paroxystic abnormalities are possible, - organo-phosphates generally give no modification despite of cholinesterases disturbances.

8. Raticides :Chloralose induces convulsive activity with significant but transitory paroxystic features,24 to 48 hours after the EEG becomes normal even during hyperpnea and photic stimulation.

9. Metals :-Pb, Hg, (chronic exposition or alimentary contamination) can induce encephalopathies with no specifically slow EEG, - Tin organo derivatives caused therapeutic accidents with encephalopathies some years ago, - Arsenical derivatives can also give encephalopathies (essentially with organo-compounds),an allergic mechanism can be noted in several cases.

PERSPECTIVES

After this brief outline we can say that the EEG is not interest to toxicology for detecting complications, following the evolution, as well as evoking the toxic. Over the last years, we have seen new toxicological pathology such as Bismuth encephalopathies, (aluminium encephalopathies are described in nephrological care unit), lithium overdosage, neuroleptic malignant syndrom and, more recently the tranquillizer withdrawal syndrom (comparable to barbiturate one). We think that EEG studies should be pursued along the lines of new medications, and industrial products. Nevertheless EEG giving only a global aspect of cerebral activity, association with animal experimentations,with biochemists and pharmacologists appears highly desirable to try to elucidate toxicological mechanisms.

Mechanisms of Toxicity and Hazard Evaluation
B. Holmstedt, R. Lauwerys, M. Mercier, M. Roberfroid eds

EVALUATION OF HAEMOPERFUSION BY COLUMN ANALYSIS

F.A. DE WOLFF[1], N.D. SMIT[1], E.J. GRÜNEWALD[2], and I.M. SCHICHT[3]
[1]Laboratory of Toxicology, [2]Department of Reanimation, and [3]Department of Nephrology, University Hospital, 2333 AA Leiden, The Netherlands

INTRODUCTION

Haemoperfusion over charcoal or resin columns is generally accepted as a valuable tool in the treatment of patients who are intoxicated with certain drugs or poisons.[1, 2, 3, 4, 5] There is, however, no unanimity for which substance haemoperfusion is an effective therapy, and for which it is not. As is often the case with new therapeutic methods, haemoperfusion is sometimes overestimated, and thought to be effective in those patients who would have recovered in a reasonable time without haemoperfusion as well.[3]

From a pharmacokinetic point of view, haemoperfusion can only be expected to be effective for drugs with a relatively low metabolic clearance and small volume of distribution.[6] This should, however, be proven for every drug in question by means of reliable laboratory methods. Measurement of serum concentrations of the poison during haemoperfusion is insufficient, since it only gives information on the disappearance from blood but not from the tissues. Therefore, the clearance by the column and the total amount of drug adsorbed to the column should be calculated. This can be done by measurement of drug levels at column inlet and outlet and at certain intervals.[2, 7] From these data, the total amount of drug adsorbed to the column can be calculated. A great advantage of this method is that column clearance can be measured as a function of time, thus providing information on the saturation of the column. A disadvantage, however, is that calculation of the amount adsorbed is dependent on the measurement of blood flow, which is often unreliable.

Therefore, the best way in our view to evaluate haemoperfusion is the measurement of the quantity of drug retained by the column material. From this quantity and from perfusion time and average serum level, the average clearance during haemoperfusion can also be calculated. In this paper, some preliminary results for five different drugs and six patients are presented.

PATIENTS AND METHODS

Patients were admitted in deep coma (grade III - IV) after taking a drug overdose for attempted suicide. Two patients took phenobarbital, one secobarbital in combination with brallobarbital and hydroxyzine (Vesparax^R), one pentobarbital, one vinylbital, and one methaqualone together with flurazepam. The latter patient died from the consequences of an aspiration pneumonia; the others recovered. Haemoperfusion over Gambro Adsorba 300 C columns via catheters which were inserted in the inferior vena cava by means of the Seldinger technique, was started as soon as a toxic serum level of the drug in question was found.

Methods. Serum concentrations of hypnotic drugs were determined according to Flanagan and Berry[8] using gaschromatography without derivatization.

Analysis of haemoperfusion columns (Gambro Adsorba 300 C) was carried out as follows. The column is opened with an iron saw and the coated charcoal granules are washed with a cold isotonic saline solution (9 g NaCl/L) to remove residual blood. The granules are placed on filter paper and dried at 80°C, and weighed. After thorough mixing, part of the granules are triturated in a mortar. Exactly 1 g of the powder is transferred into a porous thimble (Schleicher and Schüll, Extraktions-Hülsen Nr. 603) and covered with glass-wool. The thimble is placed in a Soxhlet apparatus which is fitted to a 300-ml bolt-head flask containing 150 ml chloroform to which the appropriate internal standard is added. The optimal amount of internal standard is estimated in a pilot experiment. For the determination of phenobarbital, phenylallylbarbituric acid is used as the internal standard; for secobarbital: pentobarbital, for pentobarbital: secobarbital, for vinylbital: butobarbital, and for methaqualone: phenobarbital.
The chloroform is boiled gently so as to achieve continuous extraction. After 5-6 hours, extraction is maximal.[9] The drugs are quantitated in the chloroform extract by gas chromatography as described elsewhere.[9]

RESULTS AND DISCUSSION

Patient 1, a 23-year-old man, attempted suicide by taking about 6 g of phenobarbital from his epileptic twin brother. The serum level of phenobarbital at admission was over 160 mg/L, indicating a severe phenobarbital intoxication. The treatment of choice in these cases is haemoperfusion in combination with forced alkaline diuresis (500 ml/h). In Figure 1, the course of the serum levels during treatment is shown. Three charcoal columns were used in succession during 270, 540 and 360 min, respectively. Haemoperfusion was discontinued as soon as the patient regained consciousness. Elimination half-life time during combined haemoperfusion and forced alkaline diuresis was 6-12 hrs; during forced alkaline diuresis *alone*, $t_{\frac{1}{2}}$ was 64 hrs (normal: 90-100 hrs).

The quantities of phenobarbital adsorbed to the columns, and the average clearance values, are given in Table 1.

TABLE 1

RESULTS OF COLUMN ANALYSIS FOR FIVE DIFFERENT HYPNOTICS IN SIX PATIENTS

Patient	Drug	Column no.	Haemo-perfusion time (min)	Quantity adsorbed (mg)	Average serum level (mg/L)	Average clearance (ml/min)	Average flow (ml/min)
1	phenobarbital	1	270	2180	150	54	230
		2	540	1900	99	36	210
		3	360	1130	52	60	260
2	phenobarbital	1	220	1430	96	68	260
3	secobarbital	1	720	515	20	36	100
		2	360	102	8	35	140
4	pentobarbital	1	45	51	20	57	165
		2	260	181	17	41	200
5	vinylbital	1	320	259	29	28	100
6	methaqualone	1	45	34	8	94	175
		2	180	80	10	44	125

It appears that for the three columns used for patient 1, there is a relationship between clearance and flow. This demonstrates the necessity of high flow rates for effective haemoperfusion.

In order to determine the contribution of forced alkaline diuresis to treatment, renal clearance values of phenobarbital were also assayed. In the

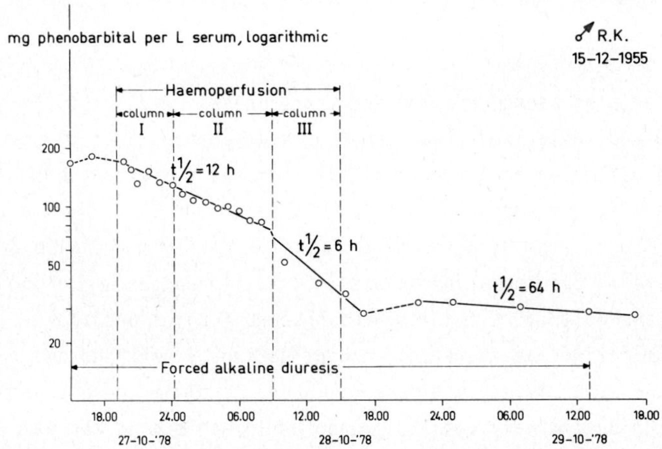

Fig. 1. Serum concentrations of phenobarbital in patient 1 during treatment.

course of 46 hours, 14 urine samples were collected. The average renal clearance of phenobarbital was shown to be 6.0 ± 3.2 ml/min (mean ± SD, n = 14), normal being 0.7 - 4.5 ml/min.[10] In Figure 2, the relationship between renal clearance of phenobarbital and urine production is shown. From this Figure it can be seen that forced alkaline diuresis, indeed, contributes to the elimination of phenobarbital: the higher the diuresis, the more phenobarbital is cleared from the plasma.

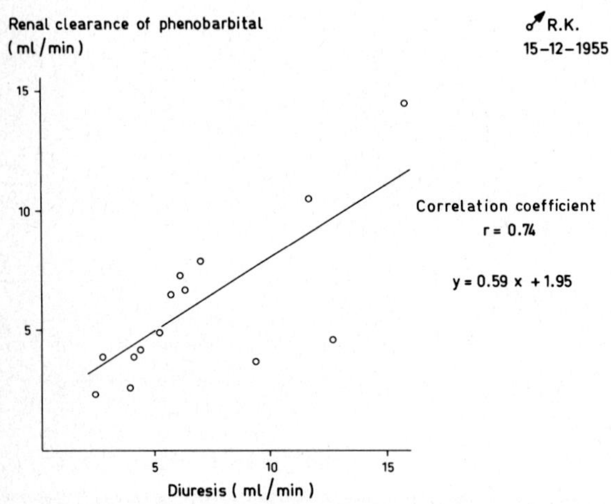

Fig. 2. Relationship between renal clearance of phenobarbital and diuresis in patient 1.

In Table 2, the results of haemoperfusion and forced alkaline diuresis for patient 1 are compared and summarized. From these data it appears that haemoperfusion is much more effective than forced alkaline diuresis in the treatment of severe phenobarbital overdosage.

In Table 1, the haemoperfusion data for the other five patients are also given. All patients were in deep coma and showed potentially dangerous serum levels at admittance (above 100 mg/L for long-acting barbiturates and above 25 - 30 mg/L for medium-acting barbiturates), except patient 6, who showed comparatively low methaqualone levels but whose clinical condition necessitated haemoperfusion. From the preliminary results presented in Table 1 it can be seen that the average column clearance values are all in the same order of magnitude for the hypnotic drugs investigated so far, and that there is a tendency that column clearance is dependent on the blood flow over the column. Further research is necessary to compare the method for evaluation of haemoperfusion proposed by De Groot, Maes *et al.*[2] with the present method.

From the data presented here it may be concluded that column analysis is a simple and reliable method to determine both the quantity of the drug adsorbed to the column material, and the average volume of plasma cleared per unit of time by the haemoperfusion column.

TABLE 2

COMPARISON OF EFFECTS OF HAEMOPERFUSION AND FORCED ALKALINE DIURESIS FOR PATIENT 1 (phenobarbital)

	Duration (hrs)	Quantity removed (g)	Average clearance (ml/min)
Alkaline forced diuresis	46	0.89	6
Haemoperfusion	19.5	5.21	50

REFERENCES

1. Widdop, B., Medd, R.K., Braithwaite, R.A., Rees, A.J., Goulding, R. (1975) Arch. Toxicol. 34, 27.
2. De Groot, G., Maes, R.A.A., van Heyst, A.N.P. (1977) Neth.J.Med. 20, 142.
3. Crome, P., Hampel, G., Vale, J.A., Volans, G.N., Widdop, B., Goulding, R. (1978) Br. Med. J. I, 174.
4. Külpmann, W.R., Oellerich, M., Blume, U., Schmidt, E., Barthels, M. (1978) Klin. Wochenschr. 56, 1171.
5. Winchester, J.F. and Gelfand, M.C. (1978) Drug Metab. Rev. 8, 69.
6. Iversen, B.M., Willassen, Y., Bakke, O.M. (1978) Lancet I, 388.
7. Tiess, D. and Osten, B. (1978) Dtsch. Gesund.-Wes. 33,1244.
8. Flanagan, R.J. and Berry, D.J. (1977) J. Chromatog. 131, 131.
9. De Wolff, F.A. and Smit, N.D. (1980) Arch. Toxicol. 43, 233.
10. Seyffart, G. (1977) Poison Index: dialysis and haemoperfusion in poisonings. Fresenius Foundation, Bad Homburg.

Mechanisms of Toxicity and Hazard Evaluation
B. Holmstedt, R. Lauwerys, M. Mercier, M. Roberfroid eds

COMPARISON OF HEMOPERFUSION AND HEMODIALYSIS CLEARANCES DURING COMBINED AND PROLONGED TREATMENT OF SEVERELY POISONED PATIENTS

GERT A. VERPOOTEN[1], AUBAIN HEYNDRICKX[2], PIERRE ZACHEE[1], MARC E. DE BROE
[1] Dept. Nephrology-Hypertension, University of Antwerp, Belgium
[2] Dept. Toxicology, R.U.G., Gent, Belgium

INTRODUCTION

The use of hemoperfusion (HP) and hemodialysis (HD) in the treatment of severe poisoning is still a matter of debate [1, 2]. Even if one decides for extracorporeal epuration, precise guidelines for the use of one of the available methods does not exist. We developped a method using the combined HP - HD for the treatment of patients with severe poisoning [3, 4]. This paper describes our first results of the HP-, HD-and overall clearance of several drugs.

MATERIALS AND METHODS

Combined HP - HD treatment was performed using a coated charcoal column (Adsorba 300 C, Gambro) and a capillary kidney placed in series. The blood flow through the system was held constant at 200 ml/min. The dialysate flow through the capillary kidney was 500 ml/min.

Blood samples were taken simultaneously from the inflow and outflow lines of the column and dialyzer (points A, B and C in Fig. 1) in syringes containing lithium-heparin (Sarstedt, Herent, Belgium) and stored at 4° C for further analysis.

Whole blood concentrations of barbiturates, carbromal and meprobamate were determined by gas liquid chromatography[5], methaqualone by a slight modification of a thin layer chromatography [6]. CCl_4, C_2Cl_4 and thallium were measured by gas liquid chromatography.

The clearance of the charcoal column, the dialyzer and the overall extracorporeal system was calculated with the following formule :

$$\text{clearance} = \frac{C_i - C_o}{C_o} \times Q_B$$

C_i and C_o : drug concentrations at the inflow and outflow line

Q_B : blood flow = 200 ml/min.

The estimated quantity extracted by the procedure was calculated as

C_m x clearance HP-HD x t

C_m : mean drug concentration during the HP - HD treatment

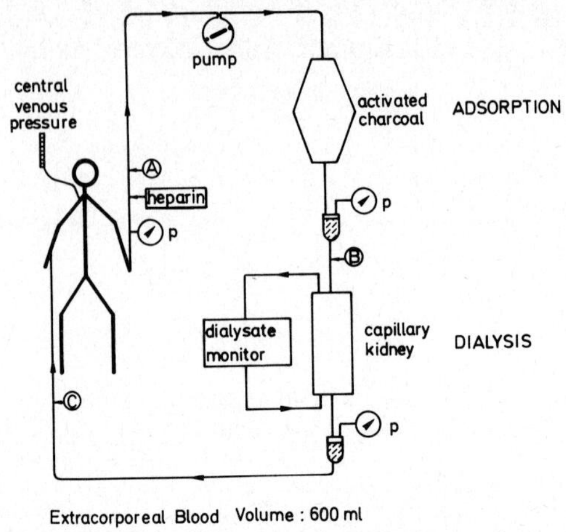

Fig. 1. Schematic representation of the hemoperfusion - hemodialysis procedure Blood samples are taken simultaneously at the points A, B and C.

RESULTS

The mean clearances obtained for the different drugs and the number of determinations and duration of treatment are listed in Table I.

TABLE I

CLEARANCE OF DIFFERENT DRUGS DURING HEMOPERFUSION (HP) - HEMODIALYSIS (HD) TREATMENT

Drug	Number of Clearance Studies	Duration of Treatment (h)	Clearance (ml/min; mean ± S.E.M.)		
			HP	HD	HP + HD
Amobarbital	8	23	122±4	17±5	129±10
Butobarbital	11	13	84±7	99±5	142±4
Hexobarbital	3	6	152	95	181
Phenobarbital	5	18	103±5	40±17	125±6
	8	23	117±3	55±9	141±3
	2	8	135	42	159
	3	7	122	-	-
Secobarbital	6	23	124±3	17±4	125±4
Carbromal	5	18	94±7	51±14	121±6
	2	8	93	-	-
Meprobamate	9	30	87±7	100±15	145±9
Methaqualone	4	20	53±4	115±8	137±5
CCl_4	4	6	55±13	10±4	59±16
	5	7	75±19	30±7	92±16
C_2Cl_4	4	6	39±4	13±6	47±5
	5	7	64±12	1±1	65±12
Thallium	5	4	133±8	47±12	150±5

Figure 2 shows the evolution of the clearances of six drugs during the treatment. For these drugs there is no tendency for lowering of the HP clearance even after prolonged treatment.

CCl_4 and C_2Cl_4 have rather lower clearances. We observed in two patients, intoxicated by a mixture of CCl_4 and C_2Cl_4, a progressive decrease in HP-clearance.

The HP clearance of thallium is three times superior to the HD clearance of this drug.

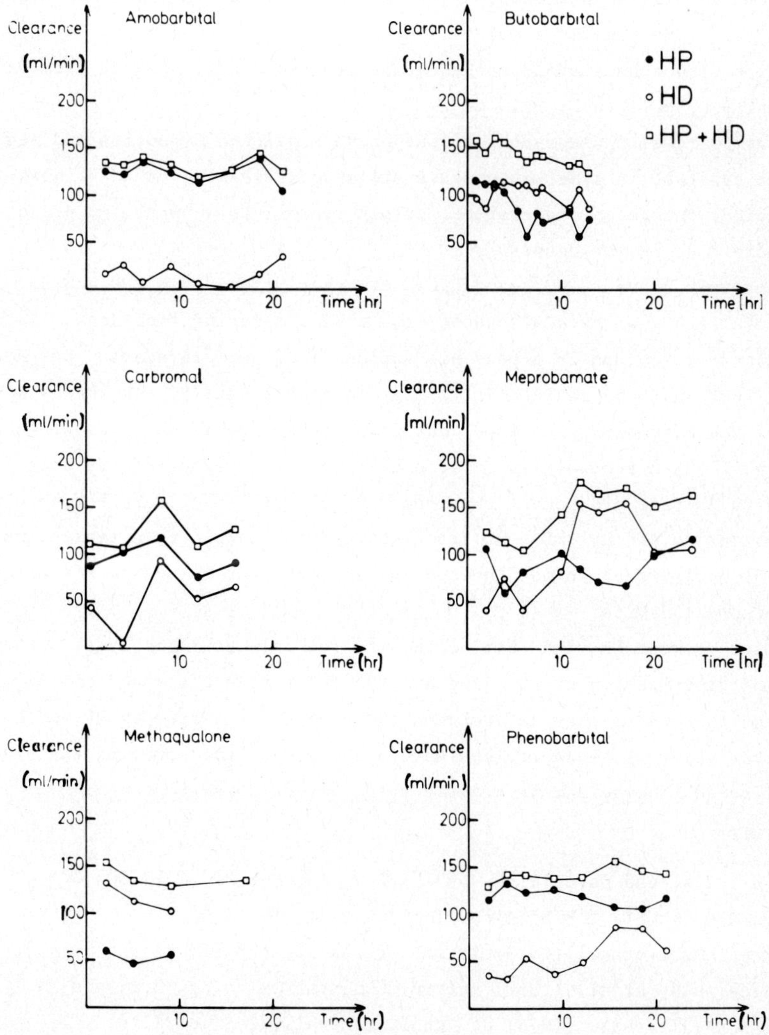

Fig. 2. The hemoperfusion (HP), hemodialysis (HD) and overall clearances (HP-HD) of six drugs are shown in function of time.

DISCUSSION

In the literature numerous reports concerning hemoperfusion and hemodialysis clearances of different drugs can be found. These clearances are however difficult to compare since they were obtained under different conditions. In this paper we report the comparison of hemoperfusion and hemodialysis clearances obtained simultaneously in the same patients for different drugs.

In the group of barbiturates the overall HP - HD clearances are rather constant ($\pm$ 150 ml/min). The respective contribution of HP and HD however is variable. In particular butobarbital and hexobarbital have high HD clearances. In most cases the clearance value of hemoperfusion are higher than those of hemodialysis. Meprobamate and methaqualone are two drugs, however, removed more efficiently by HD than by HP.

The hemoperfusion clearances of the above mentioned hypnotics and sedatives remained constant in time, even after prolonged treatment up to 30 hours. In our opinion, change of the charcoal column every 3 to 4 hours, as proposed by some authors [7], is not necessary.

The organic solvents CCl_4 and C_2Cl_4 are poorly removed by HP and HD. Moreover the clearances have a tendency to level off during treatment. Saturation of the charcoal column is a possible explanation, but degradation of the membrane that surrounds the charcoal particles is also possible. The heavy metal thallium has a good HP clearance, but is also dialyzable to a lesser extent. This high clearance however results only in a 14 % removal of the drug from the patient (a 25 year old woman, who took 100 mg thallium sulfate 5 hrs before admission) during a 4 hrs HP - HD treatment. This example illustrates the fact that a high clearance is not the only parameter determining the efficiency of an extracorporeal device.

It must be kept in mind that besides the clearance of the drug, the apparent volume of distribution of the drug and the total body clearance of the drug are also important parameters determining the removal of a drug by HP and/or HD.

Further study is needed to evaluate the value of the combined and prolonged hemoperfusion - hemodialysis treatment for severe poisoning.

REFERENCES

1. Lorch, J.A. and Garella, S. (1979) Ann. Intern. Med. 91, 301-304
2. Medd, R.K. et al. (1973) Arch. Toxicol., 31, 163-174
3. De Broe, M.E. et al. (1979) Artif. Organs, 3, 188-190
4. De Broe, M.E. et al. (1980) Intern. Congres Toxicology Brussels
5. Thomas, J.J. et al. (1978) J. Annal. Toxicol., 2, 219-225
6. Heyndrickx, A. and De Leenheer, A. (1969) Eur. J. Toxicol., 2, 56-58
7. Vale, J.A. et al. (1975) Br. Med. J., 1, 5-9

Mechanisms of Toxicity and Hazard Evaluation
B. Holmstedt, R. Lauwerys, M. Mercier, M. Roberfroid eds

PROGNOSIS AND TREATMENT OF METHANOL INTOXICATION

R.L.LINS[1], P. ZACHEE[1], M. CHRISTIAENS[1], F.VAN DE VIJVER[1], L.DE WAELE[2], P.SANDRA[3]
M.E.DE BROE[1].

1. Dept.Nephrology-Hypertension, University of Antwerp, Belgium.
2. Dept.Toxicology RUG, Gent, Belgium.
3. Lab.Org.Chemistry, RUG, Gent, Belgium.

INTRODUCTION

Methyl alcohol (wood alcohol), although a poison with high oral and inhalation toxicity, is still used in many preparations like antifreeze, paint removers, denatured alcohol and printing solutions[1].

The final outcome of the patients intoxicated with methanol is difficult to predict[2,3]. Recently the degree of metabolisation of methanol as measured by formic acid serum concentrations was proposed as one of the important factors determining the amount of the anion gap and subsequent acidosis observed in this patients, and prognosis[4].

This paper describes our own experience of severe methanol poisoning in four patients. All were treated by a combination of hemoperfusion (HP) and hemodialysis (HD).

METHODS

Methanol, ethanol and formic acid were determined in serum, erythrocytes and whole blood by gaschromotography[5,6].

Patients were treated by a combination of HP and HD as earlier described[7,8]. In this method a cellulose coated actived charcoal (Adsorba 300 C Gambro, Sweden) and a capillary kidney Nephros 16F160 (Organon Technika, Belgium) are used with a single pass delivery system, (Unimat Bellco, Italy). Bloodflow in the extracorporeal circuit was 120-200 ml/min. Blood samples for determination of methanol, ethanol and formic acid were taken before the charcoal column, between the charcoal column and the artificial kidney, and after the artificial kidney.

The clearance of the charcoal column and the dialyzer was calculated with the following formula :

clearance = $\frac{C_i - C_o}{C_i}$ X QB were C_i and C_o = drug concentration at inflow and outflow of devise, and QB = blood flow.

The estimated quantity extracted by the procedure is calculated as Cm X clearance HP-HD X t, were Cm is the calculated mean concentration during the HP-HD treatment.

CASE REPORTS

Case 1 R.S.

A 29 year old man, with known ethyl alcohol abuse for at least 4 years, is admitted after ingestion of 250 ml methanol, and an unknown quantity of ethanol. Most of the methanol was taken a few hours before admission, but drinking started 2 days earlier.

There was slight confusion, agitation and spots before the eyes. On clinical examination there was hyperventilation, blood pressure was 150/80, pulse rate was 80/min., arterial blood pH was 7.12, PCO_2 10 mmHg, PO_2 128 mmHg, bicarbonate 3.3 mEq/l, and anion gap 35 mEq/l.

Lactic acid was 22 mg/100 ml (normal value 6-16), pyruvic acid 0.4 mg/100 ml (normal value 0.4-0.6). The blood methanol level was 138 mg/100 ml, the ethanol level was 91 mg/100 ml and formic acid 33 mg/100 ml. The optic fundi were normal.

Ethanol and intravenous sodiumbicarbonate (1100 mEq in 15 hours) were administrated. HP-HD treatment was started and continued for 9 hours. The methanol level decreased to 38 mg/100 ml (T 1/2 = 4 hrs). There was complete recovery of the patient without sequelae.

Case 2 E.R.

A 29 year old engineer, with ethyl alcohol abuse since 15 years, was admitted after drinking 300 ml methanol, during a period of 3 days. On admission there was mental confusion, agitation and desorientation. Clinical examination revealed hyperventilation and tachycardia. Blood pressure was 170/95 mmHg. Arterial blood pH was 7.23, PCO_2 22 mmHg, PO_2 109 mmHg, plasma bicarbonate 8.8 mEq/l, anion gap 38 mEq/l, methanolemia 475 mg/100 ml, formic acid 81 mg/100 ml; ethanol was not detectable in the plasma.

Treatment with ethylalcohol, sodiumbicarbonate (600 mEq during the first 12 hrs) and HP-HD, during 12 hours, was started immediately. The methanol level decreased to 49 mg/100 ml. (T 1/2 = 3.2 hrs). There was complete recovery of the patient without sequelae.

Case 3 Y.B.

A 22 year old Russian sailor ingested a large quantity of ethanol, and afterwards about 250 ml methanol. Aproximately 30-35 hours later he was found unconscious. On admission he was in coma stage IV, with cyanosis, hypoventilation and shock. Pulse rate was 60/min, body temperature 31° C. Arterial blood pH was 6.66, PCO_2 65 mmHg, PO_2 75 mmHg, bicarbonate 7.5 mEq/l and the anion gap was 36.5 mEq/l.

Lactic acid was 98 mg/100 ml, pyruvic acid 0.9 mg/100 ml. The serum level of methanol was 163 mg/100 ml of ethanol 78 mg/100 ml, of formic acid 82/100 ml Optic fundi were normal.

Treatment consists of intubation, artificial ventilation, dopamine, intravenous ethanol and bicarbonate (1100 mEq during the first 24 hours). HP-HD treatment was continued during 24 hours. After 16 hours of dialysis methanolemia was zero. An isoelectrical E.E.G and circulatory arrest on bilateral carotidal angiography were noted. Treatment was arrested.

Case 4 A.G.

A 38 year old Russian sailor ingested also 250 ml methanol in comparable conditions as mentioned in case 3. His clinical condition on admission was analogue to case 3 : coma stage IV, shock, hypoventilation, body temperature 32° C, pulse rate 140/min. Arterial blood pH was 6.65, PCO_2 37 mmHg, PO_2 176 mmHg, bicarbonate 3.9 mEq.l, anion gap 39 mEq/l. Lactic acid was 97 mg/100 ml, pyruvic acid 1.2 mg/100 ml, methanolemia 167 mg/100 ml, ethanolemia 76 mg/100 ml, formic acid 59 mg/100 ml. Optic fundi showed hemorrhages.

Intubation, artificial ventilation, intravenous ethanol, sodiumbicarbonate, dopamine and HP-HD were started and continued during 24 hours. Methanolemia was zero after 16 hours. Again an isoelectrical E.E.G. and circulation arrest on bilateral carotidal angiography were noted. Treatment was arrested.

RESULTS

The pertinent clinical and biochemical data in our four patients are shown in table 1. The delay between ingestion and admission varied considerably, and was not exactly known. Total ingested amount and serum bicarbonate on admission, are comparable. Plasma levels of methanol and ethanol were in the same range in three of the four patients. The fourth patient had a serum level of methanol which was considerably higher, he took no ethanol.

TABLE 1

PERTINENT ANAMNESTIC, CLINICAL AND BIOCHEMICAL DATA ON ADMISSION

Patient/sexe	Age/yrs	Methanol ingestion ml	Time interval	Grade of coma (0-IV)	BP	PH	HCO_3^- mEq/l
1. R.S. ♂	29	± 250	a few hrs (?)	0	150/80	7.1	3.3
2. E.R. ♂	49	300	3 days (?)	0	170/80	7.2	8.9
3. Y.B. ♂	22	± 250	30 hrs (?)	IV	60/	6.6	7.5
4. A.G. ♂	38	± 250	30 hrs (?)	IV	60/	6.6	3.9

	Methanol mg%[x]	Ethanol mg%[x]	Formic Acid[x] mg%	Final outcome
1. R.S.	138	91	33 mg%	Survived
2. E.R.	475	0	81 mg%	Survived
3. Y.B.	163	78	82 mg%	Deceased
4. A.G.	167	76	59 mg%	Deceased

[x] Methanol, ethanol and formic acid concentration in the serum before start of HP-HD.

All had formic acid serum concentration clearly above 10 mg/100 ml. Optic fundi were normal or atypical. Treatment with alkali, ethanol and HP-HD was comparable in the four patients, but two died and two survived.

The combined HP-HD treatment was started since there were insufficient data on possible concomittent drug ingestion and as part of a systematic study evaluating the effect of HP-HD on different drugs. Evolution of the serum methanol levels are shown in figure 1.

Extraction during this treatment was between 50-60 mg methanol. The clearance of methanol by the charcoal column was negligible in all four cases (table 2), while the artificial kidney has a high methanol clearance value. The same results are observed with formic acid. The clearance values were only limited by blood flow in the extracorporeal circuit. The two patients who survived were followed after the initial acute phase. There were no ophtalmologic disturbances.

DISCUSSION

After ingestion, methanol is partly excreted unchanged by the lungs and the kidney, and partly metabolised to formaldehyde and formic acid[9,10].

The toxicity of methanol is considered to be due to its metabolites, explaining

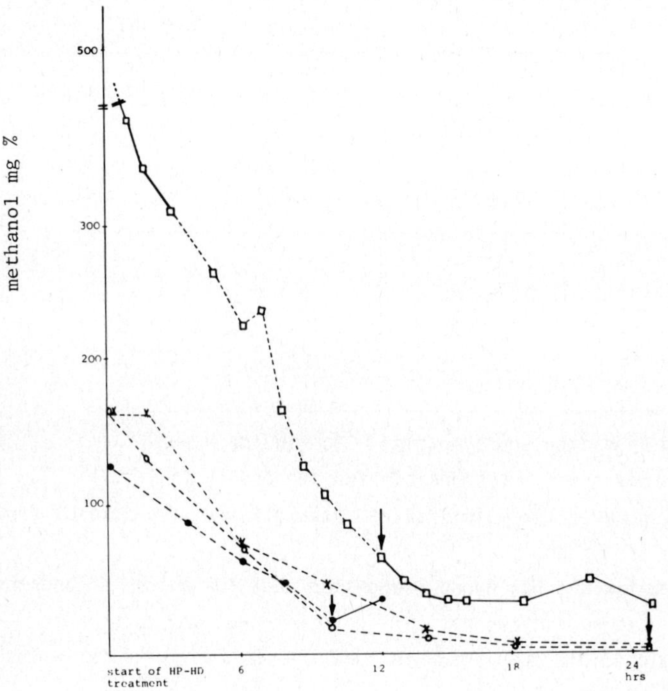

FIGURE 1

METHANOLEMIA THE FIRST 24 HRS AFTER ADMISSION ↓ = end of HP-HD treatment

●—● RS, □—□ ER, ○—○ YB, ×—× AG

TABLE 2

CLEARANCE (ml/min) OF METHANOL BY THE CHARCOAL COLUMN AND ARTIFICIAL KIDNEY

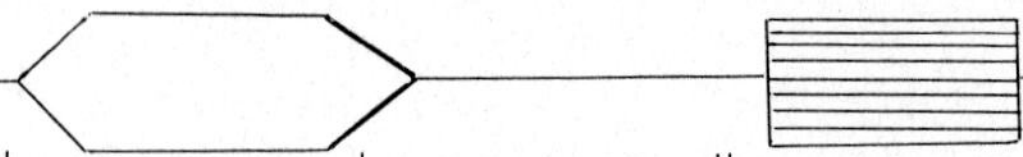

	charcoal		kidney	
	methanol	formic acid	methanol	formic acid
1. R.S.	neglig.	—	174	—
2. E.R.	neglig.	neglig.	200	77
3. Y.B.	neglig.	neglig.	150	105
4. A.G.	neglig.	neglig.	120	120

the interval between ingestion and symptoms[11-13]. In the monkey it was shown that formic acid is responsible for the ocular toxicity[14-16].

In human subjects however there is lack of information on the role of formic acid in the toxicity of methanol.

Very recently McMartin and his group[4] suggested that the anion gap and the subsequent acidosis observed in two patients with methanol poisoning was entirely due to formic acid accumulation in their serum. Our results in four patients however clearly show that formic acid is not the only factor contributing to the increased anion gap and acidosis (table 3). Even if the lactic and pyruvic acid concentrations are taken into account the anion gap is not filled up to normal values. Other factors must contribuate to this important accumulation of anions.

The degree of metabolic acidosis has been considered as an important factor determining the prognosis of methanol poisoning. Mortality has also been correlated with ingestion of more than 30 ml of methanol, blood levels of

TABLE 3

ANION GAP OBSERVED IN THE FOUR PATIENTS

Rest = Anion gap - (Lactic Acid + Formic Acid)

	Na^+	K^+	Cl	HCO_3^-	Anion Gap	Lactic Acid	Formic Acid	Rest
					mEq/liter			
1. R.S.	132	4.3	98	3.3	35.0	2.4	7.2	25
2. E.R.	137	5.3	95	9	38.3	—	17.3	21
3. Y.B.	140	4.0	100	7.5	36.5	10.8	17.7	8
4. A.G.	142	4.5	103	4.5	39	10.7	12.8	15.5

more than 100 mg/100 ml or a formic acid serum level of more than 10 mg/ 100 ml[3,4,12]. Although all this "bad outcome" criteria were fullfilled in our four patients only two died. Even the serum levels of formic acid could not be correlated with mortality. First other metabolites could be responsible for toxicity and for acidosis as is suggested by our results. Secondly, differences in further oxidation of formic acid to carbon dioxide, operating through folate-dependent reactions, are possible[17].

It is clear that irreversible brain damage can occur within 12-24 hours, with high doses of methanol. Subsequent correction of acidosis, ethanol infusion and hemodialysis can be ineffectual as is shown in two of our patients and already described by Gonda[3].

The most important factor in therapy is prompt and sustained hemodialysis, until plasma methanol level decreases below 25 mg/100 ml, combined with ethanol and alkali therapy. Hemodialysis must be started if more than 30 ml methanol is ingested, if bicarbonate is less than 10 mEq/l or methanol plasma level is more than 50 mg/100 ml. We can definitely state that the use of hemoperfusion over activated charcoal has no place in the treatment of methanol poisoning.

REFERENCES

1. Dreisbach, R.H (1977) Handbook of Poisoning, ninth edition, Lange Medical Publications, Los Altos, California, pp. 159-161.
2. Chew, W.B. et al (1946) JAMA, 130, 61-64.
3. Gonda, A. et al (1978) Am. J. Med., 64, 749-758.
4. McMartin, K.E. et al (1980) Am. J. Med., 68, 414-418.
5. Heyndrickx, A. et al (1969) Pharmac. T. België, 46, 86-101.
6. Sandra, P. Personal Communication.
7. De Broe, M.E. et al (1978) Artif. Organs, 3, 188-190.
8. De Broe, M.E. et al (1980) Intern. Congres Toxicology, Brussels 1980.
9. Bartlett, G.R. (1950) Am. J. Physiol., 163, 614-618.
10. Röe, O. (1955) Pharmacol. Rev., 7, 399-412.
11. Bennett, I.L. et al (1953) Medicine (Baltimore), 32, 431-463.
12. Cowen, D.L. (1964) Ann. Intern. Med., 61, 134-135.
13. Keyvan-Larijarni, H. and Tannenberg, A.M. (1974) Arch. Intern. Med., 134, 293-296.
14. Hayreh, M.S. et al (1977) Arch. Ophtalmol., 95, 1853-1858.
15. Martin-Amat, G. et al (1977) Arch. Ophtalmol., 95, 1847-1850.
16. McMartin, K.E. et al (1977) J. Pharmac. Exp. Ther., 201, 564-572.
17. Billings, R.E. and Tephly, T.R. (1979) Bioch. Pharmac. 28, 2985-2991.

Mechanisms of Toxicity and Hazard Evaluation
B. Holmstedt, R. Lauwerys, M. Mercier, M. Roberfroid eds

SODIUM NITROPRUSSIDE: COMPARISON OF THE ANTIDOTAL EFFECT OF HYDROXOCOBALAMIN AND SODIUM THIOSULFATE IN RABBITS⁺

J. PILL*, P. ENGESER*, M. HÖBEL*, and V.A.W. KREYE**
Department of Pharmacology*, and IInd Department of Physiology**, University of Heidelberg, D-6900 Heidelberg (Fed. Rep. of Germany)

INTRODUCTION

Sodium nitroprusside (SNP) is a powerful antihypertensive when infused iv., but may be highly toxic on overdosage since in vivo 5 CN^- groups are released from each molecule. Sodium thiosulfate (TS) by supplying sulphur for the rhodanase reaction, and hydroxocobalamin (B_{12a}) by directly binding CN^-, are potent antidotes to CN^-, and hence also to SNP[1,2,3,4]. In rabbits, we have compared the antidotal effects of TS and B_{12a} when given as bolus injections, or by infusion simultaneously with a toxic dose of SNP. For this purpose, their effect on the acid-base balance and on survival was studied.

METHODS

In heparinized New Zealand rabbits (2-3 kg b.w.), infusions and injections were made into the ear veins, and blood samples were withdrawn from the central ear artery for blood gas analyses. SNP, TS, and B_{12a} were dissolved in distilled water; in the case of SNP and TS, the solutions were corrected for crystal water, and in the case of B_{12a}, for bound water and impurities (i.e. 20% of weight; J.P. IX). The volumes given for infusions were 0.6 ml/kg·h (SNP,TS) or 2.23 ml/kg·h (B_{12a}), and those for bolus injections of TS and B_{12a} were 1.5 ml/kg.

RESULTS

Comparison of bolus injections of TS and B_{12a} in acute SNP intoxication

The infusion of 7.5 mg SNP/kg·h, i.e. the $LD_{100;61min}$[2], for 40 min led to a severe metabolic acidosis which was maximal 70 min after the start of the SNP infusion. Subsequently, those rabbits that had survived the acute SNP intoxication (4 of 7 animals) recovered gradually, but slowly, from the metabolic acidosis (Fig. 1). When 20.8 mg TS/kg, i.e. a SNP/TS molar ratio of

⁺Supported by the German Research Foundation within SFB 90 "Cardiovascular System".

1:5, was injected as a bolus immediately after cessation of the SNP infusion (min 40), the animals showed a much less marked metabolic acidosis, and recovered rapidly; 110 min after the start of the SNP infusion, pH and base excess did not differ significantly any more from the control values (Fig. 1). Higher doses of TS (1:10 and 1:20) had no greater antidotal potency.

In contrast to what would be exspected the bolus injection of B_{12a} (SNP/ B_{12a} molar ratio 1:5) had no advantage over TS as an antidote in acute SNP intoxication. Whereas the course of the pH and base excess values ran in parallel during the first 100 min of the experiment, in the subsequent phase of observation the base excess values remained considerably lower after B_{12a} than after TS (Fig. 1). When a greater bolus of B_{12a} (1:10) was injected, its antidotal effect was equal to that of TS 1:5.

Comparison of the antidotal effects of TS and B_{12a} infused together with SNP

As shown before[2], the infusion of 7.5 mg SNP/kg·h ($LD_{100;61min}$) was tolerated for 4 h without obvious signs of a metabolic acidosis when TS was infused simultaneously at a SNP/TS molar ratio of 1:5. The parallel infusion of B_{12a}

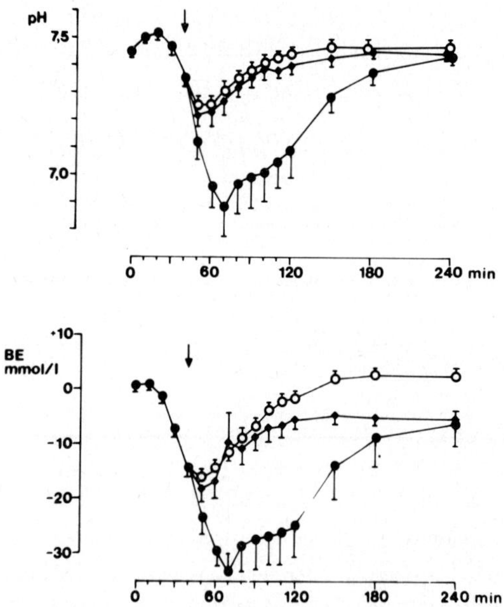

Fig. 1. Effects of bolus injections of TS (o—o ↓; 20.8 mg/kg; i.e. a SNP/TS molar ratio of 1:5; n = 6), and B_{12a} (◆—◆ ↓; 147.3 mg/kg; i.e. 1:5; n = 7) on the arterial blood pH and base excess (BE) changes induced by an infusion of 7.5 mg SNP/kg·h for 40 min. ●—● Effects of an iv. infusion alone (n = 7). $\bar{x} \pm$ S.E.

1:5 had a similar beneficial effect on the blood pH, but after 4 h, i.e. at the end of the experiment, the base excess was significantly lower than with the parallel infusion of TS 1:5 (-12.9 ± 1.0 mval, $\bar{x}$ ± S.E., n = 7; and -6.8 ± 0.8 mval, n = 10, resp.; t = 2.3041, $2P < 0.05$). In addition, 3 of 7 animals of this group died in the subsequent 24 h period suggesting that the antidotal effect of B_{12a} was inferior to that of TS. This assumption was further substantiated when lower doses of TS and B_{12a} (SNP/antidote molar ratio 1:4) were infused in parallel with SNP (Fig. 2); whereas with TS 1:4 signs of a metabolic acidosis were negligible, blood pH and base excess fell steadily with B_{12a} 1:4. A severe metabolic acidosis had developed at the end of the infusion period, and 9 of 10 animals had died during this period or the subsequent 24 h.

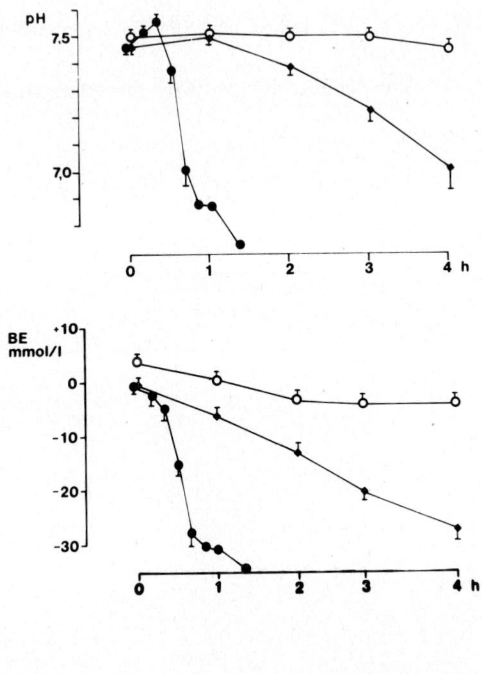

Fig.2. Effects of an iv. infusion of SNP (●—●; 7.5 mg/kg·h; n = 6) alone, and in parallel with infusions of TS (○—○; 25 mg/kg·h, i.e. a SNP/TS molar ratio of 1:4; n = 10), and B_{12a} (◆—◆; 177 mg/kg·h; i.e. 1:4; n = 10), respectively, on the arterial blood pH and base excess (BE) in rabbits. $\bar{x}$ ± S.E.

SUMMARY AND CONCLUSIONS

After the induction of an acute SNP intoxication in rabbits, the bolus injection of TS and B_{12a} at a SNP/antidote molar ratio of 1:5 was equally effective in reducing the early signs and severity of the metabolic acidosis, whereas during the subsequent observation period the base excess with B_{12a} as an antidote was found to be lower than with TS. When the two antidotes were given in parallel with a highly toxic dose of SNP, TS proved to be definitely superior to B_{12a}. We suggest that for clinical purposes, SNP should always be administered in combination with TS (1:5). Also, it would be desirable that brands of SNP-TS mixtures be marketed to make SNP a safer drug.

REFERENCES

1. Smith, R.P. and Kruszyna, H. (1974) J. Pharmacol. exp. Ther., 191, 557-563.
2. Höbel, M., Kreye, V.A.W. and Pill, J. (1978) Klin. Wochenschr., 56 (Suppl. I), 147-152.
3. Kreye, V.A.W., Raithelhuber, A. and Höbel, M. (1976) Naunyn-Schmiedeberg's Arch. Pharmacol. (Suppl), 293, R66.
4. Posner, M.A., Rodkey, F.L. and Tobey, R.E. (1976) Anesthesiology, 44, 330-335.

LEGISLATIVE, SCIENTIFIC AND SOCIOECONOMIC CONSIDERATIONS UNDERLYING TOXICOLOGY TESTING OF NEW CHEMICALS

Symposium chairmen: S.L. Friess, M. Fondu and P. Recht

© 1980 Elsevier/North-Holland Biomedical Press
Mechanisms of Toxicity and Hazard Evaluation
B. Holmstedt, R. Lauwerys, M. Mercier, M. Roberfroid eds

REGULATORY ISSUES IN TOXIC SUBSTANCES CONTROL LEGISLATION

J. Clarence Davies
The Conservation Foundation, 1717 Massachusetts Avenue, N.W., Washington, D.C. 20036

In the late 1960's both scientific discoveries and unfortunate incidents drew attention to a new type of environmental problem which acquired the label "toxic substances." The label was not very precise but generally included both heavy metals and industrial organic compounds. Toxic substances tended to differ from the more traditional environmental pollutants in several respects: they could produce adverse effects even when produced in quite small amounts; the effects were frequently long-term and irreversible; and control of toxics could not be limited to any single environmental medium because human exposure typically could occur through air, water, consumer products, or in the workplace.

The concern about toxic substances led to demands for public policies that could deal with the problem. In 1969 I wrote: "The dangers posed by chemicals and metals represent a vast, unexplored set of problems . . . what is needed is a Federal agency with responsibility for determining the health effects of all such substances, setting standards for human exposure to them, registering and approving new chemicals, and monitoring the course of such substances in the environment, thus tracing the sources of human exposure."[1] In 1969 Switzerland passed a law on trade in toxic substances. In 1970 the U.S. Council on Environmental Quality began drafting what eventually, in 1976, became the Toxic Substances Control Act.

Japan approved a Chemical Substances Control Act in 1973 and Sweden passed toxics legislation in the same year. In 1974 Canada approved an Environmental Contaminants Act, the Organization for Economic Cooperation and Development (OECD) adopted a recommendation that member states evaluate the effects on man and the environment of chemicals before the chemicals were commercialized, and the Batelle Institute in Geneva completed a study for the European Economic Community (EEC) on the feasibility of a system for evaluating chemicals before their commercial introduction. The French passed a toxics law in 1977, but delayed its implementation until 1979 hoping that it could be coordinated with action by the EEC. In September 1979 the EEC Council of Ministers finally approved a directive to the member states (79/831/EEC) regarding testing and notification of new chemicals. The directive is generally known as the Sixth Amendment Directive because it is in the form of a sixth amendment to a 1967 Council directive.

The U.S. Toxic Substances Control Act (TSCA) (15 USC 2601-2629) and the EEC directive are now the two major regulatory frameworks for evaluating new chemicals. I shall briefly discuss the provisions of each as they relate to the testing and evaluation of new chemicals.

PROVISIONS OF TSCA

TSCA is a complex law, almost 50 pages in length. Its complexity derives not so much from its length as from the intricate interrelationship among the different sections of the act. Any summary of TSCA's provisions must thus be an oversimplification.

The act covers testing and regulation of both new and existing chemicals. However, its most important goal is to generate information and take action to prevent the initial manufacture of new chemical products that would pose an unreasonable risk. "Unreasonable risk" is the criterion for most of the regulatory actions that the Environmental Protection Agency (EPA) Administrator can take under the act.

Section 5 of TSCA requires manufacturers or processors to notify EPA at least 90 days before manufacturing a new chemical. If EPA takes no action within the 90 days the chemical can be manufactured. EPA is authorized to extend the initial 90-day review period for an additional 90 days. The notification that the manufacturer or processor submits to EPA must include, insofar as such information is known to the person submitting the notice or is reasonably ascertainable: 1) the common or trade name, the chemical identity, and the molecular structure of the chemical; 2) the proposed uses of the chemical; 3) reasonable estimates of the amount of the chemical to be manufactured for each use; 4) a description of the byproducts resulting from the manufacture, processing, use or disposal of the substance; 5) estimates of the number of workers who will be exposed to the chemical and the duration of the exposure; 6) the manner or method of disposal of the chemical, and 7) a description of any other reasonably ascertainable data concerning the environmental and health effects of the substance.[2]

Under the act a new chemical is defined as any chemical substance not included in the inventory of existing substances which the EPA Administrator is required to compile and keep current. The initial inventory was published in May 1979. As additional chemicals go through the notification process they are added to the inventory so that subsequent manufacturers of the same chemical do not have to give notification. Significant new uses of an existing chemical may be subjected to the notification process, but EPA has not yet issued regulations defining what constitutes a significant new use.

Section 4 of TSCA gives the EPA Administrator broad authority to require testing of either new or existing chemicals. If he determines that a substance may pose an unreasonable risk or that it will enter the environment in substantial quantities or that there may be substantial human exposure to the substance, he may promulgate a rule requiring testing of the substance. Such a rule can cover categories of chemicals as well as individual compounds, and the categories could be based on types of uses, production volume, or other dimensions aside from chemical structure. The first Section 4 testing rule proposed by EPA proposed testing of chloromethane and chlorinated benzenes for oncogenic and teratogenic effects.

PROVISIONS OF THE DIRECTIVE

The EEC directive deals with notification and testing of new chemicals. It does not cover control of chemicals except for labeling and packaging requirements. It also does not deal with existing chemicals, and its definition of what is a new chemical and which new chemicals must meet the notification requirements differs markedly from the provisions of TSCA.

A new chemical under the directive is a chemical marketed after September 18, 1981. Whereas TSCA requires notification prior to manufacturing a new chemical, the directive requires notification prior to marketing. Thus a new chemical manufactured by a firm for its own use must be notified under TSCA but not under the EEC directive. The directive also excludes polymers and substances marketed only for research and analysis purposes. Substances marketed in quantities of less than one ton per year per manufacturer are subject to the notification requirement but are exempted from the testing requirements contained in the directive. The directive thus contains a number of important exemptions which TSCA does not. However, the directive is more encompassing than TSCA in one very significant respect. Under TSCA once a notification has been filed for a chemical, the chemical is included in the inventory and subsequent manufacturers can produce the chemical without notification. This is not the case under the EEC provisions. The directive requires that each new manufacturer of a new chemical must conform to the notification requirements. In other words, a new chemical remains a new chemical forever, unlike the TSCA system where a new chemical becomes an old chemical after it has first been manufactured.

Annex VII of the EEC directive describes in some detail the tests that must be performed on a new chemical. These include tests for LD_{50}, skin irritation, eye irritiation, skin sensitization, a 28-day sub-acute toxicity test, two short-term mutagenicity tests, acute toxicity for fish and for daphnia, and tests for environmental degradation. The tests must be conducted according to methods recommended by the competent international bodies when such recommendations exist. An escape clause from the base-set requirements is provided, the annex stating that, "If it is not technically possible or if it does not appear necessary to give information, the reasons shall be stated."

Annex VIII of the directive describes in general terms two higher-level sets of tests above the base set. Level One includes additional studies on fertility, teratology, and mutagenicity; a ninety-day or longer sub-chronic test; and a variety of additional ecotoxicology studies. Level Two includes longer-term studies on both chronic human effects and ecotoxicology. The relationship between the results of base-set testing and the need to conduct higher level tests is unclear, but each of the higher levels is conditioned on a level of production volume, the so-called "step plan." Level One studies may be required when production of a chemical by a manufacturer reaches 10 tons per year or a cumulative total of 50 tons. Level Two tests are triggered by production volume of 1,000 tons per year or 5,000 tons cumulatively.

IMPLEMENTATION OF EEC DIRECTIVE

Implementation of the EEC directive is dependent on passage of legislation by each of the nine EEC member nations. Each nation has until September 1981 to enact legislation that follows the contents of the directive.

Although the directive provides a common framework, it is likely that each national law will differ in important respects from the laws passed by the other common market countries. For example, although the directive is clearly based on notification before _marketing_, it appears likely that the Dutch will follow the example of the U.S. and require notification before _manufacturing_ a chemical. If one assumes that the directive is a set of minimum requirements, then the Dutch proposal, being more encompassing, is not a violation of the directive.

Some of the other aspects of the national legislation will also undobutedly create diviersity within the EEC. For example, the directive does not deal at all with existing chemicals. The Danish law passed in May 1979 (before final approval of the directive) states: "The provisions applying to a new chemical substance shall also apply to a chemical substance which before October 1, 1980, has been sold in or imported to this country, if, after this date, it is sold or imported for significantly altered purposes or in significantly increased quantities."[3] A parallel provision is contained in the 1977 French law. The June 1979 draft law of the Federal Republic of Germany authorizes the Federal Government to place on the same level as new substances, by means of a statutory order, such old substances and groups of substances as appear questionable with respect to health hazards or protection of the environment. It would not be surprising if each nation dealt differently with the subject of existing chemicals. There may be similar diversity with respect to the details of the test requirements, where the burden of proof lies for showing that a test is not required for a particular chemical, and other aspects of the directive. Even if the statutory language enacted by the member nations is uniform and consistent with the directive, there will undoubtedly be significant national differences in how the laws are actually interpreted and applied.

The OECD has taken a strong interest in toxics testing and control. Following a high-level April 1978 meeting in Stockholm, the OECD efforts to harmonize the regulation of toxic chemicals were accelerated. Currently they are organized into six areas: data requirements and testing methods, good laboratory practices, information exchange, confidentiality, economic and trade impacts, and development of an international glossary of key terms. The testing methods work is being done by six expert groups under the leadership of individual member countries. These are: physical-chemical properties (Germany), ecotoxicology (Netherlands), degradation/accumulation (Japan/Germany), long-term toxicology (U.S.), short-term toxicology (U.K.) and step-sequence testing systems (Sweden). Each of the first five expert groups has completed a draft report, and these reports are now being circulated for comment. It is likely that the results of the OECD testing efforts will be used by all or most of the EEC nations in implementing their versions of the EEC directive. They will also have a direct impact on the implementation of TSCA.

IMPLEMENTATION OF TSCA

To date the implementation of TSCA has been largely a lesson in the problems and pitfalls of translating statutory language into practical application.

This lesson has been most vividly taught by the experience under the new chemical notification provision of TSCA, Section 5, which went into effect July 1, 1979. As of February 22, 1980, 61 premanufacturing notifications had been received by EPA. Only 29--less than half--contained any effects data whatsoever. None contained chronic studies and only 17 contained the results of short-term screening tests. Only a few of the notices contained specific information about exposure and almost none contained information about ecotoxicity. As the EPA Administrator summarized in a letter to Senator Muskie, "There is no doubt that the general lack of adequate information is contrary to the Congressional intent in passing Section 5 and that it contradicts industry's oft-expressed view of how it conducts its premanufacture activities."[4]

Despite this experience, EPA, as of April 1980, had taken no action under Section 5(e) of the act which covers notifications where EPA finds that the available information is insufficient to evaluate the health and environmental effects of a chemical. Given that action has not been taken against companies filing notifications that contain no health or environmental data, and given that the more testing a company does the more likely it is to provide evidence that a chemical poses an unreasonable risk, the act may have the effect of discouraging companies from testing new chemicals, exactly the opposite effect from what was intended.

The implementation of Section 4 of TSCA, which authorizes EPA to require testing of new or old chemicals, has been almost as discouraging. Before the EPA Administrator can promulgate a testing rule the law requires him to make a formal finding that the chemical to be tested either may present an unreasonable risk or may be anticipated to enter the environment in substantial quantities or that there may be substantial or significant human exposure to the substance. He must also find that there are insufficient data and experience to determine or predict the effects of the chemical. The agency has interpreted these findings to require, among other things, the agency to conduct an exhaustive literature search before issuing a testing rule on a chemical. The result has been that many months and as much as a million dollars may be spent to issue a rule for a major chemical. In some cases it would be less expensive for the agency to do the testing itself than to provide the support material it considers necessary to require the manufacturer to do the testing. In any case, the agency's interpretation of the law has severely limited the number of testing rules which can be issued.

The problems with Section 4 and 5 may be partially remedied over the coming months. Several efforts are underway to explore whether there is a more efficient way to issue Section 4 testing rules. With respect to Section 5 new chemical notifications, EPA has said that it will issue testing guidelines which will not be legally binding but will at least make generally known what information can reasonably be expected to be contained in a pre-manufacture notification. The agency is also preparing several 5(e) orders delaying manufacture until more information is provided. It is possible, but not likely, that the combination of testing guidelines and 5(e) actions will result in adequate notifications. If the agency ever untangles itself from the legal problems of Section 4, the Section 4 testing rules could result in more adequate testing of new chemicals, but this is unlikely to happen any time in the near future.

The best solution to the perverse incentives now provided by Section 5 may well be for the U.S. to adopt the EEC approach. This would entail a requirement for a base set of tests to be performed on new chemicals and a partial exemption from Section 5 notification requirements for chemicals initially produced in amounts less than one ton. Although logically distinct, the base set requirement and the low-volume exemption are economically, administratively, and politically inseparable. A base set requirement without the exemption would be a major impediment to innovation, would be economically very damaging to small companies, and might flood EPA with an unmanageable amount of data. A small-volume exemption without the testing requirement would be meaningless because there is nothing to be exempted from.

This solution would guarantee that at least a minimum of toxicological information was submitted for the larger volume new chemicals. It would focus EPA's attention on the chemicals likely to pose a greater risk, because the higher the production volume the higher environmental and human exposure is likely to be, other things being equal. Volume is, of course, not the only non-testing indicator of risk, but Section 4 could be used to require testing of small-volume chemicals that may pose an unreasonable risk. Finally, by making U.S. requirements similar to those of the EEC, the proposal would significantly reduce the chances that toxics regulation will interfere with international trade.

CHEMICAL TESTING AND INTERNATIONAL TRADE

Aside from new chemical notification requirements, several other aspects of chemical testing regulations pose difficult issues with important ramifications for international trade. Three issues of particular importance are control of imports, trade secrets, and determination of unreasonable risk.

Both TSCA and the EEC directive define new chemicals to include imports. To the extent that the inclusion of imports is limited to bulk shipment of chemicals these provisions do not pose any particular problem themselves. They do pose a problem when applied to the importation of goods or articles containing chemicals. On the one hand it is unreasonable and impractical to require an importer of clothing or automobiles or almost any other finished good to know the chemical constituents of the product and thus to be able to ensure that the constituents have conformed to the relevant chemical control requirements. On the other hand, to exclude imported articles from the relevant requirements would place domestic manufacturers at an economic disadvantage and would also allow the possibility that unreasonable chemical risks would be domestically introduced by imports. For example, if the U.S. did not regulate articles a foreign manufacturer could import into the U.S. children's sleepwear containing the carcinogen Tris. Not only would a significant hazard be introduced, but the foreign manufacturer might be able to sell his goods more cheaply than domestic U.S. manufacturers by using a chemical which was prohibited to domestic manufacturers.

There are no really good solutions to the dilemma of regulating imported articles. A selective approach will probably have to be adopted, requiring disclosure of certain known hazards. But a selective strategy will require close international coordination if the controls are not to be construed as barriers to international trade.

An even more acute and certainly more general disclosure problem relates to protection of trade secrets. The EEC directive only requires member states to forward a summary of the test results on new chemicals to other states and the EEC Commission. The directive also states that, "Member states and the Commission shall ensure that any information concerning commercial exploitation or manufacturing is kept secret."[5] In contrast, TSCA requires that the actual test data be published by EPA in the Federal Register, a daily government publication distributed to the public. European manufacturers are quite fearful that any trade secret information which they give to EPA will fall into the hands of their competitors. Some European manufacturers have threatened to stop exporting their products to the U.S. because of the threat that secret information will be disclosed.

The trade secret issue is very complex and affects all aspects of toxic substances control. The European governments tend to be much more sympathetic to tight protection of trade secrets than does the U.S. With respect to test data on new chemicals, the trade secret question is compounded by the question of whether subsequent manufacturers should reimburse the original manufacturer of a new chemical for use of the original manufacturer's test data. Under the EEC scheme such reimbursement is necessary, under TSCA it is not unless the testing is required under Section 4 of the act. Despite these difficulties, the problem is not intractable. It should be possible to work out a satisfactory reimbursement system. Most test data can be made public without seriously jeopardizing trade secrets, and the rights of the original developer of the data can be protected through coding or an affidavit or some other device to prevent the data from being used for regulatory purposes by other manufacturers without permission.

All of the regulatory control actions under TSCA are keyed to the existence of an "unreasonable risk," a term which the act is careful not to define. The EEC directive, being oriented primarily to notification, not control, contains no equivalent term. But undoubtedly the national laws to implement the directive will have to use some equivalent term if they are to serve the goal of actually reducing chemical hazards.

Space does not allow an adequate discussion of how unreasonable risk should be determined.[6] But it is clear that the decision to regulate a chemical must involve a balancing or trade-off between the risks and benefits of use of the chemical. It is also clear that the balance frequently will be struck differently in different nations. This may be because of differences in cultural attitudes or political pressures. It may also be because of substantive differences. Consider, for example, the benefits of DDT in a country where malaria is a major problem and DDT is the major available weapon to combat the disease, as compared with a country where DDT is used to slightly increase cotton crop yields and cotton is already produced in surplus amounts. It should not be surprising that DDT is considered essential in the first country but is deemed an unreasonable risk in the second country.

International uniformity in defining unreasonable risk and in many other aspects of toxics control is unreachable and probably undesirable. But international cooperation and communication are essential. Toxics laws in all the industrialized nations are at an early stage, and both TSCA and the EEC directive will evolve in perhaps unforeseeable directions in the coming months and years. But it is amply clear now that Europe and the U.S. have much to learn from each other in dealing with chemical regulatory issues. A process of mutual learning and adjustment is necessary if adequate control of toxic substances is to be achieved.[7]

NOTES

1. Davies, J. Clarence, The Politics of Pollution, first ed. (New York, Pegasus, 1970), pp. 198-199.
2. TSCA, Sections 5(d)(1) and 8(a)(2).
3. Denmark, Act. No. 212 of May 23, 1979 on Chemical Substances and Products, Section 11, subsection 3.
4. Letter from Douglas M. Costle to Senator Edmund S. Muskie, March 18, 1980.
5. Article 7, Section 3.
6. For the author's views on the subject see Davies, et al., "Determining Unreasonable Risk Under the Toxic Substances Control Act," Washington, D.C., The Conservation Foundation, 1979.
7. For further elaboration of the issues covered in this paper see Gusman, et al., "International Issues in Notification and Control of Chemicals," Washington, D.C., The Conservation Foundation and The Institute for European Environmental Policy, 1980 (forthcoming).

© 1980 Elsevier/North-Holland Biomedical Press
Mechanisms of Toxicity and Hazard Evaluation
B. Holmstedt, R. Lauwerys, M. Mercier, M. Roberfroid eds

TIER TESTING SYSTEMS IN TOXICOLOGY AND DECISION-MAKING CRITERIA FOR THEIR USE

B. D. ASTILL, H.B. LOCKHART, J. B. MOSES, A. NASR, R. L. RALEIGH, and C. J. TERHAAR

Health, Safety, and Human Factors Laboratory, Eastman Kodak Company, Rochester, New York 14650, U.S.A.

INTRODUCTION

There is a clear and pressing need for schemes that organize, relate, and evaluate information about chemical hazards to health and the environment in a systematic manner. Such schemes should identify the types of information needed to evaluate the hazards involved, and should enable the user to select the types of testing needed to define the hazard. The schemes should also relate intended uses to testing requirements, and should provide some means for the user to decide when information or testing is sufficient. In particular, such schemes should be free from mandatory requirements; rather, they should allow for judgment in the selection of appropriate tests. Any scheme evolved to meet these needs should also permit the prediction of likely testing requirements from an inspection of the available information, even though the information may be incomplete or fragmentary.

A scheme for the evaluation of chemical hazard to health and the environment attempting to meet these requirements, is presented in this article. The scheme sets up four basic categories requiring information. Within each category, criteria are established to define that category. Each criterion is evaluated numerically. By summing the numerical values within a category, scores for the four basic categories are obtained. The scores are combined to yield final scores for Health Hazard and for Environmental Hazard. These scores are then used as decision points or triggers in a hierarchical assembly of health and environmental tests. A final score can be used as a guide to determine if the existing information is adequate to define the hazard, or if more testing is required. The final score also indicates what the extent of additional testing might be. Inherent in the scheme are requirements for information so that judgments can be made about the most appropriate tests within a level of testing. On completion of any additional testing, the scheme provides for re-evaluation to confirm the original score or to obtain a new one. Thus, a decision can be made to test further, or to establish that the available information is sufficient for evaluation.

CATEGORIES AND CRITERIA

The Toxic Substances Control Act provides a useful guide to the categories of importance in making risk assessments. Four categories of information as required in this scheme are:

M_H - The Magnitude of health exposure

M_E - The Magnitude of environmental exposure

E_H - The Effects of an exposure on human health

E_E - The Effects of an exposure on the environment

Categories M_H and M_E may be regarded as approximations to the dose, or exposure concentration. Criteria for these categories should, therefore, be chosen to define these entities in a usable manner. It is desirable to introduce quantification for these criteria such that a rating of intensity or severity can be made. Summation of such ratings provides a total score for a category. One useful numerical rating system relies upon two boundaries; the upper boundary defines the lower maximum intensity limit for a criterion and the lower boundary defines the upper minimum limit. These boundaries establish a rating system of three levels of "intensity", 1, 2, and 3 in ascending order.

The criteria chosen to define the magnitude of the health exposure are summarized in Table 1.

The quantity of a chemical manufactured annually is of significance because it represents the maximum possible amount to which a population may be exposed. The boundaries selected for quantities manufactured are realistic in terms of annual production volumes in the chemical industry. The second M_H criterion uses a lower boundary of 1,000 and an upper boundary of 1,000,000 for people exposed. These values approximate the range of population size between a moderate sized industrial plant and a large city. A lower score for a smaller number of people exposed does not imply a lesser degree of concern for the individual who is a member of a small population. In a large population there is greater opportunity for variations in susceptibility, and in some cases it is not possible to control exposures to a chemical as well as for a small population. The level of information needed to determine the hazard is thus greater for a larger than for a smaller population.

TABLE 1

CRITERIA FOR MAGNITUDE OF HEALTH EXPOSURE (M_H)

		Rating
Production in pounds*/yr	$<1 \times 10^6$	1
	$1 - 100 \times 10^6$	2
	$>100 \times 10^6$	3
Number of people exposed	<1000	1
	$1000 - 1 \times 10^6$	2
	$>1 \times 10^6$	3
Duration of exposure	<200 hours/yr	1
	200 - 2000	2
	>2000	3
Populations exposed: In-plant or manufacturing; consumer; general public:		
	Single population	1
	Two populations	2
	Three populations	3

*lb x 0.45 = kg

The lower boundary for duration of exposure reflects the situation of an individual in the workplace; 200 hours would be four consecutive weeks of working day exposure. The upper boundary for duration of exposure reflects the difference between an individual in the workplace and a consumer or member of the general population. Finally, three distinct populations can usually be identified with regard to the manner of exposure and the extent exposure can be controlled. These are: 1) a single working group in a single factory, 2) two or more work populations, and 3) the general public. The preceding criteria can be applied to each of these population groups, and indeed, each could be treated as a separate category.

The criterion chosen to define the magnitude of the environmental exposure are summarized in Table 2. The boundaries chosen for amounts discharged are at least an order of magnitude lower than those chosen for annual production volume. This reflects the consideration that, in general, chemicals are produced to be used rather than to be wasted. The lower boundary for the number of sites of discharge reflects the possibility of one manufacturer with a number of plants handling a given chemical, or of a small citys discharge situation, or one chemical used by a limited number of manufacturers. The upper boundary reflects the discharge situation for a chemical used over a fairly wide geographical area. The frequency of discharge distinguishes between an infrequent or sporadic occurrence for the lower boundary, and a common occurrence for the upper boundary.

TABLE 2

CRITERIA FOR MAGNITUDE OF ENVIRONMENTAL EXPOSURE (M_E)

		Rating
Amount discharged in pounds*/yr	$<1 \times 10^5$	1
	$1 \times 10^5 - 5 \times 10^6$	2
	$>5 \times 10^6$	3
Number of sites of discharge	<25	1
	25 - 2500	2
	>2500	3
Frequency of discharge in times/yr	<5	1
	5 - 25	2
	>25	3
Dwell time after discharge Half-life in days	<1	1
	1 - 7	2
	>7	3

*lb x 0.45 = kg

In addition to criteria establishing quantity, extent, and frequency of a discharge, an important additional concern is the length of time a chemical may remain in the environment. A criterion for duration or dwell time, expressed as half-life in days, is included to meet this concern. Boundaries are chosen to reflect the distinction between readily degradable or transformable substances and those showing a considerable environmental stability or persistence.

A scoring system for health effects based on assessments of specific effects, such as hepatotoxicity, mutagenicity, and neurotoxicity, is too complicated to be readily usable. The criteria should be stated in general terms, and those selected are summarized in Table 3. The rat oral LD_{50} was selected since it is clearly desirable to know the lethality of a chemical, and the oral LD_{50} is the basis of some commonly used classifications of relative toxicities. The lower boundary for the LD_{50} defines a "highly toxic" substance, and the upper boundary is a commonly accepted value for substances of moderate or little lethality. It is convenient to distinguish between immediate and prolonged effects in assessing the health effects of chemicals. Immediate effects are those following an exposure within a short time. The amount of exposure may range from a low dose or concentration to an acute non-lethal dose. Prolonged or delayed effects may result from a single or a few short duration exposures, or may result from continuous or prolonged intermittent exposures.

TABLE 3

CRITERIA FOR HEALTH EFFECTS (E_H)

		Rating
LD_{50} (P.O., rats) mg/kg	> 500	1
	50 - 500	2
	< 50	3
Immediate effects	None	1
	Reversible	2
	Irreversible	3
Prolonged effects	None	1
	Reversible	2
	Irreversible	3

A further distinction can be made between reversible and irreversible effects. The boundaries for the effects criteria are between no effects and reversible effects, and between reversible and irreversible effects. A chemical would receive a rating of 1 in the absence of any effects. If the effect produced was a moderate skin (or eye) irritation, the rating for immediate effects would be 2, since irritation is usually reversible. If destructive skin or eye damage occurred, the rating for immediate effects would be 3. Similar considerations apply in rating prolonged systemic effects.

The criteria for the effects of chemicals on the environment define areas that have become, by consensus, of the most concern. These are summarized in Table 4. The compatibility of a chemical with secondary waste treatment may be considered the chemical's effect on the performance of secondary waste treatment micro-organisms. A quantitative measure of this effect, referred to as the 5-hour IC_{50}, is the concentration of test chemical inhibiting metabolic rate of such micro-organisms by 50 percent in five hours. Experience with this test has provided an upper boundary of 5,000 mg/l for chemicals producing essentially no effect, and a lower boundary of 250 mg/l for those chemicals producing marked effect on waste treatment micro-organism metabolism.

The criterion for aquatic toxicity is derived from the aquatic concentration lethal to 50 percent of the test species in 96 hours (96 hr. LC_{50}). The boundaries chosen are 100 mg/l for substances not likely to be lethal to fish, and 10 mg/l for substances highly lethal to fish.

An adequate indicator of bioconcentration potential may be provided by the octanol/water partition coefficient of the chemical. Boundaries for this criterion are 100 for chemicals of little or no bioconcentration potential, and 10,000 for chemicals of considerable bioconcentration potential.

TABLE 4

CRITERIA FOR ENVIRONMENTAL EFFECTS (E_E)

		Rating
Compatibility with waste treatment, five hour IC_{50}, mg/l	>5000	1
	250 - 5000	2
	<250	3
Aquatic Toxicity (fish) LC_{50}, mg/l	>100	1
	10 - 100	2
	<10	3
Bioconcentration Potential (octanol/water distribution coefficient)	<100	1
	100 - 10,000	2
	>10,000	3

The collection and assessment of the above information and the assignment of scores is facilitated by using a worksheet. The worksheet lists the various criteria and provides spaces for their tabulation and rating. Summation of ratings then gives the final health and environmental scores. The worksheet allows the user to estimate ratings regardless of the quality or availability of information. The value of a final score is considerably enhanced when precise data on use of a chemical and its biological effects are available. Predictions from chemical structure, human experience, and professional intuition aid in the evaluation worksheet for screening purposes, and for guidance to the type of testing that may be needed. The worksheet is also a useful checklist for required information. The final summed health and environmental scores as decision points in a testing scheme will be described later.

HIERARCHICAL TESTING

Several levels of information and testing are necessary for health and environmental hazard assessment and these are listed in Table 5.

Baseline information is obtained before any program of testing is started. This information includes approximations of the quantities manufactured and disposed, product application and function, and the type, extent and duration of exposure in scoring for M_H and M_E. The completeness of such information will usually depend on the stage of development or use of the product.

Baseline information also includes biological and environmental activity estimated from inspection of the chemical structure. While quantitative structure activity relationships are presently restricted to a few areas of pharmacological activity, a number of general relationships are accepted. Baseline information also includes the results of the literature searches for health, biological and environmental effects.

TABLE 5

INFORMATION AND TESTING LEVELS

Base Line Information

- Quantities manufactured and disposed
- Exposure estimates
- Product function and application
- Structure activity correlation
- Literature search

Level I
- Physicochemical information
- Health and environmental screening

Level II
- Basic toxicology and environmental tests

Level III
- Subacute exposures and intermediate environmental testing

Level IV
- Long term health and environmental effects

In some cases baseline information may be complete enough for hazard assessment, particularly where previous toxicity studies are available from the literature. Where biological testing is indicated, tests to be considered are most conveniently arranged in three levels:

Level I: Physicochemical Tests and Health and Environmental Screening

This level of testing is conveniently divided into physicochemical and biological testing. Physicochemical screening tests include descriptions of physical state, fundamental properties of the molecule including but not restricted to molecular weight and melting point, solubilities and reactivity as expressed by pH and pKa, corrosivity, and purity. It is prudent to perform physicochemical and biological testing with properly characterized materials similar to those intended for use in commerce. The tests in Level I are neither mandatory nor comprehensive; the selection of tests should depend on the test chemical and its proposed uses.

Commonly selected health and environmental screening tests are the range finding LD_{50}, skin, and eye irritation, fish LC_{50}, and the BOD_5/COD ratio.

The baseline information and the health and environmental screening in Level I may provide adequate data for assessments of the hazard for relatively small volume chemicals, and for chemical intermediates that are not isclated.

In particular, when a chemical used in commerce is completely enclosed for its function, information obtained up to and including Level I may be sufficient for risk assessment.

Level II: Basic Toxicology and Environmental Tests

This level of testing is intermediate between acute tests and subchronic or 90-day feeding studies, and also provides more precise environmental information. Examples of these tests are summarized in Table 6. One or more of these studies should be based on the type of exposure anticipated.

TABLE 6

LEVEL II: BASIC TOXICOLOGY AND ENVIRONMENTAL TESTS

Basic Toxicology Testing

- (Level I plus 2 week feeding or inhalation with clinical chemistry, hematology and pathology)
- Repeated skin application test

In vitro mutagenesis battery

Environmental Tests

- Activated sludge effects
- Photodegradation $T_{\frac{1}{2}}$
- Biodegradation $T_{\frac{1}{2}}$
- Plant growth and germination effects
- Octanol/H_2O and Soil H_2O Partition Coefficients

Level III: Subchronic Exposures and Intermediate Environmental Testing

Suggested health effects and environmental tests at level III are summarized in Table 7.

TABLE 7

LEVEL III: SUBCHRONIC EXPOSURES AND INTERMEDIATE ENVIRONMENTAL TESTING

Health Effects

- Ninety-day rodent feeding or inhalation study
- Fertility studies
- Teratology
- $T_{\frac{1}{2}}$ in rodents; metabolites

Environmental Effects

- Nitrification inhibition
- Algal toxicity
- Fourteen to twenty-one day biodegradation
- Short term simulated fate study
- Egg-fry (larval) fish studies
- Bioconcentration factor

Level IV: Long-Term Health and Environmental Tests

The final level of testing includes biological and environmental tests that may be recommended for evaluation of high volume compounds of widespread dispersion. These suggested studies are summarized in the following Table.

TABLE 8

LEVEL IV: LONG TERM HEALTH AND ENVIRONMENTAL EFFECTS

Health Effects

- Two-year rodent study
- Three-generation reproductive performance
- Teratology
- Pharmacokinetics in test and target species

Environmental Effects

- Biodegradation products identification
- Soil interaction tests
- Long-term aquatic studies

It is clear that tests selected from Level IV may require a substantial commitment of resources and time. A sequential scheme of the type described in this article provides information that could be of great assistance in deciding whether to perform Level IV tests. Level IV testing is presumably most appropriate when the use of a material in commerce is so widespread that there is a need to be certain that such use is not a matter of concern to health or the environment, or that such testing will enable conditions of use to be properly defined.

It should be emphasized here that none of the tests at any level of testing is mandatory. Only the most appropriate test(s) should be made. Other more appropriate tests may be made at the discretion of the investigator. All available baseline data and prior information should be used to make decisions regarding the appropriateness of planned studies.

DECISION MAKING

This scheme divides the process of hazard assessment into two parts, i.e. tabulation and organization of information and data and hierarchical ordering of tests for environmental and health effects. The key requirement is, therefore, the relation between the numerical scoring of the data and the four levels of testing. The following relationship between scores and levels of testing was derived by the process of trial and error.

Level of Testing	Sum of Health or Environmental Score
I	Less than or equal to 9
II	10 - 13
III	14 - 17
IV	Equal to or greater than 18

The health or environmental score may be used independently tc arrive at a level of testing. For example, it is possible to have a health score of between 10 and 13 and an environmental score of greater than 18. Under such circumstances the level of testing for health effects would be II, and for environmental effects would be IV.

The apparent discrepancy in boundaries for each level of testing, e.g.for Level I is 9 and the lower level for Level II is 10, is deliberate. The discrepancies were introduced to permit judgment in selecting the test level, since in fact, there may not be clear-cut distinctions between levels of testing. Assignment to a level by a score does not imply all tests in that level would be required, but they should be selected as appropriate to the use or discharge of the chemical in question.

The scheme is employed for hazard assessment in the following manner:

(i) Assemble information

(ii) Tabulate and rate information using a worksheet

(iii) Obtain scores for health or environmental categories by summation of ratings

(iv) Apply scores to obtain testing levels for health and environment

(v) Select and perform appropriate tests and evaluate the results

(vi) Tabulate results of testing and obtain revised ratings

(vii) Obtain new scores, and

(viii) Reassess level of testing

The flow-chart indicates a suggested use of the scheme for premanufacturing notification under Section 5 of the U.S. Toxic Substances Control Act. For example, steps (i) through (iv) above may place the chemical in Level II. Examination of Level II may indicate that information from certain tests may be needed to complete the assessment. If on completing the tests the score still remains within the boundaries for Level II, a judgment may be made that the information on health and environmental effects would be adequate for premanufacturing notification purposes. Alternatively, the results of testing may take the new score outside the upper boundary of Level II. In that event, additional tests may need to be selected. The flow-chart can be used independently for health or environmental scoring.

COMMENTS

Experience with a very wide range of industrial chemicals has shown that a scheme of this type possesses a number of useful attributes. It is first and foremost an organized and systematic way to evaluate exposure, effects, data, and information. In addition, it provides a quantitative assessment of the criteria involved, not encumbered by complicated systems of weighting for various factors. In this sense a score for health or environment is readily broken down into identifiable components.

The scheme is readily adaptable to information retrieval systems, and corresponding modifications or changes in criteria ratings are easily interpolated. The scheme relates the type and scope of testing to conditions of use, exposure, and disposal, and permits for flexibility in judgment in the selection of testing. While the scheme separates health and environmental testing, it requires that health and environmental concerns be examined at the same time. The scheme is a valuable adjunct in integrating testing requirements with research and development needs since it yields early identification of testing needs. It is of particular value in both cost and time control because it can be used to prevent unnecessary or inappropriate testing. By the early assessments of toxicity, the scheme is of value for chemicals under investigation for research and development. Chemicals which may pose a high degree of potential hazard can be identified early so that the selection of feasible substitutes can be initiated. As indicated, the scheme can be used to respond to changes in production volume or discharge pattern since testing levels can be reassessed under changed conditions. The scheme also distinguishes between unisolated intermediates, isolated intermediates, final compounds and manufacturing processes in the selection of appropriate testing.

DECISION MAKING FLOW CHART

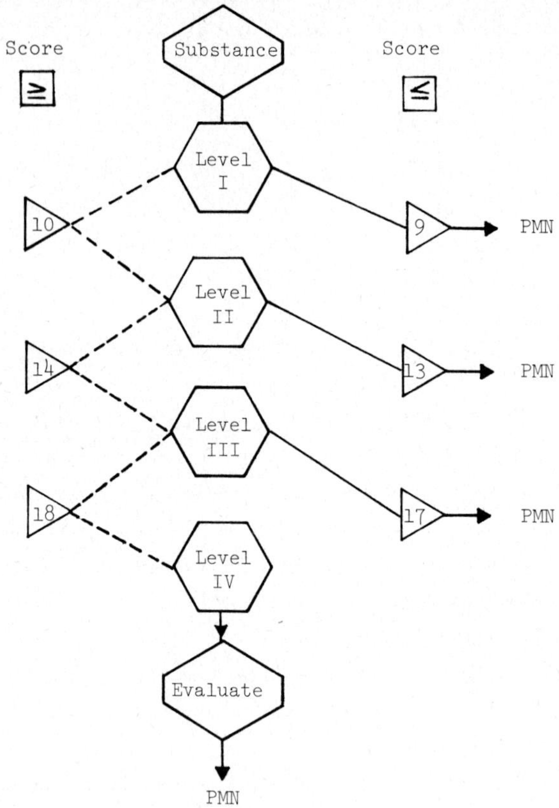

PMN = Premanufacturing Notification

This paper is based in part on Astill, B.D., et al., "Sequential Testing for Risk Assessment", Environmental Risk Analysis for Chemicals, R. A. Conway, Ed., Van Nostrand Reinhold Co., 135 West 50th Street, New York, N.Y. 10020 (to be published in 1980).

Mechanisms of Toxicity and Hazard Evaluation
B. Holmstedt, R. Lauwerys, M. Mercier, M. Roberfroid eds

TOXICITY TESTING, HAZARD ASSESSMENT AND DATA QUALITY ASSURANCE FOR CHEMICAL REGULATORY PURPOSES

PETER R. B. NOEL
Huntingdon Research Centre, Huntingdon, England.

During the last 30 to 40 years, there have been phenomenal developments in at least parts of the chemical industry, as a result of basic research, development, production techniques and marketing. At the same time there has been an increasing awareness of associated risk to (mainly) human beings and, therefore growing demands for greater assurance of reasonable safety.

The assessment of safety has, I suggest, gone through three phases of development to date. Firstly, there was a period of *increasing awareness*, when highly reputable companies began testing their products for safety and toxicity (and the first governmental intervention occurred through the FDA). The second phase was precipitated by the after-effects of thalidomide when, perhaps by *public intervention*, governmental authorities were established to make independent assessments as to whether products should be marketed or not. These authorities were expected to review the then "present state of the art" and indicate to the industry how its assessments would be made and, therefore, indirectly the investigational work that had to be undertaken (i.e. Guidelines). Finally, we have entered the third phase, which may kindly be described as one of documentary *quality assurance*. The latter phases appear to have originated from overt *mistrust*.

The three phases are not clear-cut because (a) superimposed on all phases has been the emphasis of criticism of animal studies without attempted appreciation of the end results in practice and, in more recent times (b) the increasing awareness of indirect risk through environmental contamination

Mistrust. One fundamental premise of "the scientific method" is that all experimental work should be reproducible. The object is to eliminate the effects of chance or spurious findings, as well as protecting the reputation of "scientific proof". This led to the development of "Scientists" who jealously guarded their personal reputations. There was a tendency, therefore, to assume that any criticism was directed at individuals and suggested lack of integrity.

With the advent of *commercial research*, criticism tended to be transferred to the organisations having a vested interest in the results of the research.

A type of *general suspicion* of impersonal bodies materialised.

During phase 2, when rapid expansion of safety testing occurred, there followed an immigration into industry of medical personnel (to anticipate assessment of clinical risk); veterinarians (to assure health and protection of animals) and other specialists, who were in part responsible for the emergence of Contract Research Organisations. Such persons added an element of *professional independence*. Apparently, however, general suspicion must have grown into mistrust, particularly by those most involved in decision making, till a point was reached when they were waiting for some incident to precipitate an attempt to assure quality by enforceable means. The attempt is being made now, despite the fact that all parties are aware that *true quality is not enforceable*.

There is another face to the mistrust-coin which has been highlighted to a lesser degree, which is the mistrust of governmental authorities by industry. This, again, is based on suspicion that however reasonable may be the intentions of governmental authorities, in practice they treat "guidelines" as "regulations" and, therefore, act with unjustifiable rigidity. In this respect each country has its own problems but the end results are similar in placing industry at a disadvantage; hence the cry for unified testing requirements, and unified methods of safety assessment. Fulfilment of such demands will not, however, be sufficient unless accompanied by an openness, frankness and consultative attitude, between governments, between governmental bodies and industry, and within industrial organisations themselves.

TOXICITY TESTING

Two completely separate questions exist: (1) What testing should I do? and (2) How should I do it? The latter involves what is now called *Good Laboratory Practice* (GLP). As regards this aspect, I would like to make the following personal observations:

(i) FDA Activity

Having 'lit the fuse' it must be recognised that the FDA positively contributed to the future methodology of safety testing by introducing its "GLP Proposals" (Federal Register, November 1976). Initially, this document appeared to contain revolutionary ideas but, with hindsight, was remarkably restrained. Having established its main principles, it then discussed with, and listened to, those who would be involved. Having completed a basis for operation, it then set up a means of ensuring compliance. After a trial period, there resulted the only set of *Regulations* (Federal Register, December 1978) associated with a national agency, which was enforceable through a system which appeared to work.

(ii) Other Proposals

Initial criticism of FDA Proposals was concerned with the vagueness of wording and, therefore, fear of misinterpretation. The subsequent appearance, however, of more detailed proposals clearly demonstrated the advantage of flexible wording. Of the recently produced Proposals, those that I personally found to be most readable and satisfying came from *Canada*.

I believe that the point of greatest importance in these Canadian "GLP Standards" is that they apply to the testing of ALL CHEMICALS.

(iii) OECD Proposals

These, I believe, require particular attention, as they represent a reasonable basis for unified, *International GLP Guidelines* which, hopefully, may be ratified by individual governments without change.

(iv) *Test Guidelines*

Amongst recent Proposals are also guidelines apparently concerned with: "What should we do?" These relate mainly to industrial and environmental chemicals. Many parts of these proposals are detailed, with details varying from one set of documents to another. Most take into account the newness of safety testing to this part of the chemical industry. Disturbing, however, is the apparent inclusion of (a) fairly detailed protocols for certain types of study, and (b) procedural details which would more correctly be included in Good Laboratory Practice guidelines.

If it is believed that there are general principles which are applicable to the toxicity and safety testing of all chemicals, then I suggest that great attention should be paid to these "test guidelines" and every opportunity should be taken of responding to governmental authorities and pressurising for international agreement, perhaps through national representatives to OECD. (Unfortunately, from the only draft of such studies that I have seen to date from OECD, there seems to be uncertainty as to how to present the advisory document and how complete or definite should be its recommendations).

HAZARD ASSESSMENT

Decision making. The task of *making a decision* as to whether or not any particular chemical should be allowed to enter the human environment is now largely in the hands of *governmental authorities*. The decision has to be made when all experimental work has been completed and only documentary evidence exists. This evidence is in the form of: (i) *reports* on studies undertaken, (ii) documentation produced at the time of experimentation (*raw data*) and (iii) *co-ordinating data* which links together the various parts. The linkage will suggest possible interpretations, (a) of parts of reports/submissions, by placing data obtained into the context of what is normal in a particular laboratory, and (b) of the whole submission, by associating background knowledge, type of chemical, chemical properties to the result of *in vitro* and *in vivo* experimentation and proposed usage.

Any such authority consists of individual human beings and no one individual is likely to be expert in all aspects of a submission. The onus of providing an adequate assessment-team falls on the government concerned. Obviously, the advice of specialists must be available. Specialisation, however, narrows the field of interest and, therefore, the overall decision may be more safely left in the hands of, what I can only describe as, *experienced generalists*: those capable of taking into account various forms of bias, the limitations of experimental data, commercial objectives, background experience with similar classes of chemical and so on, in order to weigh potential benefits against risks.

The *human* element must not, however, be forgotten. The documentation with which they are faced, is usually massive in size and, therefore, the method of presentation is important. Questions may arise when reading the documents - and these should be anticipated; but not infrequently there may be no answer, no comment or the information may be elsewhere in the documentation, but not so indicated. Both searching through a large submission (to avoid being criticized for not being aware of exactly what each part contains) and requesting further information to be supplied, result in irritation to all parties and the delaying of the assessment. I suggest that the level of irritation produced, is *one measure of the quality of reports or submissions*. That such deficiencies exist can be deduced from comments in almost all GLP-documents:

e.g. Requests for *justifications*: for selection of animal species, dose levels, routes of administration, particular test procedures, etc.

e.g. Requests for *summaries, interpretation and the reaching of conclusions* for individual studies, because assessors can have no knowledge of minor differences and variations between testing facilities.

Many authorities have produced lists indicating the order in which they would like data to be presented. This is a guide and not a rigid equivalent of editorial requirements for scientific journals. Duplication of comment for the convenience of the reader is, therefore, not a sin. Jargon or ambiguous terms can be defined to aid clarity. Explanations of environmental conditions or particular situations are desirable because the assessor was not present during the experimental period.

Basic Principles. The *principles* used in making an assessment of any chemical are two-fold: (a) determine what could happen to man as a result of ingesting that chemical (*toxicity*) and (b) determine the conditions of exposure that are considered to be reasonably safe (*safety*). Taken together, a practical conclusion may be reached regarding maximum exposure conditions, which is the *hazard assessment*. To ensure that there is no suspicion of vested interest the final decisions are made by independent bodies (the authorities) but hazard assessments should be made continually throughout experimental programmes and before it is decided whether to make a submission or not. All parties are, therefore, involved.

Because we are not dealing with an exact science, another type of assessment is repeatedly necessary (to the point of making a submission): the commercial one of, immediate cost versus potential benefit or return. This cannot be ignored and will be dealt with again when considering quality assurance. It is a practical and constraining factor on purely scientific aspirations. Some of the effects produced are:

(1) The desire to know what is current thought as regards test programmes at the present time - leading to a demand for *test guidelines and their equivalents*.

(2) Acceptance in general that there is no perfect animal model. Therefore, the requirement for a minimum of two test animal species is logical. How often, however, is this the subject of criticism, but do the critics undertake metabolic investigations to decide whether there is an appropriate animal model for a particular chemical?

(3) The need to know what degree of risk is acceptable for individual chemicals - whether in terms of quantity of chemical produced per year; the emotional response to certain types of toxic effect, or the acceptance of high risk for essential chemicals such as drugs.

(4) The need to be told what is the minimum number of studies, minimum number of animal groups, minimal size of groups and minimal duration of exposure that will satisfy governmental authorities because the human population at risk is always greater than the number of experimental animals to be used.

(5) Knowledge of what importance authorities place on results relating to particular animal species. In many types of investigation, especially those which are long-term, no acceptable, logical, answer exists. Some authorities advise the use of the "rat and the dog". Others go for a "rodent and a non-rodent". All that I have met agree that there should be a means of selecting species from pharmacological and metabolic data - but no-one appears to have an overview which convinces them that the additional work undertaken would produce benefits greater than the present pragmatic method of selection.

In vitro testing and the use of non-mammalian species is highly suspect because of 'remoteness' from man. Justification for such use is, therefore, essential but extremely difficult unless a "peer review" determines value and this evaluation is accepted by authorities. Once again, therefore, there is the dilemma, with many calling for "test guidelines" and others wishing for practical/scientific evaluation. The latter has been, to date, largely in the hands of individuals and a few governmental organisations, but the increasing need for evaluation has been demonstrated more recently, by co-operative 'trials'. Such evaluations represent a new type of scientific activity, involving large expenditure with no immediate, direct return to contributors.

It is the industry who are crying out for unification of government regulations. It should be at industry-government level, that a demand is made for international investigation of test procedures (if situations such as those surrounding present mutagenicity-packages, are not to occur).

DATA QUALITY ASSURANCE

Having decided on the investigatory programme to be followed, to make a hazard-assessment, each individual study has to be undertaken. During the period of investigation, it is possible to see what is taking place at that point in time but past events, even those that occurred only a few days before, can only be determined from written or computer-stored records and the memories of those who undertook the study. The fallibility of human memory for detail needs no further comment. Whether computer-stored data is fallible has yet to be determined. The only potentially "infallible" method is documented evidence on paper or film. *Retention and preservation* of the document is, therefore, the first essential of data quality assurance.

The documented records relating to individual studies can never cover every detail and action. They are essentially a form of "note taking", which also imply that certain practices have been followed, which are "routine" for that testing facility. A second essential of data quality assurance is, therefore, the recording of such practices in the form of *Standard Operating Procedures* (SOP's). (A further essential is some form of assurance that such practices are followed).

After completion of a study, all that exists are the documentary records and certain preserved samples. The type of records kept have qualities which are unique to individual organisations and to bundle these together into book form and call it a report is clearly impractical. A separate, readable document is, therefore, required in the form of "a report" and it may be assumed that this is an accurate and complete representation of the raw data. This is achieved through another essential: *A Quality Assurance Unit*. The quality and completeness of records kept can never be determined; it is a matter of trust plus occasional checking. Some additional assurance may, however, be obtained by knowledge of, or information relating to, the *Personnel* concerned and perhaps the *Environmental Conditions* - both required by GLP.

Assurance of Quality. Assurance of quality is an immense subject in its own right, which may be (over-) simplified by separation into four aspects:

(i) Local quality control
(ii) Management commitment to producing a quality product
(iii) Guarding of scientific reputation, and
(iv) Documentary completeness and accuracy

Reference to all these aspects is evident in most GLP guidelines. The first is of concern to those with day-to-day control of laboratory activities. The second involves pride in the organisation in relation to cost. Of key importance to quality assurance is, however, the third aspect, which is the responsibility of the *Study Director*. Like other humans, Study Directors are not infallible and may have a limited expertise with regard to certain specialist aspects of individual studies. Quality Assurance therefore requires that Study Directors work as part of a *well-trained team*; have the ability to recognise their own limitations and, when necessary, will make use of *specialist/expert opinions*.

Documentary Accuracy is the foundation of GLP, on which may be built the scientific quality to be appreciated by observers. To achieve a solid foundation, GLP introduced to the Scientific Community the FDA's one new concept: the *Quality Assurance Unit:* which it defined as an individual/group, independent of the investigators, whose activities may be summarised as:

(i) Know what is going on (through Protocols and Master Schedules)
(ii) Check that what is done is that which is required to be done (through *Inspections*), and
(iii) Check that what is claimed to have been done, was done, (through *Final Report Audits*)

QUALITY ASSURANCE UNIT ACTIVITY

The QAU activities and methods used at the Huntingdon Research Centre have already been presented at another Symposium and published (Noel, P.R.B., 1979)[1]. Since that time, further experience has been gained and it is to this that I will refer here. (It should be remembered that in an organisation such as ours, the work volume in terms of number of studies is very high and, therefore, the QAU has to be relatively large, consisting of senior scientists, inspectors and clerical support, which presently totals about 15 staff).

(i) Although inspectors need not have a scientific background and may be selected for their personality and doggedness, it is essential that senior scientific staff are included in the Unit to assess the *relative importance of "errors detected"* in determining the appropriate method of ensuring correctness and follow-up. QAU activity has been welcomed by the majority of staff but will probably always remain a sensitive activity, because of a minority who dislike criticism, implied or real. (Many errors are only "apparent" but quality records or reports should remove ambiguity).

(ii) The basic activity of a QAU is essentially repetitive and thus, tends towards monotony. Any method of *introducing variety* is, therefore, beneficial. It also reduces staff turnover which is expensive in terms of time required to train and the lost efficiency during period of inexperience. Careful selection of staff is, therefore, important, especially after a short period of exposure to QAU work.

(iii) The established principle associated with the checking of microscopy data should be applied to other aspects of studies, particularly the recording of clinical signs - if an attitude is to be maintained within testing facilities that, any observation is important. Those technicians who live close to animals should be encouraged to record (sign and date) all their observations, using their own words. The animals will subsequently be examined by scientific supervisors, director or veterinarian, who collate the observations and record, in professional terms, any abnormality or diagnosis. It is the professional opinion that has to be reported subsequently - not the preliminary steps that led up to the diagnosis. Failure to include in reports these preliminary steps is, therefore, not an omission-error.

(iv) The scheduling of QAU work is not simple, and not adequately covered by the combination of Study Protocol and Master Schedule. We supplement protocols with "time sheets" which add "intended calendar dates" to the specified study events. In our experience, even this has to be supplemented or rather up-dated, nearer to each individual date, to ensure that minor rescheduling has not taken place and, therefore, the QAU staff miss an event or have a wasted journey to animal house or laboratory.

Cost of QAU Activity. On introduction of "GLP", the burning question was - How much will it cost? Although many assessments were made, I know of no reliable method that would allow such a calculation to be made. Many of the requirements involved high initial expenditure with relatively less subsequently, for maintenance and up-dating, e.g. SOP's. There were other special situations and one worth mentioning is unique to contract research organisations: the cost, in terms of time, associated with sponsor-inspections and -audits of their own studies performed on the premises of CRO's. This, of course, is additional to the normal sponsor-CRO contact concerned with scientific matters. The amount of additional time varied greatly from sponsor to sponsor depending, I believe, on how the sponsor interpreted GLP-documents. Such activity is, of course, a duplication of effort.

The presence within an organisation of an independent QAU, provides the most *easily identifiable additional expenditure* associated with the introduction of GLP. Information on "cost" is, therefore, necessary for both control and justification of such expenditure. To obtain such information, routine time-keeping (at least, over specified intervals) is considered to be essential, especially as regards study inspections and final report auditing. The data must, however, be collected under practical conditions, assuming that any deficiencies in the time-keeping system are constant, thus allowing comparison between one set of observations and another.

In recording recent information relating to HRC's QAU activities on inspections and final report audits, below - I have "misused" the data recently collected, in an attempt to indicate *actual times* and *rates of working*. It should be remembered, however, that the data is based on the total time taken to complete an activity and will thus include the effects of training new staff and also everyday practical difficulties, such as the chasing of missing documents when rat data is incomplete.

Inspections. We can now confirm that *checklists are essential* as aide-memoire, but they should not be so detailed as a - re-write of SOP's. Too elaborate checklists rob inspectors of their initiative. Secondly, total inspection of all aspects (phases) of individual studies at one time has proved to be impractical and undesirable. Three aspects of inspection techniques have to be covered: (i) observation of ongoing events and routine procedures, (ii) subsequent checking of the records relating to such observed activities and (iii) later follow-up in the same, and similar, studies of any potential errors.

Individual organisations will break down studies in different ways and the total time taken to make complete inspections of the associated events must depend on local circumstances. Inspection times for general toxicological studies have been collected, and expressed as ratios or "units of time" - each unit currently representing very nearly half-an-hour:

Pre-dosing events	1 unit
Routine animal experimentation	4 units per inspection
Laboratory investigations and records......	4 " " "
Post-mortem examinations	2 units per kill
Non-routine examinations	1 - 1.5 unit per inspection

Considering *mean total times* for relatively routine toxicological studies in a single species, the following were obtained:

4-week study	7 hours approx.
13-week "	9 hours "
26-week "	11 hours "
52-week "	18 hours "
2-year "	27 hours "

Final Report Audits. The objectives remain unchanged: the detection of errors of transcription, calculation and omission. The various steps in checking final reports have not changed, consisting firstly of assuring completeness of raw data, then subdivision of the report into parts, the checking of each part and, finally, the reporting of QAU findings on a "Report Check Form". (The last, includes recording details of individual errors).

Some parts of reports still require checking of every numerical item).

Two alternative *sample-checking* procedures are still available for use: (a) *Sequential Analysis*, the graphs being prepared from information set out by

Moroney, M.J. (1969)[2] but, in fact, this method has almost fallen into disuse because of the extra time involved in finding a number in the raw data when it has to be checked against the randomly selected value in a report; (b) *Method of British Standards Institution* (1972)[3], which allows preliminary random selection of all items to be checked with subsequent checking of each item in the most convenient order. Attempts have been made to alter the parameters associated with our selected Operating Characteristic Curve but each modification considered to date, appears to have difficulties associated, particularly when attempts are made to increase the batch size.

> Our operating parameters remain: "M. AQL = 0.4" which, in fact, is the closest to the OC curve for our selected sequential analysis. The procedure requires the checking of 315 items out of each batch of 3201-10,000 items. The acceptance rates expected for parts of reports that have 3% errors is about 1.5% but if the error rate is ½% or less, 93% would be accepted.

Our experience has shown that useful measures of QAU performance are (i) *mean time per report*, (ii) *number of hours per 100 pages* and (iii) *number of pages per hour*. Performance clearly differed according to type of study and also the size of toxicological studies. An arbitrary division of studies was made according to the size of the final report: (i) 0-100 pages, (ii) 101-300 pages, and (iii) greater than 301 pages.

Mean Times per Report:

Size Group	No. Reports	Mean No. PAGES (actual)	Mean TIME (HRS)
0-100	59	50	14
101-300	36	170	29
>301	15	700	48

Rate of Checking:

Size Group	No. Reports	HRS/100 pages	PAGES/HR
0-100	59	28.4	3.5
101-300	36	17.2	5.8
>301	15	6.8	14.6

(These figures include the checking of raw data for completeness; the division of reports into separate sections and the setting up of individual checking procedures).

Combining all the data relating to general/reproductive toxicological studies obtained from 89 recent BSI-sample checks, the overall mean results were:

(i) that it takes 2.9 hours to check 100 items, or

(ii) 34 items can be checked per hour (1.8 minutes per item).

The rate of checking *short-term studies*, generally required about 20% more time.

Comparisons between non-toxicological studies (such as metabolism, analytical chemistry, cell biology, etc.) revealed remarkable similarity to checking rates for toxicological studies:

> Comparing 27 and 59 reports respectively; 26.8 hours compared to 28.4 hours were required per 100 pages or the rate of checking was 3.7 compared to 3.5 pages per hour.

During the period analysed, the QAU was required to check one rodent toxicological report of 7,000 pages length. In this exceptional case the rate of checking was remarkably similar (within 10%) to the rate for shorter reports. It was the consistency of checking rates associated with different studies and different sizes of final reports, that gave us confidence that the information presented was of practical use.

CONCLUSION

The recent events that I have attempted to describe and comment on have, I believe, highlighted the *thought processes*, which have governed the actions of parties interested in ensuring public safety: governmental authorities, industry, testing facilities and the public themselves. If I am correct, the driving force has been - *mistrust*.

This is surely not an ideal source of motivation. That we should have reached such a state is, to say the least, disappointing. None of the parties can escape a share of the blame, because all, within recent years, have indulged in *destructive criticism* of the present-day attempts to determine risks, and assess safety.

We have to deal with an inexact, biological science. This should give an equal opportunity to criticize in a constructive way. There is some evidence at the present time that the interested parties are getting together and co-operating in a constructive manner in order to produce standards and guidelines that will be internationally recognised. Is it too much to hope, therefore, that another outcome would be the return of *trust* to the relationship between the interested parties who, in reality, *all have the same objective?*

REFERENCES

1. Noel, P.R.B. (1979). The Data Audit, Topics in Toxicology: Good Laboratory Practice, MTP Press Limited, pp. 73-93.

2. Moroney, M.J. (1969). Facts from Figures, Pub. Penguin.

3. Methods of British Standards Institution (1972). Guide to the Use of BS 6001: Sampling Procedures and Tables for Inspection by Attributes.

© 1980 Elsevier/North-Holland Biomedical Press
Mechanisms of Toxicity and Hazard Evaluation
B. Holmstedt, R. Lauwerys, M. Mercier, M. Roberfroid eds

THE INTERNATIONAL PROGRAMME ON CHEMICAL SAFETY

E.SOMERS*

WHO, Geneva

INTRODUCTION

It is self-evident that the scope and nature of our chemical environment have shown dramatic developments in the last 30 years. Some four million chemicals have been synthesized or isolated from natural products[1] : The inventory of existing chemical substances in commerce numbers about 70,000[2].
Estimates of new chemicals entering the market each year in excess of one tonne range from 200 to 1000 : it is considered that eventually 400 premanufacturing notification forms will be submitted annually under the U.S. Toxic Substances Control Act[2]. Chemical industry is a significant factor in national economies and international trade. The Secretary General of the OECD stated that in 1977 the chemical industry of member countries produced products worth over $ 300 billion.

These facts give an impression of the size of the problem. What is the impact of these chemicals on human health and the environment ? Here we have serious grounds for concern : in recent years the acute and chronic effects of chemicals have often produced drastic effects so that a succession of once esoteric chemicals have become household words in the wake of their unwelcome notoriety - dioxins, 2, 4, 5 - T, saccharin, PCBs, vinyl chloride, asbestos, mirex, mercury and so forth. Most countries have adopted systems of control, ranging from regulatory to voluntary, that attempt to cope with the health and environmental issues. The task, however, has international dimensions. Not only because the volume of trade in chemicals is large but also because a collaborative approach is needed for the evaluation of

---

* Seconded from Environmental Health Directorate, Health Protection Branch, Department National Health and Welfare, Ottawa, Canada.

the health and environmental effects of chemicals. In this manner costly duplication of national efforts to test and assess chemicals can be avoided and scarce human resources of toxicological expertise can be best husbanded.

It was with these concerns in mind that in 1977 the World Health Assembly resolved (WHA30.47) to examine the options for international cooperation with a view to accelerating and making more effective and internationally comparable the evaluation of health risks from chemicals, as well as exchanging information on new hazards, providing emergency response, and developing manpower training. Meetings of experts followed so that by 1978 the World Health Assembly resolved (WHA31.28) that to implement such a programme a Central Unit should be established at WHO Headquarters for planning and coordinating a network of national institutions that would be assigned specific tasks. It is important to note that from the outset the programme was to be based on cooperation between national institutions. In January 1979 a plan of action was endorsed by the Executive Board of WHO that established the International Programme on Chemical Safety (IPCS). The Executive Heads of UNEP, ILO, and WHO signed a Memorandum of Understanding in April 1980 whereby the IPCS became a cooperative venture of the three organizations so that the effects of chemicals on human health and the environment would be considered - for both human and non-human targets. Negotiations are currently in progress with FAO concerning their involvement. In June 1980 the IPCS became operational when the Central Unit was established at WHO Headquarters in Geneva.

Aims of IPCS

In summary the objectives of IPCS are :

i) to evaluate the effects of chemicals on human health and the environment,

ii) to develop guidelines on exposure limits of chemicals in air, food, water, and the working environment,

iii) to develop methodology for toxicity testing, epidemiological and clinical studies, and risk assessment,

iv) to coordinate laboratory testing and epidemiological studies when an international approach is appropriate ; and promote research on dose-response relations and on mechanisms of biological action of chemicals,

v) to develop information for coping with chemical accidents ; to promote technical cooperation on control of toxic substances in Member States ; and to promote training and development of manpower.

These are imposing objectives and to have any hope of success in achieving them it is essential that the necessary resources, both financial and human, are provided by Member States.

It is important to recognize that the IPCS brings together existing activities as well as initiating new ones. It is not a *de novo* activity but rather a strengthening and extension of existing work. WHO has a long and distinguished record of evaluating the safety of chemicals. For more than 20 years - in collaboration with FAO - the toxicity of food additives, contaminants, and pesticide residues in food have been assessed. In collaboration with ILO standards and permissible levels have been developed for occupational exposure. The International Agency for Research on Cancer has evaluated over 450 chemicals for carcinogenic risk to humans. With UNEP support some 17 comprehensive environmental health criteria monographs have been published (or are in press). International and European drinking water standards for chemicals were and are being developed. All of these activities will continue and be, we trust, immeasurably aided by the development of the cooperative approach under IPCS.

Organizational Structure

The relationship between the cosponsoring organizations and the managerial and advisory elements of IPCS are shown in Fig.1[3]. The key components of the IPCS structure are :

Intersecretariat Coordinating Committee
Programme Advisory Committee
Technical Committee
Central Unit within WHO
Network of Lead Institutions
Sub-network of Participating Institutions
Focal Points for IPCS

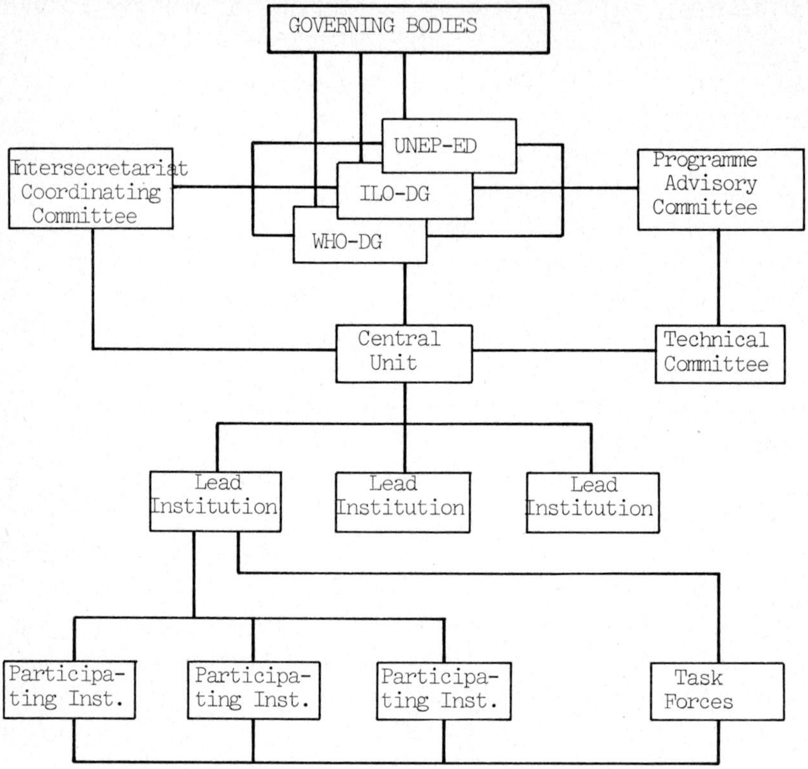

Fig.1. Joint WHO/ILO/UNEP PROGRAMME

The Coordinating Committee provides the managerial link between the cosponsoring organizations and the Central Unit. The Programme Advisory Committee advises on the policies and priorities, the work plan and budget of the IPCS while the Technical Committee, which comprises directors of lead institutions, is concerned with developing the work of the lead and participating institutions and selecting priority substances and programme topics. The latter Committee should provide the scientific leadership and direction for the programme thus ensuring that the outputs are internationally acceptable. The Central Unit is responsible for the management of the programme and implements IPCS on behalf of the cooperating organizations operating, of course, under WHO procedures. It is the nerve centre of the operation providing links, and where required support, to the programme elements.

The IPCS is based on a network of lead and participants institutions designed to achieve an organized sharing of work between different national institutions. The concept is that one lead institution should be designated - with the aid of the Programme Advisory Committee - as responsible for a particular group, or sub-group, of chemicals e.g. food colours, industrial chemicals, classes of pesticides. Lead institutions have also been designated for such activities as manpower development, emergency response, and mutagenicity testing. Internationally recognized competence in the specific field is a criterion for choice. It is implicit that lead institutions will work on those topics which are of high priority to their own governments. The relationship between lead and participating institutions will have to be developed by the Technical Committee but it may be preferable to have a flexible system whereby lead institutions co-opt participating institutions for a particular activity. The outputs from the lead institutions must be subjected to rigorous international scrutiny and evaluation as has always been the practice of the WHO Expert Committees.

Two international lead institutions have been designated. The International Agency for Research on Cancer has agreed to be the lead institution for chemical carcinogenesis, part of this work will entail an extension of the established monographs on the evaluation of carcinogenic risk, the selection of further priority chemicals, and improvements in methodology for testing chemicals. UNEP has agreed that the International Register of Potentially Toxic Chemicals (IRPTC), with the assistance of the International Referral Service (INFOTERRA) and the computerized data base of the Industry and Environment Office, should operate as the lead institution for the collection, retrieval and dissemination of information. Different operating procedures will be required for these lead institutions, which are international in authority, than for national institutions.

Regional Components

It has been intended from the outset that the WHO Regional Offices will assume a leading role particularly in the dissemination and application of results, technical cooperation, and manpower development. The European region has been particularly active for there is already in place a UNDP-supported project on chemical safety and, with the support of the Danish International Developement Agency, a joint project with Headquarters on the revision of drinking water standards. The European region is particularly interested in developing programmes on manpower training, emergency response to contingencies, and environmental health impact assessment. Other WHO regions have expressed an interest in collaborating in IPCS, in particular PAHO, and links have been proposed to the Pan American Center for Human Ecology and Health in Mexico.

Programme Outputs

Put in its simplest form : what tangible results can we expect from IPCS ? Acknowledging that some of these outputs are already extant, they can be listed :

(i) Evaluations of the health and environmental effects of new and existing chemicals : these could range from extensive monographs and criteria documents to single sheet reports,

(ii) evaluations of specific effects, such as carcinogenicity, mutagenicity, and teratogenicity, or of effects on specific organs,

(iii) guidelines on exposure limits : these can be ADI's for food additives and pesticides, or recommended levels for the working environment,

(iv) guidelines on methodology for exposure measurement, risk assessment, toxicity and epidemiological studies,

(v) information on chemical accidents, regulatory control,

(vi) response to chemicals emergencies,

(vii) advisory services for technical cooperation,

(viii) trained manpower.

Indisputably, these are ambitious goals. But the need is real and the benefits can be appreciable. An extended international evaluation of the wealth of chemicals to which we are exposed is needed by all Member States, both developed and developing. There is no doubt that for countries that cannot make such evaluations an international assessment is more acceptable than one carried out by other national authorities. The cost of testing and evaluating is so high and skilled personnel so scarce that it is incumbent on all of us to share limited resources and avoid overlap and duplication. Consistency of testing will aid comparability and acceptance of data obtained in different countries and ultimately will aid both the international trade in chemicals and the harmonization of control measures. The alarming increase in the number of accidents involving toxic chemicals demands that we all share our limited expertise and experience. The IPCS in an attempt to provide an international infrastructure to produce the outputs enumerated above.

Current Status of IPCS

The IPCS has received encouraging support from Member States. To date Canada, Japan, and Finland have signed Memoranda of Understanding with the cosponsoring organizations covering their collaboration in the IPCS and committing resources, both human and financial. Similar Memoranda of Understanding have been developed with another five countries who have made pledges in cash or kind and preliminary negotiations have been held with another six countries. Strong indications of support have been received from the Commission of the European Communities and suggestions for future collaboration with the Chemicals Programme of OECD are being developed.

With non-governmental organizations a joint WHO/SCOPE Scientific Group on Methodologies for the Safety Evaluation of Chemicals has been established. The first executive meeting will take place in July 1980 at which a study on reproductive dysfunction is to be initiated.

The Programme Advisory Committee met for the first time three months ago and determined that the highest priority objectives for IPCS for 1980-81 are : the evaluation and dissemination of scientific information, manpower training and development, and risk estimation for chemicals. Within the groups of chemicals, household products, pesticides, food additives, and industrial chemicals (particularly those in the ILO Hazard Alert System) were considered to be of immediate priority for evaluation. Lead institutions were accepted from 11 countries and the directors, or their representatives, of these institutions are to attend the first meeting of the Technical Committee in July 1980. This Committee is to develop the work plan and operation of the programme.

This, then, is where we are with IPCS. A beginning has been made to what is undoubtedly a complex and ambitious programme. Its success will rest on many factors for a nice balance will be required to achieve the desired mixture of collaboration, coordination - and perhaps even cajolery. Many disparate functions and activities will have to be knitted together. However, IPCS cannot be 'all things to all men' it must concentrate on a limited number of tangible, realizable goals. The aims and intentions of IPCS are admirable but the execution requires the support and commitment of the scientific communities in Member States. The quality of its outputs will determine whether or not that support will continue and grow.

REFERENCES

1. Maugh, Th.M.(1978) Science, 199, 162.
2. Anon.(1980) Environ.Sci.Technol., 14, 138-140.
3. Report of 1st Meeting of Programme Advisory Committee, EHE/80.10, WHO, Geneva (1980) International Programme on Chemical Safety.

Mechanisms of Toxicity and Hazard Evaluation
B. Holmstedt, R. Lauwerys, M. Mercier, M. Roberfroid eds

TOXICOLOGICAL ASPECTS OF EUROPEAN COMMUNITY LEGISLATION REGARDING NEW CHEMICALS

M.-TH. VAN DER VENNE, A. BERLIN, W. J. HUNTER, P. RECHT
Commission of the European Communities, Health and Safety Directorate, Luxembourg

I. INTRODUCTION

The sixth modification of the Directive of 27 June 1967 on the approximation of the laws of the Member States relating to the classification, packaging and labelling of dangerous substances was adopted in June 1979 by the Council which deals with new chemical substances. It is this directive that will be detailed on its toxicological aspects.

The original directive of 1967 on dangerous substances, as well as a proposal for a Directive on Major Accidents (OJ C212 of 24 August 1979) and also a Directive of the Council of 27 July 1976 (OJ L262 of 27 September 1976) relating to the limitation for putting on the market and use of certain dangerous substances and preparations, have all three underlying toxicological aspects. These are not detailed as they are for the new chemical substances and will not make part of this exposé.

2. NEW CHEMICALS

2.1 The Sixth Modification. This was approved by the Council in June 1979 and deals only with new chemical substances. The principal object of this Directive is a requirement to notify these substances to the competent authority in the Member State, at least 45 days before being placed on the market. The Commission will receive the notification dossier or a summary and will keep a list of all substances notified. The Commission also sends a copy of the notification to the other Member States. There are certain exceptions because other Community Directives apply. These are for:

- medicinal products, narcotics and radioactivie substances;
- the carriage of dangerous substances by rail, road, inland waterway, sea or air;
- foodstuffs or feedingstuffs;
- pesticides and fertilizers (as regards the notification procedure);
- substances in the form of waste;

- substances in transit which are under Customs supervision provided they do not undergo any treatment or processing.

2.2 Notification. The sixth modification establishes the principle that notification should take place in the country of manufacture or, if the substance is imported from outside the Community, in the country into which it is first imported. A notification which has been properly made in one Member State of the Community is automatically valid in other Member States. In other words, if a manufacturer or importer can show that a substance has been properly notified in the country of origin or of the first importation he is free to put it on the market in other countries of the Community. The sixth modification is thus not only designed to protect health and the environment, it is also designed to remove important barriers to trade within the Community, i.e. intra-Community trade. A manufacturer may safely project sales on a Community-wide basis without the fear that in one or more countries of the Community, his product will be blocked by regulations concerning marketing.

The notification has to include the following:

- a technical dossier supplying the information necessary for evaluating the foreseeable risks, whether immediate or delayed, which the substance may entail for man and the environment, and containing at least the information and results of the studies referred to in Annex VII (the "base set"), together with a detailed and full description of the studies conducted and of the methods used or a bibliographical reference to them;
- a declaration concerning the unfavourable effects of the substance in terms of the various uses envisaged;
- the proposed classification and labelling of the substance in accordance with the directive (Annex VI);
- proposals for any recommended precautions relating to the safe use of the substance (Annex VI).

Annex VII (the "base set") is a bundle of information which is arranged under six broad headings. the headings relate to:

(1) the identity of the substance, e.g. its chemical name, empirical and structural formula and composition, including impurities;
(2) information relating to proposed uses and estimated production and/or imports for each of the anticipated uses or fields of application;

(3) physico-chemical properties of the substance, e.g. melting point, relative density;

(4) results of toxicological studies. This is a series of tests for the assessment of acute, toxic, irritant or corrosive effects on the skin and eyes, sensitization, sub-acute effects and mutagenic effects. The acute testing foreseen includes the following points:

- Acute toxicity including LD50 derived from this acute testing via cral, dermal or inhalation administration. A minimum of two routes are foreseen for substances other than gas from one should be the oral route - the other route depending on the intended use and on the physical properties of the substance. Gases and volatile liquids should be administered by inhalation.
- Skin irritation.
- Eye irritation.
- Skin sensitization.
- The sub-acute testing is directed to a subacute toxicity 28 days.
- Mutagenicity at this level is intended as two series of short term tests - one bacteriological with and without metabolic activation, one non bacteriological.

(5) Results of ecotoxicological studies. These are for effects on organisms, i.e. acute effects on fish and acute effects on daphnia, as well as certain tests of degradation.

(6) Possibilities of rendering a substance harmless.

If it can be shown to be necessary for the evaluation of the hazard which may be caused by a substance, the competent authorities may:

- carry out such sampling as is necessary for control purposes;
- ask for further information and/or verification tests concerning the substances of which they have been notified. This may also include requesting the infromation referred to in Annex VIII earlier than provided for.

Annex VIII concerns additional information and tests. There are two levels:

- Level 1. This is for substances which reach a level for an individual notifier of 10 t/year or a total of 50 tonnes. The toxicological studies are aimed at assessing effects on fertility, teratogenic effects, sub-chronic and chronic effects, and examine in more detail mutagenic effects.

Therefore toxicological testing foresees

- a fertility study
- a teratology study
- subchronic and chronic toxicity studies
- additional mutagenicity studies linked with those already performed at the base set level.

The ecotoxicology studies are: an algal test; a prolonged test with daphnia; a test on a higher plant; a test on the earthworm; a prolonged toxicity study with fish; a test for species accumulation; a prolonged biodegradation study.

- Level 2. When the quantity of a substance placed on the market by a notifier reaches 1,000 t/year or a total of 5,000 tonnes the notifier informs the competent authority, who then draws up a programme of tests to be carried out by the notifier in order to enable the competent authority to evaluate the risks of the substance for man and the environment. The test programme includes toxicological studies that allow to watch particularly at this wide level of spreading of a chemical the following effects and more in depth when this was already considered in Level 1: chronic, carcinogenic, teratogenic effects, effects on the fertility, toxicokinetic action - acute and subacute effects in a second species.

  The toxicological studies foreseen are the following:

  - chronic toxicity study
  - fertility study
  - teratology study (both in relation to the results of the study performed at level 1)
  - carcinogenicity study
  - additional toxicokinetic studies
  - acute and subacute toxicity study on a second species when the results of level 1 indicate a need therefore.

  The following are the ecotoxicology studies: additional tests for accumulation, degradation and mobility; further bioaccumulation studies; a prolonged toxicity study with fish; an additional toxicity study (acute and sub-acute) with birds; an additional toxicity study with other organisms; an absorption-desorption study.

The authority receiving the notification has to decide on its own responsibility which information is covered by industrial and commercial secrecy. However, if a notifier considers that there is a confidentiality problem, the notifier may indicate the information which he considers to be commercially sensitive and disclosure of which might harm him industrially or commercially, and which he therefore wishes to be kept secret from all persons other than the competent authorities and the Commission. Confidential information brought to the attention either of the Commission or of a Member State has to be kept secret. Industrial and commercial secrecy does not apply to:

- the trade name of the substance;
- physico-chemical data concerning the substance in connection with Annex VII, point 3;
- the possible ways of rendering the substance harmless;
- the interpretation of the toxicological and ecotoxicological tests and the name of the body responsible for the tests;
- recommended methods and precautions.

Annex VI contains the general classification and labelling requirements for dangerous substances. The criteria for classification of the dangerous substances into very toxic, toxic and harmful is based on LD50 (oral and percutaneous) and LC50 (inhalation) values.

Category	Oral, Rat LD50 mg/kg	Dermal, rat or rabbit LD50 mg/kg	Inhalation, rat LC50 mg/1/4h
Very toxic	< 25	< 50	< 0.5
Toxic	25 - 200	50 - 400	0.5 - 2
Harmful	200 - 2000	400 - 2000	2 - 20

Reference is made also to other properties: corrosion, irritation - and effects other than acute that the testing performed in the animals according to Annex VII and VIII has evidenced (e.g. carcinogenic, mutagenic, allergenic, teratogenic, etc.). Recall is made of the phrases (R phrases) indicating special risks and safety advice (S phrases). In a total of 14 criteria for dangerous substances five are directed at safety, eight are directed at health and one is directed at the environment.

Annex V will contain the methods to be used for testing the physico chemical properties, the toxicity and the ecotoxicity, the methods are currently drafted by national experts.

3. CONCLUSIONS

Annex VI shows the use that can be made of the results of an acute toxicity testing in terms of the classification of substance.

The results of the tests on corrosion and irritation serve also for the labelling. In addition the results of other tests e.g. mutagenicity, carcinogenicity, teratogenicity can also be taken into account for the labelling. The precise function of these other tests with respect to the directive is less clearly defined.

The step sequence system takes into account the manufactured quantity of the test substance and the results of earlier testing allowing a health assessment evaluation.

To assist the Commission in carrying out evaluation of the toxicity and ecotoxicity of chemical substances, the Commission has set up an advisory Scientific Committee to examine the toxicity and ecotoxicity of chemical compounds.

© 1980 Elsevier/North-Holland Biomedical Press
Mechanisms of Toxicity and Hazard Evaluation
B. Holmstedt, R. Lauwerys, M. Mercier, M. Roberfroid eds

LIAISON WITH INDUSTRY IN THE PROVISION OF ESSENTIAL INFORMATION FOR THE MANAGEMENT OF POISONING

DR. J. B. SPOONER, M.A., M.B., B.Chir.,
Medical Director, Sterling-Winthrop Group Limited, Surbiton, Surrey, KT6 4PH, ENGLAND.

Although clinically poisoning may be attributable to a number of categories of agent, the one of greatest significance in Western Europe is the self-administered acute drug overdose. During the course of the development of new medicines, a considerable amount of data are generated for registration purposes (Table 1). As an illustration of the way in which these requirements have increased, it is worth considering the numbers of studies required for 1972 compared with those for 1979 (Table 2). Although the two products concerned are not in the same therapeutic category, the increase in the number of studies required is apparent. A significant part of the increased requirement is related to animal studies of acute and repeated dose toxicity. The former is the LD_{50} test, while the latter can vary from country to country (Table 3). The result of this increase in data requirements was for the submission to increase from 60,000 pages in 1972, to 203,000 pages in 1979. One question we ask today is whether this volume of information is of practical significance to the clinical toxicologist. In most instances, the rigorous adherence to predetermined data requirements, results in an excess of information which bears no relationship to the use of the new medicine in man.

Fancher (1) emphasised the desirability of selecting animal models for pharmacological, metabolic, pharmacokinetic and toxicological studies in which the findings would have the greatest predictive value for expectations in humans. In spite of this, the choice of species continues to be based in large part on precedent, convenience, economics and regulatory requirement. Is this really the best way of proceeding? Should a case be made for much earlier consultation between those responsible for animal toxicology within the pharmaceutical industry and clinical toxicologists? If so, how can regulatory authorities be persuaded to accept a more flexible approach to data requirements?

PARACETAMOL

With the benefits of hindsight and the resultant selectivity that can be carried out, it is worth looking at a case in which real concern on a product safety only became apparent in the clinic, even though animal toxicity studies had been carried out and yet where subsequently it was apparent that animal studies closely reflected the situation in man. A study of the toxicity of paracetamol provides such an example.

Table 4 provides a brief review of studies of the acute oral LD_{50} in the mouse for paracetamol. On the whole these are in fair agreement both in terms of the LD_{50} and the comments as to the cause of death. From this, it would be reasonable to conclude that the clinical toxicity of paracetamol is likely to be of the same order as that of aspirin and that there is nothing remarkable about the cause of death.

Similar data for oral toxicity of paracetamol in the rat is given in Table 5. The LD_{50} in this species is much higher than in the former but lends support to the view that paracetamol is likely to be of similar safety to that of aspirin.

In 1966, however, it was noted that hepatic damage was apparent in those animals which survived the initial hours after dosage, yet succumbed a day or more later. It is interesting to note that the authors of this report stated that what prompted them to look for liver necrosis was recent experience in their laboratory with liver necrosis produced by oral administration of tannic acid. They almost apologetically state that liver necrosis was noted in the title of the communication "simply because it was a rather unique feature of our findings on the acute oral toxicity of paracetamol" (7).

A brief historical digression notes that paracetamol was first synthesised in 1878 and was first studied clinically and rejected in 1893. It re-entered the clinical scene in the late 1940's and was first marketed in an analgesic mixture in 1950. It was first marketed as a single substance analgesic in the U.K. in 1956 and was included in the British Pharmacopoeia in 1963. The first published reports of hepatic necrosis in man following paracetamol overdosage were made in 1968 (8,9). Thus, by 1966, paracetamol had been on the market in the U.K. for ten years achieving widespread use and the potential hepatotoxicity had just been identified from animal investigations and clinical observation.

Over the immediately following years, interest in paracetamol and its hepatotoxicity increased as the numbers of overdose cases leading to hepatic necrosis increased. During the early 1970's, work was carried out to identify the metabolites of paracetamol and their relationship to the hepatic necrosis from overdosage. In 1974, Mitchell and co-workers, proposed that this hepatic necrosis was mediated by a toxic metabolite formed from the oxidative metabolism of paracetamol (10).

Work was also being carried out by Sterling-Winthrop Group which included studies of metabolism and of possible antidotes to the hepatotoxicity. Using a system of two dimensional thin layer chromatography, it had been possible to identify the metabolites of paracetamol and to show that qualitatively the overdose situation did not result in a change in these metabolites. The nature of these metabolites was identified and their metabolic relationship proposed. Similar studies with various animal species, demonstrated the variation in the metabolism of paracetamol. From this, it is clear that there is no exact representative of man in terms of the metabolism of paracetamol, but on the principle that the reactive metabolite following oxidation is the potentially toxic factor, the mouse appeared to present the most acceptable animal model for further study. Having confirmed the appropriateness of the mouse for studies into paracetamol toxicity, 84 single drug substances and a number of combinations of them were studied in over 4,500 animals in order to investigate possible antidotes to the hepatotoxic effect of paracetamol. A selection of the results is given in Table 6 with the products grouped according to whether they were effective, ineffective, or possibly harmful.

Reports on this work were made at the symposium held in London in 1976, which was sponsored by the Company and attended by many clinicians interested in the subject. At that symposium, initial clinical experience with cysteamine and methionine, amongst others, was reported, indicating the value of these treatments (11). A typical result of studies at that time is given in Table 7.

Since that time, further work with n-acetylcysteine has shown this to be a very effective antidote to paracetamol toxicity (12) and work continues on the prevention and treatment of hepatic toxicity of paracetamol.

This short revue of the development of knowledge of paracetamol toxicity, its understanding and management, is clearly helped by being retrospective. But, it raises a number of points pertinent to the subject under debate.

1. It took 10 years from the date of introduction to the recognition of the unusual toxic effects of paracetamol. Although the product was introduced before any regulatory authority required to give its clearance, the studies carried out were not dissimilar to those presently required. Are we any better off today in identifying potential clinically significant toxicity in new products?
2. It took eight years from the date of identifying the toxicity of paracetamol to the date of arriving at a clinically significant method of management. This happened in spite of close collaboration between the Company and at least four centres of excellence dealing with clinical toxicology.

The questions that arise are:-

1. What improvement can be made in terms of co-operation between industry and clinical toxicologists in order to identify, understand and propose appropriate treatment for the potential clinical toxicity of new pharmaceutical products?
2. Can animal studies be more specifically selected to provide relevant data to man?
3. Can these studies replace rather than add to current regulatory authority requirements?
4. Can the time scales be such as to provide relevant information at an early stage of a new drug's development?

TABLE 1

GENERAL DATA REQUIREMENTS FOR REGISTRATION OF MEDICINE IN EUROPE

SCIENCE	GENERAL REQUIREMENTS
Chemistry	Method of synthesis, physicochemical characterisation, evaluation of impurities, drug substance specification, stability.
Pharmacy	Description and formula of dosage form, method of manufacture, quality control and stability. Biological availability.
Pharmacology	Evaluation of therapeutic effect. Evaluation of secondary effects on other organs or systems.
Pharmacokinetics	Absorption, distribution, biotransformation and excretion.
Acute toxicity	LD_{50} determinations usually in two species by two routes of administration.
Repeated dose toxicity	Administration by proposed therapeutic route to two or more species to assess toxic effects.
Reproduction toxicology	Examination for embryotoxic and teratogenic effects (dosage during organogenesis). Examination for effects prior to, during and after parturition (peri-natal studies). Examination for effects on fertility and general reproduction performance.
Carcinogenicity	Administration to two or more species, e.g. mouse and rat for up to 24 and 30 months respectively, to assess carcinogenic effects.
Mutagenicity	No requirements have been finally established yet by the European national regulatory agencies.
Human pharmacology	Tolerance tests in healthy volunteers. Pharmacokinetic and therapeutic effect evaluation in patients.
Clinical studies	Evaluation of efficacy and safety in the proposed indications.

TABLE 2

REGISTRATION OF BENORYLATE AND TRILOSTANE

BENORYLATE (1972)		TRILOSTANE (1979)	
Pharmacology	17	Primary pharmacology	27
		Secondary screening	9
Pharmacokinetics	12	Pharmacokinetics	7
Acute toxicity:		Acute toxicity:	
mouse	1	mouse	1
rat	1	rat	1
		rabbit	1
		dog	1
Repeated dose toxicity:		Repeated dose toxicity:	
40 days rat	1	90 days rat	1
200 days rat	1	18 months rat	1
217 days dog (7 mths)	1	+ ancillary studies	4
		12 months monkey	1
		+ ancillary studies	2
		Carcinogenicity:	
		18 months mouse	1
		24 months rat	1
Reproduction toxicity:		Reproduction toxicity:	
teratology rat	1	teratology rat	3
teratology rabbit	1	teratology rabbit	1
		fertility male rat	1
		fertility female rat	1
		perinatal rat	1
TOTAL	36	TOTAL	65

TABLE 3

REPEATED DOSE TOXICITY STUDIES

UNITED KINGDOM	FRANCE	GERMANY
1968 CSD Guidelines	1972 Arrete (17.4.72)	1971 (Source Droit et Pharmacie)
At least two species (one of which is a non-rodent). Rat and dog or monkey are normally used. Duration - at least six months	At least two species (one of which is a non-rodent). Two studies (2-4 weeks and 3-6 months). The latter study is not necessary for single dose administration to man. Similar in wording to the EEC Directive 75/318.	Same as France (1972)
1979 DHSS Guidelines (MAIL)	Present Requirements	1979 (Source - BGA Symposium
At least two mammalian species (one of which is a non-rodent). Dosage must be 7 days/weeks. Duration of studies is related to proposed clinical use, as follows:	The Experts require repeated dose studies of at least 6 months duration.	At least two species (one non-rodent). Length of studies is related to proposed clinical use, as follows:
Clinical use — Toxicity Test Single dose — 2 weeks up to 7 days — 4 weeks 7-30 days — 3 months >30 days — 6 months		Clinical use — Toxicity Test 1-2 doses — 2-4 weeks up to 7 days — 4-6 weeks 7-30 days — 3 months > 30 days — 6 months

TABLE 4

ACUTE ORAL LD_{50} IN MOUSE

AUTHOR	YEAR	TIME(HRS.)	(MG/KG)	COMMENT
(S-Winthrop)	1950	168	1000	Respiractory arrest
Smith (2)	1958	-	610	-
		-	717	
Boxill (3)	1958	96	525	Respiratory failure
Manolov (4)	1963	72	670	-

TABLE 5

ACUTE ORAL LD_{50} IN RAT

AUTHOR	YEAR	TIME(HRS.)	(MG/KG)	COMMENT
Clark (5)	1952	48	>3200	Convulsions
Renault (6)	1956	24	4500	-
Smith (2)	1958	-	3000	-
Boxill (3)	1958	96	4400	Respiratory failure
Manolov (4)	1963	72	3000	-
Boyd (7)	1966	<24	3710	Convulsions
		>24	2-3000	Hepatic damage

TABLE 6

EFFECT OF TREATMENT ON MORTALITY RATE IN MICE AFTER PARACETAMOL (875mg/kg)

TREATMENT	DOSE (mg/kg)	ROUTE	MORTALITY % AT 7 DAYS Treated	Controls
Methionine	400	Oral	13	97
Cysteine	400	Oral	0	77
Cysteamine	200	s.c.	33	87
Glutathione	50	s.c.	54	80
Dimercaprol	30	s.c.	80	97
Hydrocortisone	5	i.p.	73	83
Promethazine	0.5	i.p.	53	47
Azathioprine	2.5	Oral	87	70

TABLE 7

	No. of Pts.	% with liver damage	% morta-lity	Mean Max AST iu/l		Mean Max Bili mmol/l	
				Survi-vors	Pts. with liver damage	Survi-vors	Pts. with liver damage
Methionine treated	17	41.2	0	469.6	1097.9	23.9	39.8
Untreated	14	100	50	2730	2730	88.6	88.6

REFERENCES

1. Fancher, O.E. (1978) Clin. Toxicol. 12:239.
2. Smith, P.K. (1958) Acetophenetidin - A Critical Biographic Review, New York: Interscience Publishers.
3. Boxill, G.C. et al (1958) J. Amer. Pharm. Ass. 47:479.
4. Manolov, P. (1963) S'Vremenna Med. 14:33.
5. Clark, B.C. (1952) Symposium on n-Acetyl p-Aminophenol, p. 23. The Institute for the Study of Analgesic and Sedative Drugs, Elkhart, Indiana.
6. Renault, H. et al (1956) Therapie 11:300.
7. Boyd, E.M. and Bereczky, G.M. (1966) Brit. J. Pharmacol., 26:606.
8. Davidson, D.G.D. and Eastman, W.N. (1966) Brit. Med. J., 2:497.
9. Thomas J.S. and Prescott, L.F. (1966) Brit. Med. J. 2:506.
10. Mitchell J.R., et al (1973) J. Pharmacol. Exper. Therap., 187:185.
11. J. Int. Med. Res. (1976) 4, Suppl. 4.
12. Prescott, L.F. et al (1977) Lancet, 2:432.

© 1980 Elsevier/North-Holland Biomedical Press
Mechanisms of Toxicity and Hazard Evaluation
B. Holmstedt, R. Lauwerys, M. Mercier, M. Roberfroid eds

TOXICOLOGY ADVISORY GUIDELINES FOR FRAGRANCE SAFETY ASSURANCE.

G. R. THOMPSON, F. H. STULTS, E. J. MORAN, K. R. TYBURCY, D. M. FORD and L. G. SCHARPF, JR.
International Flavors and Fragrances, 1515 Highway 36, Union Beach, N. J. (USA).

INTRODUCTION

Safety evaluations of fragrance formulations are complicated by the number and frequency of formulae routinely utilized. The 40-80,000 formulations in a company file, or even the 20-80 daily submissions to customers, cannot all be tested for safety assurance. Other criteria for safety assessments must be developed. Since each formulation typically contains 200-600 ingredients drawn from a library of approximately 3000 individual chemicals (diluted to 10-12,000 different solutions), composite ingredient safety assessments can be achieved by computerization once individual ingredient safety assessments have been completed. We recently reported our computerized system for simultaneously accomodating the numerous variables and dimensions associated with composite ingredient safety assessments for fragrance formulae[1]. The present report will define the five criteria utilized to achieve uniform safety for each fragrance ingredient, and define benefits derived from application of these criteria.

BASIC CRITERIA

I. Fragrance ingredient safety assessments must be based upon Skin Concentrations (i.e., actual exposure levels). Skin concentrations are related to oil Use Concentrations (UC) and oil Ingredient Concentrations (IC):

$$SC = \frac{(IC)(UC)}{100}.$$

Exposures to IC in fragrance formulations are dependent upon the UC of the formulation which, in turn, varies between products and use categories. The only constant value for comparison of potential human exposure levels to human test data is SC.

II. Safety evaluations for an ingredient in a fragrance formula must consider the total (generic) concentration of chemically equivalent materials. Since fragrance formulations are complex mixtures of many ingredients, several grades or sources of the same ingredient may be used in the formulation. Safety assessments must consider the total IC of all chemically equivalent forms of the ingredient (generic concentration) available for human exposure as in the following example for the generic Citral:

Ingredients Containing Citral	Ingredient (% Citral)	Formula IC (%)	Generic Conc. (% Citral)
Ambre 1600	0.016	10	0.0016
Bergamot 61	2.000	2	0.0400
Chloralene Savon	15.000	5	0.7500
Citral T	96.000	10	9.6000
Citral Pure Synthetic	100.000	1	1.0000
Citral Extra	100.000	5	5.0000
Citral Special	100.000	10	10.0000
Lemon Tetrarome	8.000	2	0.1600
Melonis AB-441A	1.500	5	0.0750
		50	26.6266

Safety assessments of sensitization risks associated with generic ingredient concentrations are based upon two assumptions:

1. sensitization is concentration dependent, and
2. mixtures are no more sensitizing than individual ingredients.

Recent publications by Steltenkamp et al. substantiated the concentration dependence of sensitization for three major fragrance ingredients[2,3,4]. Additionally, their reports indicated that fragrance formulations with at least one of the three ingredients did not produce more sensitization reactions in human subjects exposed to concentrations that approximated individual ingredient exposure concentrations. Opdyke[5] previously reported the absence of sensitization potential for natural fragrance oils (mixtures), and selected synthetic ("quenching") mixtures, at equivalent, or higher, concentrations than produced reactions when an individual ingredient from the mixture was applied. These observations supported application of these two assumptions.

III. Product types can be separated into risk categories. Fragrances are utilized in hundreds of different types of products, but each type of product does not necessarily represent a unique hazard for consumers. Product risk categories can be formed through the application of 10 criteria that influence risk assessment:

1. Exposure concentration
2. Duration of exposure
3. Frequency of exposure
4. Extent of body exposure
5. Region of body exposure
6. Extent of population exposure
7. Subpopulation susceptibility
8. Penetration potential
9. Misuse potential
10. Liability potential.

The following product risk categories resulted from the application of the above criteria to 18 subgroups of use categories:

1. Baby, first aid, medicinal cosmetics, personal hygiene
2. Sun screens and related products
3. Antiperspirant, deodorant
4. Aerosol, bath, body lotion/powder, cosmetic, hair, lip, soap
5. Cologne, perfume
6. Detergent
7. Animal
8. Nonbiological (not applied directly to man or animals).

IV. Ingredient safety margins should be proportional to the risk for each product. Safety margins typically reflect differences between the maximum experimental no-effect level and the exposure concentration. Classically, food additive criteria have included a 10-fold margin for interspecies variations and another 10-fold margin for intraspecies differences resulting in the overall safety margin of 100-fold. Since no-effect levels for sensitizers are usually defined in human studies, the interspecies factor is not applicable. Additionally, the breadth of risk reflected in the risk categories support multiple safety margins directly proportional to the risk, rather than a single factor. However, the 10-fold intraspecies factor provides a "benchmark" for comparing safety margins for each risk category. Reasonable safety margins above no-effect levels in definitive human dermal studies for each product risk category are proposed as follows:

Product Risk Categories	Safety Margins From No-effect	From Category #5
1. Baby, first aid, etc.	50X	10X
2. Sun	35X	7X
3. Antiperspirant, deodorant	35X	7X
4. Aerosol, bath, body lotion/powder, etc.	15X*	3X*
5. Cologne, perfume	5X	1X
6. Detergent	5X*	1X*
7. Animal	2.5X	0.5X
8. Nonbiological	1X*	0.2X*

These risk category safety margins resulted from the combined impact of the 10 risk assessment criteria described in criterion #3 above when applied to the experimental no-effect level. Safety margins of less than 10X resulted from reduced contributions from these criteria while the larger margins resulted

*Dilution factors were not included.

from increased overall contributions. Although the safety margins in risk categories #4,3,2 and 1 progressively increase, the impact upon Ingredient Concentration (IC) is minimal due to decreased product end use concentrations (UC).

V. Ingredient safety margins can be adjusted to accomodate different types of toxicological response. The safety margins defined in criterion #4 above can be effectively utilized for sensitization and photobiological responses. Other toxicological effects may warrant additional safety factors as indicated for the cologne/perfume risk category:

	Cologne/Perfume Safety Margins
1. Topical responses (sensitization, photobiologic effects)	5X
2. Materials absorbed through the skin and producing reversible target organ effects (i.e., liver, kidney, etc.)	100X
3. Materials absorbed through the skin producing irreversible target organ effects (i.e., CNS changes, reproductive effects, etc.)	$\geq$1000X
4. Materials producing genetic effects, carcinogenicity and/or mutagenicity	$\geq$10,000X (or even no usage)

Safety margins associated with the most hazardous response would serve as the baseline for defining permitted exposure levels. Extension of these cologne/perfume safety factors to other risk categories would warrant accomodation of the additional safety margins between risk categories (i.e., reversible effects become 1000X for baby products). Additionally, individual risk category safety margins can be increased as warranted by experimental data. For example, the sun category safety margin could be increased to 70X for known phototoxicants. In short, the safety margins can be standardized for each type of toxicological response.

BENEFITS

1. Standardizes industry safety guidelines. Application of standardized safety criteria will not only enable the fragrance industry to provide even safer products, but will also simplify safety evaluations, streamline creativity, decrease operational costs and minimize the need for enhanced governmental scrutiny of our industry.

2. Reduces the possibility of commercial crises. Utilization of the toxicology Advisory Guidelines (TAG) criteria provides documented evidence of safety for economically important materials that might otherwise experience

unwarranted attacks based upon questionable data. Additionally, adverse publicity, or even product recalls, resulting from improper use of an ingredient can be minimized by application of these criteria.

3. Openly defines the scientific validity of fragrance safety criteria. TAG will assure the continuation of a history of safe use for fragrance ingredients. Public definition will encourage scientific peer review that should accelerate development of new information and improved criteria.

4. Diminishes prospects for additional government regulations. Several governments are considering additional regulations for controlling the safety of fragrances and fragrance ingredients. The voluntary release of scientifically defensible safety guidelines would encourage cooperation from these governments.

REFERENCES

1. Thompson, G. R., et al. (1980) Toxicological Guidelines for Automatic Evaluation of Fragrance Ingredients in Formulations. I. Contact Sensitization, Society of Toxicology, presentation #397, March 9-13, 1980.
2. Steltenkamp, R. J., et al., Hydroxycitronellal - A Survey of Consumer Patch Test Sensitization, Food and Cosmetics Toxicology, in press.
3. Steltenkamp, R. J., et al., Citral - A Survey of Consumer Patch Test Sensitization, Food and Cosmetics Toxicology, in press.
4. Steltenkamp, R. J., et al., Cinnamic Alcohol - A Survey of Consumer Patch Test Sensitization, Food and Cosmetics Toxicology, in press.
5. Opdyke, D. L., (1976) Inhibition of Sensitization Reactions Induced by Certain Aldehydes, Food and Cosmetics Toxicology, Vol. 14, No. 3, pp. 197-198.

METABOLISM AND HEPATOTOXICITY

© 1980 Elsevier/North-Holland Biomedical Press
Mechanisms of Toxicity and Hazard Evaluation
B. Holmstedt, R. Lauwerys, M. Mercier, M. Roberfroid eds

UDP-GLUCURONOSYLTRANSFERASE ACTIVITY OF CULTURED CELLS *IN SITU* AND *IN VITRO*

JASWANT SINGH and FRIEDRICH J. WIEBEL
Institut für Toxikologie umd Biochemie, Abteilung für Toxikologie, Gesellschaft für Strahlen- und Umweltforschung, 8042 Neuherberg/ München (Federal Republic of Germany)

INTRODUCTION

The present studies are part of a larger effort concerned with the activity and regulation of xenobiotic-metabolizing enzymes in established cultures of toxicological interest[1-5]. One of the major pathways for the detoxification of reactive chemicals is their conjugation with glucuronic acid. In the following we describe the activity in cultured cells of the UDP-glucuronosyltransferase (GT), which has partially been characterized by the specificity toward its aglycons (e.g. 1-naphthol, 3 hydroxybenzo(a)-pyrene, p-nitrophenol)[6] and has been variously labeled as 'GT-I'[6] or 'late fetal' GT form[7].

MATERIALS AND METHODS

Cell cultures. The source of the cell lines and their culture conditions have been previously described[2]. Cells approaching confluency were used.

GT assay. After 2 washes with phosphate-buffered saline, cells were collected by gentle scraping, centrifuged at low speed and used as a source of the enzyme[2]. GT activity toward the substrate 3-hydroxybenzo(a)pyrene (3-OH-BP) was determined according to Singh and Wiebel[3]. UDP-glucuronic acid (UDPGA) was measured by a recently described fluorometric assay[4].

In situ GT activity. Cells were grown in 60x15 mm plastic plates at 37°C and medium was changed 24 hrs before the experiments. 3-OH-BP (final 50 uM) was added in methanol (final 0.5%) to triplicate plates. After 7.5 and 15.0 min the medium was removed and cells were scraped in cold water (1.0 ml/plate). Aliquots of medium and cell suspensions were analysed for the presence of 3-OH-BP conjugates by spectrofluorometry[3].

The identity of the conjugates was established by enzymatic hydrolysis and high pressure liquid chromatography[5].

RESULTS AND DISCUSSION

As shown in Table 1, <u>in vitro</u> GT activity varied by a factor of 10 between the cell lines tested. The level of activity in H-4-II-E cells was about the same as that in homogenates of rat liver[8]. No activity was detectable in V79, C81, or NC37BaEV cells. Exposure to benz(a)anthracene induced GT activity about 2-fold in H-4-II-E and 3T3/BALB cells. The degree of activation by the non-ionic detergent Brij-58 ranged from 1.2- to 6-fold in the different cell lines (cf. Fig. 1 and [5]). In its level of activity, degree of induction and activation, GT activity in the various cell lines resembles that in mammalian tissues.

In the presence of detergent the dependency of <u>in vitro</u> GT activity on UDPGA followed Michaelis-Menten kinetics with an apparent K_m of 0.2 mM (Fig. 1). However, in the absence of detergent, the kinetics were non-linear. With near saturating

TABLE 1

UDP-GLUCURONOSYLTRANSFERASE IN CELLS IN CULTURE: BASAL ACTIVITY AND INDUCIBILITY

Cell Lines	nmol BP-3-glucuronide formed/min/mg protein[a] untreated	BA-treated[b]
H-4-II-E, hepatoma, rat	1.15	1.76
RAG, renal adenoma, BALB/C mouse	0.97	1.00
BHK21 (C13), kidney, Syrian hamster	0.35	0.31
3T3/BALB, fibroblasts, mouse	0.18	0.40
L-A9, fibroblasts, C3H/An mouse	0.17	0.23
A-549, pulmonary carcinoma, human	0.12	0.14
V-79, lung, Chinese hamster	< 0.005	< 0.005
C-81, fibroblasts, cat	< 0.005	< 0.005
NC37BaEV, lymphoblastoid, human	< 0.005	< 0.005

[a]GT activity in freshly collected cells was determined without detergent.

[b]Cell cultures were treated with benz(a)anthracene (5 ug/ml medium, DMSO final 0.1%) for 48 hrs.

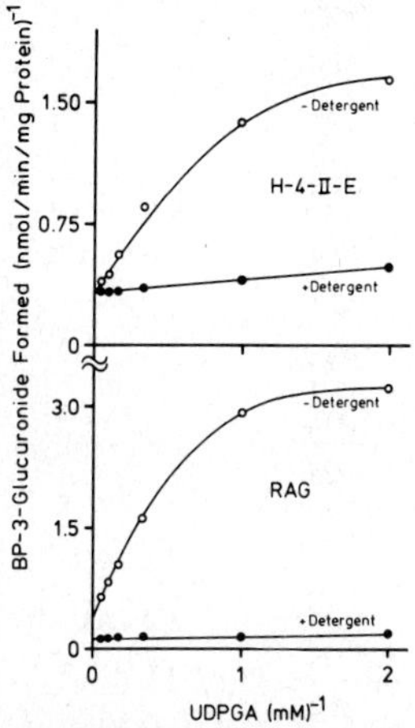

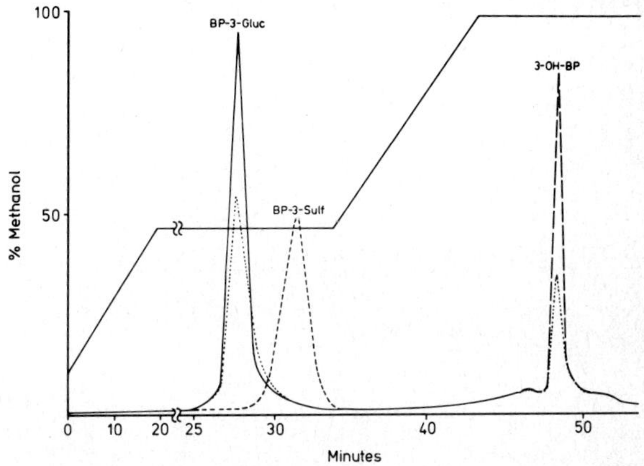

Fig. 1: Double reciprocal plot for GT dependency on UDPGA. GT activity in freshly collected cells was determined in the absence or presence of Brij-58 (0.0125%).

Fig. 2: HPLC analysis of 3-OH-BP conjugates. Aliquots of medium and cells exposed *in situ* to 3-OH-BP (50 uM) were analysed by reverse phase HPLC[5]. Gradient ——//—— ; conjugates formed *in situ* ·····; reference compounds: 3-OH-BP —— —— ; BP-3-glucuronide ———— ; BP-3-sulfate -----.

concentrations of UDPGA (20 mM), the V_{max} approached that found in the presence of detergent. At concentrations greatly exceeding the physiological level, UDPGA may act like a chaotropic agent and induce conformational changes in the membranes increasing the number of active enzyme sites available to UDPGA.

HPLC analysis of the total water soluble metabolites of 3-OH-BP formed *in situ* indicated that in H-4-II-E cells (Fig. 2) as well as in RAG and A549 (data not shown), BP-3-glucuronide is the only detectable conjugate. As shown in Table 2, GT activities in intact cells were similar to the *in vitro* activities when the latter were measured at UDPGA concentrations occuring in the intact cells. These results suggest that the enzyme in intact cells is operative in its "latent" form. It is also apparent from the data that changes in UDPGA concentrations at the "physiological" levels modified the velocity of the *in vitro* reaction to a minor degree. A tenative analysis of the reaction kinetics showed that the intracellular UDPGA concentrations were about 3 times above

TABLE 2

COMPARISON OF *IN SITU* AND *IN VITRO* GT ACTIVITY: DEPENDENCY ON UDP-GLUCURONIC ACID

	nmol BP-3-glucuronide formed/min/mg protein							
	In Vitro						In Situ	
	UDPGA (mM)							
CELL LINES	0.065	0.125	0.25	0.5	1.0	3.0		
H-4-II-E	-	0.58	0.68	0.81	0.90	1.20	0.96	(0.5 mM)[a]
A-549	-	0.07	0.11	0.13	0.15	0.18	0.12	(1.40 ")
RAG	0.23	0.30	0.41	0.48	0.60	1.0	0.40	(0.40 ")
BHK	0.08	0.10	0.14	0.19	0.30	0.40	0.10	(0.08 ")
V79	-	-	-	-	-	<0.005	0.005	(0.09 ")

[a]Numbers in parentheses give the intracellular UDPGA concentrations. They were estimated from the UDPGA content[4] and the cell volumes determined according to Baur *et al.*[9].

the apparent Km_{UDPGA} in the various cell lines except in BHK cells which exhibited only a 2-fold difference. Thus, although UDPGA is present in the cells at less than saturating concentrations, the co-factor is not likely to be a major regulatory determinant for GT in intact cells.

REFERENCES

1. Wiebel, F.J., Brown, S., Waters, H.L. and Selkirk, J.K. (1977) Arch. Toxicol. 39, 133-148.
2. Wiebel, F.J. and Singh, J. (1980) Arch. Toxicol. 44, 85-97.
3. Singh, J. and Wiebel, F.J. (1979) Analyt. Biochem. 98, 394-401.
4. Singh, J., Schwarz, L.R. and Wiebel, F.J. (1980) Biochem. J. (in press).
5. Singh, J. and Wiebel, F.J. (in preparation).
6. Bock, K.W. and Lilienblum, W. (1979) Biochem. Pharmacol. 28, 695-700.
7. Wishart, G.J (1978) Biochem. J. 174, 485-489.
8. Wiebel, F.J., Pawlak, A. and Singh, J. (1980) Fine-needle aspiration biopsy of the rat liver, Pergamon Press, Frankfurt, pp. 39-47.
9. Baur, H., Kasperek, S. and Pfaff, E. (1975) Hoppe-Seyler's Z. Physiol. Chem. 356, 827-838.

© 1980 Elsevier/North-Holland Biomedical Press
Mechanisms of Toxicity and Hazard Evaluation
B. Holmstedt, R. Lauwerys, M. Mercier, M. Roberfroid eds

IN VITRO COMPARATIVE BIOACTIVATION OF ALIPHATIC HALOGENATED HYDROCARBONS

I. GLENN SIPES AND A. JAY GANDOLFI

Toxicology Program, University of Arizona, Tucson, AZ 85724

INTRODUCTION

Man is exposed to halogenated hydrocarbons (HHC) from his conception to his death. As many of these compounds are suspected of being carcinogenic[1], tests to confirm or deny their reactivity or carcinogenicity are now of ultimate importance. The interaction of reactive intermediates with cellular components has correlated well with the toxicity and/or carcinogenicity of many agents, thus the elucidation of the reaction of metabolic intermediates of HHC with cell components and the correlation of binding to toxicity is a necessary emphasis in understanding and counteracting their toxicity[2]. The objective of this investigation was to compare the rat hepatic microsomal bioactivation of twelve HHC by measuring their covalent interaction with tissue macromolecules.

MATERIALS AND METHODS

Chemicals. Uniformly ^{14}C-labeled CCl_4(1), $CHCl_3$(2), CH_2Cl_2(3), CH_3I(4), $CBrCl_3$(5), CCl_2CHCl(6), CHClCHCl(7), CH_2ClCH_2Cl(8), CH_2BrCH_2Br(9), $CHCl_2CH_2Cl$(10), CCl_3CH_3(11), and $^{14}CF_3CHClBr$(12) were obtained at greater than 99% radiochemical purity from New England Nuclear Corp. or California Bionuclear Corp. Chemical purity as checked by gas chromatography in our laboratory was 97-99%.

Animals. To induce the microsomal cytochrome P-450, male Sprague-Dawley rats were treated with phenobarbital (PB, 0.1% w/v in their drinking water for 10 days), Aroclor 1254 (500 mg/kg IP five days before sacrifice), or 3-methylcholanthrene (3-MC, 50 mg/kg IP two days before sacrifice).

Microsomal Preparation. Rats were sacrificed by cervical dislocation and hepatic microsomes prepared as previously described[3]. The microsomal pellet was suspended in 50 mM Tris-HCl pH 7.4 buffer and frozen at -70°C. The frozen microsomes retained activity for several weeks as evidenced by the stability of the CO-difference spectra of cytochrome P-450 and aminopyrine N-demethylase activity.

Incubation. To obtain optimum binding to microsomal protein and lipids, HHC were incubated with 10 mg hepatic microsomal protein, while for binding to DNA, optimum conditions were 1-3 mg microsomal protein and 5 mg calf thymus

DNA. Incubations were performed in 12 ml tubes with Teflon-lined screw caps in the presence of a NADPH generating system[3]. Boiled microsomes were used for background, non-enzymatic binding levels. The incubation system was flushed with N_2 or O_2 four times prior to addition of ^{14}C-labeled substrates. In one set of experiments, glutathione (GSH) was added to the incubation to a final concentration of 1 mM prior to the addition of the HHC substrate. ^{14}C-labeled HHC were diluted with unlabeled compound and ethanol so that the addition of 2 μl of the diluted substrates to the incubation mixture (2 ml) would result in 2 μmoles of substrate with 1 μCi radioactivity. Immediately following the addition of ^{14}C-labeled HHC the tubes were sealed and incubated with shaking for appropriate time periods.

Macromolecule Isolation. Incubations were stopped by the addition of cold ethanol and the extraction technique of Sipes et al.[3] was used to isolate and exhaustively extract the microsomal protein and lipid. Aliquots of the extracted protein and lipid were counted for radioactivity and assayed for protein and lipid phosphorous[3].

The incubations for binding to DNA were stopped by placing samples on ice and adding two volumes of -20°C ethanol followed by centrifugation (1000 x g 20 min) to pellet protein and DNA. This procedure was repeated and then the resulting pellet resuspended in 5 ml of buffer (10 mM Tris: 10mM EDTA: 10 mM NaCl pH 7.9). The samples were then transferred into dialysis bags along with 0.5 ml of 20% sodium dodecyl sulfate (SDS) and two mg of Pronase. The bags were incubated overnight at 37°C in 1.5 liters of the above buffer containing 2% SDS with at least one change of buffer. The contents of the bag were mixed and extracted twice for two hours with 10 ml $CHCl_3$/isoamyl alcohol (24:1). The top aqueous layers were mixed with 10 ml 0.1 M saline in 90% ethanol and allowed to set at 4°C for 60 minutes. The precipitated DNA was spooled on a glass rod and redissolved with gently shaking in 3 ml of 10 mM Tris, pH 7.4 buffer. Samples are then taken for radioactive counting and determination of DNA content by UV absorption[4].

RESULTS

The initial objective of this study was to determine which atmosphere, O_2 or N_2, permitted the optimum bioactivation of each HHC. Only CCl_4(1), $CBrCl_3$(5), $CF_3CHClBr$(12) and CH_3I(4) required a N_2 atmosphere for optimum bioactivation and subsequent covalent binding of the reactive intermediates to lipid, protein and DNA. All subsequent studies were performed under the optimum atmosphere for the particular HHC. Pretreatment of rats with PB or Aroclor 1254, increased the amount of HHC covalently bound to microsomal lipid and protein. The *in vitro* binding of CH_3I(4), which does not require enzymatic bioactivation, was unaffected by pretreatment of the animals with inducing agents. Little, if any, effect on the bioactivation of the various HHC was observed when microsomes from animals pretreated with 3-MC were used in the incubations. Table 1 compares the *in vitro* covalent binding of various HHC to microsomal protein, lipid and DNA when the incubations were performed under optimal conditions. Incubations were performed for 15 min. for the binding to lipid or protein, since the bioactivation was linear for this time. Longer times (60 min.) were necessary to maximize the amount of covalent binding of HHC to DNA.

The HHC could be divided into three groups relative to their bioactivation and subsequent binding to microsomal protein. The least reactive group included CH_2Cl_2(3) and the CHClCHCl(7). The middle group is delineated by CCl_4(1) and $CF_3CHClBr$(12). The most reactive group includes CH_2BrCH_2Br(9), $CBrCl_3$(5), and $CHCl_2CH_2Cl$(10). Many of the HHC were bioactivated and bound to microsomal lipids far more than previously demonstrated. The rates of bioactivation and binding to lipids could not be grouped as easily as those to protein and a much wider range in binding was observed (Table 1). The HHC yielding the greatest binding to lipid were $CBrCl_3$(5), $CHCl_2CH_2Cl$(10) and CCl_4(1). The presence of 1 mM GSH greatly inhibited the binding of $CHCl_3$(2), CCl_2CHCl(6), CH_2ClCH_2Cl(8), CH_2BrCH_2Br(9), $CHCl_2CH_2Cl$(10). The effect was most dramatic with those HHC bioactivated in an O_2 atmosphere. In the studies for measuring covalent binding of HHC to DNA, CH_2BrCH_2Br(9), $CBrCl_3$(5), $CHCl_3$(2), CCl_4(1), $CCl_2CHCl_2CH_2Cl$(10) bound in this order from 0.52 to 0.35 nmoles/mg DNA. The other organohalogens bound around 0.1 nmole/mg DNA to almost non-detectable levels. Some nonenzymatic binding was evident with $CBrCl_3$ and CCl_2CHCl. Subsequent treatment of the isolated DNA with Pronase did not release the bound radioactivity.

DISCUSSION

These studies were designed to determine if the degree of *in vitro* microsomal bioactivation of the HHC correlated with their known toxicities and to determine if protein, lipids and DNA could serve as nucleophiles for the electrophilic reactive intermediates. In general there was good correlation between the degree of covalent binding to protein and/or lipids and the hepatotoxic potential of the HHC. However, it is not possible to extrapolate

TABLE 1.

IN VITRO MICROSOMAL BIOACTIVATION AND COVALENT BINDING OF ORGANOHALOGENS TO PROTEIN, LIPID, AND DNA

Microsomes were obtained from rats treated with PB and incubations were performed under optimum atmosphere (O_2 or N_2). Values have been corrected for background binding.

Organohalogen[a]		Protein[b]		Lipid[c]		DNA[d]
CCl_4	(1)	5.3±1.2	2.4[e]	37.5±7.2	2.2[e]	.39±.08
$CHCl_3$	(2)	14.7±3.8	2.2	10.3±2.7	2.1	.46±.13
CH_2Cl_2	(3)	0.2±0.1	2.0	0.2±0.1	3.1	.01±.00
CH_3I	(4)	7.2±2.8	0.8	0.1±0.1	1.0	.01±.01
$CBrCl_3$	(5)	20.3±7.6	1.6	49.5±24.2	1.7	.51 ±.18
CCl_2CHCl	(6)	2.4±1.0	2.1	8.0±0.9	1.3	.36±.08
CHClCHCl	(7)	0.1±0.1	1.6	0.2±0.1	3.3	--
CH_2ClCH_2Cl	(8)	1.5±0.4	6.0	0.9±0.2	3.5	.04±.02
CH_2BrCH_2BR	(9)	28.2±6.0	2.4	4.0±1.9	4.2	.52±.14
$CHCl_2CH_2Cl$	(10)	18.9±2.7	5.3	41.7±5.2	8.2	.35±.07
CCl_3CH_3	(11)	1.5±0.7	1.2	6.5±4.2	0.6	.05±0.1
$CF_3CHClBr$	(12)	1.2±0.6	2.6	3.6±1.4	3.5	.08±.01

a. Numbers in parentheses used to identify compound.
b. Values are mean ± SD for at least 8 determinations. Expressed as nmoles bound/mg protein/15 minutes.
c. Values are mean ± SD for at least 8 determinations. Expressed as nmoles bound/micromole lipid phosphorous/15 minutes.
d. Values are mean ± SD for at least 5 determinations. Expressed as nmoles bound/mg DNA/60 minutes.
e. Underlined numbers are the ratio of binding to proteins and lipids for phenobarbital: control microsomes

directly from binding obtained in this *in vitro* system to toxicity obtained in the whole organism, since the *in vitro* system was designed to obtain maximum binding. In the intact liver protective mechanisms may be available which are absent in the *in vitro* microsomal assays. In addition, microsomal enzyme induction is a critical factor for the initiation of liver injury by many HHC and other xenobiotics. Thus, it is likely that *in vitro* binding would overestimate the hepatotoxic potential.

Several results obtained in this study can illustrate this over estimation. If the *in vitro* binding of CCl_4(1) and $CHCl_3$(2) to protein is compared, one could conclude that $CHCl_3$ is a more potent hepatotoxin. This is generally not the case. $CHCl_3$(2) is a threshold toxin. Only when liver GSH levels are depleted does the true toxic potential of $CHCl_3$(2) become apparent.[5] In PB-treated rats, reactive metabolite(s) of $CHCl_3$(2) rapidly deplete GSH[5] and the hepatotoxic potential of $CHCl_3$(2) equals or exceeds that of CCl_4(1). Another interesting example is $CHCl_2CH_2Cl$(10), generally considered a weak hepatotoxin. The covalent binding of this HHC equaled that of the extremely potent hepatotoxin, $CBrCl_3$. Again, $CHCl_2CH_2Cl$ is a threshold toxin requiring enzyme induction coupled with GSH depletion for expression of toxicity.[6] This is exemplified by the 5-8 fold increase in binding when microsomes from PB-treated rats were used and the inhibitory effect of GSH. Although such studies may result in overestimation of toxic potential, they can also provide direction to determine critical factors that can potentiate toxicity. A good example was the observation that the binding of halothane is markedly enhanced when incubations are performed under N_2.[7] This observation led to elucidation of the reductive component of halothane biotransformation and development of animal models of halothane hepatotoxicity.[8]

The results obtained support the hypothesis that cytochrome P-450 catalyzes the bioactivation of these HHC. Microsomes from PB-treated rats were generally 2-6 times more active than those from control rats. However, it should be emphasized that other pathways may also mediate the bioactivation of selected HHC. For example GSH transferases may result in the bioactivation of CH_2Cl_2(3), CH_2ClCH_2Cl(8) and CH_2BrCH_2Br(9)[9]. Since microsomes from 3-MC treated rats were about equal to control microsomes in bioactivation potential, cytochrome P-448 is of minor importance in the bioactivation of this class of toxins. In fact, 3-MC pretreatment often results in protection from the hepatotoxic effects of certain HHC.[10]

The binding to DNA was greatest for those HHC that are suspected or known carcinogens[12] such as CH_2BrCH_2Br(9), $CHCl_3$(2), CCl_4(1) and CCl_2CHCl(6). The binding of these HHC to DNA was low relative to that obtained for lipids and protein and tended to reflect their binding to these macromolecules. Considerable effort was expended to insure the extracted DNA was free of associated protein. Whether or not binding of these HHC to DNA is the mechanism of carcinogenesis is unknown. Since these HHC result in tissue injury, it can be argued that their carcinogenicity is the result of an epigenetic mechanism. Compounds such as $CF_3CHBrCl$(12), the widely used anesthetic, and CH_2Cl_2(3), a replacement solvent for other HHC, had only minute amounts of radioactivity associated with the isolated DNA. To date these compounds have not been shown to be carcinogenic. The carcinogenic potential of the other HHC is less well established.

In summary this study presents an *in vitro* model system for the comparative bioactivation of organohalogens which may be a viable tool in directing studies to determine the putative carcinogenicity and/or toxicity of a variety of organohalogens. The system is optimized in order to favor bioactivation by utilizing highly active hepatic microsomes and the preferred atmosphere and by eliminating competing detoxification pathways. Further work is needed to clarify bioactivation pathways and similar studies should be performed using microsomes from extrahepatic tissues, since many of these HHC produce toxicity in a number of tissues.

ACKNOWLEDGEMENTS: Supported by NIH Grant CA 21820. The expert assistance of J.R. MacDonald, A. DiRenzo and Mary Neron is gratefully acknowledged.

REFERENCES

1. Weisburger, E.K. (1977) Environ. Health Perspect. 21, 7-16.
2. Mitchell, J.R., Nelson, S.D., Thorgeirsson S.S., McMurtry, R.J. and Dybing, E. (1976) Prog. in Liver Disease 5, 259-279.
3. Sipes, I.G., Podolsky, T.L., Brown, B.R., (1977) Environ. Health Perspect, 21, 171-178.
4. Marmur, J. (1961) J. Biol. Chem. 3, 208-218.
5. Docks, E.L. and Krishna, G. (1976) Exp. Mol. Pathol. 24, 13-22.
6. MacDonald, J.R., Gandolfi, A.J., Sipes, I.G., (1980) Fed. Proc. 39(3), 999.
7. Uehleke, H., Hellmer K.H., Tabarelli - Poplwski, 5. (1973) Naunyn - Schmiedebergs Arch. Exp. Path. Pharmak. 279, 39-52.
8. McLain, G.E., Sipes, I.G., Brown, B.R. (1979) Anesthesiology 51, 321-326.
9. Rannug, U., Sundrall, A. and Ramel C. (1978) Chem.-Biol. Interactions 20, 1-16.
10. Reid, W.D., Christie, B., Eichelbaum, M. and Krishna, G. (1971) Exp. Mol. Pathol. 15, 363-372.
11. IARC Monographs on the evaluation of the Carcinogenic Risk of Chemicals to Humans 1979, 20, 1-609.

© 1980 Elsevier/North-Holland Biomedical Press
Mechanisms of Toxicity and Hazard Evaluation
B. Holmstedt, R. Lauwerys, M. Mercier, M. Roberfroid eds

THE HEPATOBILIARY TOXICITY OF PENICILLIC ACID, A CARCINOGENIC MYCOTOXIN

P. K. CHAN AND A. W. HAYES
Department of Pharmacology and Toxicology, University of Mississippi Medical Center, Jackson, Mississippi 39216, U. S. A.

ABSTRACT

Penicillic acid (PA), a carcinogenic mycotoxin, causes generalized hepatic necrosis in the mouse. The hepatotoxicity of PA was substantiated by the fact that PA 1) increased pentobarbital sleeping time, 2) decreased pentobarbital metabolism both *in vivo* and *in vitro*, 3) decreased hepatic reduced glutathione (GSH) with more than 80% depletion of GSH at the highest dose, 4) elevated serum transaminase activities and bilirubin level, and 5) increased sulfobromophthanlien (BSP) and idocyanine green (ICG) retention. PA-induced biliary dysfunction was evidenced by depression of ICG biliary excretion in both mice and rats. Acute toxicity of PA was increased by pentobarbital and 3-methylcholanthrene (3MC) pretreatment but decreased by SKF 525A. Cysteine protected against PA toxicity, while diethylmaleate (DEM) pretreatment increased PA toxicity. While cystiene pretreatment protected PA-treated mice against depletion of hepatic GSH, against elevation of SGPT and SGOT and against increased BSP and ICG retention, DEM pretreatment enhanced these effects. Phenobarbital, but not 3MC pretreatment, potentiated the elevation of SGPT; neither pretreatment had an effect on PA-induced hepatic GSH depletion. Therefore, PA toxicity may be elicited via an active metabolite. *In vitro* PA-GSH reaction suggested that PA could react with GSH both nonenzymatically and enzymatically. A mechanism for the toxicity of PA is proposed.

INTRODUCTION

Penicillic acid (PA), an α, β-unsaturated conjugated lactone, is produced by several food-borne fungi[1]. Since the discovery of its carcinogenicity in experimental animals[2, 3, 4] and its subsequent isolation from agricultural products[5, 6, 7, 8, 9], PA has been considered a potential environmental health hazard for man. In addition to its carcinogenicity, PA is hepatotoxic in experimental animals. For example, PA caused generalized hepatocyte necrosis in mice[10] and sinusoidal congestion in canine liver[11]. Furthermore, morphologic damage occurred in cultured hepatocytes treated with a PA concentration as low as 1×10^{-5} M[12]. Studies were undertaken to examine the hepatobiliary toxicity of PA, and to delineate its mechanism of toxicity.

MATERIAL AND METHODS

The purity (>99%) of PA, a gift from Dr. Alex Ciegler, U.S.D.A., was determined by melting point and infra-red and nuclear magnetic resonance spectroscopy. High resolution mass spectral analysis confirmed compound identity.

Animal treatment. PA was dissolved in normal saline for injection. Cysteine (150 mg/kg) in saline and diethylmaleate (DEM) in corn oil (0.3 ml/kg) were injected ip 5 and 30 min prior to PA administration, respectively. Sodium phenobarbital or sodium pentobarbital (75 mg/kg daily for 3 days) and 3-methylcholanthrene (3MC) (20 mg/kg for 4 days; or 50 mg/kg for 3 days) were given to mice for enzyme induction; PA was given 24 hr after the last dosing. SKF 525A was given 45 min prior to PA administration. Control animals received normal saline or corn oil.

The LD50 of PA in mice was estimated by the method of Weil[13]. Pentobarbital sleeping time was determined by administrating a challenge pentobarbital dose (60 mg/kg) and measuring the time between the losing and regaining of the righting reflex of the animals. Blood pentobarbital levels were determined by the method of Goldbaum[14]. The 9000 g supernatant fraction was used for *in vitro* metabolism of pentobarbital as described by Boulus *et al.*[15] with modification[16].

Reduced glutathione (GSH) levels were determined by the fluorometric method of Cohn and Lyle[17] as modified by Hissin and Hiff[18]. Oxidized GSH levels were determined as described by Hadley *et al.*[19]. SGPT and SGOT activities and serum bilirubin levels were measured colorimetrically with assay kits from Sigma Chemical Co. (St. Louis, MO, USA). BSP and ICG levels were assayed as described[20, 21].

Biliary excretion of ICG was examined by cannulating the common bile duct of mice after the gall bladder was ligated. Biliary excretion of ICG in rats was examined by cannulating the common bile duct. ICG was injected iv via the tail vein in mice or the femoral vein in rats.

PA in the *in vitro* PA-GSH reaction studies was analyzed by the high pressure liquid chromatographic procedure as described by Chan *et al.*[23].

Statistical analysis was performed using Student's unpaired t-test or weighted least squares of the 2 x 2 factorial (in a complete randomized design experiment) analysis of variance[22] with the Statistical Analysis System (SAS) computer program. The level of significance was chosen as $\alpha < 0.05$.

RESULTS AND DISCUSSION

PA increased pentobarbital sleeping time in a dose dependent manner (Fig. 1). The half-life of pentobarbital in the blood was prolonged in PA-treated mice (Fig. 2). *In vitro* metabolism of pentobarbital was inhibited competitively by

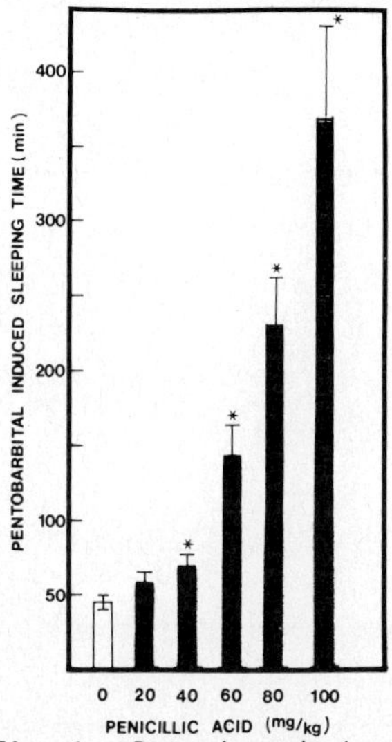

Fig. 1. Dose-dependent effect of penicillic acid on pentobarbital-induced nacrosis determined at 48 hr.

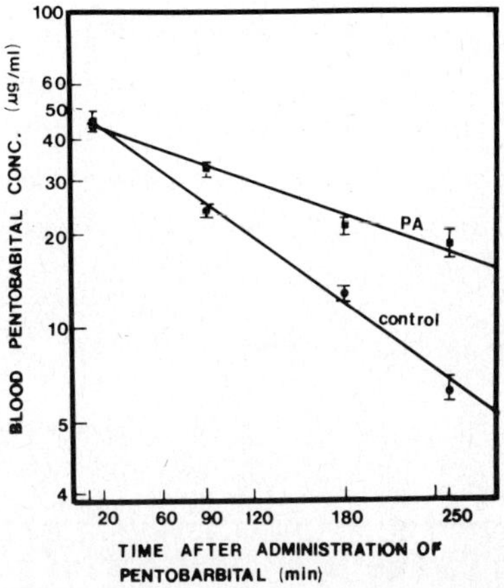

Fig, 2. Effect of penicillic acid (PA) (80 mg/kg) pretreatment on the biological decay of pentobarbital (60 mg/kg) in blood.

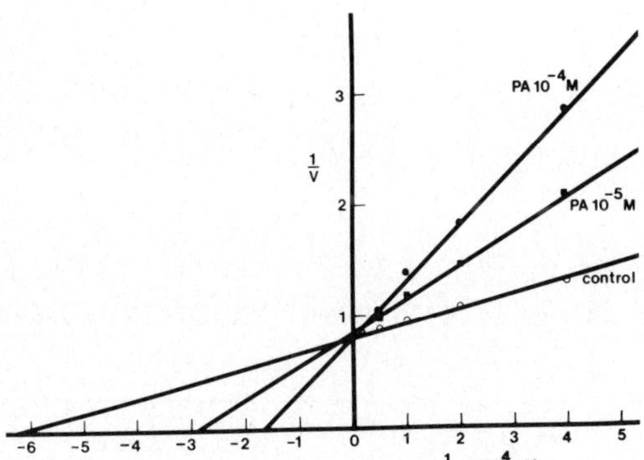

Fig. 3. Lineweaver-Burk Plot of the *in vitro* effect of penicillic acid (PA) on pentobarbital metabolism.

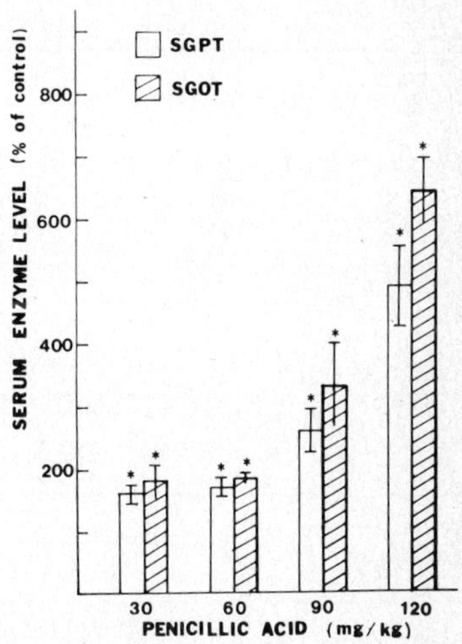

Fig. 4. Dose dependent increase in serum glutamic-pyruvic (SGPT) and glutamic-oxalacetic (SGOT) transaminase activities determined 24 hr after administration of penicillic acid.

PA (Fig. 3). SGPT and SGOT activities, indicators of hepatic injury, were elevated in PA-treated mice (Fig. 4). Furthermore, the serum bilirubin level in PA-treated mice was increased (Table 1). PA increased plasma BSP and serum ICG concentrations (Table 2). These results substantiated the hepatotoxicity of penicillic acid. Furthermore, hepatic GSH was depleted more than 80% when determined 45 min after a 240 mg/kg dose of PA was given (Fig. 5). Oxidized GSH and extra-hepatic GSH were not affected (data not presented).

TABLE 1

EFFECTS OF PENICILLIC ACID ON SERUM BILIRUBIN IN MALE MICE GIVEN PENICILLIC ACID

DOSE (mg/kg)	Time (hr)	Direct Serum[a] Bilirubin, mg/100 ml	Total Serum[a] Bilirubin, mg/100 ml
0.0	—	.355 ± 0.01	.554 ± 0.02
30	24	.530 ± 0.07[b]	.714 ± 0.05[b]
90	24	.525 ± 0.06[b]	.780 ± 0.34[b]
90	48	.670 ± 0.14[b]	1.20 ± 0.15[b]

[a]Each value represents the $\bar{X}$ ± S.E. of 3 to 4 animals

[b]Significant at p < 05. ND: Not done

TABLE 2

EFFECTS OF PENICILLIC ACID ON PLASMA AND SERUM RETENTION OF SULFOBROMEPHTHALAIN (BSP) AND INDOCYANINE GREEN (ICG)

Dose (mg/kg)	Time (hr)	15 min plasma[a] BSP (μg/ml)	30 min plasma[a] BSP (μg/ml)	15 min serum[a] ICG (μg/ml)
0.0	—	19.31 ± 1.9	10.8 ± 3.6	18.0 ± 0.2
30	24	ND	14.18 ± 1.8	18.0 ± 0.7
90	2	ND	27.8 ± 2.7[b]	38.0 ± 0.1[b]
90	24	72.6 ± 14.3[b]	ND	56.0 ± 0.4[b]
90	48	ND	88.9 ± 21.8[b]	139.0 ± 1.1[b]

[a]Each value represents the $\bar{X}$ ± S.E. of at least 3 animals

[b]Significant at p <0.05. ND: Not done

Biliary dysfunction also was observed in PA-treated mice and rats. Pretreatment with a single LD50 dose of PA (90 mg/kg, ip) resulted in depression of total biliary excretion of ICG in both species (Table 3). This depression was dose and time dependent. A 42% and 57% decrease in biliary excretion of ICG was observed in rats and mice 48 and 72 hr after PA treatment, respectively.

The acute toxicity of PA was increased by the enzyme inducers, pentobarbital and 3MC, but decreased by the enzyme inhibitor, SKF 525A (Table 4). Cysteine pretreatment protected mice against PA acute toxicity, and DEM, an GSH depletor, potentiated PA toxicity. These results suggested that PA toxicity may be elicited via an active metabolite and that GSH may be involved in the detoxification of PA *in vivo*.

This suggestion was supported by the fact that (1) cysteine pretreatment reversed and DEM pretreatment potentiated PA-induced depletion of hepatic GSH, elevation of SGPT and the increase in serum ICG retention (Tables 5, 6), and (2) phenobarbital pretreatment but not 3MC, potentiated PA-induced elevation of SGPT. However, phenobarbital, 3MC and SKF 525A had no significant effects on PA-induced depletion of hepatic GSH.

TABLE 3

THE EFFECTS OF PENICILLIC ACID (PA) ON BILIARY EXCRETION OF ICG IN MICE AND RATS

	% Administered ICG Dose Excreted[a]	
	Mice	Rats
Control Normal Saline	40.8 ± 2.8 (17)	50.7 ± 4.5 (6)
PA (90 mg/kg)		
12 hr	33.4 ± 3.3 (3)	N.D.
24 hr	31.7 ± 4.8 (4)	30.0 ± 4.0[b] (5)
48 hr	28.7 ± 3.2[b] (6)	29.3 ± 6.0[b] (5)
72 hr	17.3 ± 5.7[b] (4)	46.0 ± 6.3[b] (3)
96 hr	42.5 ± 5.0 (3)	N.D.
PA (30 mg/kg)		
48 hr	46.9 ± 4.1 (3)	50.0 ± 4.0 (3)
72 hr	N.D.	44.8 ± 3.9 (3)

[a] Total amount of ICG excreted in 24 min and 15 min in mice and rats, respectively.

[b] Significantly different from control at $p < 0.05$.
Number in the brackets represents the number of animals.
N.D. = Not done.

The PA-GSH reaction, studied *in vitro* by HPLC analysis, demonstrated that PA can react with GSH both enzymatically and nonenzymatically (Fig. 6).

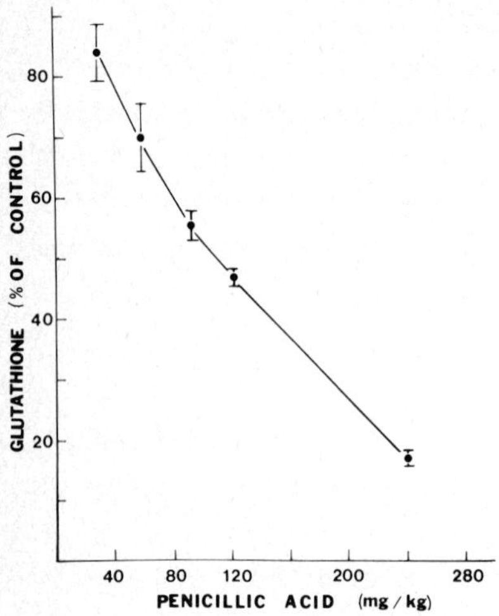

Fig. 5. Depletion of hepatic reduced glutathione determined 45 min after administration of penicillic acid.

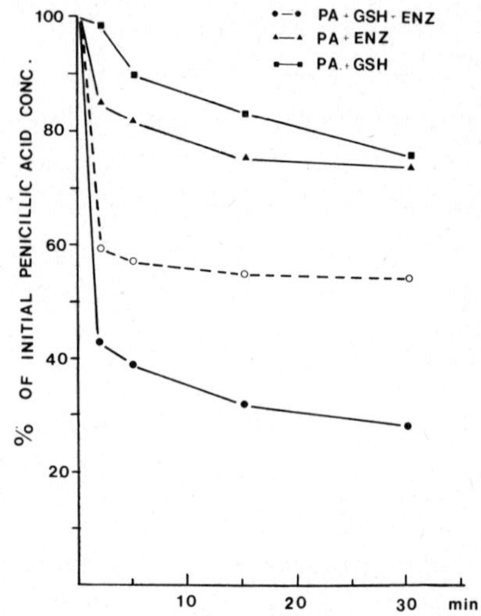

Fig. 6. *In vitro* penicillic acid (PA) and glutathione (GSH) reaction. 9,000 g mouse liver homogenate was used as enzyme source (ENZ). Dotted line represents GSH dependent PA enzymatic reaction corrected for non-enzymatic and nonspecific reaction.

TABLE 4

EFFECTS OF PENTOBARBITAL, 3-METHYLCHOLANTHRENE, SKF-525A, DIMETHYL MALEATE, AND CYSTEINE ON THE ACUTE TOXICITY OF PENICILLIC ACID (PA)

Pretreatments	Total animals	LD50[a] (mg/kg)	CI (mg/kg)
Normal Saline	80	90.00	105.3-76.86
Cysteine (150 mg/kg 5 min before PA)	45	(None died even at 202.5 mg/kg)[b]	
Cysteine (150 mg/kg 20 min after PA)	40	90.00	110.5-76.86
Diethly maleate (0.3 ml/kg 30 min before PA)	40	49.74[c]	56.96-43.46
SKF-525A	20	170.00[c]	246.9-166.0
3-Methylcholanthrene	40	55.32[c]	64.63-47.37
Pentobarbital	40	53.17[c]	63.04-44.78

[a]Calculated by Weil's (1952) table. [b]Five animals were in the 202.5 mg/kg group
[c]Significantly different ($p < 0.05$) from normal saline-pretreated groups.

TABLE 5

EFFECT OF PENICILLIC ACID (PA), CYSTEINE AND DIETHYLMALEATE (DEM) ON HEPATIC REDUCED GLUTATHIONE (GSH) LEVEL AND ON SERUM GLUTAMATE-PYRUVATE TRANSAMINASE (SGPT) ACTIVITY.[a]

	GSH (μmole/g) PA (mg/kg)		SGPT (unit/ml) PA (mg/kg)	
	0	90	0	90
Saline	4.79	2.51	20.75	48.50
Cysteine (150 mg/kg)	5.36	4.61	29.00	28.25
Corn Oil	4.97	2.69	22.3	48.50
DEM (0.3 ml/kg)	2.76	1.25	25.3	156.50

[a] Hepatic GSH and SGPT activities were determined 45 min and 24 hours after PA administration, respectively. Each value represents the mean of 4 animals.

Data were analyzed by 2 x 2 factorial complete randomized design weighted least square analysis of variance.

TABLE 6

EFFECT OF PENICILLIC ACID (PA), CYSTEINE AND DIETHYLMALEATE (DEM) TREATMENT ON SERUM INDOCYANINE GREEN (ICG) RETENTION.

	15 min serum ICG concentration (μg/ml)[a] PA (mg/kg)	
	0	90
Saline	19.8	112.8
Cysteine (150 mg/kg)	17.7	17.6
Corn Oil	18.1	60.7
DEM)0.3 ml/kg)	17.3	406.1

[a] Each value represents the mean of 4 animals. ICG retention was determined 48 hours and 12 hours after PA administration in cysteine and DEM pretreated animals, respectively. Data were analyzed by 2 x 2 factorial complete randomized design weighted least square analysis of variance.

To help explain these observations, we have proposed the metabolic scheme illustrated in Fig. 7. This scheme assumes that all reaction rates follow first order kinetics. PA can either bind nonenzymatically to (1) GSH at the α, β conjugated double bond or at the olefenic group to form a nontoxic adduct[10], or PA can be biotransformed to (2) an active metabolite which can either be deactiviated by GSH to (3), form other GSH adducts or (4) bind to a macromolecule and thus induce toxicity. It is obvious that if GSH were depleted as in the case of DEM pretreatment, that the active metabolite would accumulate and toxicity would increase. The opposite effect would be expected if the GSH level were maintained by cysteine when given prior to PA administration. On the other hand, the PA-induced depletion of GSH should not be changed greatly in enzyme-induced animals although toxicity was increased in the former group, and decreased in the later group. This probably was because any change in PA-induced GSH depletion in the enzymatic pathway would be balanced by opposite changes in the nonenzymatic pathway. However, increasing the rate of active metabolite formation would probably increase the rate of toxic metabolites binding to macromolecules by the minor pathway. By the same token, the opposite effect would be expected when the activation process is inhibited.

Data were analyzed by 2 x 2 factorial complete randomized design weighted least square analysis of variance.

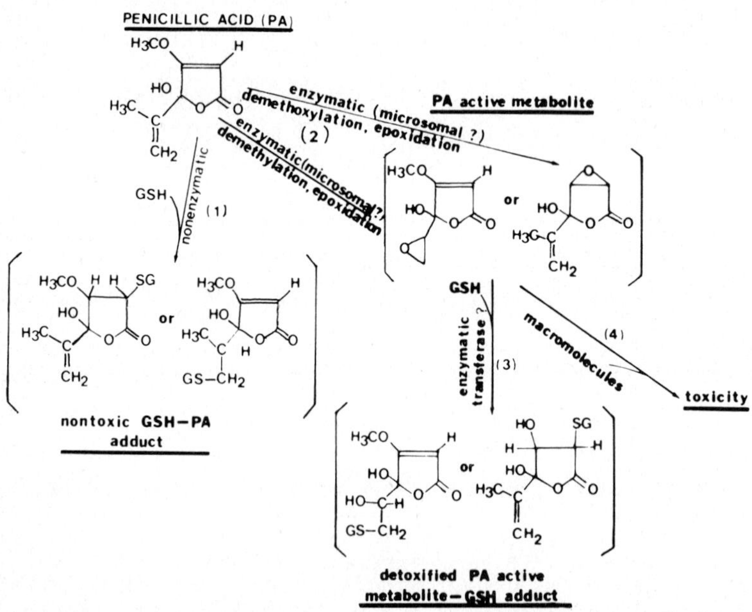

Fig. 7. Schmatic of proposed pathway for activation and detoxification of penicillic acid in male mice.

TABLE 7

EFFECT OF PENICILLIC ACID (PA), PHENOBARBITAL (PHENO.), 3-METHYLCHOLANTHRENE (3MC), AND SKF 525A TREATMENT ON HEPATIC REDUCED GLUTATHIONE (GSH) LEVELS AND SERUM GLUTAMATE-PYRUVATE TRANSAMINASE (SGPT) ACTIVITY.[a]

	GSH (μmole/g)		SGPT (units/ml)	
	PA (mg/kg)		PA (mg/kg)	
	0	90	0	90
Saline	5.01	2.89	19.3	48.5
Pheno.	5.41	3.11	25.0	99.0
Corn Oil	4.71	2.65	22.0	48.5
3MC	5.17	2.54	39.3	43.0
Saline	5.68	2.89		
SKF 525A	4.04	3.16		

[a] Hepatic GSH and SGPT activities were determined 45 min and 24 hours after the administration of PA. Each value represents the mean of 3 animals.

ACKNOWLEDGMENTS

This work was supported by ES-02191 and ES-01351. Mr. Chan was supported by Training Grant ES-07045.

REFERENCES

1. Scott, P. M. (1978) Mycotoxic Fungi, Mycotoxins and Mycotoxicoses. An Encyclopedia Handbook, eds. D. Wyllie and L. G. Morehouse, Marcel Dekker, Inc., New York and Basel. Vol. 1, p. 311.
2. Dickens, F. and Jones, H. E. H. (1961) Brit. J. Cancer, 15, 85-95.
3. Dickens, F. and Jones, H. E. H. (1963) Brit. J. Cancer, 17, 100-108.
4. Dickens, F. and Jones, H. E. H. (1965) Brit. J. Cancer, 19, 392-403.
5. Kuntzman, C. P. and Ciegler, A. (1970) Appl. Microbiol., 20, 204-207.
6. Pero, R. W., Harven, D., Owens, R. G. and Snow, J. P. (1973) J. Chromatogr., 65, 501-506.
7. Bacon, C. W., Sweeney, J. G., Robbins, J. D. and Burdick, C. (1973) Appl. Microbiol., 26, 155-160.
8. Thorpe, C. W. and Johnson, R. L. (1974) J. Assoc. Offic. Anal. Chem., 57, 861-865.

9. Snow, J. P., Lucas, G. B. Harven, R. W. and Owens, R. G. (1972) Appl. Microbiol., 24, 34-36.

10. Ciegler, A., Mintzlaff, H. J., Weisledes, D. and Listner, L. (1972) Appl. Microbiol., 24, 114-119.

11. Hayes, A. W., Unger, P. D. and Williams, W. L. (1977) Ann. Nutr. Aliment. 31, 711-722.

12. Umeda, M. (1971) Japan J. Exp. Med., 41, 195-207.

13. Weil, C. S. (1952) Biometrics, 8, 249-261.

14. Goldbaum, L. R. (1952) Anal. Chem., 24, 1604-1613.

15. Boulos, B. M., Short, C. R., and Davis, L. E. (1970) Biochem. Pharmacol., 19, 723-732.

16. Chan, P. K., Reddy, C. S. and Hayes, A. W. (1980) Toxicol. Appl. Pharmacol., 52, 1-9.

17. Cohn, V. H. and Lyle, J. (1960) Anal. Biochem., 14, 434-440.

18. Hissin, P. J. and Hiff, R. (1976) Anal. Biochem., 74, 214-226.

19. Hadley, W. M., Bousquet, W. F. and Miya, T. S. (1974) J. Pharma. Sci., 63, 57-59.

20. Kutob, S. D. and Plaa, G. L. (1962) J. Appl. Physiol., 17, 123-125.

21. Caesar, J., Shaddon, S., Chiaduaski, L., Guevara, L. and Sherlock, S. (1961) Clin. Sci., (London) 21, 43-57.

22. Draper, N. R. and Smith, H. (1966) Applied Regression Analysis, John Wiley and Sons, Inc., New York, pp. 77-81.

23. Chan, P. K., Siraj, M. Y. and Hayes, A. W. (1980) J. Chromatogr., 194, 387-398.

© 1980 Elsevier/North-Holland Biomedical Press
Mechanisms of Toxicity and Hazard Evaluation
B. Holmstedt, R. Lauwerys, M. Mercier, M. Roberfroid eds

HEXACHLOROBENZENE AND 2,4,5,2',4',5'-HEXACHLOROBIPHENYL - A COMPARISON OF THEIR DISTRIBUTION, BIOTRANSFORMATION AND PORPHYRINOGENIC ACTION IN FEMALE RATS

GÜNTER KOSS, SIGRID SEUBERT, ANDREAS SEUBERT, MANFRED HERBERT, WOLFGANG KORANSKY AND HELMUT IPPEN
Institute of Toxicology and Pharmacology, Pilgrimstein 2, D-3550 Marburg; Clinic of Dermatology, v.-Sieboldstr. 3, D-3400 Göttingen (Federal Republic of Germany)

INTRODUCTION

Hexachlorobenzene (HCB) and 2,4,5,2',4',5'-Hexachlorobiphenyl (Hexa-CB) belong to those xenobiotics which because of their porphyrinogenic action in animals and man are of toxicologic importance[1,2]. In an animal experiment we compared their pharmacokinetic behavior and porphyrinogenic action with the aim of obtaining more information about the mechanism of inducing porphyria.

RESULTS

Body weight gain, distribution and biotransformation

During the experiment, in which 2 groups of rats received 177 µmoles/kg HCB or Hexa-CB every second day for 10 weeks, the body weight gain of these animals did not differ from that of controls. Examination of the tissues revealed a comparatively high content of Hexa-CB in the adipose tissue, a similar content of both compounds in the liver and more HCB than Hexa-CB in blood (Table 1).

Both substances are excreted in unchanged and metabolized form. So far 2 metabolites of Hexa-CB were isolated, both have phenolic groups. One of them is identical with the already known hexachlorobiphe-

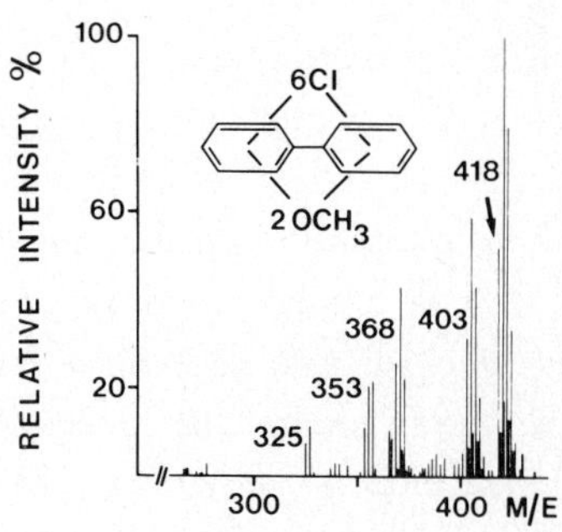

Fig. 1. Mass spectrum and proposed formula of a metabolite (as methyl ether) of Hexa-CB isolated from the feces of female rats.

TABLE 1

Content of HCB and Hexa-CB in the tissues of female rats after oral administration of 177 µmoles/kg of either substance every other day for 10 weeks, and the content of porphyrins in the liver 24 hrs after the last treatment[a]

	Administration of		
	HCB[b]	Hexa-CB	Oil
Body weight:			
start of experiment	135 ± 5g	127 ± 6g	132 ± 4g
end of experiment	210 ± 10g	205 ± 7g	216 ±15g
Substance content in			
adipose tissue	39 ± 14[c]	55 ± 22	-[d]
liver	1.4±0.1	1.3±0.4	-
blood	0.6±0.3	0.1±0.01	-
Total liver porphyrins[e]	20 ± 10[f]	710 ± 60	0.7 ± 0.2

[a] All methods used in this experiment are described elsewhere[3-5].
[b] Each treatment group consisted of 4 animals.
[c] µmoles/g wet tissue.
[d] Not determined.
[e] The liver was not perfused prior to porphyrin analysis.
[f] nmoles/g wet tissue.

nylol[6]. The other metabolite contains apart from 6 chlorine atoms additionally 2 OH-groups (Figure 1).- HCB is converted to a comparatively large number of metabolites. We identified chlorophe - nols and sulphur containing compounds. The chlorophenols have either one or two hydroxyl groups. One of these phenols also contains sulphur (Figure 2). To the sulphur containing metabolites belong mercapturic acids, free thiophenols, thioanisoles, sulphoxides and sulphones[3,4,7,8].

On the basis of amounts of the

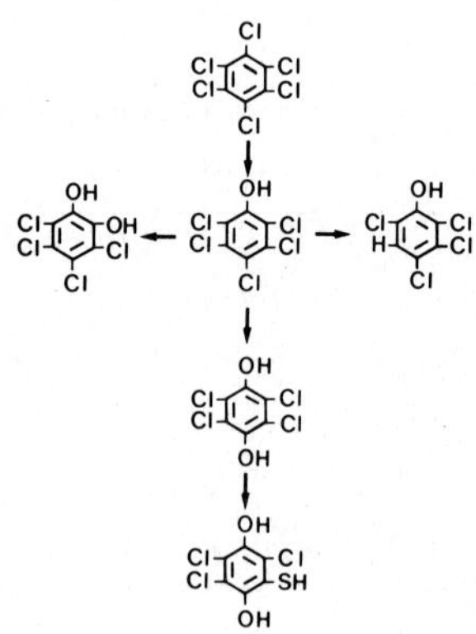

Fig. 2. Proposed metabolic pathway of the formation of chlorophenols from HCB in rats.

unchanged substances and their metabolites in the excreta we estimated the biotransformation rate of HCB to be 40% and of Hexa-CB to be about 10%. Therefore, HCB and Hexa-CB differ both in the storage and extent of their metabolism.

Porphyrinogenic action

Numerous findings obtained so far support the thesis that the metabolic conversion of HCB is a prerequisite for inducing porphyria[5]. In regard to this thesis, we compared the porphyrinogenic action of HCB with that of Hexa-CB, which differ in their extent of biotransformation. Contrary to the expectation, however, we observed in the liver of the Hexa-CB treated animals a 30-40 times higher porphyrin content than in the liver of the rats dosed with HCB (Table 1). Despite their relatively low liver porphyrin values, the HCB treated animals excreted more porphyrins with the urine (84 $\pm$ 60 nmoles/day) than the animals which received Hexa-CB (56 $\pm$ 38 nmoles/day). In the porphyrin distribution pattern of the liver and urine of the rats treated with HCB and Hexa-CB, uroporphyrin (60 - 65%) and heptacarboxyporphyrin (34 - 39%) predominated, while in untreated animals mainly copro- and protoporphyrin are present. Almost similar was the amount of 5-aminolevulinic acid (8 µmoles/day) and porphobilinogen (2 µmoles/day) in the urine of both treatment groups. The controls excreted 0.1 and 0.2 µmoles/day, resp., of either porphyrin precursor.

DISCUSSION

From the different concentration rates of both compounds in the blood, liver and adipose tissue (Hexa-CB = 1:13:550; HCB = 1:2:65) it is concluded that Hexa-CB possesses a more pronounced lipophilicity than HCB. In view of the contamination of man, this observation is considered to be of importance, since very often its total body burden is calculated on the basis of the drug content in blood, which can easily be sampled.

The comparatively high liver porphyrin content and the limited porphyrin excretion via the urine in the Hexa-CB treated rats is remarkable. Obviously, these animals retain the porphyrins to a greater extent than the rats which received HCB. Since Hexa-CB like HCB leads to morphologic liver tissue alterations[9,10], we conclude that the porphyrin accumulation is closely associated with the impairment of this organ. However, the cause of this accumulation is not known.- Our previous studies had shown a connection between the biotransformation of HCB and the predominance of uro- and heptacarboxyporphyrin in the distribution pattern of the liver porphyrins[5]. Accordingly, conversion products of HCB are thought to cause the inhibition of the uroporphyrinogen decarboxylase. Whether metabolites of Hexa-CB are also involved in the inhibition of the enzyme, is not known as yet.

It is concluded, that the extent of porphyria may not be recognized by analysing the urine, but can be by estimating the porphyrin content in the liver. The comparison of the liver content of porphyrins with both inducing substances indicates a more pronounced porphyrinogenic action of Hexa-CB.

ACKNOWLEDGEMENTS

This study was supported by the Deutsche Forschungsgemeinschaft and by P.G. Unna-Stiftung.- The authors thank Mrs. J. Seidel and Miss. B. Würminghausen for skillful assistance.

REFERENCES

1. DeMatteis, F., Prior, B.E. and Rimington, C. (1961) Nature (Lond.) 191, 363-366.
2. Vos, J.G., Strik, J.J.T.W.A., VanHolsteyn, C.W.M. and Penning, S. (1971) Toxicol. Appl. Pharmacol. , 20, 232-240.
3. Koss, G., Koransky, W. and Steinbach, K. (1976) Arch. Toxicol. 35, 107-114.
4. Koss, G., Koransky, W. and Steinbach, K. (1979) Arch. Toxicol. 42, 19-31.
5. Koss, G., Seubert, S., Seubert, A., Koransky, W., Kraus, P. and Ippen, H. (1980) Internat. J. Biochem. (in press).
6. Sundström, G., Hutzinger, O. and Safe, S. (1976) Chemosphere, 4, 249-253.
7. Jansson, B. and Bergman, A. (1978) Chemosphere, 3, 257-268.
8. Renner, G., Richter, E. and Schuster, K.P. (1978) Chemosphere, 8, 663-668.
9. Böger, A., Koss, G., Koransky, W., Naumann, R. and Frenzel, H. (1979) Virchows Arch. A Path. Anat. Histol., 382, 127-137.
10. McKinney, J.D., Chae, K., Gupta, B.N., Moore, J.A. and Goldstein, J.A. (1976) Toxicol. Appl. Pharmacol., 36, 65-80.

Mechanisms of Toxicity and Hazard Evaluation
B. Holmstedt, R. Lauwerys, M. Mercier, M. Roberfroid eds

EFFECTS OF DIETARY VITAMIN A (RETINOL) ON THE REDUCTION OF HEPATIC RETINOL STORAGE CAUSED BY 2,3,7,8-TETRACHLORODIBENZO-p-DIOXIN

TUULA THUNBERG AND ULF G. AHLBORG
Department of Toxicology, Karolinska Institutet, and National Laboratory of Environmental Medicine, P.O. Box 60 400, S-104 01 Stockholm (Sweden)

INTRODUCTION

Recent compilations of epidemiological data have estimated that environmental factors are responsible for the major part of human cancer. Chemicals, both manmade and naturally occurring, are probably the main causative agents. Furthermore, constituents in food seems to represent important factors in cancerogenesis. Cancer is a multifactorial disease and its development will be dependent on the interaction between initiating, promoting, and inhibiting agents that reaches man through food and environment.

One essential component in food, vitamin A (retinol), has been demonstrated to possess an inhibitory effect on initiation[1,2] and on promotion[3].

The highly toxic contaminant in many industrial chlorophenol preparations, 2,3,7,8-tetrachlorodibenzo-p-dioxin (TCDD), has recently been demonstrated to severly affect the organism's ability to store retinol[4]. Hepatic storage of retinol was studied

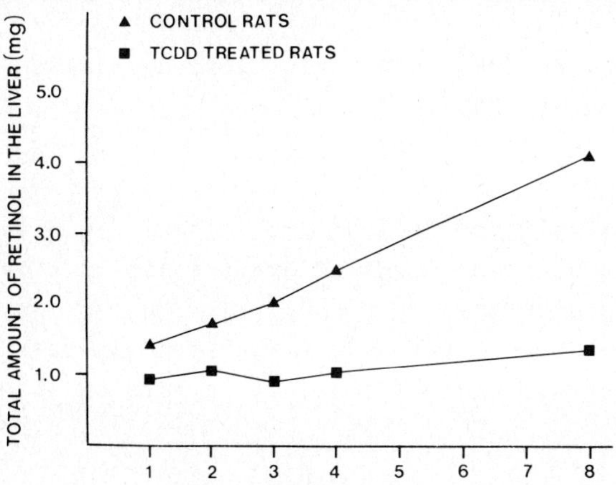

Fig. 1. Total amount of retinol in the liver of Sprague-Dawley rats during an 8 week experiment. From Thunberg et al. 1979.

in rats during an 8 week period, and it was found that 10 µg/kg of TCDD in a single oral dose inhibited the storage of retinol as compared to control rats (Fig. 1.). TCDD has also been demonstrated to induce many enzyme systems, e.g. dechlorination[5] and glucuronidation[6].

The purpose of the present experiment was to study how dietary levels of retinol affect the effects of TCDD on retinol storage and UDP-glucuronosyltransferase (UDPGT) activity.

MATERIALS AND METHODS

Male Sprague-Dawley rats were treated with TCDD and kept on varying diets for 4 weeks according to Table 1.

TABLE 1
EXPERIMENTAL DESIGN

Retinol content of diet, mg/kg	Single oral dose of TCDD, µg/kg bodyweight 0	0.1	1.0	10
	Number of rats in each group			
1.2	10	10	10	10
3.0	10	10	10	10
6.0	10	10	10	10

Hepatic retinol levels and UDPGT activities were determined according to Thunberg et al., 1980[7].

RESULTS

Body weight gain was significantly lower in all animals given the highest TCDD-dose but no other signs of overt toxicity were evident in the TCDD-exposed animals.

A dose-dependent increase in liver weight was found in rats on diets with low or high retinol content, but not in rats on standard diet.

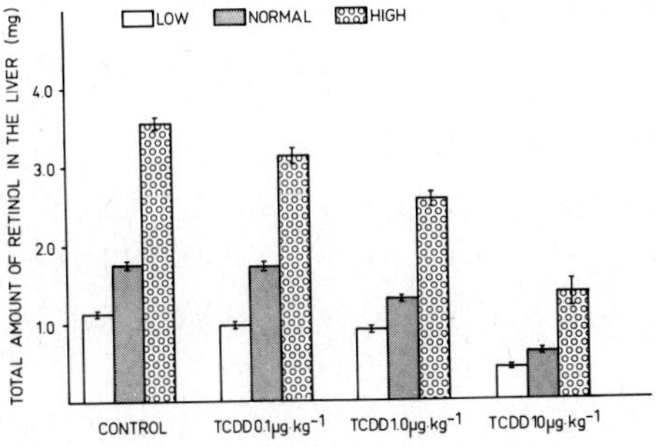

Fig. 2. Total amount of retinol in the liver of control and TCDD-treated rats 4 weeks after administration.[x]

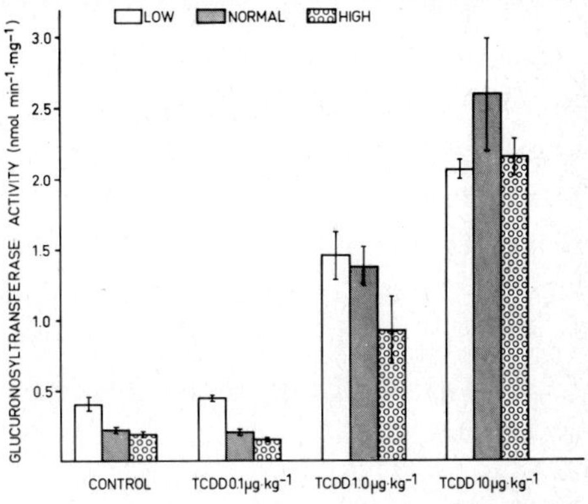

Fig. 3. Hepatic UDPGT activity in control and TCDD-treated rats 4 weeks after administration.[x]

Upon analysis of hepatic retinol, it was found that both retinol concentrations and total amounts of retinol stored decreased in a dose-dependent manner. The total amount of retinol stored is demonstrated in Figure 2. For the animals given 10 μg/kg of TCDD, the high retinol diet was not enough to ensure a retinol concentration or a total storage comparable to that of untreated rats kept on standard diet.

Figure 3 demonstrates the UDPGT activity in the different experimental groups. A significant effect of TCDD is obvious at 1.0 and 10.0 μg/kg of TCDD and regardless of the diet. However, in all but the groups treated with the highest TCDD-dose, the UDPGT activity is significantly related to the retinol level in the diet, the activity being highest in the groups kept on the diet with low retinol content.

DISCUSSION

The present study confirms the earlier finding that TCDD affects the storage of retinol in the liver[4]. This effect is dose-

[x] From Thunberg et al. 1980.

dependent and appears already at a single oral dose of 0.1 μg/kg. Hepatic UDPGT, which plays a central role in the metabolism of retinol, is demonstrated to be induced in inverse proportion to the level of hepatic retinol. This supports the hypothesis that the effect of TCDD on retinol, at least partly, may be the result of a higher rate of retinol conjugation and excretion.

The data from the different dietary levels of retinol demonstrate that the effect of TCDD partly can be compensated. This indicates that, within the dose range and time period studied, no effect on the storage capacity of the liver occurs.

Retinol has been demonstrated to have an inhibitory effect on microsomal oxidative processes, which are involved in the formation of reactive metabolites[1]. Our findings that UDPGT activity is influenced by the level of retinol in the diet is further confirmation of the inhibitory potency of retinol. A low dietary retinol level may thus result in a more rapid metabolism of several compounds, but also in a higher rate of excretion due to increased conjugation. The somewhat contradictory results achieved in studies of the influence of vitamin A on cancer promotion may thus be dependent on the balance between these processes.

ACKNOWLEDGEMENTS

This work was supported by grants from the Swedish Environment Protection Board (7-403/78-79).

REFERENCES

1. Hill, D.L. and Shih, T. (1974) Cancer Res., 34, 564-570.
2. Busk, L. and Ahlborg, U.G. (1980) Toxicology Letters in press.
3. Sporn, M.B., Dunlop, N.M., Newton, D.L. and Smith, J.M. (1976) Federation Proc., 35, 1332-1338.
4. Thunberg, T., Ahlborg, U.G. and Johnsson, H. (1979) Arch. Toxicol., 42, 265-274.
5. Ahlborg, U.G. and Thunberg, T. (1978) Arch. Toxicol., 40, 55-61.
6. Lucier, G.W., McDaniel, O.S., Hook, G.E.R. and Fowler, B.A. (1973) Environ. Health Perspect., 5, 199-209.
7. Thunberg, T., Ahlborg, U.G., Håkansson, H., Krantz, C. and Monier, M. (1980) Arch. Toxicol. in press.

Mechanisms of Toxicity and Hazard Evaluation
B. Holmstedt, R. Lauwerys, M. Mercier, M. Roberfroid eds

CHANGES IN RAT LIVER MORPHOLOGY AND METABOLIC ACTIVITIES AFTER EXPOSURE TO CHLORINATED PARAFFINS

ODD G. NILSEN*, RUNE TOFTGÅRD** AND HANS GLAUMANN***
*Department of Pharmacology and Toxicology, School of Medicine, University of Trondheim, Norway. **Department of Pharmacology and Department of Medical Nutrition, Stockholm and ***Department of Pathology, Huddinge Hospital, Karolinska Institute, Sweden

INTRODUCTION

Chlorinated paraffins (CP) are extensively used in lubricants, cutting oils, paints, rubber and plastics. No satisfactory analytical methods are available for their quantitative determination. Except for low acute toxicity, very few data are available on the biological effects of these compounds. Chlorinated paraffins are often used as substitutes for PCB's. Since PCB's cause changes in the morphology and enzymatic activities in the liver, an examination has been made of the effects of the various chlorinated paraffins (defined by their carbon chain length and chlorine content) on rat liver.

MATERIALS AND METHODS

Male Spraque-Dawley rats of 300 g were given chlorinated paraffins in corn oil in doses of 1 g per kg body weight i.p. once daily for four days for investigations on liver microsomal metabolic activities and in doses of 1 g per kg body weight on day 1, 4 and 6 for morphological analysis of the liver. The animals were killed by decapitaion on the 5th and 7th day respectively, allowing only free excess to water during the last night. Cytochrome P-450 was determined according to Omura and Sato[1] and the O-deethylation of 7-ethoxyresorufin according to Prough et al.[2]. Phenol fraction I and II in the high pressure liquid chromatographic separation of benzo(a)pyrene (B(a)P) were eluted with the same retention times as 9-hydroxy- and 3-hydroxy-B(a)P respectively[3]. SDS polyacrylamide gel electrophoresis were performed on slab gels using a discontinuous buffer system[4].

For morphological analyses rat livers were perfused through the portal vein with 3% glutaraldehyde containing 0.1 M cacodylate buffer and 0.1 M sucrose. Processing for electronmicroscopy was performed according to standard procedures.

The Student´s t-test was used and p-values less than 0.05 were considered significant.

TABLE 1

EFFECTS[a] OF CHLORINATED PARAFFINS[b] ON RAT LIVER WEIGHT AND LIVER MICROSOMAL ACTIVITIES[c]

Substance	Liver weight / body weight	nmol P-450 / mg protein	O-deethylation of 7-ethoxyresorufin
CP-149	0.048±0.002[d]	0.65±0.07	80±6
CP-159	0.046±0.002[d]	0.73±0.09[d]	39±5[d]
CP-171	0.042±0.001[d]	0.71±0.05[d]	37±4[d]
CP-350	0.038±0.001[d]	0.62±0.08	84±6
CP-549	0.034±0.001	0.65±0.08	86±13
Control	0.034±0.001	0.55±0.07	80±8

	Benzo(a)pyrene					
	9,10-diol	4,5-diol	7,8-diol	phenol I	phenol II	quinon
CP-149	12± 2	79±22[d]	22±3[2]	25± 8[d]	156±17[d]	91±15[d]
CP-159	17±10	105± 8[d]	19±6[d]	35±17[d]	127± 8[d]	148±10[d]
CP-171	13± 2	145±21[d]	18±4[d]	11± 5	128±22[d]	136±15[d]
CP-350	12± 4	43±11[d]	5±3	11± 4	73±21	44±14[d]
CP-549	23± 5	38± 2[d]	7±6	40±12[d]	241±50[d]	60±14[d]
Control	15± 5	25± 4	8±3	13± 2	86±14	15± 6

[a] Mean values ±SD are given. n=4.
[b] I.p. injections of 1 g/kg once daily for four days. CP-149, CP-159 and CP-171 denote C_{10-13} paraffins containing 49, 59 and 71% of chlorine respectively. CP-350 and CP-549 denote C_{14-17} and C_{18-26} paraffins containing 50 and 49% of chlorine respectively.
[c] Expressed as pmol metabolite/mg protein, min.
[d] Significantly different from control. $p<0.05$.

RESULTS AND DISCUSSION

Table 1 demonstrates that chlorinated paraffins with short length of their carbon chain (C_{10-13}) and different degree of chlorination exert a more profound effect on rat liver weight, content of liver microsomal cytochrome P-450 and liver microsomal enzymatic activities when compared to paraffins with a higher length of the carbon chain (C_{14-26}). Higher degree of chlorination of the C_{10-13} paraffins was correlated with increased formation of B(a)P-4,5-diols and content of microsomal cytochrome P-450. However, the elevation of the liver to body weight ratio and the O-deethylation of 7-ethoxyresorufin were inversly correlated to the degree of chlororination. An increase in the two specific forms of cytochrome P-450 with molecular weights of 50 000 and 54 000, identified by electrophoresis, and the increased formation of B(a)P-4,5-diols, show that chlorinated paraffins display much of the same characteristics as phenobarbital[3]. The decreased metabolism of 7-ethoxyresorufin indicate that CP-159 and CP-171 at the same time inhibit other metabolic steps associated with the cytochrome P-450 enzyme system.

CP-149 caused a significant proliferation of the smooth ER, whereas CP-549 had only a modest effect (Fig. 1). It should be noted that both paraffins increased the total microsomal concentration of cytochrome P-450 to the same extent. The proliferation of smooth ER was increased most extensively by the compounds with

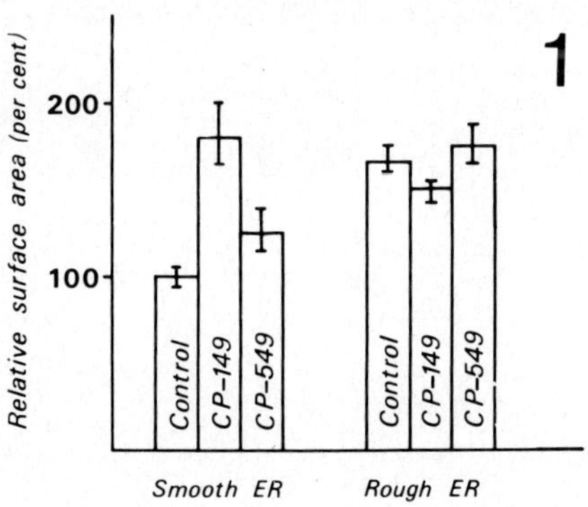

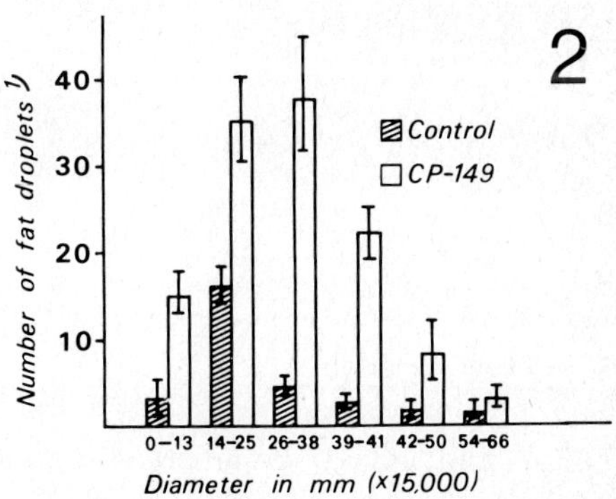

Fig. 1. Effect of CP-149 and CP-549 on the surface area of the smooth and rough ER. 40 randomly chosen pictures taken from periportal areas of 3 control and 4 experimental animals were analyzed. The surface area for smooth ER was 3.0 m^2/gram of liver (=100%).

Fig. 2. Relative numbers and size of fat droplets in control and CP-149 treated rats 1) Per 12 micrographs.

shorter chain length. CP-149 and 159 gave rise to increased occurrence of cytoplasmic lipid droplets (Figs. 2 and 3). These lipid droplets can not be exported out of the cell but must be degraded intracellularily. This conclusion is based on the increased numbers of forming autophagosomes and lysosomes containing lipid material with clear sign of degradation of the fat droplets (Fig. 4). CP-149 exposure resulted in increased numbers and size of peroxisomes as well as mitochondria and occasionally also in formation of mega mitochondria (Fig. 5).

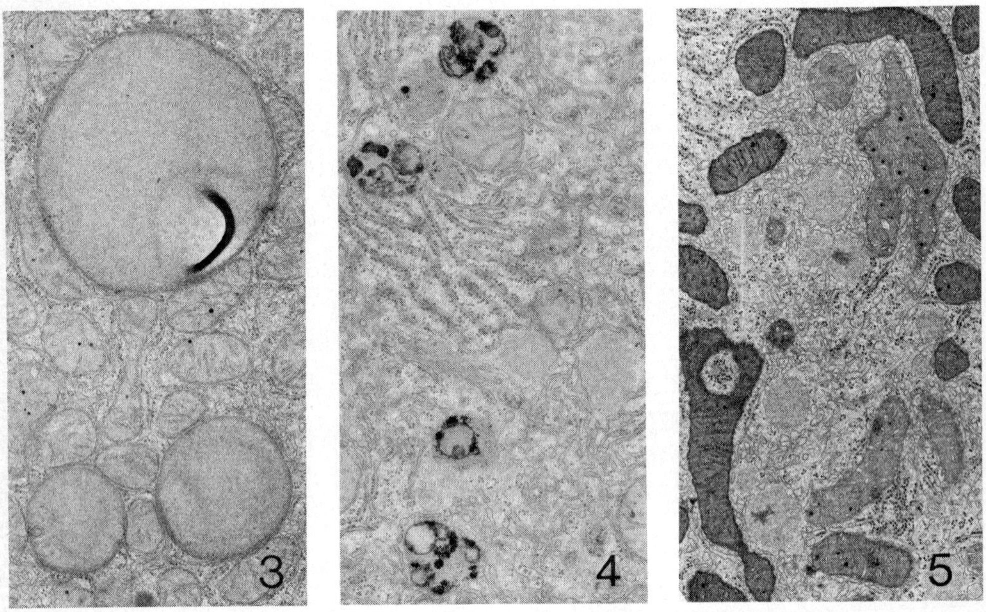

Figs. 3, 4 and 5. Electron micrographs depitced to illustrate lipid droplets (3), lysosomes containing partially degraded lipid material (4) and large mitochondria and numerous peroxisomes (5).

ACKNOWLEDGEMENTS

This study was supported by the Swedish Work Environment Health Fund, the Swedish Cancer Society and the Norwegian Research Council for Science and the Humanities.

REFERENCES

1. Omura, T. and Sato, R. (1964) J. Biol. Chem. 239, 2370-2378.
2. Prough, R.A., Burke, M.D. and Mayer, M.T. (1978) Methods of Enzymology, vol III, Academic Press, New York, pp. 372-377.
3. Toftgård, R., Nilsen, O.G., Ingelman-Sundberg, M. and Gustafsson, J.-Å. (1980) Acta Pharmacol. Toxicol. 46, 353-361.
4. Laemmli, U.K. (1970) Nature (Lond.) 227, 680-685.

© 1980 Elsevier/North-Holland Biomedical Press
Mechanisms of Toxicity and Hazard Evaluation
B. Holmstedt, R. Lauwerys, M. Mercier, M. Roberfroid eds

WHOLE BODY DISTRIBUTION OF ^{3}H LEVAMISOLE IN RATS AND MICE

P.BENARD - C. BRUNET* - M. CAZIN* - J.P. BRAUN - V. BURGAT-SACAZE - A.G.RICO
Ecole Vétérinaire Laboratoire de radioéléments et d'études métaboliques
31076 Toulouse Cedex France
* Université de Lille II - Faculté de Pharmacie - Laboratoire de Pharmacodynamie 59045 Lille Cedex France

INTRODUCTION

Levamisole is an antinematodal drug because of its broad range of activity in numerous species. So it is widely used in veterinary and human medicine[1]. In recent years, it has been studied for its beneficient effects in chronic and recurrent infectious, particulary in patients with immunodeficiency syndromes (rheumatoid arthritis, some types of cancer certain infectious diseases)[2]

Before studying its mode of action as an immunostimulant agent we studied the metabolism using ^{3}H labelled levamisole. The first of the metabolic studies was autoradiography, performed to identify concentrations of radioactivity in various organs in the whole body of rats. The aim of this paper is to present results obtained by whole body autoradiography in rats and mice given (^{3}H) levamisole.

MATERIALS AND METHODS

Labelled compound: Tritium labelled S(-) 2,3,5,6 tetrahydro 6 phenyl imidazo (2,1 b) thiazole or levamisole was purchased through the Commissariat à l'Energie Atomique (Saclay-France) in an ethanolic solution. The specific activity was 17 $Ci.mol.^{-1}$

Animals Charles River CD Cobs rats weighing 50g and C 3 H black mice weighing 20 g were given 2.5 mg/kg of (^{3}H) levamisole, the activity thus delivered being 1 m Ci/Kg. They were sacrificed 30 min, 1 hr, 4 hr, 8 hr, 16 hr, 24 hr, 48 hr, 72 hr, 96 hr and 8 days after treatment.

Technique All animals were killed with ether and frozen directly on a microtome stage by rapid immersion in a freezing medium. A 10 % aqueous solution of carboxy methyl cellulose was used as a mounting mediuma, which formed a firm support all around the animal when frozen. Whole body sagittal sections (thickness = 20 µm) were then cut with a PMV 450 semi-automatic microtome according to ULLBERG's technique; after they were collected, sections were allowed to dry by storage overnight at -20°C in the cryostat. Dried sections were then pressed directly against a rapid film (Ultrofilm ^{3}H)[3-5]. It is single coated with a thin layer of relatively large sized crystals. As this film lacks an anti-scratch layer, it allows easily tritium registration. The films were stored in a light tight bag at -30°C. At the end of a six months exposure period, the section and the film were separated. The former was stained (Mayer's haematoxylin) for histological examination, the latter was developed, fixed and rinsed. All operations were performed in well defined and controled conditions to produce autoradiograms that could be compared.

RESULTS

Results are given for mice, in Figure 1. In both species, the highest activity was detected 30 minutes after treatment. Then it decreased quickly to trace amounts which are still present in the blood stream 8 hours after the administration.

The same kinetics are observed for the organs. The liver concentrates the highest activity in both species as soon as 30 min after oral administration. It is noteworthy that trace amounts are always present in this organ 4 days after the administration. In mice, an important fraction of radioactivity is eliminated by the bile.

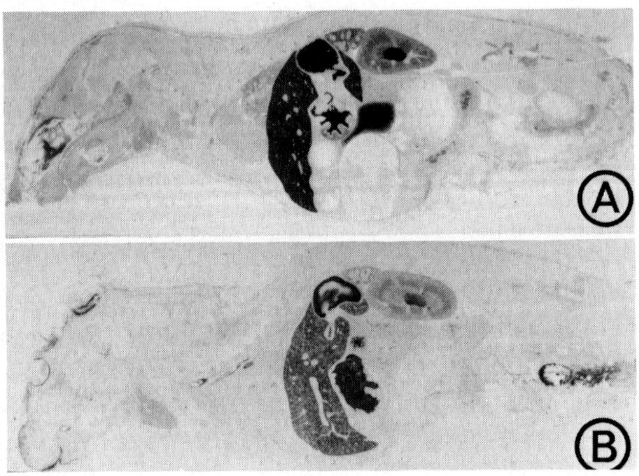

Fig. 1. Whole-body autoradiograms of mice after oral administration of (^{3}H)levamisole. Black areas correspond to radioactivity. A= 30 minutes; B= 2 hours . The highest uptake occurs in the liver, the kidney, the urine and the melanin.

The kidney radioactivity is lower than the hepatic one. In this organ, the distribution of the isotope is rather homogenous with a higher activity in the corticomedullary junction and the medulla. The radioactivity does not persist in this organ after the 24th hour.

In the other organs, low activities are present in melanin-containing organs as demonstrated by results obtained on black mice. When studying enlargement of a whole body autoradiogram, it was demonstrated a high uptake of labelled metabolites in the uveal tract(Fig 2), the skin, hair follicles, etc.... In pregnant mice, a low radioactivity is found in the fetal body 30 min after treatement. At this time, a low uptake occurs in the retina. On animal sacrificed 4 hours after the oral administration, only trace amounts are found in the fetal body except in the uveal tract which binds high activity.

DISCUSSION

From the above results, it appears that the distribution of radioactivity is rather similar in rats and mice. Several considerations are important for metabolic, toxicological and pharmacological purposes.

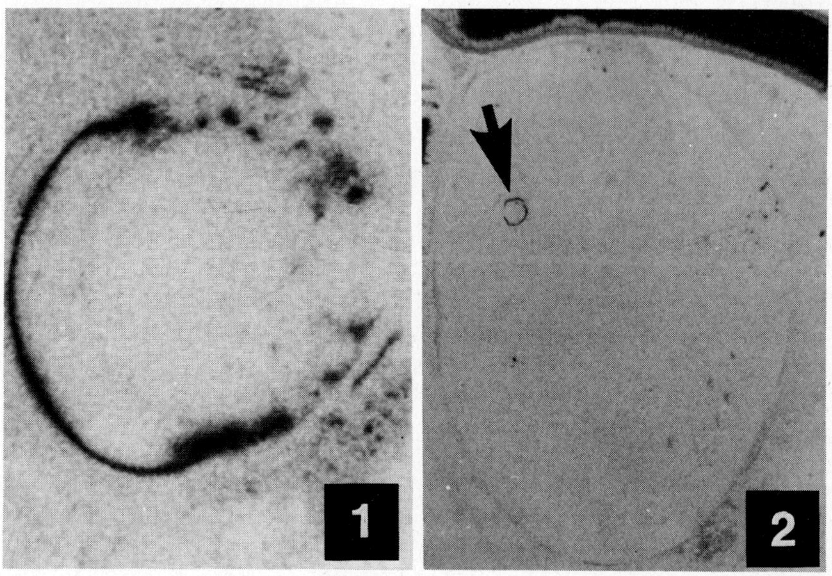

Fig. 2. Details of autoradiograms of mice injected with (^{3}H)levamisole and sacrificed 2 days (1) and 4 hours (2) later. Note the high uptake in the uveal tract (1) of the adult mouse and (2) of the fetus (arrow).

From a metabolic point of wiew, this study suggests that the kinetics of incorporation of radioactivity in all the organs is very rapid. However, the distribution in the different organs is rather different when considering albinos rat or pigmented mice. In coloured mice, an important uptake occurs in melanin containing tissues. This fixation is persistent as tritium is still bound to the uveal tract 4 days after the administration. As fetal melanin also binds radioactivity, these observations suggest that at least one metabolite has a high affinity for melanin. It seems now important to investigate the consequences of this affinity.

This study also demonstrate that the thymus gland does not fix high activities. However, trace amounts oftritium are present in this organ during 8 hrs after the administration either in adult mice or in young rats (50g). This low fixation could confirm the hypothesis about the mode of action of levamisole. GOLDSTEIN[6] has suggested that it could act by mimicing of the thymopoïetin, a thymic hormon, to produce its immunoregulatory effects.

REFERENCES

1 MEYER JONES,L., BOOTH,N.H. and Mc DONALD, L.E. (1977), Veterinary Pharmacology and Therapeutics, The Iowa State University Press, Ames, pp 1-1380.

2 JANSSEN, P.A.J. (1976), The levamisole story, Jucker E., Basle and Stuttgart, pp 347-383.

3 ULLBERG, S. (1954), Acta Radiol. suppl.118, pp 1-110.

4 ULLBERG, S. (1977), Science Tools. Special issue, 2, pp 1-31.

5 LARSSON, B. and ULLBERG, S. (1977), Acta Pharmacol. Toxicol., 41, suppl. 1, pp 48-49.

6 GOLDSTEIN, G. (1978), J. Rheumatol., 5, suppl. 4, pp 143-148.

© 1980 Elsevier/North-Holland Biomedical Press
Mechanisms of Toxicity and Hazard Evaluation
B. Holmstedt, R. Lauwerys, M. Mercier, M. Roberfroid eds

THE METABOLISM OF 2-BROMO-[1-^{14}C]ETHAN-1-AMINE (BEA): A MODEL COMPOUND FOR INDUCING RENAL PAPILLARY NECROSIS (RPN)

P.H. BACH, R. CHRISTIAN*, J. BAKER* and J.W. BRIDGES
Department of Biochemistry and Institute of Industrial and Environmental Health and Safety, University of Surrey, Guildford, and *Ciba-Geigy Research, Horsham, (England).

INTRODUCTION

Renal papillary necrosis (RPN) in man has often been associated with the long-term abuse of analgesics. This lesion has, however, proved difficult to reproduce experimentally[1], thus the molecular pathogenesis has remained obscure.

The induction of RPN (within a few days) by a *single dose* of 2-bromo-ethan-1-amine HBr(BEA) was first reported in 1913[2] and the morphological changes that follow the administration of this compound have since been described at both the light[3] and electron microscopic[4] level. BEA undergoes spontaneous cyclisation (under certain circumstances) to form the alkylating agent ethyleneimine (EI)[3], which has long been known to cause RPN[5]. It is generally assumed that BEA causes RPN *via* the formation of EI, but the pathogenesis for neither compound is known, and only limited metabolic studies on EI in the rat have thus far been reported[6].

MATERIALS AND METHODS

Synthesis of labelled BEA

2-Bromo-[1-^{14}C]ethan-1-amine HBr (BEA) was synthesised[7] (purity >98%, specific activity 210.2 kBq/mg; 44.4 MBq/mmol) from [2-^{14}C]ethan-1-ol-2-amine HCl (Radiochemical Centre).

Animals, dosing and label collection

Male Wistar rats 200-250 g were housed in Metabowls (Jencons) for the 24 h preceding the start of the investigation. BEA was dissolved in physiological saline immediately prior to use and administered by injection or by gavage at the dose and activity shown below. Exhaled air was drawn out of the Metabowl and through two traps, (a) 1N-HCl (for exhaled amines) and (b) 2N-NaOH (for CO_2). Spontaneously voided urine was collected at 4, 8 and 12 h, then at 24, 48 and 72 h. Faeces and the contents of both types of breath traps were collected every 24 h for 72 h.

Bile and urine were collected into preweighed vials from anaesthetised rats (Pentobarbitone sodium, 60 mg/kg) where both the bile duct and bladder had been cannulated. The urethra had been tied off in all cases to prevent loss of urine *via* this route. BEA was administered iv *via* the exposed external right jugular vein. Specimens were collected hourly for 5 h, the containers re-weighed, a measured aliquot removed for LSC and the final loss of weight used to estimate total activity and volume.

Measuring radioactivity

Radioactivity recovered in urine, faeces and bile, and the HCl and NaOH traps were counted using a detergent-based liquid scintillation cocktail system and correcting for quenching using an internal standard.

Wholebody autoradiography

Rats were dosed with 50 mg/kg BEA (148 kBq per rat) ip and killed 1 and 2 h later by cervical dislocation, then frozen in hexane at -70°C. Wholebody autoradiographs were prepared using standard techniques .

Analysis of metabolites

Pooled samples of urine and of bile were taken to dryness by rotary evaporation at <40°C (there was no loss of radioactivity), dried under vacuum and the polar metabolites extracted into methanol from the urine and bile residues (>95% recovery). TLC plates were spotted with this extract under a stream of pure dry N_2, run and autoradiographed for three months.

Chromatography was undertaken on two supports (I) Silica gel 60 (Merck - 0.2 mm on aluminium sheets - not heat activated) or (II) Cellulose MN 300 (Anachem, Luton - 0.5 mm). The solvent systems were (a) propan-2-ol-ammonium hydroxide (33% m/v)-water (90:8:2, v/v), (b) methanol saturated with NH_3 vapour, (c) chloroform-methanol (9:1, v/v), and (d) propan-2-ol-ethanol - 1N-HCl (3:3:2, v/v) .

Functional amine groups were vizualised on TLC plates, under UV light, after spraying with fluorescamine (2.5 mg/ml acetone).

RESULTS

Almost 70% of the dose was recovered in the urine in 72 h with small amounts in faeces and breath (Table 1). Up to 30% of the dose was excreted in the urine of cannulated animals in 5 h and up to 8.1% was recovered from the bile in the same time.

TABLE 1

RECOVERED ^{14}C EXCRETED FROM NON-ANAESTHETISED RATS

Mean Sum Percentage of Radioactivity Recovered

Dose mg/kg	Route	Urinary 12 h	Urinary 24 h	Urinary 72 h	Exhaled 24 h	Exhaled 72 h	Faecal 24 h	Faecal 72 h	Total 0-72 h
50[a]	ip	52.1	63.8	68.0	4.9	5.4	1.8	2.3	75.7
100[a]	po	34.6	54.2	66.3	3.4	4.4	2.6	3.3	74.0
100[b]	sc	49.8	64.5	70.0	2.8	3.4	2.2	2.7	76.1

[a]Mean for 3 rats, 74-111 kBq
[b]1 rat, 296 kBq

Radio-labelled BEA derived material was vizualised most strongly in the bladder, in the kidneys and less so in the liver. In addition, there was labelled material in the stomach and in the caecum.

A minimum of 6 urinary metabolites (3 with functional amine groups) and 5 bile metabolites (3 with amine groups) were discernible on the TLC autoradiograms (chromatographic system I a). None of the bile or urine metabolites behaved chromatographically the same as BEA or ethanolamine and there were no common metabolites in the bile and urine based on R_f and amine reaction.

DISCUSSION

An understanding of the molecular pathogenesis of BEA-induced RPN will provide an essential foundation in understanding how a similar lesion develops as a response to chronic analgesic abuse. Although it has been much investigated as a model papillotoxic chemical the metabolism and distribution of BEA has not previously been reported.

Intraperitoneally administered BEA is rapidly and completely absorbed (it was absent from the peritoneal cavity after 1 hour) and its distribution was confined largely to the kidney, bladder and liver. No less than half of the expired radio-label had entered intermediate metabolism and had been converted to CO_2. The nature of the rapidly excreted volatile basic component has not, as yet, been identified. Up to 8% of the parenterally administered dose was excreted in the bile of anaesthetised rats, but only 2 to 3% was recovered in the faeces. This significant biliary excretion and enterohepatic circulation is unexpected for a compound of low molecular weight (125.0) where even its glucuronic acid conjugate would be expected to be excreted *via* the kidney.[8]

The high intra-gut concentration of the intraperitoneally administered dose shows an important contribution to BEA absorption by stomach wall secretion. The prominent biliary excretion could, in part, be explained by an augmentation caused by a flux from both the peritoneal cavity and the liver. Significant stomach, caecal and large and small intestine recoveries of ^{14}C were found following an ip dose of labelled EI, however, neither bile recoveries nor autoradiographic distribution were reported[6].

The urinary clearance of BEA was faster, and its recovery more complete, than was reported for EI (urine recovery 50 to 60%[6]), but exhaled and faecal recoveries of labelled material were similar. In common with the previously reported studies on EI[6] we found several BEA metabolites in urine, the molecular structures for which have not yet been elucidated. About one percent of a volatile alkylating agent (assumed to be EI) was recovered in the urine of the rats studied by Wright and Rowe[6], but we have not been able to show the urinary excretion of EI *per se* after BEA had been administered to rats.

Many of the metabolic parameters for BEA and EI are similar and we cannot, at this stage, preclude cyclisation *in vivo*. Any EI thus formed would quickly react with physiological macromolecules, or perhaps micromolecular nucleophiles, one of which may be the 'proximate' papillotoxin. Work is in progress to identify the metabolites of BEA with a view to testing this hypothesis. We cannot, however , exclude the possibility that trace concentrations of BEA enter the nephron where they are converted into EI in an ionic environment and at a pH that facilitates the direct alkylation of macromolecules and produce a cytotoxic effect on specific functional areas of tubular epithelial or medullary interstitial cells, thus causing RPN.

ACKNOWLEDGEMENTS

PHB was supported, in part, by the South African Medical Research Council.

REFERENCES

1. Rosner, I. (1976) C.R.C. Rev. Toxicol., 4, 331-352.
2. Oka, A. (1913) Virchows. Arch. Path. Anat. Physiol., 214, 149-160.
3. Murray, G. *et al* (1972) Amer. J. Pathol., 67, 285-302.
4. Hill, G.S. *et al* (1972) Amer. J. Pathol., 68, 213-234.
5. Davies, D.J. (1970) J. Pathol., 101, 329-332.
6. Wright, G.J. and Rowe, V.K. (1967) Toxicol. Appl. Pharmacol., 11, 575-584.
7. Bach, P.H. and Bridges, J.W. (1980) in preparation.
8. Smith, R.L. (1973) Excretory Function of Bile. Chapman-Hall, London, p22.

Mechanisms of Toxicity and Hazard Evaluation
B. Holmstedt, R. Lauwerys, M. Mercier, M. Roberfroid eds

DETECTION OF CHEMICAL-INDUCED PORPHYRIA IN MAN. POSSIBILITIES IN BIOMONITORING OF EXPOSURE TO CHEMICALS.

STRIK, J.J.T.W.A.
Dept. of Toxicology, Agricultural University, De Dreijen 12,
6703 BC Wageningen, The Netherlands.

Hepatic porphyria in man is a disorder of porphyrin metabolism which also can be caused by exposure to certain halogenated hydrocarbons and some miscellaneous compounds (1). A number of these substances are known for their common use in industry and agriculture or because of their reputation as environmental contaminants. In human accidental or industrial exposure the occurrence of hepatic porphyria has been reported to be caused by vinylchloride (2), hexachlorobenzene (3), brominated biphenyls (4) and tetrachlorodibenzodioxin (5). Many more compounds are shown to be porphyrinogenic in tissue culture of chick embryo liver cells or in animals (1).

In clinical cases in man the condition of hepatic porphyria is usually associated with a considerable increase in the total amounts of porphyrins, especially uroporphyrin and heptacarboxylic porphyrin, excreted in the urine (6). The molecular mode of action of porphyrinogenic chemicals has not yet been elucidated. For a review of the possible molecular mode of action see Debets and Strik (7). However, there is evidence that inhibition of the enzyme uroporphyrinogen decarboxylase fulfils an essential role in the onset of chemical-induced porphyria, resulting in an increase of accumulation in the liver and excretion of uro- and heptacarboxylic porphyrin. A qualitative change in the excretion pattern of urinary porphyrins provides an indicator for chemical-induced disturbance in the pathway of heme synthesis. The proportion of porphyrin metabolites containing eight and seven carboxylic groups is increased relative to those containing six, five and four of these groups.

In this study the urinary porphyrin excretion was studied of citizens who were supposed to be exposed to chemicals released into the air by industrial activities.*

---

*Full papers are in preparation.

A. In a pedigree of 66 persons of a family living in the TCDD contaminated area of Seveso (Italy) and outside (a few hundred kilometers away) urinary porphyrin analysis was performed to detect a possible genetical TCDD evoked predisposition for two reported clinical cases of porphyria cutanea tarda (PCT). Sampling of urine took place in October - November 1978. Urine was stored frozen until analysis.

B. From June - November 1979 urine was collected from 49 children from 2 - 7 years old, who live near an industrial district (see map). Five days the wind was blowing from South-East. During these days the children were supposed to be exposed by wind from the industrial area. One day the wind originated not from that area.
Urinary analysis performed were:
total porphyrins (8), porphyrin pattern (9) and creatinine (10).
A normal urine is supposed to contain less than 5% heptacarboxylic porphyrin and 70% coproporphyrin out of the total present.

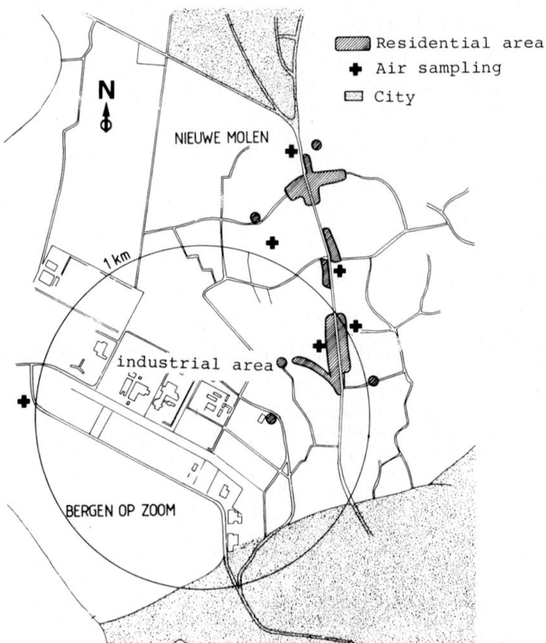

Localisation of industrial area and residential area of the children

Results.

A. In the possibly TCDD exposed group (25 persons) 25% had a total porphyrin level between 200 and 400 μg/l. In the control group (41 persons) 13% had a porphyrin level between 200 and 400 μg/l.
Five out of eight persons of the TCDD exposed group, mostly men, consumed more than 0.5 l wine a day and had a urinary porphyrin level exceeding 200 μg/l. In the control group 5 out of the 17 persons drinking more than 0.5 l a day had an increased total porphyrin excretion.
In the possibly TCDD exposed 63% abnormal urinary porphyrin patterns were found versus 19% in the control group.

B. Total porphyrin excretion of all the children during the sampling days was not significantly different (figure 1; t-test $p > 0.05$). Interference of age and sex did not influence the total porphyrin data. On the contrary,

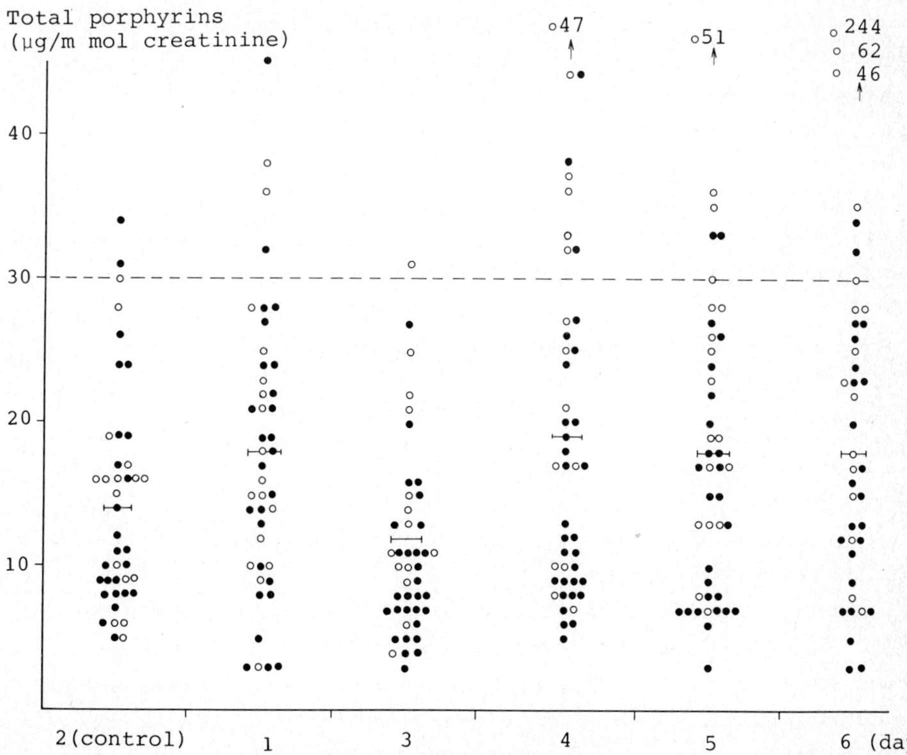

Fig. 1. Total urinary porphyrins of children living near an industrial district (see map)

the total porphyrins in urine of the children who live near a heavy traffic road (indicated by O) are significantly higher compared to the children who live elsewhere (indicated by ●) (wilcoxon; $p < 0.05$). This was observed on day three, four, five and six. The porphyrin patterns of urine collected on day two, three and five, showed no abnormal porphyrins. However, the coproporphyrin content was in the range of 80 - 90%.

Discussion.

Total porphyrins

In the possibly TCDD exposed group (25 persons) 25% had a total porphyrin level between 200 and 400 µg/l. In the control group (41 persons) 13% had a porphyrin level between 200 and 400 µg/l.

Increased total porphyrin levels may also be found after heavy alcohol consumption (11). Five out of eight persons, mostly men, consumed more than 0.5 l wine a day. These persons belonging to the possibly TCDD exposed group indeed had a urinary porphyrin level exceeding 200 µg/l. In the control group 5 out of the 17 persons drinking more than 0.5 l wine a day had an increased total porphyrin excretion.

The total porphyrin content in urine of children who lived near a heavy traffic road were higher compared to the children who lived elsewhere. Especially the coproporphyrin fraction in all their urine was increased (90% versus 70% in "normal" adults). Responsible for this could be lead originating from leaded gasoline. More additional evidence for this hypothesis could be collected by measuring zinc protoporphyrin, δ-aminolevulinic dehydratase (ALAD) and lead levels in blood and comparing the urinary porphyrin excretion.

Porphyrin pattern

In the possibly TCDD exposed group far more (63% versus 19% in the control group) abnormal porphyrin patterns appeared. A predisposition in connection with an aggrevating factor of alcohol or TCDD exposure may give rise to the two PCT cases in the family.

In a group of persons from Michigan, exposed to the porphyrinogenic compound PBB, it has been found that 47% of these people had an abnormal porphyrin pattern. In a control group from Wisconsin 6% of these people had an abnormal porphyrin pattern (4). In a group of industrial workers exposed to hexachlorocyclopentadiene, allylchloride, epichlorohydrin or endrin the urinary porphyrin patterns all showed to be normal (12). In a Japanese group of 21 persons (16

Yusho patients and 15 controls) without any indications for porphyria 10% of them showed abnormal urinary porphyrin patterns (13). It has been found in an Italian (Seveso) group of 115 persons possibly exposed to TCDD an incidence of 50 to 100% of abnormal porphyrin patterns (14). On the contrary, rabbits kept in some low TCDD contaminated areas of the Seveso regio did not show any histological or biochemical liver or kidney damage, particularly no porphyria (15).

Concluding remarks.

Total porphyrins

From different studies (4, 12, 13, 14) it seems that up to ± 200 μg/l excretion of total urinary porphyrins is normal. So far no real abnormal high total porphyrin levels were found in the studies mentioned.

Porphyrin pattern

In control groups an incidence of up to 19% abnormal porphyrins is reported. In young people and children the incidence of abnormal porphyrin patterns is much lower or none. So it seems that a higher incidence of more than 20% abnormal urinary porphyrins may be indicative for exposure without any indications for symptoms or illnesses to porphyrinogenic compounds. Unknown other factors and possibly age, sex, alcohol or oestrogens also play a role in evoking the incidence of abnormal porphyrin patterns.

Acknowledgement: The author is very grateful for the technical assistance provided by the Technological Department, the drawings by C. Rijpma and M. Schimmel and the photography by A. van Baaren of the Biotechnion of the Agricultural University. The laboratory assistance of Miss E.G.M. Harmsen, M.M.T. Janssen, J.P.H. Linssen and G.J.M. Brouwer is greatly appreciated.

References.

1. Strik, J.J.T.W.A., F.M.H. Debets and G. Koss, Chemical Porphyria in R.D. Kimbrough (Ed.), Halogenated biphenyls, terphenyls, naphthalenes, dibenzodioxins and related products, Elsevier/North-Holland, Amsterdam, 1980.

2. Lange, C.E., H. Block, G. Veltman and M. Doss, Urinary porphyrins among PVC workers, in: Porphyrins in Human Diseases, M. Doss (Ed.), Karger, Basel, 352 (1976).

3. Cam, C. and G. Nigogosyan, J. Amer. Med. Assoc. 183 (1963) 88.

4. Strik, J.J.T.W.A., M. Doss, G. Schraa, L.W. Robertson, R. von Tiepermann and E.G.M. Harmsen, Coproporphyrinuria and chronic hepatic porphyria type A found in farm families from Michigan (U.S.A.) exposed to polybrominated biphenyls (PBB), in Chemical Porphyria in Man, J.J.T.W.A. Strik and J.H. Koeman (Ed.), Elsevier/North-Holland, Amsterdam, 1979, p. 29.

5. Bleiberg, J., M. Wallen, R. Brodkin and J.L. Aplebaum, Arch. Derm. 89 (1963) 793.

6. Doss, M., Porphyrins and Porphyrin precursors, in Clinical Biochemistry, Principles and Methods, vol. 11, M. Curtius and M. Roth (Ed.), De Gruyter, Berlin 1974.

7. Debets, F.M.H. and J.J.T.W.A. Strik, An approach to elucidate the mechanism of hexachlorobenzene-induced hepatic porphyria, as a model for the hepatotoxicity of polyhalogenated aromatic compounds (PHA's), in Chemical Porphyria in Man, J.J.T.W.A. Strik and J.H. Koeman (Ed.), Elsevier/North-Holland, Amsterdam 1979, p. 181.

8. Harmsen, E.G.M. and J.J.T.W.A. Strik, Total porphyrin analysis in urine, in Chemical Porphyria in Man, J.J.T.W.A. Strik and J.H. Koeman (Ed.), Elsevier/North-Holland, Amsterdam 1979, p. 211.

9. Strik, J.J.T.W.A. and E.G.M. Harmsen, Urinary porphyrin pattern analysis, in Chemical Porphyria in Man, J.J.T.W.A. Strik and J.H. Koeman (Ed.), Elsevier/North Holland, Amsterdam 1979, p. 213.

10. Gorter, E. and W.C. de Graaff, Klinische Diagnostiek, Stenfert Kroese, Leiden, 7th ed. 1955, p. 440.

11. McEwin, R., Med. J. Austr. Aug. 25 (1973) 398.

12. Nagelsmit, A., P.N. van Vliet, W.A.M. van der Wiel-Wetzels, M.J. Wielaard, J.J.T.W.A. Strik, C.F. Ottevanger and N.J. van Sittert, Porphyrins as possible parameters for exposure to hexachlorocyclopentadiene, allylchloride epichlorohydrin and endrin, in Chemical Porphyria in Man, J.J.T.W.A. Strik and J.H. Koeman (Ed.), Elsevier/North-Holland, Amsterdam, 1979, p. 55.

13. Strik, J.J.T.W.A., H. Kip, T. Yoshimura, Y. Masuda and E.G.M. Harmsen, Porphyrins in urine of Yusho patients, in Chemical Porphyria in Man, J.J.T.W.A. Strik and J.H. Koeman (Ed.), Elsevier/North-Holland, Amsterdam, 1979, p. 63.

14. Centen, A., J.J.T.W.A. Strik and A. Colombi, Coproporphyrinuria and chronic hepatic porphyria type A found in people from Seveso (Italy) exposed to 2, 3, 7, 8-tetrachlorodibenzo-p-dioxin (TCDD), in Chemical Porphyria in Man, J.J.T.W.A. Strik and J.H. Koeman (Ed.), Elsevier/North-Holland, Amsterdam, 1979, p. 75.

15. Strik, J.J.T.W.A. and J.M.F. de Wit, Int. J. of Biochem. (in press).

METALS

Mechanisms of Toxicity and Hazard Evaluation
B. Holmstedt, R. Lauwerys, M. Mercier, M. Roberfroid eds

EXCRETION OF METALS INTO THE INTESTINE; A COMPARATIVE STUDY IN RATS

S.G. SCHÄFER AND W. FORTH

On the intestinal excretion of metals into the gastrointestinal tract (GIT) is often referred to in literature; however, until now, no systematic investigation is available. Therefore, after i.v. application of Rb, Sr, Zn, Cd, Hg, Bi, Pb, Co, Cu, and Tl the metal excretion from blood across the mucosal epithelium into the lumen of jejunum- and colon-segments as well as by bile was measured.

MATERIALS AND METHODS

In adult male rats (Urethan 1.25 g/kg) the blood supply of the kidneys was tied off. Jejunal segments were prepared starting with the flexura duodenojejunalis; colonic segments were prepared starting with the valvula ileocoecalis. The intestinal segments were ligated and connected by silicon tubings with storage vials by which the segments were perfused with small volumes (4-5 ml) of saline. During the experiments the rats were placed on a temperated ($37^{o}C$) platform, to which a battary of temperated storage vials was attached. The niveau of the platform could be moved up and down against a second battary of temperated storage vials. The intestinal segments were perfused by the up and down movements of the platform (5/minute).

The amount of metal excretion into the intestine was calculated from the concentration of the radioactively labeled metals and the actual volume of the perfusion fluid. The volume was measured using ^{3}H- or ^{14}C-polyethylene-glycole-4000 (PEG-4000) as an unabsorbable marker.

In a second series of experiments the excretion of the metals by bile was measured. The ductus choledochus of anesthetized rats

TABLE 1

EXCRETION OF METALS AFTER INTRAVENOUS APPLICATION ACROSS THE MUCOSAL EPITHELIUM, BY BILE AND BY THE KIDNEYS.

		Excretion into gut and bile[1)]			Excretion by kidneys			
		% of the dose per 1 hr			% of the dose	% of the dose	dose	species
metal	dose µmoles/kg	gut	bile	total		per 1 hr	µmoles/kg	
Zn	3.7	0.340	0.19	0.53	0.20/24 h	0.01	-	rat (9)
Cd	3.7	0.0710	0.40	0.47	0.08/ 9 h	0.005	2.2	rat (8)
Hg	3.7	0.310	0.14	0.45	0.80/24 h	0.04	3.0	rat (2)
Bi	3.7	0.580	0.35	0.93	16/4/ 3 h	5.5	-	rat (11)
Pb	3.7	0.310	0.49	0.80	24 / 24 h 5.8/24 h	1.00 0.25	5.0 2.4	rat (3) rat (1)
Co	3.7	0.029	2.21	2.24	63.5/72 h	0.90	-	rat (5)
Cu	3.7	0.115	0.37	0.49	0.46/24 h	0.02		rat (2)
Sr	3.7	1.61	0.55	2.16	18.8 /24 h	0.80		mouse (7)
Rb	3.7	3.13	0.08	3.21	27.2 /30 d	0.04	-	man (10)
Tl	1.85	8.87	0.073	8.94	35.61/14 d	0.11	-	rat (6)

1) The excretion of the metals in the entire small intestine was calculated on the basis of the jejunal values obtained experimentally. Length of either jejunum and ileum: 35 cm; since the surface of the ileum amounts to half of that of the jejunum, the jejunal values were divided by 2. Length of duodenum: 10 cm. The excretion of the metals into the colon was calculated per 18 cm length.

was canulated by PVC-tubes. The bile was collected in periods of 20 minutes for two hours.

RESULTS AND DISCUSSION

The experiments were carried out using two doses of metals: 3.7×10^{-10} and 3.7×10^{-6} moles/kg b.w.. For the sake of simplicity only the results of the higher dose are given in the table. In the table the excreted amounts of the metals into the gut lumen and by bile are summarized. Furthermore, the table contains the amount of metals excreted by the kidneys as far as they could be found in literature. When calculating the excreted amount of metals for the entire length of the intestine, the total length of the jejunum and duodenum of 45 cm was assumed. The metal excretion in jejunum and duodenum was assumed as being identical. The ileal excretion of metals was calculated as being half of that of the jejunum excretion since the surface of the ileum mucosa amounts to half of that of the jejunum (4).

The entire length of the colon was assumed as being 18 cm. The calculated values of the metal excretion into the entire gut were summed up with the amount of metals excreted by bile resulting the total amount of metal excretion into the GIT. These results can be compared with data from literature on the metal excretion by the kidneys.

Referring to the excretion into the GIT the metals can be divided into three groups:

(1) metals which are mainly excreted by the kidneys: Co, Bi.

(2) metals which are excreted in equal parts by the kidneys and into the GIT: Pb

(3) metals for which the excretion into the GIT exceeds that by the kidneys: Rb, Sr, Zn, Cd, Hg, Cu, and Tl.

On the basis of the results presented here no information is available on the mechanism by which the metals are excreted either across the mucosa epithelium or by bile into the GIT. However, following the concentration in plasma and in the perfusion fluid of the intestinal segments, Rb and Tl are secreted against a concentration gradient across the mucosa epithelium. A transport against a concentration gradient was also observed for the secretion of Sr, Rb, Cu, Cd, and Bi.

Since the blood supply of the kidneys was tied-off, the results may be misleading as far as the role of the GIT as excretory organ is concerned under normal conditions. However, for some metals the GIT-including bile-must be considered as an important way of excretion of metals. In order to evaluate the significance of metal excretion into the GIT for possible therapeutic purposes it is necessary to know the nature of the excreted metal compounds and their possible reabsorption during the passage along the intestinal canal.

Supported by a grant of the DFG Fo 58/7

REFERENCES

1. Castellius, N. and Aloj, S. (1964) Brit. J. Industr. Med. 21, 308-314
2. Cikrt, M. (1973) Arch. Toxicol. 31, 51-59
3. Conrad, M.E. and Barton, J.C. (1978) Gastroenterology, 74, 731-740
4. Fisher, R.B. and Parsons, D.S. (1950) J. Anatomy 84, 272-282
5. Greenburg et al. (1947) J. Biol. Chem. 147, 749-756
6. Henning, C.H. (1979) Diss., Fachbereich Biologie, Ruhr-Universität Bochum
7. Humphreys, E.R. et al. (1972) Second Int. Conf. on strontium metabolism, Glasgow and Strontian, 12-19 Aug. 1972
8. Kiyozumi, M. and Kojima, S. (1978) Chem. Pharm. Bull. 26, 3410-3415
9. Methfessel, A.H. and Spencer, H. (1973) J. Appl. Pharmacol. 34, 63-67
10. Ray, C.T. et al. (1955) J. Lab. Clin. Med. 45, 408-430
11. Russ, G.A. et al. (1975) Rad. Res. 63, 443-454
12. Schäfer, S.G. (1979) unpublished data

© 1980 Elsevier/North-Holland Biomedical Press
Mechanisms of Toxicity and Hazard Evaluation
B. Holmstedt, R. Lauwerys, M. Mercier, M. Roberfroid eds

PERMEABILITY OF THE LUNG TO INHALED HEAVY METALS

D. B. MENZEL, S. J. WILLIAMS, J. A. GRAHAM, F. J. MILLER and D. H. GARDINER
Duke University Medical Center, Departments of Pharmacology and Medicine, Durham, NC 27710, U. S. Environmental Protection Agency, Health Effects Research Laboratory, Research Triangle Park, NC 27711, U. S. A. and Universität Tübingen, Pharmakologisches Institut, Tübingen, D-7400, FRG.

INTRODUCTION

The presence of Ni- and Co-bearing compounds in the atmosphere is largely the result of the combustion of fossil fuels by man. Crude oil and coal contain traces of these and other heavy metals which, on combustion, are converted to a variety of oxides and sulfides. Nickel carbonyl occurs as well. The heavy metal content of fly ash, the inorganic residue from combustion of coal and oil released into the air, is roughly inversely proportional to the aerodynamic diameter of the particles. Ni, for example, is concentrated by 4 times in the respirable particles. Cigarette smoking can also increase the exposure to heavy metals especially Ni. Inhalation of Ni has been associated with cancer in man. The ability of the lung to remove these metals may be of importance in their biological effects, especially carcinogenesis. We report here a comparative study of the rates of removal of these metals at doses similar to those encountered environmentally by man.

METHODS AND MATERIALS

The permeability of the lung to ^{60}Co and ^{63}NI was determined <u>ex vivo</u> using isolated, ventilated and perfused rat lungs (IVPL)[1]. The lungs were perfused with Krebs-Henseleit buffer (pH 7.40, 37°) containing 4% bovine serum albumin, 5 mM glucose and 0.5 mM Na_2EDTA. Perfusion was maintained at 24 mm Hg until the lungs were free of blood and then perfused at a constant flow of 10 ml/min. The perfusate was kept saturated with 5% CO_2-95% O_2. Lungs were ventilated by negative pressure (-3 to -15 cm H_2O, Vt=1.5 or 2 cc, 80 breaths/min). $NiCl_2$ and $CoCl_2$ solutions were instilled intratracheally in 100μl of isotonic sucrose, pH 7.4, to measure removal from the airways. Uptake from the vasculature was measured by perfusion with Krebs-Henseleit without EDTA or albumin containing ^{63}Ni of ^{60}Co at the concentrations indicated. Flow was maintained at 2 ml/min in the absence of albumin.

Unidirectional uptake was estimated by the use of blue dextran (5mg/ml) as a vascular marker[2].

The removal of Ni and Co from the airways _in vivo_ was determined at fixed intervals after instillation of 100 ul of isotonic sucrose containing $^{63}NiCl_2$ or $^{60}CoCl_2$ at the indicated concentrations[2].

RESULTS

The removal of Ni and Co from the IVPL was found to follow first order kinetics up to 90 min. Ni caused an initial increase in the removal of Ni from the lung. Co had no effect on its own permeability and neither did nitrate or sulfate in prior experiments. The initial alteration in permeability to Ni was proportional to the starting Ni concentration and was not an artifact of the method. The first order rate constants for removal of Ni and Co are set out in Table 1, indicating that the removal was by diffusionally controlled processes.

TABLE 1

REMOVAL OF Ni AND Co FROM THE AIRWAYS OF THE PERFUSED RAT LUNG

Dose (nmol/lung)	Rate Constant of Removal ($X10^{-3}min^{-1}$) (N=4; Mean $\pm$ S. E.)	
	Ni	Co
1	0.71 $\pm$ 0.17	8.72 $\pm$ 1.00
10	1.31 $\pm$ 0.20	10.30 $\pm$ 1.90
100	2.40 $\pm$ 0.17	9.59 $\pm$ 0.11

Removal of Ca or Mg from the perfusate profoundly altered the rate of removal of Ni from the lung but had no effect on the removal of Co. At a dose of 10 nmol/lung, the removal of Ni was 12.8 times faster in Ca and Mg free perfusate, 5.2 times faster in Ca free, and 2.82 times faster in Mg free medium. In all cases the perfusate was maintained isotonic by the addition of sucrose.

A comparison of the _ex vivo_ and _in vivo_ methods is shown in Table 2. The rate of removal of Ni _in vivo_ was also independent of the dose over a 127 fold range in dose, supporting the concept that removal is diffusionally controlled. The values for the two methods compare well, although the _in vivo_ method is more limited.

TABLE 2

REMOVAL OF Ni FROM THE AIRWAYS OF THE RAT IN VIVO AND EX VIVO

Dose (nmol/lung)	Rate Constant of Removal ($X10^{-3}min^{-1}$; Mean ± S. E.) Ex Vivo (N=4, at each dose)	In Vivo (N=12, at each dose)
1	0.71 ± 0.17	2.07 ± 0.22
10	1.31 ± 0.20	1.40 ± 0.35
127	2.40 ± 0.17	2.30 ± 0.59

A plot of effluent radioactivity and blue dextran from lungs perfused with both Ni and Co showed that these ions had a volume of distribution greater than the vascular marker, blue dextran. Over the supply rates of 0.01 to 10 μmol/min of Ni, the unidirectional uptake was proportional to the concentration of Ni in the perfusate. Similarly, over the supply rates of 0.1 to 3.0 μmol/min of Co, the unidirectional uptake was also proportional to the Co concentration. Both ions are taken up from the vasculature by diffusionally controlled processes. The rate of uptake of Co was 1.5 times that of Ni. At equilibrium the extraction ratios for both ions were also independent of the supply rates.

Non-linear regression analysis of the wash-out curves of Ni and Co from the lungs indicated two components. The faster represented the wash-out of the vasculature, while the slower represented the diffusion of Ni or Co from extravascular space. The process was diffusionally controlled also and the same as the rate of uptake, suggesting that the permeability of the capillary membranes are symmetrical.

Determination of dry weight to wet weight ratios in all lungs demonstrated that these kinetic data were not due to the movement or bulk flow of water since no differences could be detected between control and experimental lungs.

DISCUSSION

The oxidation state and chemical composition of Ni and Co compounds in the air is not known at present. The divalent oxidation state, therefore, serves as a good model for assessment of the ability of the lung to remove these metals once deposited within the airways or taken up from the vasculature. The pulmonary removal process for both Co and Ni is diffusionally controlled. The rate of removal is slow compared to sulfate (100 times faster) or to

Na^+ (5 times faster). These experiments do not delineate the site of removal, but the lymphatic and tracheobronchial circulation or the macrophage and mucocilliary pathways do not seem to contribute much since these are severed or blocked in the IVPL and no major differences were detected between the *in vivo* and *ex vivo* rates.

Ni, but not Co, shares the same channels as Ca and Mg, but we do not know if Ni affects intracellular Ca or Mg concentrations. Ni may also share the same intracellular binding sites as Ca and Mg. Given the important role of Ca in smooth muscle contraction and general cellular function, these observations suggest a possible mechanism for Ni toxicity and carcinogenesis. We report elsewhere in this Congress that Ni also inhibits the cytochrome P_{450}-dependent O-demethylase of the lung. Perhaps more importantly, large arterial-venous differences were observed on perfusion and only a small fraction of both Co and Ni were removed. The tenacious binding of Co and Ni may be particularly important in assessing the air pollution hazards of particulate Ni and Co in urban air.

ACKNOWLEDGEMENTS

This work was supported in part by the A. von Humboldt Stiftung, EPA Grant R806337, NIH Grant ES01859 and a Fogarty Fellowship. The kind support of Professor M. Siess made this work possible.

REFERENCES

1. Charles, J. M., et al. (1977) Toxicol. Appl. Pharmacol. 41, 91.
2. Pickett, R. D., et al. (1975) J. Pharmacol. Exp. Therap. 194, 545.

© 1980 Elsevier/North-Holland Biomedical Press
Mechanisms of Toxicity and Hazard Evaluation
B. Holmstedt, R. Lauwerys, M. Mercier, M. Roberfroid eds

SUBCHRONIC EFFECTS INDUCED BY NiO-INHALATION IN WISTAR RATS

C.H. WEISCHER[1], H. OLDIGES[2], D. HOCHRAINER[2], W. KÖRDEL[2] ([1]present address: Schmidtbonnstr. 8, 53 BONN 1, BRD; [2]Fraunhofer-Institut für Toxikologie und Aerosolforschung, Grafschaft, BRD)

INTRODUCTION

Nickel is a constituent of urban air probably deriving from engine exhaust and fuel combustion. According to SUNDERMANN et al. (1) nickel enters the body via four routes: 1) orally, 2) by inhalation, 3) percutanously and 4) by parenteral route. As there is only a little information on the inhalation toxicity of NiO we intended to get some details of the effects on clinical, clinico-chemical and histopathological parameters induced by a subchronic NiO-inhalation in Wistar rats.

Further we were interested to compair the results with those obtained after a subacute NiO-inhalation of a previous study (WEISCHER, C.H., et al., 1980) (2).

MATERIAL AND METHODS

For the inhalation experiments 3 groups of virgine female Wistar rats (strain: TNO W 74) were continuously exposed to NiO-aerosols in the concentrations of 200, 400 and 800 $\mu g/m^3$ respectively, over a period of 120 days, 24 hours a day (except for daily 10-20 min. interruptions for cleaning of the inhalation chambers and feeding). Each group consisted of 9 or 10 rats. In addition 10 control rats were kept in normal air. The animals were housed in a fully climatized room, and they had free access to water. To minimize oral nickel uptake, new uncontaminated food (Ssniff[R]) was offered in the evening only. Every morning the remaining food was taken away. At the end of experiments 0.5 to 1.5 ml urine was collected in a PVC tube and thereafter blood was taken from the carotid artery under ether anesthesia from each animal.

The following clinical and clinico-chemical parameters were studied: wet weights of lungs, liver and kidneys; in blood: erythrocytes, leukocytes, hematocrit, hemoglobin, MCV; in serum: alkaline phosphatase, urea, bilirubin, glucose, SGOT and SGPT; in urine: creatinine, alkaline phosphatase, urea, protein and glucose.

The Ni-concentrations in lungs, liver, kidneys, spleen and pancreas were determined. The same organs were studied histopathologically. We studied the IgG-content in serum using the method according to O.J. BJERRUM et al. (3). The immunoelectrophoretic run was done with 2V/cm for 18 hours.

The results were statistically analysed using the Test of KRUSKAL and WALLIS and the rank Test of WILCOXON, WHITNEY and MANN. The inhalation device and the inhalation procedure were the same as used and described by OBERDÖRSTER et al. (4), PRIGGE (5) and WEISCHER et al. (2).

RESULTS

The following parameters were significantly increased: the relative wet weight of lungs in all exposed groups ($p \leq 0.002$) erythrocytes in the group receiving 800 $\mu g/m^3$ ($p \leq 0.01$) (s.fig.1); activity of alkaline phosphatase in urine in all exposed groups ($p < 0.05/p < 0.01$) (s.fig.2); activity of SGOT in the groups receiving 400 and 800 $\mu g/m^3$ ($p < 0.01/p < 0.05$) (s.fig.1).

Significantly reduced were the following parameters: the growth rate (body weight increament); relative wet weights of kidneys ($p < 0.01$) in all exposed groups ($p < 0.01$) (s.fig.2); leucocytes in the groups receiving 400 and 800 $\mu g/m^3$ ($p < 0.01$) (s.fig.1); MCV only in the group receiving 800 $\mu g/m^3$ ($p < 0.01$); glucose in urine in the groups receiving 200 and 400 $\mu g/m^3$ ($p < 0.01$).

Hemoglobin, hematocrit, alkaline phosphatase in serum, urea in serum and in urine, glucose in serum, relative protein in urine, bilirubin in serum, SGPT, relative wet weights of livers, and Ni-content in pancreas were not significantly changed.

The IgG-content in serum was increased in the groups receiving 400 and 800 $\mu g/m^3$.

The Ni-concentrations in lungs, livers and kidneys were significantly increased in all groups and in spleen in the groups receiving 400 and 800 $\mu g/m^3$ (s.fig.3). The histopathological investigations showed in a different degree in single or in all exposed animals respectively the following alterations: Severe leasions in lungs (such as thickened septa, multiple foci of macrophages, chronic emphysema, peribronchial infiltration of round cells, areas with granular protein-containing material, edema, and in kidneys granular degeneration of tubuli. In our study a subchronic NiO-inhalation induces in rats lesions in lungs, liver and kidneys, as seen before after an intoxication by an other heavy metal (5).

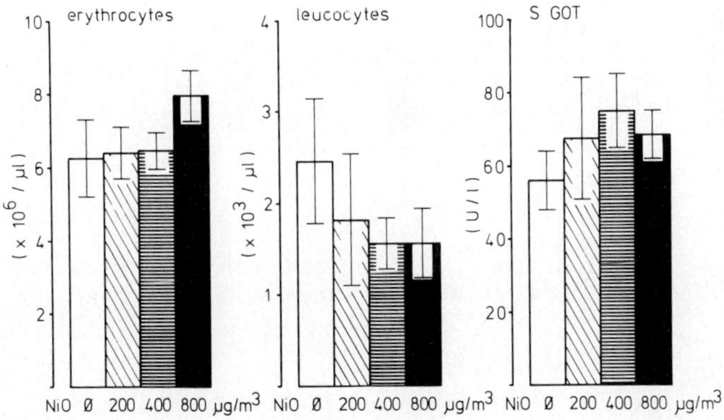

Fig. 1. Effects of a subchronic NiO-inhalation in wistar rats. Effects on clinical, clinico-chemical parameters.

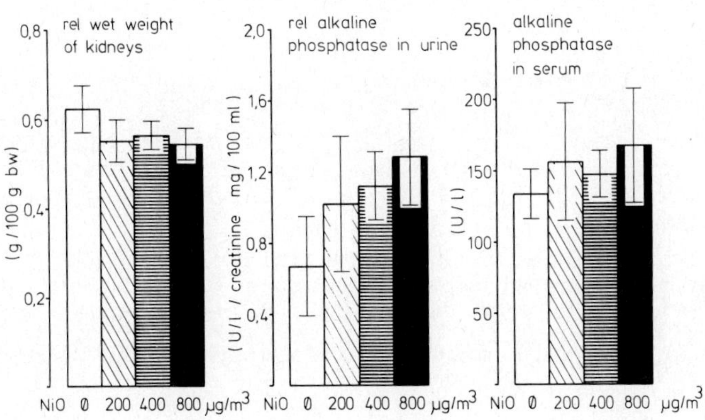

Fig. 2. Effects of a subchronic NiO-inhalation in wistar rats. Effects on clinico-chemical parameters.

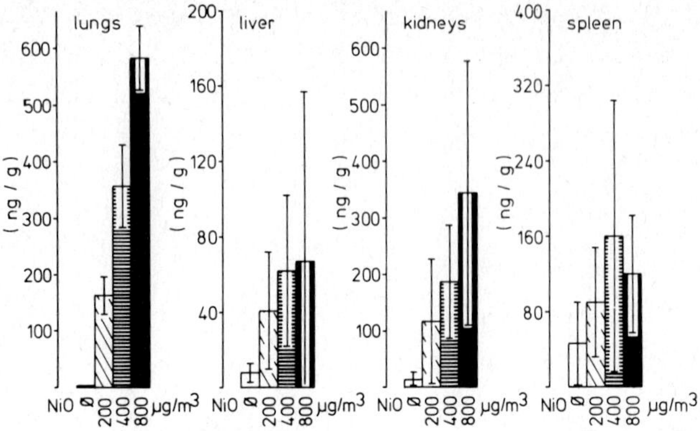

Fig. 3. Effects of a subchronic NiO-inhalation in wistar rats. Ni-concentrations in lungs, liver, kidneys and spleen.

ACKNOWLEDGEMENT

The authors wish to express their appriciation to Prof. Dr. Mohr, Hannover, for the histological examination, to J. Greve, N. Hennecke and J. Schmidt for theirskilful technical assistance.

REFERENCES

1. Sunderman, F.W. jr., Coulston, F., Eichhorn, G.L., Fellows, J.A. Mastromatto, E., Reno, H.T., Samitz, M.H. (1975) Nickel, a report of the Community on Medical and Biologic Effects of Environmental Pollutants. National Academy of Sciences. Washington, D.C., USA.

2. Weischer, C.H., Kördel, W., Hochrainer, D. (1980) Effects of oral administration of $NiCl_2$ and of NiO-inhalation in Wistar rats. (Zbl. Bakt. Hyg. I. Orig. B., in press).

3. Bjerrum, O.J., Ingild, A., Løwenstein, H., Weeke, B. (1973) in: A mannual of quantitative Immunoelectrophoresis edited by: N.A. Axelsen, J. Krøll, and B. Weeke, Universitetsforlaget, Oslo, p. 145-148.

4. Oberdörster, G., Baumert, H.P., Hochrainer, D., Stöber, W. (1979) The clearance of cadmium aerosols after inhalation exposure, Amer. Ind. Hyg. Assoc. J., 40, 443-450.

5. Prigge, E. (1978) Early signs of inhalative Cadmium uptake in rats. Arch. Toxikol. 40, 231-247.

Mechanisms of Toxicity and Hazard Evaluation
B. Holmstedt, R. Lauwerys, M. Mercier, M. Roberfroid eds

METABOLIC PATTERNS OF LOW AND TOXIC DOSES OF THALLIUM IN THE RAT

[1]E.SABBIONI, [1]E.MARAFANTE, [1]J.RADE, [2]A.DI NUCCI, [2]C.GREGOTTI and [2]L.MANZO
[1]Chemistry Division, Commission of the European Communities, Joint Research Centre, Ispra Establishment, 21020 Ispra (Varese), Italy and [2]Institute of Pharmacology II, School of Medicine, University of Pavia, 27100 Pavia, Italy

INTRODUCTION

Toxic health hazards from excessive exposure to thallium compounds have been recognized for a long time. Gastrointestinal and cardiovascular disorders, peripheral and central nervous system damages and alopecia have been reported as typical features of the acute or chronic intoxications by thallium-containing cosmetics and rodenticides[1,2]. While governmental regulations have strongly limited acute thallotoxicosis in most developed countries, increasing concern stems from the potential adverse health effects of the long term low level exposure to thallium delivered into the environment from various anthropogenic sources, such as coal burning power plants, copper, lead and zinc smelters, combustion of fuel oil and potash-derived fertilizers[3]. The present industrial uses of thallium are too limited to cause generalized pollution, but localized pollution accidents have been reported[4].

Most available data on thallium toxicity are derived from human poisonings or from animal experiments in which high concentrations of thallium were used. As a consequence, the effects of prolonged exposure to minute amounts of thallium are still unknown, and no studies have been reported on the metabolic fate of the different chemical forms of thallium occurring in the environment.

In the biogeochemical cycle thallium largely occurs as thallous ion, but the presence in the environment of inorganic Tl^{3+} as well as of organothallium species has been demonstrated. Speciation studies on thallium in seawater and freshwater have shown this element to exist primarily as cationic or neutral Tl(III) complexes in equilibrium with atmospheric oxygen. Human population may also be exposed to trivalent Tl_2O_3 and Tl^{3+} in the acidic smelter fumes from pyrites used for phosphate fertilizer production. In addition, evidence has been obtained that thallium can be biomethylated by bacteria to form dimethylthallium. This process requires Tl(III) ions and involves methylcorrinoid derivatives such as methyl B_{12} capable of transferring carbanion methyl groups[5].

This paper describes the disposition and intracellular distribution of thallium administered to rats over a range of doses from acute toxic ones down to fractions of picograms. Inorganic monovalent and trivalent Tl ions, as well as

TABLE II - ^{201}Tl CONTENT OF RAT TISSUES AFTER DIFFERENT DOSES OF THALLOUS IONS[a]

Tissue	Thallium content (% dose)			
	dose (μg Tl/rat)			
	0.00004	2	20	2000
Kidneys	4.65±0.5	5.65±0.8	5.10±0.6	4.90±0.55
Liver	1.70±0.3	2.16±0.4	2.60±0.5	2.80±0.15
Testes	1.10±0.8	1.22±0.3	1.70±0.3	1.30±0.15
Lung	0.20±0.06	0.20±0.04	0.26±0.03	0.40±0.01
Heart	0.20±0.08	0.28±0.05	0.20±0.05	0.47±0.02
Muscle[b]	28.35±8.1	27.54±2.43	33.21±4.86	40.98±4.86
Brain	0.23±0.05	0.23±0.01	0.31±0.01	0.27±0.09
Blood[c]	0.34±0.17	0.34±0.17	0.34±0.17	0.51±0.34

[a]Animals sacrificed 16 hrs after i.p. administration. Mean ± S.D. of 5 experiments. [b]Estimated to be 30% of b.w. [c]Calculated for blood volume of 63 ml/kg

indicated by the presence of appreciable levels of ^{201}Tl radioactivity in the stomach and intestine, as well as the prolonged retention of thallium in organs such as kidney, testis, heart and brain.

Negligible differences in the distribution pattern of ^{201}Tl were found in tissues of rats given different doses of monovalent thallium ions. 16 hrs after injection, the tissue content of thallium in rats given 2000 μg Tl/rat were similar to those found in the animals receiving doses as low as 4×10^{-5} μg Tl/rat (Table II). In addition, no dose-related differences in the intracellular distribution of thallium were found in liver and testis (Table III). 16 hrs after

TABLE III - INTRACELLULAR DISTRIBUTION OF THALLIUM

subcellular fraction	thallium content (% total homogenate) dose, μg Tl^{+}/rat			
	0.00004	2,000	0.00004	2,000
	liver		testis	
Nuclei	33.5±4.9	37.4±1.3	24.1±3.3	29.5±1.8
Mitochondria	10.7±2.5	7.9±1.6	10.0±2.0	11.8±1.1
Lysosomes	8.8±1.7	8.5±1.3	9.3±1.1	6.7±1.8
Microsomes	9.7±0.9	5.8±0.8	8.4±0.9	3.5±1.0
Cytosol	37.3±2.1	30.4±2.8	48.2±6.4	48.5±2.5

16 hrs after the i.p. administration of thallium. n= 4 experiments

DISCUSSION

In laboratory animals, the LD_{50s} of both the inorganic Tl(I) and Tl(III) compounds for all administration routes fall in the range of about 5 to 70 mg/kg. The normal human daily intake seems to be lower than 2 μg, and absorption of 5-6 fold higher amounts of thallium, i.e. 150-180 ng/kg/day is thought to occur in the proximity of coal fired power plants [3,7].

In this study the metabolic pattern of different thallium species was examined in the rat following the administration of doses ranging from acute toxic doses to minute amounts, very likely close to the levels of environmental exposure.

The results obtained confirmed the extensive diffusion and retention of thallium in tissues including brain, heart, skeletal muscle and testis, that is in the main targets of Tl toxicity.

The ability of Tl(I) to activate the membrane (Na + K)ATPase is thought to play a primary role in the movements of the thallous ion in mammalian tissues as well as in its K-like tendency to intracellular accumulation[3]. The uptake and concentration of thallium in tissue cells specialized for cation transport such as kidney and salivary glands give further support to this assumption.

Besides the prolonged retention by tissues, other factors including enteral recycling and tubular reabsorption, likely contribute to the extremely slow removal of thallium from the body, as is generally observed in acute poisoning. Indeed, thallium was found in urine and feces even 5 months after the ingestion of a single toxic dose[8].

Results of this study also indicated that the metabolic pattern of thallium in the rat is independent of the dose absorbed, and that the mechanisms determining the disposition and tissue and cell concentration of thallium operate both at toxic and at extremely low doses. These findings suggest the possibility of thallium accumulation under circumstances causing the continuous absorption of this element in some quantity.

Inorganic monovalent and trivalent thallium species exhibited similar distribution patterns in rat tissues. Dimethylthallium seemed to be poorly absorbed by the intestine, but a similar intracellular distribution of ^{201}Tl was found in animals treated with inorganic Tl(I) and Tl(III) species or dimethylthallium. This suggests an identical metabolism of the monovalent and trivalent forms, i.e. the biochemical conversion of these forms into a single chemical species. At present, however, the form and valence status of thallium in the organism is still unknown.

Intrinsic biological activity of thallous ions is suggested by the ability organic dimethylthallium have been examined.

METHODS

The preparation of the different forms of ^{201}Tl-labelled thallium compounds and analytical controls have been previously described[5,6]. Male Sprague Dawley albino rats weighing 190-200 g were injected intraperitoneally with 0.00004, 2, 20 or 2000 μg/rat of thallium sulphate in 0.25 ml of saline, plus 1.85 Mbq (50 μCi) of ^{201}Tl in the same chemical form. Additional groups of animals were treated with an olive oil suspension of ^{201}Tl-labelled dimethylthallium bromide by gavage,3.15 mg/rat,or with 0.25 ml solution of ^{201}Tl-labelled inorganic Tl(III) ions by intraperitoneal or oral route, at doses of 2 μg/rat and 3.15 mg/rat, respectively. The animals were sacrificed at various time intervals after treatment and ^{201}Tl levels in blood and tissues were measured.

Liver, kidneys and testes were homogenized in cold 0.25 M sucrose 10 mM Tris Cl, and subcellular fractions were obtained by differential centrifugation. ^{201}Tl radioactivity was measured in blood, organs and subcellular fractions by an automatic counting Packard 3520 equipped with a 2 x 1 in. NaI(Tl) crystal.

RESULTS

Table I shows representative results of the rat tissue distribution of ^{201}Tl after i.p. treatment with 2 μg Tl/rat as thallous ions. Rapid uptake of thallium in the kidney, heart and salivary glands was observed. 2 hrs after injection, average thallium concentrations of 0.4, 0.5 and 0.6 per cent of dose/g tissue were found in liver, pancreas and skeletal muscle, respectively. Results also pointed out the sustained excretion of thallium into the intestinal lumen, as

TABLE I - DISTRIBUTION OF ^{201}Tl IN RAT TISSUES

Tissue	thallium content (%dose/g)		
	2h	40h	192h
Kidney	2.57±0.16	4.43±0.44	2.50±0.68
Heart	0.63±0.07	0.37±0.03	0.96±0.06
Salivary glands	0.42±0.03	0.39±0.18	0.30±0.02
Brain	0.02±0.002	0.16±0.02	0.15±0.03
Testes	0.20±0.01	0.69±0.12	0.68±0.22
Stomach	0.68±0.28	0.43±0.03	0.27±0.03
Small intestine	1.46±0.32	0.95±0.02	0.35±0.04

Dose: 2 μg/Tl rat as thallous ions by i.p. route; n=5 rats per group ± S.D.

TABLE IV - DISPOSITION AND RENAL INTRACELLULAR DISTRIBUTION OF DIFFERENT THALLIUM SPECIES

		Tl^{+}	Tl^{3+}	Dimethyl-Tl
		thallium content (% dose)		
tissue distribution	Kidneys	6.80±1.00	6.10±0.8	0.56±0.16
	Liver	3.80±0.25	2.90±0.3	0.12±0.02
	Testes	3.70±0.32	3.90±0.51	0.07±0.004
	Salivary glands	1.21±0.22	1.32±0.07	0.02±0.006
	Heart	0.65±0.14	0.51±0.19	0.06±0.002
	Brain	0.57±0.02	0.75±0.09	0.02±0.003
		thallium content (% total kidney homogenate)		
intracellular distribution	Nuclei	26.1±2.6	26.5±3.9	23.2±3.5
	Mitochondria	9.7±2.1	10.8±2.8	10.6±1.5
	Lysosomes	14.6±2.4	18.5±3.2	15.6±2.9
	Microsomes	9.0±2.4	8.1±2.2	8.4±2.1
	Cytosol	40.6±3.3	36.1±4.4	42.2±5.3

Rats sacrificed 16 hrs after oral administration of 3.15 mg Tl/rat as ^{201}Tl-labelled inorganic Tl(I) or Tl(III) ions, or dimethylthallium. n=5 experiments.

administration, the highest ^{201}Tl content was found in nuclei and in the post-microsomal fraction. 8-12 per cent of cellular thallium was present in mitochondria.

Close similarities in the metabolic patterns of thallium were also observed after oral or intraperitoneal administration of the inorganic monovalent or trivalent thallium species. The same analogies in the disposition and intracellular distribution of inorganic Tl(I) and Tl(III) shown in Table IV (16 hrs after oral administration of 3.15 mg Tl/rat) were found at other time intervals after dosing, as well as in experiments in which lower doses were given to rats. 16 hrs after the oral administration of dimethylthallium, ^{201}Tl retention in tissues was found to be 1-2 orders of magnitude lower than in the animals treated with the inorganic thallium species, and extremely low or non-measurable amounts of ^{201}Tl were detected 40 hrs after ingestion and subsequently. However, a quite similar intracellular distribution pattern of thallium was observed in liver and kidney of animals given the organic or inorganic Tl^{3+} species.

of Tl(I) to substitute for potassium, with a higher affinity than this ion, in the activation of the (Na + K)ATPases and other K-requiring enzyme systems and cell functions[3]. Competitive inhibition by Tl(I) of both the influx and efflux of K^+ in rat liver mitochondria was also observed in recent studies[9], and it may be postulated that in the presence of thallous ions a relative deficiency of potassium in K-specific sites for which Tl^+ has a higher affinity occurs, leading to alterations of mitochondrial biochemical pathways where potassium plays a specific role[10]. On the other hand, while experimental evidence of the biochemical activity of trivalent thallium has been obtained, the uptake of Tl(I) by yeast mitochondria and the formation of Tl(III) in the cristate mitochondria indicate that oxidation of thallium in vivo can take place[5].

REFERENCES

1. STEVENS, W. et al. (1974) Int. J. Clin. Pharmacol. Ther. 10, 1-22.
2. RICHELMI, P. et al. (1980) Arch. Toxicol. 43, 321-325.
3. SABBIONI, E. and MANZO, L. (1980) in Advances in Neurotoxicology, L. Manzo ed., Pergamon Press, Oxford, pp. 249-270.
4. PRINZ, B. et al. (1979) Staub-Reinhalt. Luft. 39, 457-462.
5. SABBIONI, E. et al. (1980) Sci. Total Environ., in press.
6. BONARDI, M. (1980) Radiochem. Radioanal. Letters, 42, 35-44.
7. SMITH, I.C.H. and CARSON, B.L. (1977) Trace Metals in the Environment. Thallium. Ann Arbor Science Publ., Ann Arbor, pp. 1-394.
8. OEHME, F.W. (1972) Clin. Toxicol. 5, 151-167.
9. DIWAN, J.J. and LEHER, P.H. (1977) Biochem. Soc. Trans. 5, 203-205.
10. GOMEZ-POUYOU, A. and TUENA de GOMEZ-POUYOU, M. (1977) J. Bioenergetics 9, 91-102.

© 1980 Elsevier/North-Holland Biomedical Press
Mechanisms of Toxicity and Hazard Evaluation
B. Holmstedt, R. Lauwerys, M. Mercier, M. Roberfroid eds

EXCESSIVE THALLIUM ABSORPTION AMONG A POPULATION LIVING NEAR A THALLIUM EMITTING CEMENT PLANT

A.BROCKHAUS, R.DOLGNER, U.EWERS, H.WIEGAND, I.FREIER, E.JERMANN and U.KRÄMER
Med. Institut für Umwelthygiene, Gurlittstr. 53, D-4000 Düsseldorf (W.-Germany)

INTRODUCTION

Thallium has not been regarded as an environmental pollutant so far although considerable amounts of thallium are emitted by coal burning power plants and certain industries such as nonferrous metal plants [1]. A special case of a local environmental pollution by thallium was discovered, however, at Lengerich (W.-Germany) in August 1979. An inspection of the production process proved that the emission of thallium was caused by a thallium containing residue of pyrite roasting which was added as a ferric oxide additive to the crude powdered lime stone for the production of special sorts of cement [2,3]. The use of this additive was stopped in August 1979.

In several successive studies performed in September - December 1979 we have investigated the thallium exposure of the population living near the cement plant by analyzing the thallium concentration in urine and hair samples. Results of the first epidemiological survey performed in September 1979 are reported in this paper.

METHODS

Population. The population living near the cement plant was invited publicly to participate in the investigation. 1265 persons (1 to 85 yr old; mean age 40.0 yr; 517 males, 748 females) participated in the first survey. A questionnaire designed to yield informations on some personal data as well as on nutrition habits, health, and socioeconomic status was applied to each person.

Urine and Hair Sampling. From each person a 24 h urine sample was taken. For conservation 5 ml HNO_3 (65%) were added to an aliquot of 95 ml of each urine sample. Hair samples were taken from the back of the head.

Thallium Analysis in Urine and Hair. Thallium content of urine (TlU) and hair samples (TlH) was determined by electrothermal atomic absorption techniques (Perkin Elmer, Model 400 and 5000, atomic absorption spectrophotometer equipped with a graphite furnace atomizer, Perkin Elmer, Model HGA 500).

TlU: 5 ml of urine were evaporated to dryness and mineralized with 1.3 ml HNO_3, H_2SO_4, $HClO_4$ (2:2:1; v/v). The residue was diluted with 13 ml H_2O and the solution adjusted to pH 9 - 9.5 by the addition of 10 ml ammonium citrate (1 M; pH 10.5). Thallium was extracted with APDC/MIBK *.

TlH: Hair segments (2 cm) proximate to the root were washed with Triton X (1%), water, acetone, and ether. The washed hair samples (~40 mg) were dried (120 °C; 2 h), weighed and ashed with a low temperature plasma asher (International Plasma Corp., Hayward, Cal. USA). The residue was dissolved in 0.5 ml H_2SO_4 (6%; v/v) and the solution adjusted to pH 9 - 9.5 by the addition of 0.22 ml aqueous NH_3 solution (25%). Thallium was extracted with APDC/MIBK.

RESULTS

Urine Analyses. A frequency distribution of the TlU-concentrations found is shown in Fig. 1. Compared to 31 control persons with no excessive thallium absorption (mean TlU: 0.43 µg/l; range: 0.1 - to 1.2 µg/l) a considerable part of the study population showed markedly increased TlU-concentrations. TlU-concentrations were not

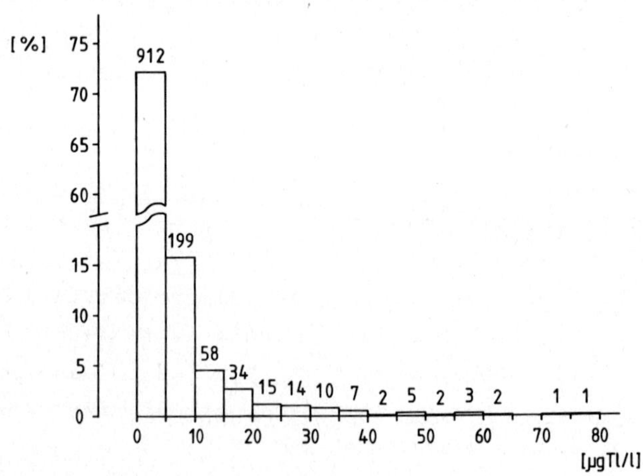

Fig. 1. Frequency distribution of Tl-concentrations in 24 h urine samples of a population (N=1265) living near a Thallium emitting cement plant.

* ammonium pyrrolidine dithiocarbamate/methyl isobutyl ketone

influenced by factors such as sex, age, and smoking habits. Data could be pooled, therefore, for further statistical analyses.

Hair Analyses. A frequency distribution of TlH-concentrations is shown in Fig. 2. Compared to the "normal" thallium content in human hair (about 10 ng/g [4,5]) a considerable part of the study population exhibited markedly increased TlH-concentrations. TlH-concentrations ranged up to 600 ng/g.

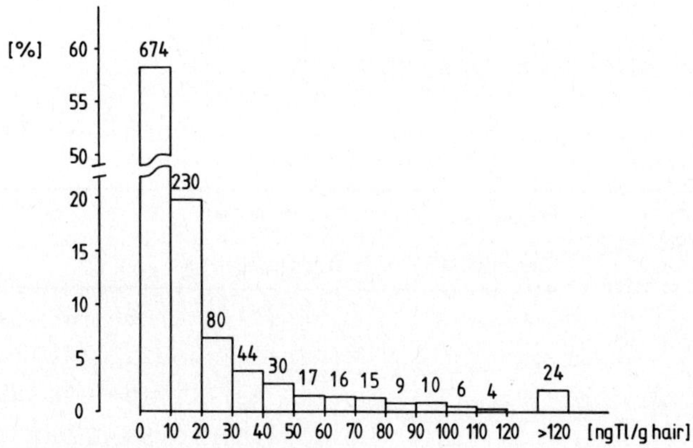

Fig. 2. Frequency distribution of hair thallium levels (TlH) of a population (N=1159) living near a thallium emitting cement plant.

Routes of Thallium Absorption. The study population was divided into two groups: group A consisted of persons consuming vegetables and fruits grown in private gardens; group B consisted of persons not consuming food grown in private gardens. Persons in groups A and B were subdivided according to the distance between their homes and the cement plant. Mean TlU-concentrations calculated for the various subgroups are given in Table 1. Results show: (a) persons consuming food grown in private gardens near the cement plant exhibit significantly higher TlU-concentrations than persons in group B; (b) mean TlU-concentrations of persons in the subgroups of A decrease with increasing distance between their homes and the cement plant; (c) no such correlation can be evaluated for persons in the subgroups of B.

From these data it can be concluded that the consumption of vegetables and fruits grown in private gardens near the cement plant has to be regarded as the main cause of excessive thallium absorption. As was demonstrated by chemical analyses of soil and vegetation [2,3] these gardens were polluted by airborne thallium containing dust. Since subjects of group B exhibited TlU-concentrations similar to the "normal" urinary thallium levels of the control persons it may further be concluded that thallium intake via the drinking water as well as a pulmonal resorption of airborne thallium did not play a significant role in explaining excessive thallium absorption.

TABLE 1

MEAN TlU-CONCENTRATIONS OF A POPULATION LIVING NEAR A THALLIUM EMITTING CEMENT PLANT

Group A: persons consuming food grown in private gardens; group B: persons not consuming food grown in private gardens.

Distance between home and cement plant (km)	µg Tl/l (number of persons) group A	group B	T	df	P
<1	3.95 (527)	0.76 (11)	4.88	536	<0.001
1 - <2	2.45 (430)	0.46 (11)	5.22	439	<0.001
2 - <3	1.74 (124)	0.63 (6)	2.39	128	<0.05
≥3	1.10 (106)	0.60 (13)	3.53	25.2	<0.05

Health Effects. According to the individual TlU-concentrations found the subjects were divided into three groups (I: < 2 µg/l; II: 2-20 µg/l; III: > 20 µg/l). Frequencies of health disorders as indicated by the completed questionnaires were calculated for these groups. Results show an increasing prevalence of certain neurological and neurovegetative disorders such as sleep disorders, visual disorders, tiredness, weakness and nervousness with increasing TlU-concentrations. No correlation could be found between increasing TlU-concentrations and a prevalence of other symptoms such as gastro-intestinal disorders, skin reactions, hair falling-out and alopecia.

REFERENCES

1. Smith, I.C. and Carson, B.L. (1977) Trace Metals in the Environment, Vol. 1 Thallium, Ann Arbor Science Publ.Inc., Ann Arbor, Mich. USA .
2. Prinz, B. et al. (1979) Staub Reinhalt. Luft 39, 457 - 462 .
3. Ministerium für Arbeit, Gesundheit und Soziales Nordrhein-Westfalen (Ed.) (1980) Umweltbelastung durch Thallium, Düsseldorf, W.-Germany .
4. Weinig, E. and Zink, P. (1967) Arch. Toxikol. 22, 255 - 274 .
5. Geilmann, W. et al. (1960) Biochem. Z. 333, 62 - 70 .

Mechanisms of Toxicity and Hazard Evaluation
B. Holmstedt, R. Lauwerys, M. Mercier, M. Roberfroid eds

METABOLISM OF ORALLY INGESTED CADMIUM IN HUMANS

ZAHIR A. SHAIKH* AND J. CRISPIN SMITH†

Department of Pharmacology and Toxicology, University of Rochester School of Medicine and Dentistry, Rochester, New York 14642 (U.S.A)

There is very little published data on the gastrointestinal absorption of cadmium. Balance studies in humans using non-radioactive cadmium reported rather high absorption. Based on average daily intake and excretion of cadmium and on tissue cadmium content in autopsy samples, it has been estimated that the absorption is less than 10% and that the biological half-time of cadmium is of the order of 10-30 years[1].

Using isotopic cadmium (^{115m}Cd), Miettinen and co-workers[2,3], Yamagata et al.[4], and Valberg and co-workers[5,6], reported that the average absorption is indeed less than 10%. However, values as high as 22-30% were observed in some cases. In one of the studies higher absorption was explained on the basis of iron-deficiency anemia[6].

Following an oral dose of ^{115m}Cd, one to five subjects in the above mentioned studies were monitored for as long as 100 days (Table 1). Whole-body half-time estimates were made in these subjects and a value of about 100 days was reported. This was rather short as compared to the half-time of several years calculated by Friberg et al.[1]

The present study was initiated shortly after the reports from Meittinen's group[2,3] to compare the gastrointestinal absorption of cadmium in males and females and also to validate the short half-time reported by these investigators. For this purpose, in addition to ^{115m}Cd, an isotope of cadmium with longer half-life (^{109}Cd) was employed. Liver and kidney areas were monitored to observe the translocation of cadmium from the liver to the kidneys reported in animals[1]. A summary of the preliminary results was published earlier[7].

MATERIALS AND METHODS

Seven male and five female volunteers participated in the study. The experimental protocol was approved by the institutional committees on investigations involving human subjects and on human use of radioactive isotopes. The

*Present address: Division of Toxicology, Department of Radiation Biology and Biophysics.

†Present address: Institute of Environmental Health, University of Cincinnati Medical Center, Cincinnati, Ohio 45267

dose of cadmium was prepared in beef kidney cortex homogenate essentially as described by Rahola et al.[2,3] Five milliliters of homogenate (1 g kidney) containing 5-10 μCi ^{115m}Cd or ^{109}Cd and 50 μg cadmium as $CdCl_2$ was ingested by each person. This was followed by drinking about 450 ml milk.

The whole-body counting facility of the University of Rochester is described elsewhere[8]. Radioactivity in whole-body was measured in standard chair geometry by a 4" X 8" NaI crystal detector. Measurements were made immediately after ingestion of the dose and at periodic intervals thereafter. In addition to whole-body radioactivity measurements , liver and left kidney were also monitored by positioning the detector directly above these regions while the person was lying supine (liver) or prone (kidney). These measurements were not started, however, until most of the unabsorbed dose was eliminated.

Individual fecal excretions were collected in plastic containers. After dilution with water, each fecal sample was homogenized and an aliquot was assayed for radioactivity in a well-type gamma counter.

TABLE 1

PUBLISHED REPORTS ON THE ABSORPTION AND BIOLOGICAL HALF-TIME OF ^{115m}Cd IN HUMANS

Investigators	N	Duration Of Study (Days)	Dose (μg Cd)	Absorption[a] (%)	Half-Time (Days)
Rahola et al.[2]	5(5)[b]	57	100	4.7- 7.0	130
Rahola et al.[3]	5(5)	92	100	4.7- 7.0	100
Yamagata et al.[4]	2	3	-	7.0-30.0	-
McLellan et al.[5]	14(1)	94	25	0.7-15.6	100
Flanagan et al.[6]	22(3)	100	25	0.5-22.0	93-202

[a]Absorption estimates are based on whole-body counting except in the case of Yamagata et al.[4] who reported it as dose minus total excretion during 3 days.

[b]Numbers in parentheses indicate the number of total subjects that were followed for the entire length of the study to obtain half-time estimates.

RESULTS

A large part of the ingested radiolabeled cadmium was excreted in feces within the first 7 days (Fig. 1). However, measurable excretion of the unabsorbed dose continued for 2-4 weeks. Urinary excretion was negligible. Recovery of cadmium in the feces was quite variable, mainly due to lack of complete collection of the feces during the first week.

Whole-body retention was monitored in the subjects for 56-808 days. The retention curve of a subject who was observed for the longest time period is shown in Fig. 2. Best fit to the data was obtained using three exponentials. The three components of the curve had half-times of 1.58, 33.7 and 9605 days (26.3 years), respectively. The slow component, which did not become well-defined until after 200 days, accounted for 2.5% of the initial whole body counts. This was considered to be an estimate of minimum absorption. Cadmium in liver and kidney did not deplete appreciably and showed apparent half-times of several years. No accumulation of ^{109}Cd was seen in the kidney with time.

Table 2 summarizes the estimates of cadmium absorption in male and female subjects. In males the absorption ranged between 1.1 and 4.1%. The highest absorption estimate was obtained in a subject who was monitored for only 56 days. If this subject had been observed for at least 200 days, the estimated absorption would have been considerably lower. Of the five females, three had absorption values very similar to those of the males (Table 2). The remaining two absorbed 5.1 and 7.0% of the dose, respectively. These two subjects appeared to have iron-deficiency anemia since they had low serum ferritin levels.

DISCUSSION

The observation that a major part of the unabsorbed cadmium is excreted

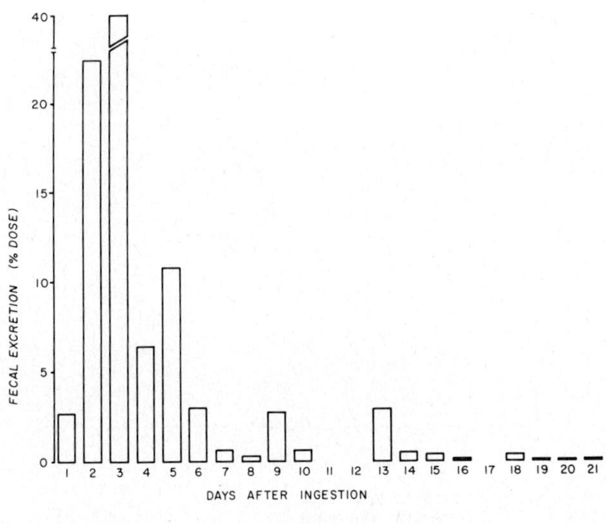

Figure 1. Elimination of cadmium in the feces of a male subject (No. 3).

TABLE 2

ESTIMATES OF ABSORPTION BASED ON THE WHOLE-BODY MEASUREMENTS

Subject No.	Sex	Age	Observation Period (Days)	Absorption (%)
1[b]	M	25	56	4.1
2	M	27	205	3.0
3	M	29	183	2.8
4	M	31	263	1.5
5	M	22	338	1.1
6	M	18	476	2.2
7	M	25	808	2.5
8	F	21	190	1.4
9	F	28	423	1.5
10	F	21	493	1.6
11[c]	F	21	553	5.1
12[c]	F	23	529	7.0

[a] Ratio of counts in slow component extrapolated to zero-time and initial whole body counts.
[b] Received ^{115m}Cd. All others were given ^{109}Cd.
[c] Serum ferritin less than 10 ng/ml.

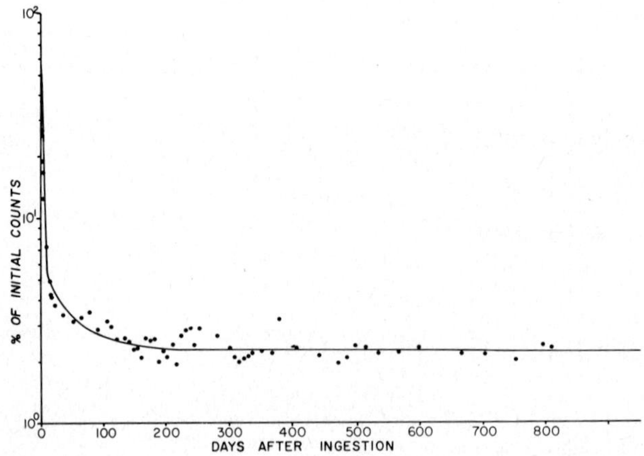

Figure 2. Whole-body retention curve of cadmium in a male subject (No. 7).

during the first few days is in agreement with earlier reports by others[2-6]. Similarly, continued fecal excretion of cadmium during the next 2-4 weeks was also noted by Rahola et al.[2,3], McLellan et al.[5], and Flanagan et al.[6] From the report by McLellan et al.[5] it appears that the transit time of cadmium in the gastrointestinal tract is longer than that of chromium, which is also poorly absorbed. It is possible that the long transit time is not only due to mixing in the colon but also due to uptake of cadmium by the mucosal cells.

Absorption was estimated in the same manner as by other investigators[2,3,5,6]. The values are somewhat lower than the mean values reported by others. The difference may be due to the differences in slopes of the slow component. In both males and females the absorption was less than 5% except in two cases with iron-deficiency anemia. Flanagan et al.[6] also pointed out the importance of iron metabolism in cadmium absorption.

The fast component in the whole-body curve (half-time=1.58 days) reflects the bulk of unabsorbed dose that appears in feces shortly after ingestion. Rahola et al.[2] had estimated the half-time of this component to be 1.8-3.2 days. A second component in the whole-body curve (Fig. 2) with intermediate half-time is mainly due to continued elimination of unabsorbed cadmium as well as excretion from the exchangeable pool of the body as mentioned above. It may also be partly due to redistribution of cadmium within various tissues.

In the whole-body elimination curve, the most important observation is that the half-time of the slow component is definitely not 100-200 days as reported by others[2-6]. The reason why other investigators reported short half-times was the fact that their studies were not carried out for long enough periods of time, as can be seen in Fig. 2, where a 26.3 year terminal half-time was observed. The previously reported longest observation period was 100 days[6]. If we had stopped monitoring our subject as early as day 200, a terminal whole-body half-time of approximately 270 days would have been erroneously concluded. Even for our longest whole-body monitoring period of 808 days, the scatter in the data is such that the predicted terminal half-time of 26.3 years is not significantly different from the infinite half-time, consistent with complete retention of a fraction of the dose. While complete retention of any of the dose is inconsistent with what is generally believed about cadmium metabolism, the implication of our study is that one would have to have a highly refined whole-body counter, the output of which is independent of any geometric effects of cadmium location and redistribution within the body. Furthermore, one would have to monitor the subjects for an inordinate period of time in order to determine the "true" terminal whole-body half-time to any significant degree.

ACKNOWLEDGEMENTS

The research was supported by Public Health Service Grants ES 01247 and ES 01248. Technical assistance of J. Keller, T. Hanley, P. Weiss, and E. Lasselle is greatfully acknowledged. The authors are indebted to Doctors R. Kilpper, G. Forbes, D. Webber and J. Hursh for their help at various stages of this project.

REFERENCES

1. Friberg, L., Piscator, M. and Nordberg, G.F. (1974) Cadmium in the Environment, CRC Press, Cleveland.
2. Rahola, T., Aaran, R. and Miettinen, J.K. (1972) Assessment of Radioactive Contamination in Man, Int. Atomic Energy Agency, Vienna, pp. 553-562.
3. Rahola, T., Aaran, R. and Miettinen, J.K. (1973) Health Physics Problems of Internal Contamination, Akademiai Kiado, Budapest, pp.213-218.
4. Yamagat, N., Iwashima, K. and Nagai, T. (1975) Bull. Inst. Publ. Health (Tokyo), 24, 1-6.
5. McLellan, J.S., Flanagan, P.R., Chamberlain, M.J. and Valberg, L.S. (1978) J. Toxicol. Environ. Health, 4, 131-138.
6. Flanagan, P.R., McLellan, J.S., Haist, J., Cherian, M.G., Chamberlain, M.J. and Valberg, L.S. (1978) Gastroenterology, 74, 841-846.
7. Shaikh, Z.A. and Smith, J.C. (1978) Toxicol. Appl. Pharmacol., 45, 306.
8. Directory of Whole-body Radioactivity Monitors (1970) Int. Atomic Energy Agency, Vienna, pp. 1-4.

© 1980 Elsevier/North-Holland Biomedical Press
Mechanisms of Toxicity and Hazard Evaluation
B. Holmstedt, R. Lauwerys, M. Mercier, M. Roberfroid eds

SEX-LINKED DISTRIBUTION OF CADMIUM, ZINC AND COPPER IN TISSUES OF CADMIUM-TREATED RATS

SILVIA GABOR and ZOE ANCA
Institute of Hygiene and Public Health, Pasteur street 6, Cluj-Napoca (Romania)

INTRODUCTION

In spite of numerous studies dealing with Cd toxic properties, there are a few and still uncertain data concerning the influence of sex on Cd metabolism, although sex is considered to be a contributing factor to the Cd toxicity[1,2]. The data available în the literature evidenced that females generally accumulate higher Cd concentrations in their body and organ tissues, as compared with the males[3,4]. A number of reports indicate that Cd toxicity, at least partly, may reside in its interference with the normal metabolism of trace essential elements[5]. Therefore, it is assumed that one of the earliest signs of Cd toxicity may be a disturbance in the metabolism of essential trace metals[6,7].

The present experiment aimed at demonstrating sex differences in the pattern of Cd accumulation as well as of essential metals, Zn and Cu distribution under repeated administration and subsequent withdrawal from Cd.

MATERIALS AND METHODS

Male and female rats of the Wistar strain weighing between 18o-2oo g were used. $CdCl_2$ was injected subcutaneously at a dose of 1 mg/kg b.w. twice a week. At the end of the 6 weeks the animals were sacrificed and the organs (liver, kidney, pancreas, adrenals, testes and ovary) were removed for Cd, Zn, and Cu content measurements. The remainig rats were withdrawn from Cd, killed after a time interval of 6 weeks and their organs subjected to metal determinations. After dry ashing of tissues at 45o^{o}C, the concentrations of metals were determined on a Perkin Elmer Model 3o3 atomic absorption spectrophotometer.

Results are expressed as means ± SD or as percent of control values. Significant differences between the means were statistically evaluated using Student's "t" test, taking $p < 0.05$ to be level of significance.

RESULTS AND DISCUSSION

Cd distribution in organs of male and female rats is presented in tables 1 and 2.

TABLE 1
ORGAN DISTRIBUTION OF CADMIUM (µg/g dry tissue) IN MALE RATS

Animals	liver	kidney	pancreas	adrenals	testes
			I Cadmium for 6 weeks		
Control	0.43±0.11	1.15±0.12	0.03±0.04	0.45±0.23	0.03±0.05
Cd	585±66.6[a]	285±23.1[a]	66±3.8[a]	35±4.2[a]	15±3.2[a]
			II 6 weeks after cadmium withdrawal		
Control	0.23±0.06	0.79±0.03	0.07±0.03	0.16±0.03	0.04±0.00
Cd	571±83.9[a]	161±17.6[a]	79.9±8.4[a]	17.8±3.6[a]	4.8±0.6[a]
II vs I	-3%	-44%	+21%	-50%	-32%

Each value represents the mean ±SD of four-five rats
a significantly different from control at $p < 0.01$

TABLE 2
ORGAN DISTRIBUTION OF CADMIUM (µg/g dry tissue) IN FEMALE RATS

Animals	liver	kidney	pancreas	adrenals	testes
			I Cadmium for 6 weeks		
Control	0.47±0.09	1.55±0.48	0.06±0.02	0.01±0.02	0.00
Cd	601±93.9[a]	235±47[a]	73.8±10.5[a]	35±3[a]	23.8±0.9[a]
			II 6 weeks after cadmium withdrawal		
Control	0.27±0.04	0.74±0.08	0.10±0.04	0.07±0.02	0.06±0.0
Cd	571±126[a]	215±55.8[a]	80.7±7.2[a]	18.5±4.3[a]	11±2.3[a]
II vs I	-5%	-9%	+9%	-48%	-47%

Each value represents the mean ±SD of four-five rats
a significantly different from control at $p < 0.01$

It can be seen that after 6 weeks of treatment there is an increased Cd content in all organs as compared with the control.

As it was expected, the liver and the kidney were the major sites of Cd deposition in males as well as in females followed by pancreas, adrenals, testes and ovary. A sex-linked difference was noticed in the distribution of Cd in ovary and testes with a much greater retention in ovary, up to 58% of testes. Sex differences were more evident 6 weeks after the withdrawal of animals from Cd. In female the concentration of metal amounted to 33% of male values in kidney and to 129% in ovary.

Effect of Cd administration on the Zn profile is shown in tables 3 and 4

TABLE 3

ORGAN DISTRIBUTION OF ZINC (μg/g dry tissue) IN MALE RATS

Animals	liver	kidney	pancreas	adrenals	testes
			I Cadmium for 6 weeks		
Control	131±4.1	133±28.9	120±23.1	135.0±54.8	225.6±9.7
Cd	353±49.7[a]	157±18.7	178±13.7[a]	97.1±15.2	234.4±13.3
			II 6 weeks after cadmium withdrawal		
Control	106±22.7	78.6±7.2	68.7±14.5	56.2±11.5	173±17.9
Cd	273±21.5[a]	121±7.3[a]	107±23.7[a]	64.9±12.5	171±6.5
II vs I	-25%	+63%	-33%	?	?

Each value represents the mean ±SD of four-five rats

a significantly different from control at $p < 0.01$

We note distinctive differences between sexes in Zn redistribution, induced by Cd. Thus, at the end of the 6 weeks of Cd treatment, Zn concentrations in male liver and pancreas were significantly higher than those of control, while in females those of liver, kidney and adrenals. When we examine Zn profile of animals withdrawn from Cd, sex difference was more pregnant. Male belonging to this group showed a significant increase of Zn in liver, kidney and pancreas, and female disclosed significantly higher amounts in kidney, pancreas and ovary.

TABLE 4

ORGAN DISTRIBUTION OF ZINC (μg/g dry tissue) IN FEMALE RATS

Animals	liver	kidney	pancreas	adrenals	ovary
			I Cadmium for 6 weeks		
Control	137±12.0	132±8.3	149±60.0	45.4±15.5	70.4±14.7
Cd	354±86.6[a]	165±22.9[a]	175±55.7	83.6±17.9[a]	96.0±33.3
			II 6 weeks after cadmium withdrawal		
Control	118±13.6	86.9±17.5	105±16.7	49.3±4.1	76.4±5.1
Cd	258±86.6[a]	134±5.9[a]	125±23.0	68.6±4.6[a]	93.6±6.5[a]
II vs I	+10%	+42%	-24%	-4%	-35%

Each value represents the mean ±SD of four-five rats
a significantly different from control at $p < 0.01$

TABLE 5

ORGAN DISTRIBUTION OF COPPER (μg/g dry tissue) IN MALE RATS

Animals	liver	kidney	pancreas	adrenals	testes
			I Cadmium for 6 weeks		
Control	11.9±4.1	13.1±1.0	3.5±0.4	4.2±0.6	9.8±1.6
Cd	17.0±0.6[b]	26.1±5.0[a]	3.5±0.1	4.9±1.1	11.4±1.8
			II 6 weeks after cadmium withdrawal		
Control	9.6±2.6	13.9±2.9	2.9±0.2	4.4±0.4	7.7±0.2
Cd	14.4±2.6[a]	26.0±5.0[a]	2.9±0.3	4.0±2.2	8.4±1.1
II vs I	-6%	-8%	-18%	-19%	-56%

Each value represents the mean ±SD of four-five rats
a significantly different from control at $p < 0.01$
b significantly different from control at $p < 0.05$

Lack of sex difference in Cu retention at the end of 6 weeks of Cd treatment was evident. In both sexes liver and kidney accumulated significantly higher amounts of Cu, compared with the control. After 6 weeks of withdrawal from Cd, the increase was significant in all female organs, while in males only in liver and kidney (tables 5 and 6).

TABLE 6

ORGAN DISTRIBUTION OF COPPER (μg/g dry tissue) IN FEMALE RATS

Animals	liver	kidney	pancreas	adrenals	ovary
			I Cadmium for 6 weeks		
Control	13.5±1.4	14.3±2.5	2.9±0.7	3.3±0.4	3.3±0.8
Cd	17.2±2.5[b]	26.9±3.8[a]	3.3±0.5	4.4±0.6	4.5±1.0
			II 6 weeks after cadmium withdrawal		
Control	11.1±1.3	17.9±2.5	3.4±0.2	3.1±0.3	3.5±0.3
Cd	21.0±4.7[a]	37.7±0.9[a]	3.9±0.3[b]	4.0±0.4[a]	4.6±0.8[b]
II vs I	+67%	+57%	+25%	-18%	-9%

Each value represents the mean ±SD of four-five rats
a significantly different from control at $p < 0.01$
b significantly different from control at $p < 0.05$

Our results show that sex takes an important part in the retention of Cd, and in Zn and Cu imbalance. We found quantitative and qualitative differences in the responses of males and females to Cd accumulation, and Zn and Cu redistribution. The effect of Cd on Zn and Cu metabolism was greater in the female organs, and Cd accumulated to a higher extent in the female tissues compared with males. The increased Cd retention in females (kidney and ovary) could be the result of a better biosynthetic apparatus for thioneins in females[8]. It is also possible that the observed reduced Cd retention in males might probably due to the presence of male sex hormones[9,10]. The more elevated uptake of Cd, Zn and Cu in tissues is generally believed to be a result of their binding to thioneins. Several researchers have presented convincing evidence that the metallothioneins are involved in heavy metal detoxification[11]. Our data on sex differences in the Cd toxicity confirm that female tolerate higher does of Cd probably due to enhanced protective mechanisms. What effects induces the redistribution of Zn and Cu in body tissues remain to be further elucidated.

REFERENCES

1. Friberg, L., Piscator, M., and Nordberg, G.F. (1971) Cadmium in the Environment CRC Press, Cleveland, Ohio.
2. Murthy, L., Rice, D., and Petering, H.G. (1978) Trace Element Metabolism in Man and Animals vol.3, M. Kirchengessner Ed., Univ. München, Germany.
3. Junko-Matsubara, K., and Machita, K. (1975) Environ. Res. lo, 29-38.
4. Sumino, K., Hayakawa, K., Shibata, T., and Kitamura, S. (1975) Arch. Environ. Health, 3o, 487-494.
5. El-gazzar, R., Boyle, J., Cornicelli, J., and Petering, H.G. (1978) Biochem. Pharmacol. 27, 2ool-2oo8.
6. Petering, H.G., Choudhury, H., and Stemmer, K.L. (1979) Environ. Health Perspect. 28, 97-lo6.
7. Julshamn, K., Utne, F., and Braekkan, O.R. (1977) Acta Pharmacol. Toxicol. 41, 515-524.
8. Stonard, M.D., and Webb, M. (1976) Chem.Biol.Interact. 15, 349-363.
9. Schnell, R.C., Means, J.R., Roberts, S.A., and Pence, D.H. (1979) Environ. Health Perspect. 28, 273-279.
lo. Kello, D., Dekanić, D., and Kostial, K. (1976) Arch. Environ. Health, 3o-33.
11. Nordberg, G.F. (1976) Dose-Response Relationship of Toxic Metals. Elsevier Scientific Publishing Company Amsterdam - Oxford - New York.

Mechanisms of Toxicity and Hazard Evaluation
B. Holmstedt, R. Lauwerys, M. Mercier, M. Roberfroid eds

COMPARISON OF BONE LESIONS IN CHRONIC CADMIUM POISONING AND VITAMIN D-DEFICIENCY

KŌJI NOGAWA and ETSUKO KOBAYASHI
Department of Hygiene, Kanazawa Medical University, Uchinada-machi,Ishikawa-ken (Japan)

Purposes and Methods

The following experiment was undertaken to clarify whether cadmium can cause osteomalacic bone changes or not, and to elucidate the relationship between chronic cadmium poisoning and vitamin D deficiency.

Seventy female wistar rats, weighing approximately 100 g, were used for this experiment. As shown in Table 1, the rats were separated into eight groups according to levels of vitamin D in the diet and cadmium-administered methods (oral and subcutaneous administration). The experiment was discontinued at 500 days and the rats were examined histologically and biochemically.

Results

The results are summarized in Table 2. Histologic investigation of the femurs revealed the same pathological changes in vitamin D-deficient control groups(Fig. 2) and in the cadmium-treated groups(Fig. 3). The main findings were osteoid tissue formation, thickening of cortex, increase in numbers of osteoblasts and osteoclasts, abnormality of subchondral ossification and fibrosis.

These findings indicate osteomalacic bone changes. Osteoid tissues are clearly identified by their intense eosinophilia(Figs. 2 and 3) in sections fixed with cyanuric chloride. It should be noted that cadmium-treated, vitamin D-adequate group 6(Fig. 3) showed the same findings as those of vitamin D-deficient control groups(Fig. 2), although vitamin D-adequate control group (Fig. 1) did not show any pathological findings.

Renal lesions in cadmium-treated groups were localized in tubules and the glomeruli were almost normal. The pathological alterations of tubules were more severe in vitamin D-deficient group than in vitamin D-slightly deficient group.

The conclusion of the present work is that cadmium exposure over long periods could induce the same findings in bone as those of vitamin D dificiency.

Acknowledgement

The authors thank Dr.F.Konishi for the histological examination.

Table 1 Experimental Condition for Each Group

Group No.	V.D		Cd Oral[c]	Cd Inj.[d]	Number of rats Initial	Number of rats Final
1	Adequate	(++)[a]	-	-	6	5
2	Slightly deficient	(+)[b]	-	-	6	5
3	Deficient	(-)	-	-	6	3
4	Slightly deficient	(+)[b]	+	-	10	3
5	Deficient	(-)	+	-	10	6
6	Adequate	(++)[a]	+	+	10	5
7	Slightly deficient	(+)[b]	+	+	12	6
8	Slightly deficient	(+)[b]	-	+	10	4

a : Vitamin D_2 was added to the control diet at the rate of 2.5 I.U/100gm of the diet for 80 days and 5 I.U/100gm of the diet for 420 days

b : Vitamin D_2 was added to the control diet at the rate of 0.5 I.U/100gm of the diet for 80 days and 1.0 I.U/100gm of the diet for 420 days

c : Cadmium was added as cadmium chloride to the control diet in a concentration of 10mg Cd/100gm of the diet

d : A 0.5ml cadmium chloride solution(300μg Cd/ml) was injected subcutaneously 22 times during the experiment

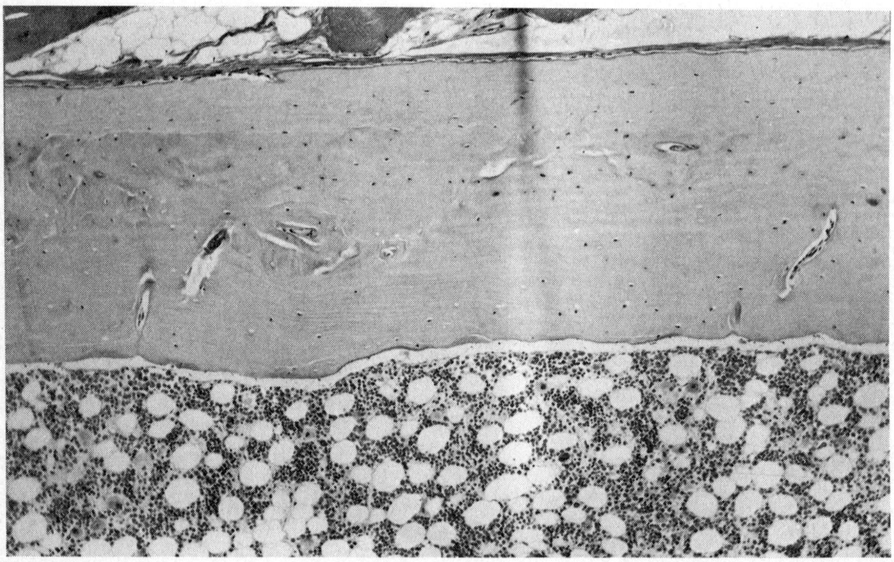

Fig.1 Cortical osseous tissue of femur: Group 1(Vitamin D-adequate control rat)

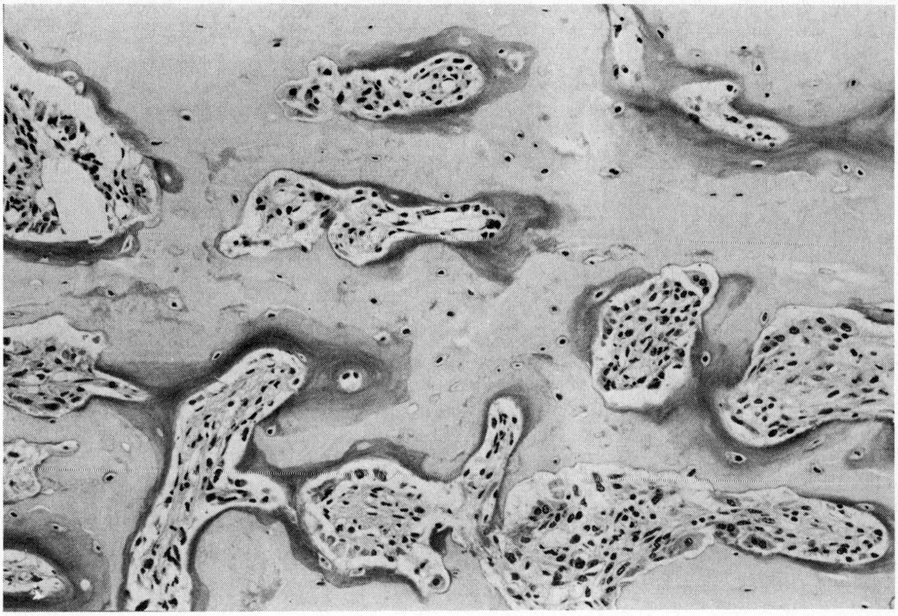

Fig.2. Cortical osseous tissue of femur: Group 2(Vitamin D-slightly deficient control rat)

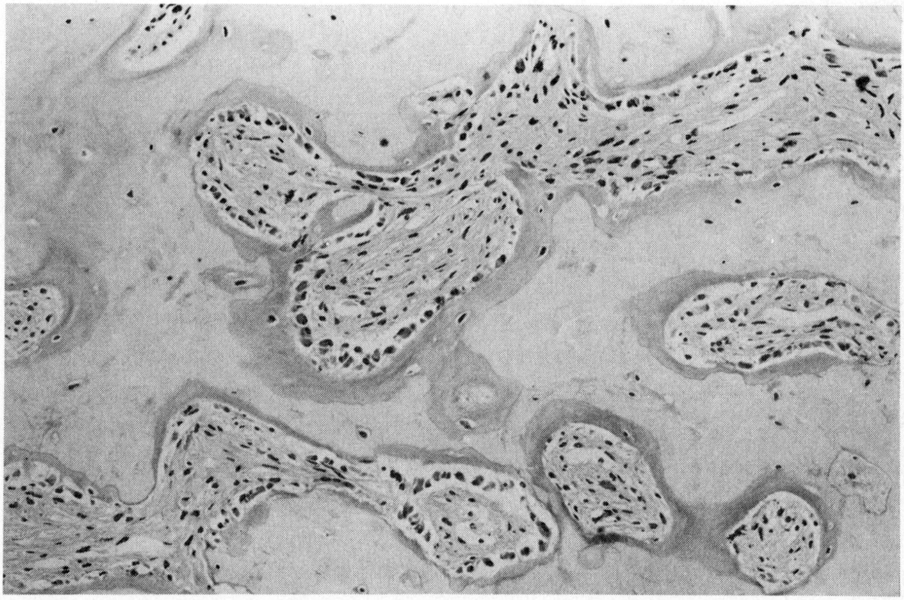

Fig.3. Cortical osseous tissue of femur: Group 6(Vitamin D-adequate,cadmium-treated rat)

Table 2 Histologic Investigation of Femurs

Group No.		Rat No.	Femur T	Ob	Oc	O	S	Fi
1		1	-	-	-	-	-	-
	Cd Oral -	2	-	-	-	-	-	-
	Cd Inj. -	3	-	-	-	-	-	-
	V.D ++	4	-	-	-	-	-	-
2		5	+	+	+	-	-	-
	Cd Oral -	6	++	+	+	±	-	+
	Cd Inj. -	7	+	++	+	+*	±	+
	V.D +	8	++	+++	++	+	+	++
3	Cd Oral -	9	+	+	±	-	±	-
	Cd Inj. -	10	++	+	+	±	-	+
	V.D -	11	+	±	+	-	-	-
4	Cd Oral +	12	++	++	+	±	+	+
	Cd Inj. -	13	++	++	++	+*	+	±
	V.D +	14	++	++	+	+*	+	±
5		15	++	++	+	±*	+	+
	Cd Oral +	16	+	+	+	±	+	+
	Cd Inj. -	17	++	+	+	-	±	±
	V.D -	18	++	++	+	+	+	+
		19	+	+	+	-	±	±
		20	++	++	++	+	+	+
6		21	++	+++	+	+	+	++
	Cd Oral +	22	++	+++	++	+	+	++
	Cd Inj. +	23	+	±	+	-	-	±*
	V.D ++	24	+	+	+	±	-	+
		25	++	++	+	-	±	+
7		26	++	+	+	±	±	±
	Cd Oral +	27	++	++	+	±	+	+
	Cd Inj. +	28	++	++	+	+	±	+
	V.D +	29	+	++	+	±	+	+
		30	++	+++	++	+	+	+
		31	++	++	+	+	±	+
8		32	++	+	±	±	±	±
	Cd Oral -	33	+	+	±	-	-	-
	Cd Inj. +	34	++	+	+	±	±	±
	V.D +	35	++	++	+	±	±	±

Group :As in Table 1
- :Denotes no effect ± :Denotes insignificant effect
+ :Denotes slight effect ++ :Denotes intermediate effect
+++ :Denotes strong effect * :Focal effect

Femur T : Thickening of cortex, Increase of trabecula
Ob : Increase in number of osteoblast
Oc : Increase in number of osteoclast
O : Osteoid formation
S : Abnormality of subchondral ossification
Fi : Fibrosis

© 1980 Elsevier/North-Holland Biomedical Press
Mechanisms of Toxicity and Hazard Evaluation
B. Holmstedt, R. Lauwerys, M. Mercier, M. Roberfroid eds

THE INFLUENCE OF ARSENITE ON THE INTERACTION BETWEEN SELENITE AND METHYL MERCURY

JAN ALEXANDER
Institute of Occupational Health, P.O. Box 8149, Dep. Oslo 1
Norway

INTRODUCTION

Selenite is known to antagonize the toxic effects of methyl mercury[1,2], to influence the organ distribution and to inhibit the biliary excretion of this metal compound[3]. Arsenite decreases the toxicity of selenite and has been found to inhibit methylation of selenide and strongly promote the biliary excretion of selenium[4,5]. Arsenite has earlier been found to increase the protective effect of selenite on methyl mercury induced toxicity in japaneese quails[6]. The mechanisms by which selenite influences methyl mercury toxicity and toxicokinetics is not fully understood[2]. The effects of arsenite alone and in combination with selenite on methyl mercury induced toxicity was studied in a cell culture model. The effect of arsenite in the biliary excretion of selenium and methyl mercury was studied and also the effect of arsenite and selenite in combination on the biliary excretion of methyl mercury. Bile from animals treated with the various substances were fractionated by gel filtration. In addition the organ distibution of selenium and methyl mercury was investgated.

MATERIALS AND METHODS

Rat Morris hepatoma cells, (dr. K. Gautvik, Oslo) cultured as described earlier[2] were used in the study. The experiments started 4 days after seeding. New medium with additions were given to the cells after 3 days and they were harvested after another 2 days. Cell growth was estimated by the amount of cell protein. Protein, glucose- and lactate uptake were determined as described elsewhere[2]. Female rats from Møllegaard, Copenhagen weighing about 250 grams were used for the animal experiments. They were fed a commercial pellet diet. The bile was collected as described earlier[3]. $CH_3{}^{203}HgCl$ (4µmol/kg) were given i.v. whereas selenite-^{75}Se and arsenite were administered i.p. In the organ distribution studies arsenite was given 10 min. prior to selenite which were given 15 min. prior to CH_3HgCl. The animals were killed after one hour. The mercury and selenium content of the organs, bile samples and fractions were determined in a γ- scintilation counter. Gel-filtration studies were done on a Sephadex -G-15 (Pharmacia, Sweden) column (40 cm x 2.6 cm) eluted with 0.1 M Tris-HCl, pH 8.0, 0.5M NaCl. Fractions of 1 ml were collected. For this purpose the bile was sampled on ice. The liver was removed after one hour and homogenized as described elsewhere[7].

RESULTS

Methyl mercury (4µM) inhibited the cell growth and causes an increased uptak of glucose and lactate from the medium (fig.1). No influence on growth, glucose- and lactate uptake was seen with arsenite (1µM) and selenite (0,5µM) alone or in combination. In the presence of selenite alone the effects of methyl mercury were partly counteracted whereas arsenite alone had no effect and even enhanced the increase in glucose uptake. However, combined, arsenite pontentiated the protective effects of selenite (fig.1).

Arsenite (10µmol/kg) greatly promoted the biliary excretion of selenite (0,5µmol/kg) (fig.2). The same amount of arsenite had no effect on the biliary excretion of methyl mercury (4µmol/kg) and did not prevent the inhibitory effect of selenite (0,5µmol/kg) on methyl mercury excretion in the bile. The effect of selenite was even slightly enhanced (fig.3). By gel filtration studies selenium in bile was found to eluate corresponding to the protein fraction and to complexes with one and two molecules of glutathione (GSH). Methyl mercury appeared as reported earlier[7] bound to protein(s) and one molecule GSH. In a separate assay selenite eluted as a peak different from the protein or the selenium-GSH complexes. When arsenite was given the increase in selenium excretion was predominantly as the complex with one molecule GSH. In the liver supernatant both selenium and methyl mercury were mostly protein bound (fig.4).

Arsenite (10µmol/kg) did not influence the slight changes in the organ distribution of methyl mercury (4µmol/kg) caused by selenite (0.5 µmol/kg). However, at the same time, arsenite treatment reduced the liver and brain content of selenium wheras blood and lung content were increased. (not shown).

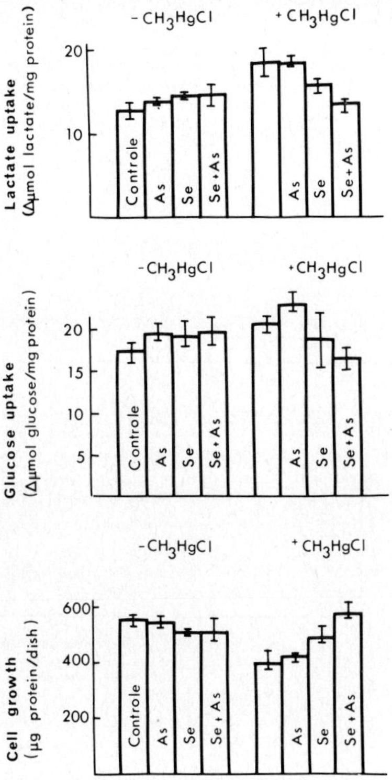

Fig.1. Effect on hepatoma cell-growth, glucose- and lactate uptake of arsenite(1uM), selenite (0.5uM) and methyl mercury (4uM) alone and in the various combinations. Mean values with range of 4 dishes are shown. (For details see text)

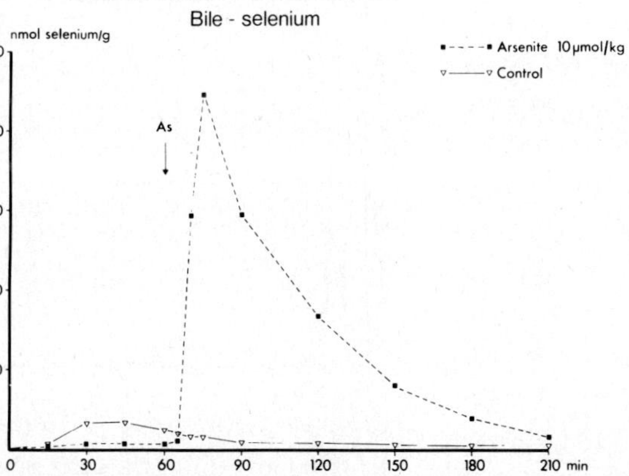

Fig.2.

Fig.2. Each value represents the selenium concentration during the interval ending at the time indicated for the sample. The curves represent one treated rat and one controle rat which are characteristic for the results in 4 treated rats and 4 control rats.

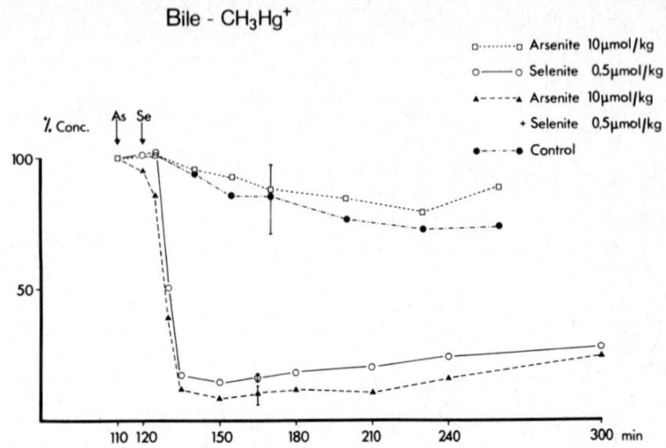

Fig.3. Each value represents the mean mercury concentration and range during the interval ending at the time indicated for the sample. The concentration at 110 min. was set to 100% for each rat. Nine rats were used in the control group and four in each of the treated groups.

DISCUSSION

The mechanism of the interaction between selenite and methyl mercury is not known. One explanation is formation of methyl mercury selenide complexes which has recently been demonstrated in biological systems[8,9]. The potentiating effect of arsenite in the preventive effect of selenite could be explained by inhibited methylation of selenide and thereby increased amounts of selenides available to form complexes with methyl mercury. However, the small amounts of selenite compared to methyl mercury needed for protection presumes involvement of specific compartements for acception of this hypothesis[2]. Another explanation is that arsenite will lead to a decrease in production of methylated selenides which have been found to be highly toxic in the presence of mercuric compounds[10].

It seems evident from the gelfiltration studies that selenium in bile occur bound to GSH and proteins. This is in accordance with the described

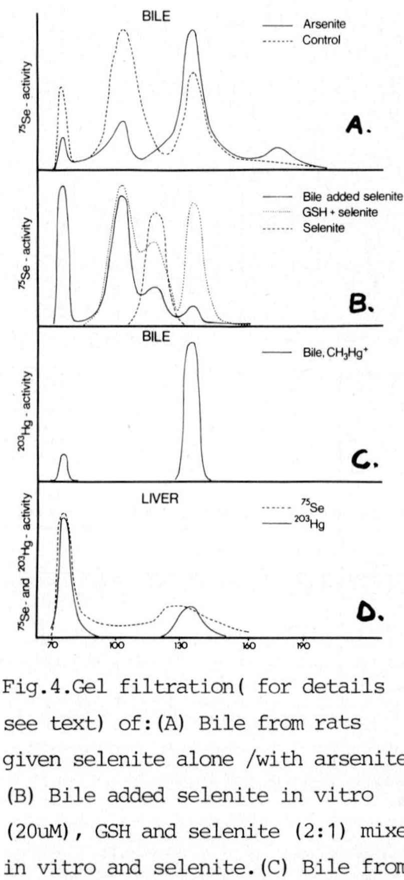

Fig.4.Gel filtration(for details see text) of:(A) Bile from rats given selenite alone /with arsenite. (B) Bile added selenite in vitro (20uM), GSH and selenite (2:1) mixed in vitro and selenite.(C) Bile from rat given CH_3HgCl.(D) Liver from rat given bothselenite and CH_3HgCl.

metabolism of selenite of which the first 4 steps can also proceed non-enzymically[5]:

$$H_2SeO_3 \xrightarrow{1} GSSeSG \xrightarrow{2} GSSeH \xrightarrow{3} H_2Se \left[\xrightarrow{5} \begin{matrix} (CH_3)_2Se \\ (CH_3)_3Se^+ \end{matrix} \right] \quad (H_2Se \xrightarrow{4} \text{proteinSe})$$

This reaction can also proceed in bile in vitro which contains about 3mM GSH[7]. Arsenite treatment probably leads to accumulation of selenium-GSH metabolites in the liver when the selenide methylation system is inhibited. These metabolites are excreted in bile. In spite of this effect on the selenium excretion into bile, the effect of selenite on methyl mercury excretion is still present. This further support that selenium specifically affects one of the steps in the excretion if methyl mercury, either by forming selenide complexes occupying the methyl mercury available for excretion (i.e. in a certain compartment) or by inhibiting the transfer of methyl mercury form the protein mercaptides to GSH[3].

The reduced amounts of selenium found in the brain after arsenite treatment might be due to decreased formation of dimethylselenide which are lipofilic. Other results indicate that this metabolite might be rapidly cleared from the brain. The increased kidney content of selenium found after arsenite treatment[4] might be due to increased biliary excretion of Se-GSH metabolites formed which are subsequently partly reabsorbed and taken up by the kidney in a similar way as methyl mercury[3]. We did not record increased kidney content of selenium after arsenite treatment in this study, probably because of too short exposure time for selenite.

ACKNOWLEDGEMENTS

I wish to thank Dr. T. Norseth for valuable discussions. The skillfull tecknical assistence of Mrs. Nordhagen, Mrs. Løken and Mrs. Goffeng Bay is highly appreciated. This work was supported by Borregaards forskningsfond.

REFERENCES

1. Ganther, H.E. et al (1972) Science, 175, 112-114
2. Alexander, J. et al (1979) Acta pharmac. et toxic, 45, 379-386
3. Alexander, J. and T. Norseth (1979) Acta pharmac. et. toxic, 44, 168-176
4. Levander, O.A. and L.C. Argrett (1969) Toxic. Appl. Pharm,

14, 308-314

5. Hsieh, H.S. and H.E. Ganther (1977) Biochem, Biophys Acta, 497, 205-217
6. El - Berganni, M.M. et al (1975), Poultry. Sci., 54, 1756-1757
7. Refsvik. T. and T. Norseth (1975), Acta pharmac, toxic, 42, 135-141
8. Magos, L. et al (1979) Chem, -Biol.Interact., 28, 359-362
9. Naganuma, A. and Imura, N. (1980) Res. Com. Chem. Path. Pharm, 27, 163-173
10. Diplock, A.T. (1976) CRC, Critical Rev. Toxicol., 4, 271-329

Mechanisms of Toxicity and Hazard Evaluation
B. Holmstedt, R. Lauwerys, M. Mercier, M. Roberfroid eds

INTERFERENCE OF INADEQUATE OXYGENATION IN HEMATOFLUOROMETER ZINC-PROTOPORPHYRIN READINGS

S. TELIŠMAN, V. KARAČIĆ, J. MECZNER, D. PRPIĆ-MAJIĆ
Institute for Medical Research and Occupational Health, M. Pijade 158, P.O. Box 291, YU-41001 ZAGREB (Yugoslavia)

INTRODUCTION

Erythrocyte protoporphyrin concentration is considered a very useful biological indicator of effect in monitoring occupational exposure to inorganic lead. Its main advantage is that it reflects integrated exposure over a longer period, yielding better correlation with effects of chronic lead exposure (blood hemoglobin[1,2], behavioural test scores[3]) in comparison with blood lead, which (although more specific for lead absorption) reflects mainly recent exposure. Protoporphyrin concentration in peripheral blood gives a better indication of the metabolically active (chelatable) fraction of the total lead body burden, it persists at high levels relatively longer than blood lead, and gives better information of past lead exposure. This test is therefore very useful in assessing average chronic lead exposure, particularly in circumstances of variable exposure, when the single protoporphyrin value is far more representative than that of the other characteristic indicators which reflect mainly recent exposure, are more prone to day-to-day variations (PbB, ALAD, ALAU, CPU)*, or are less sensitive in the range of occupational exposure limit values (ALAU, CPU). However, the protoporphyrin test is significantly less useful in detecting recent excessive lead exposure, for, if considered alone, it may lead to a false negative assessment of lead absorption[4]. In order to overcome this disadvantage, the protoporphyrin test should be considered simultaneously with another sensitive indicator reflecting recent lead exposure (PbB and/or ALAD). Due to the fact that protoporphyrin in peripheral blood and blood lead do not follow the same dynamic pattern, one should expect to find sometimes a very poor or quite insignificant correlation between these two indicators, particularly within population groups which are not homogenous with regard to the onset, duration, and intensity of lead exposure, or the time elapsed since past lead exposure[5].

Contrary to erythrocyte protoporphyria, where protoporphyrin mainly exists

---

* Abbreviations: blood lead (PbB), erythrocyte δ-aminolevulinic acid dehydratase (ALAD), urinary δ-aminolevulinic acid (ALAU), urinary coproporphyrin (CPU).

in its free form, at increased lead absorption or in iron deficiency it is not free but chelated with zinc to form zinc-protoporphyrin (ZPP). Numerous analytical methods have been used for the assessment of lead exposure. Some of them measure ZPP, others total erythrocyte protoporphyrin - traditionally called "free" erythrocyte protoporphyrin (FEP), or total erythrocyte porphyrins (EP). Basically, it is not crucial whether ZPP, FEP, or even EP is measured since about 90% of the total erythrocyte porphyrins consist of protoporphyrin caused by lead absorption. However, because of essentially different methods (using either whole blood or erythrocytes for analysis, different standards for calibration, and measuring different constituents) which yield significantly different numerical values, there is an urgent need for a standardization of the methodology. A simple portable ZPP-hematofluorometer which allows instant reading by use of a minute amount of unprocessed blood offers such a possibility. In order to ensure comparable data by this atractive method, which yields highly significant correlations with other more sophisticated protoporphyrin methods, possible interferences have to be quantified.

This paper deals with the influence of increased blood carboxyhemoglobin (COHb) concentrations on hematofluorometer ZPP readings.

MATERIALS AND METHODS

Heparinized venous blood samples from workers occupationally exposed to lead were taken for analysis. All determinations were carried out on the day of the blood collection, before and following the exposure to carbon monoxide *in vitro*. CO was generated by the reaction of concentrated formic and sulphuric acids (p.a.) with subsequent absorption of possible trace quantities of CO_2 in a 40% solution of potassium hydroxide. ZPP was measured by means of a Bell-Aviv hematofluorometer calibrated in mmol ZPP/mol Hb (CV<3%), and %COHb by the method of Commins and Lawther[6] (CV<3%). Mean values of duplicate analyses were used for calculations.

RESULTS

Original ZPP_o and $COHb_o$ values together with corresponding ZPP_i and $COHb_i$ values obtained after *in vitro* exposure of blood samples to carbon monoxide are presented in Table 1. Due to the wide range of initial ZPP values, the relationship between the relative decrease in ZPP $(\frac{ZPP_o - ZPP_i}{ZPP_o})$ and the increase in COHb ($COHb_i - COHb_o$) is presented in Fig.1.

Due to the fact that the ZPP-hematofluorometer measures the ratio between the zinc-protoporphyrin fluorescence and the absorption of light by oxyhemoglo-

TABLE 1

THE INFLUENCE OF INCREASED COHb CONCENTRATION IN BLOOD ON HEMATOFLUOROMETER ZPP READINGS

Concentrations before ($COHb_o$ and ZPP_o) and after ($COHb_i$ and ZPP_i) *in vitro* exposure of blood to carbon monoxide.

% COHb		mmol ZPP/mol Hb	
$COHb_o$	$COHb_i$	ZPP_o	ZPP_i
1.5	82.9	1.67	1.24
2.0	6.1	3.32	3.16
1.0	1.4	2.34	2.31
	24.5		2.05
	58.2		1.75
0.4	43.8	1.80	1.41
	60.3		1.27
	74.8		1.24
1.9	18.9	1.64	1.49
	52.9		1.30
	78.7		1.19
0.5	9.8	2.18	1.87
	34.4		1.71
	70.0		1.59
0.3	2.4	1.94	1.84
	10.2		1.77
	20.7		1.66
	40.6		1.50
0.6	10.8	1.67	1.50
	23.9		1.33
	73.7		1.18
0.5	20.3	1.34	1.13
	30.5		1.08
0.8	6.1	1.46	1.37
	35.8		1.18
	53.6		1.11

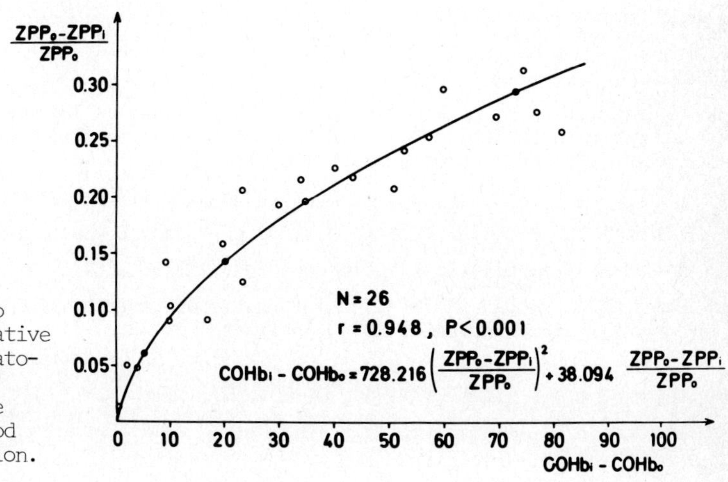

Fig. 1.

The relationship between the relative decrease in hematofluorometer ZPP readings and the increase of blood COHb concentration.

bin, complete oxygenation of the blood hemoglobin is required. Despite a very careful oxygenation of the blood in the course of the hematofluorometric measurement (by thorough stirring of the blood drop in contact with air oxygen on the instrument's glass slide), it was obvious that the drying of the blood film prevented complete oxygenation at increased COHb levels. The decrease in maximal ZPP readings was highly correlated with the increase of COHb and the relationship was non-linear corresponding to aprox. 6, 9, and 14% decrease of the original ZPP for the increase of 5, 10, and 20% COHb, respectively. The curved rather than linear relationship was probably due to the exponential decrease in blood COHb concentration during the oxygenation on the blood on the instrument's glass slide, which yielded correspondingly lower actual COHb values at the time of the maximal ZPP readings.

The influence of inadequate oxygenation on hematofluorometer ZPP readings was previously observed by Grandjean and Lintrup[2] and Alessio et al.[7], who found significantly higher (on average 30% and 50%, respectively) values in capillary blood compared to venous blood. However, such a difference was not found by Grunder and Moffit, Jr.[8], who oxygenated the samples by stirring and spreading the blood on the instrument's glass slide during hematofluorometric measurement. Our results indicate a significant influence of increased COHb concentration on hematofluorometer ZPP readings. Even though the decrease in ZPP is very small, it should be taken into account when establishing lead exposure limits expressed by ZPP concentration, particularly in workers exposed to both lead and carbon monoxide (foundries, smelters, etc.) and/or heavy smokers. Complete elimination of the influence of an increased COHb concentration is possible only by separate agitation of the blood sample with oxygen prior to hematofluorometric measurement.

REFERENCES

1. Telišman, S. and Prpić-Majić, D. (1979) Proceedings International Conference Management & Control of Heavy Metals in the Environment, London 18-22 September 1979, CEP Consultants Ltd, Edinburgh, pp. 62-65.
2. Grandjean, P. and Lintrup, J. (1978) Scand.J.Clin.Lab.Invest., 38, 669-675.
3. Valciukas, J.A. et al. (1978) Int. Arch. Occup. Environ. Health, 41, 217-236.
4. Beritić, T. et al. (1977) J. Occup. Med. 19, 551-557.
5. Beritić, T. et al. (1978) 19th International Congress on Occupational Health, Dubrovnik 25-30 September 1978, Abstracts, p. 38.
6. Commins, B.T. and Lawther, P.J. (1965) Brit. J. Ind. Med., 22, 139-143.
7. Alessio, L. et al. (1978) Med. Lavoro, 69, 563-575.
8. Grunder, F.I. and Moffit, Jr., A.E. (1979) Amer. Ind. Hyg. Assoc. J., 40, 686-694.

Mechanisms of Toxicity and Hazard Evaluation
B. Holmstedt, R. Lauwerys, M. Mercier, M. Roberfroid eds

NEUROGENIC COMPONENTS IN CARDIOVASCULAR REACTIVITY OF CHRONICALLY LEAD-EXPOSED RATS

MARCO CARMIGNANI[(°)], PAOLO BOSCOLO[(°°)], PAOLO MARCHETTI[(°)] and A. IANNACCONE[(°°)]
Departments of Pharmacology[(°)] and Occupational Medicine[(°°)], Catholic University School of Medicine, Via Pineta Sacchetti 644, 00168 Rome (Italy)

INTRODUCTION

It is debatable whether lead exposure may induce hypertension and degenerative vascular diseases. However, lead has been reported to affect the kallikrein-kinin, renin-angiotensin-aldosterone and adrenergic systems[1,2].

Nervous functions are primarily affected in lead-exposed humans and animals[3]. Nevertheless, there is no evidence, to date, that lead exposure may affect the cardiovascular function acting also by nervous system mediated mechanisms.

In this preliminary study we assess the effects of chronic lead-exposure on cardiovascular function considering the possible role of both neurogenic and/or humoral action mechanisms.

MATERIALS AND METHODS

Animals. Sixteen adult male Sprague-Dawley rats, randomly divided into two groups, were fed a standard laboratory diet. Treated group was exposed for 160-180 days to lead (as acetate) in deionized drinking water at the concentration of 50 μg/ml.

Cardiovascular determinations. The animals were anesthetized with i.p. injected sodium pentobarbital (40 mg/kg) and a tracheal cannula was inserted. Polyethylene catheters were placed in a femoral artery and a femoral vein. The systemic blood pressure (BP), BP maximum rate of rise (dP/dt max), heart rate and standard limb II electrocardiogram were continuously monitored on a Beckman type RM Dynograph recorder. A derivative computer was used for dP/dt.

Protocol. After a stabilization period of at least 30 min, bilateral carotid occlusion (BCO) was performed (30 sec) at 2 cm below the bifurcation. The sensitivity (gain) of the baroreflex arc was assessed by the method described by Smyth et al.[4], considering the mean of several test injections of i.v. phenylephrine (20 μg/kg). Dose-response relationship was then determined for i.v. injections of increasing doses (with 2.0 ratio) of norepinephrine (0.25 - 1 μg/kg), epinephrine (0.125 - 1 μg/kg), angiotensin I (0.25 - 1 μg/kg), angiotensin II (0.25 - 1 μg/kg) and bradykinin (0.075 - 0.300 μg/kg). Finally, gradual doses of i.v. hexamethonium (0.625, 1.25, 2.5 mg/kg) were tested on cardiovascular parameters before and after selective vagotomy carried out at the neck below the nodose ganglion. Each of the following tests was not made until the parameters had returned to the values preceding the BCO and had stabilized. Blood samples were collected at the end of experiments and blood lead levels were determined by atomic absorption spectrometry.

Linear regression and analysis of variance (baroreflex sensitivity) and Dunnett's t test for multiple comparison were used.

RESULTS

No significant difference between control and exposed animals could be seen either in growth and in body weight or in general appearance. However, lead-exposed rats were more aggressive and difficult to handle than controls.

Blood lead levels were (mean ± SE) 13.6 ± 3.2 μg/100 ml in control and 38.4 ± 3.6 μg/100 ml in exposed animals ($P<0.001$).

Lead-treated rats showed (mean ± SE) both systolic (183 ± 6 mmHg) and diastolic (138 ± 6 mmHg) BP values significantly increased ($P<0.001$, $P<0.005$) in relation to those of control animals (127 ± 5 and 97 ± 3 mmHg, respectively). Also dP/dt max of exposed rats appeared to be significantly increased (9125 ± 178 mmHg/sec; $P<0.01$) when compared with that of controls (6375 ± 249 mmHg/sec).

Baroreflex gain was decreased in the lead-exposed group, reaching a mean value of 1.62 msec/mmHg,which differs (df = 1:96, F = 43.84, $P<0.01$) from the control one (4.54 msec/mmHg).

The effects of BCO on systolic and diastolic BP and on dP/dt max were strongly reduced in lead-exposed rats; on the other hand, no significant difference was found for heart rate (Table 2).

The systo-diastolic BP and dP/dt max changes induced by some of the tested doses of designated drugs are presented in Table 1. No significant difference in heart rate values was noted for each of the agonists studied. In the exposed animals the responses to norepinephrine and angiotensin II were increased with a dose-dependent effect, while those to angiotensin I and bradykinin were unchanged. The diastolic hypotension induced by the lower doses of epinephrine (0.125 and 0.150 μg/kg) was greater in exposed that in control rats. On the other hand, the increase of both systolic and diastolic BP values and of dP/dt max observed with higher doses of epinephrine was not significantly affected by the lead exposure.

As shown in Table 2, the ganglion blocking drug used (hexamethonium) was

TABLE 1

CARDIOVASCULAR RESPONSES OF CONTROL AND LEAD-TREATED[a] RATS FOLLOWING I.V. INJECTION OF DESIGNATED DRUGS[b]

DRUGS μg/kg		BLOOD PRESSURE (mmHg) SYSTOLIC		DIASTOLIC		dP/dt MAX (mmHg/sec)	
		Control	Treated	Control	Treated	Control	Treated
Norepinephrine	1	+48 ± 2	+63 ± 4**	+41 ± 4	+51 ± 3*	+1063 ± 90	+2250 ± 74**
Epinephrine	0.125	+ 6 ± 2	-11 ± 2**	- 7 ± 2	-26 ± 3**	+ 905 ± 81	+1252 ± 62**
	1	+41 ± 3	+44 ± 4	+31 ± 3	+35 ± 5	+1653 ± 96	+1603 ± 62
Angiotensin I	0.50	+44 ± 3	+41 ± 3	+25 ± 4	+23 ± 5	- 547 ± 40	- 583 ± 46
Angiotensin II	0.50	+47 ± 4	+70 ± 6**	+40 ± 3	+69 ± 5**	- 468 ± 49	- 721 ± 53**
Bradykinin	1.50	-28 ± 4	-26 ± 3	-30 ± 3	-23 ± 2	- 550 ± 43	- 538 ± 35

[a] See text in Materials and Methods.
[b] Values represent mean changes ± SE (n = 8).
**P<0.01, *P<0.05 indicate significantly different from control.

TABLE 2

CARDIOVASCULAR RESPONSES OF CONTROL AND LEAD-TREATED[a] RATS TO BILATERAL CAROTID OCCLUSION (B C O), TO I.V. HEXAMETHONIUM (HEX; 2.5 mg/kg), TO VAGOTOMY AND TO I.V. HEX AFTER VAGOTOMY [b].

GROUPS	BLOOD PRESSURE (% change) SYSTOLIC	DIASTOLIC	dP/dt MAX (% change)	HEART RATE (% change)
CONTROL				
B C O	+ 34 ± 2	+35 ± 2	+39 ± 2	+ 7 ± 1
Hex	- 25 ± 3	-29 ± 1	-30 ± 2	- 7 ± 1
Vagotomy	+ 16 ± 3	+17 ± 2	+14 ± 2	+ 9 ± 1
Hex after vagotomy [c]	- 43 ± 2**	-39 ± 2*	-27 ± 1	-32 ± 2***
LEAD-TREATED				
B C O	+16 ± 1***	+15 ± 1***	+20 ± 2*	+ 4 ± 1
Hex	-52 ± 4**	-63 ± 5*	-53 ± 3***	-13 ± 1*
Vagotomy	+ 6 ± 1*	+10 ± 1*	+ 9 ± 1	+ 3 ± 1
Hex after vagotomy [c]	-46 ± 5	-57 ± 6	-49 ± 5	-10 ± 2

[a] [b] See Table 1.
[c] Compared with the responses to Hex obtained in the same group.
***P<0.001, **P<0.01, *P<0.05 indicate significant differences.

able to induce systemic hypotension, bradycardia and reduction of dP/dt max which were much stronger in lead-exposed animals. Thus, the vagotomy increases the hexamethonium effects only in the control group, while it is ineffective in the treated rats. Similarly, the vagotomy , by itself, is followed by a significant increase of systemic BP higher in control than in lead-exposed rats.

DISCUSSION

In our experimental conditions, chronic lead exposure is able to induce hypertension and increase of cardiac inotropism without significant changes in heart rate. On the whole, previous results are consistent with the hypothesis that chronic lead exposure may cause sympathetic hyperactivity and baroreflex hyposensitivity. On the other hand, our results do not exclude the possibility that lead may also reduce the vagal parasympathetic activity. In this regard, lead has been reported to induce in rats hypofunction of cholinergic parameters[5].

Our experiments show that lead exposure induces in rats specific alterations of the cardiovascular reactivity to physiological agonists. The observed potentiation of the cardiopressor responses to norepinephrine (dose-related) and the increase of diastolic hypotension induced by low doses of epinephrine might be explained by assuming a lead-dependent vascular hypersensitivity to both alpha and beta stimulation. Thus, lead-induced increase of cardiovascular responses to angiotensin II agrees with our preliminary observations suggesting a lead-inhibitory effect on the angiotensin-I-converting enzyme activity.

Our results demonstrate that (besides humoral factors) neurogenic components are specifically involved in the cardiovascular alterations of rats with lead-induced hypertension, though we are unable at this stage to evaluate their relative role.

REFERENCES

1. Boscolo, P. et al. (1979) The Role of Occupational Exposure to Toxic Metals on the Development of Hypertension. In: Management and Control of Heavy Metals in the Environment, Perry R., Ed., CEP Consultant,Ltd., Edinburgh, pp. 325-328.
2. Williams, B.J. et al. (1977) Toxicol. Appl. Pharmacol., 40, 407-413.
3. Valciukas, J.A. et al. (1978) Science, 201, 465-467.
4. Smyth, H.S. et al. (1969) Circulation Res., 24, 109-121.
5. Carroll, P.T. et al. (1977) Biochem. Pharmacol., 26, 397-402.

Mechanisms of Toxicity and Hazard Evaluation
B. Holmstedt, R. Lauwerys, M. Mercier, M. Roberfroid eds

EFFECT OF ORAL ZINC INTAKE ON THE BIOLOGICAL EFFECT OF LEAD

MOHAMED ABDULLA
Unit for Community Care Sciences at Dalby and Research Department 2, University Hospital, S-221 85 Lund (Sweden)

INTRODUCTION

Although metal poisoning from lead, mercury, cadmium, arsenic, etc. as a human health hazard has been recognized for centuries, the prophylactic aspects of trace elements that are known to be essential for human nutrition have evoked interest only during the last few years. At present it is being recognized more and more, that mineral nutrition and mineral supplementation are playing important role against the hazards of environmental exposure to toxic metals. This is especially true as regards a few essential micronutrients such as iron, zinc, magnesium and selenium. In the past, toxic effects of heavy metals were studied very often separately and accordingly little attention was directed to the consequences of the simultaneous presence and interaction of other elements with similar chemical properties and electronic configuration. Because the toxicity of heavy metals in biological systems is mainly reflected by the inhibition of enzymes concerned with the regulation of normal metabolic functions, it is relevant to consider the antagonistic effect of essential elements on enzyme inhibition caused by metal poisoning. The activity of most metallo-enzymes present in normal cells can be altered or modified by the competitive displacement of the metal at the active site by another toxic or essential element. Most divalent metals are known to interact in competitive mechanism(s) involving the active site(s) of several enzymes. Enzyme kinetic studies can thus effectively be used to evaluate the interaction between different metals at the cellular level.

Recent studies have indicated that dietary zinc provides protection against the toxicity of lead[1,2,3]. Our own studies have shown that parenterally administered zinc in animals provide protection against the biological effects of acute and chronic poisoning by lead and cadmium[4,5]. In our studies, we have measured the activity of delta-aminolevulinic acid dehydratase (ALAD) in red blood cells to evaluate the antagonism between lead and zinc. Earlier studies have shown that the lead-induced inhibition of ALAD can be antagonized by zinc[6]. The present study in healthy human subjects has been conducted to investigate the effect of oral zinc intake on ALAD activity in erythrocytes and lead in blood.

MATERIALS AND METHODS

Three separate studies have been carried out to investigate the influence of oral zinc intake on ALAD activity. In the first study, seven healthy adults consumed 2.07 mmol zinc/day for 12 weeks and five subjects, of the same mean age, received a placebo for the same period. In the second study, six healthy adults consumed 1.38 mmol zinc/day for 12 weeks; and finally in the third study seven persons consumed 0.69 mmol zinc/day for the same period. Blood samples were collected prior to, during, and after the experimental period. On an average, 10 different blood samples were collected. ALAD activity measurements were made within four hours of blood sampling by the European Standardized Technique[7]. Haematological measurements were made within 20 hours of blood sampling. Zinc, copper, magnesium, calcium, and lead were measured by atomic absorption spectrophotometry after necessary pretreatment of the blood samples. Alkaline phosphatase activity measurements in granulocytes were made by a standard method. And the activity of DNA repair enzymes in lymphocytes was measured according to a method described by Pero *et al.*[8].

RESULTS

In the first study, we observed that the ALAD activity in erythrocytes started to increase after two weeks of zinc intake, reached peak levels after six weeks, and remained constant thereafter. Along with the increase in the enzyme activity, there was an increase in plasma zinc levels when compared with the placebo group. Similar trends were observed in the other two investigations, although the increase were not as high as those which were found in the first study. In the second and third studies, we measured the plasma copper levels and found that, along with the rise in plasma zinc, there was a reciprocal decrease in copper levels, and the copper/zinc ratio in the plasma reached a significantly low level towards the end of the experimental period. In the last two studies, we also measured the increase of zinc in erythrocytes together with measurements of whole blood lead levels. Our results indicated that lead levels in whole blood decreased 20 - 30% after 4 weeks of zinc intake along with an increase of zinc in erythrocytes and an increase in ALAD activity. We also observed an increase in the activity of granulocyte alkaline phosphatase in the third study together with an increase of zinc in granulocytes. The DNA reapir studies done in the second and third groups showed that the repair activity increased significantly after the zinc intake. The significance of this finding is difficult to interpret at the present. Fig. 1 and 2 show part of the results.

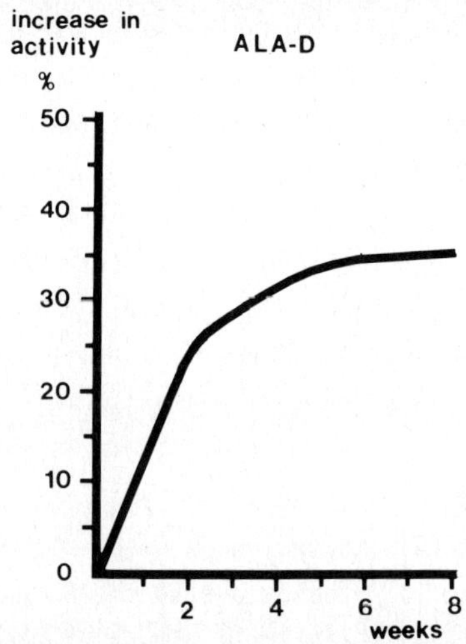

Fig. 1. ALAD activity in erythrocytes after zinc intake.

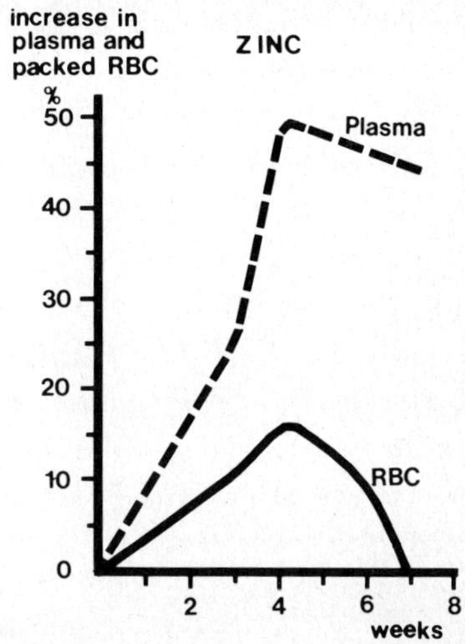

Fig. 2. Zinc in plasma and erythrocytes after zinc intake.

DISCUSSION

In recent years, oral zinc therapy has been shown to have beneficial effects on several clinical conditions. In experimental studies, both oral and parenteral administrations of zinc in humans and in several animal species have been shown to improve certain clinical conditions, such as retarded growth, abnormalities in reproduction, and impaired hair growth associated with zinc deficiency. The beneficial effect of zinc against cadmium poisoning is well known today. In spite of the remarkable advances in zinc biochemistry and nutrition during the past few decades, little is known regarding the mechanism(s) involved in the absorption and distribution of the element. Even less is known as regards the interaction between zinc and other trace elements with similar properties at the intestinal and cellular levels. Zinc absorption and transfer to the vascular system are related to the synthesis of metallothionine in the enterocytes[9]. It appears that the zinc which is not transferred to plasma from enterocytes is specifically bound to metallothionine, the synthesis of which is proportional to the dietary intake of zinc. Metallothionine is also known to bind other divalent metals such as copper, cadmium, and probably lead. When the dietary intake of zinc is high in the gastrointestinal tract, it appears that the absorption of the above metals is reduced along with an increased fecal excretion.

Recently, Cerklewski and Forbes[1] reported that optimal and superoptimal dietary intake of zinc reduced the absorption of lead. This was later confirmed by El-Gazzar *et al.*[2]. Some years ago, Willoughby *et al.*[10] showed that the clinical symptoms of lead poisoning in the foal could be prevented by administring zinc. In 1977, Thomassino *et al.*[11] reported a clinical case of acute lead poisoning that could be partially counteracted by the administration of zinc. Papaioannou *et al.*[3] in 1978 showed that dietary zinc supplementation and vitamin C could reduce blood lead levels in battery workers. From all of these studies, it appears that the protection conferred by zinc in lead poisoning is effective both at the intestinal level and at the cellular level.

The average daily intake of zinc from prepared foods in Sweden and other industrialized countries is 8 - 10 mg as compared with the recommended allowance of 12 - 15 mg[12]. One reason for this low intake is probably due to the increased consumption of refined foods. In order to achieve a beneficial effect of zinc against heavy metal poisoning, it would appear that it is necessary to increase the bio-availability of zinc by effective modification of the diet.

REFERENCES

1. Cerklewski, F.L. and Forbes, R.M. (1976) J. Nutr., 106, 689-696.
2. El-Gazzar, R.M., Finelli, V.N., Boiano, J. and Petering, H.G. (1978) Toxicol. Letters, 1, 227-234.
3. Papaioannou, R., Sohler, A. and Pfeiffer, C.C. (1978) Orthomol. Psych., 7, 2, 94-106.
4. Haeger-Aronsen, B., Abdulla, M. and Schütz, A. (1976) Arch. Environ. Health, 31, 215-220.
5. Abdulla, M., Svensson, S. and Nordén, Å. (1979) Proceedings, Management and Control of Heavy Metals in the Environment, London, Sept.79 pp.179-182
6. Abdulla, M. and Haeger-Aronsen, B. (1974) Symposium on Zinc. Proceedings, Zederfeldt (Ed.) pp. 115-121.
7. Berlin, A. and Schaller, K.H. (1974) Z. Kli. Chem. Klin. Biochem., 12, 389-390.
8. Pero, R.W., Bryngelsson, C., Mitelman, F., Nordén, Å. and Thulin, T. (1976) Proc. Natl. Acad. Sci., 73, 2496-2500.
9. Cousins, R.J. (1979) Nutr. Rev., 37, 4, 97-103.
10. Willoughby, R.A., Mac Donald, E., McSherry, B.J. and Brown, G. (1972) Can. J. Comp. Med., 36, 348-359.
11. Thomasino, J., Zuroweste, E., Brooks, S., Petering, H., Lener, S. and Finelli, V. (1977) Arch. Environ. Health, 32, 244-247.
12. Abdulla, M., Svensson, S. and Nordén, Å. (1979) Scand. J. Gastroent., 14, 52, 168-171.

BIOLOGICAL MONITORING OF CHILDREN LIVING IN THE VICINITY OF A LEAD SMELTING PLANT*

D. PRPIĆ-MAJIĆ, B. MATIJEVIĆ, V. KARAČIĆ and A. KERŠANC
Institute for Medical Research and Occupational Health, M.Pijade 158,
P.O.B.291, 41001 ZAGREB (Yugoslavia)

INTRODUCTION

The children who live in communities near a lead smelting plant are at permanent health risk owing to the continuous undue lead exposure through lead contaminated air, soil and food. Most of them were even born with a higher lead body burden through the increased prenatal lead exposure from mothers living in the same area. In such population the biochemical control of exposure is necessary in order to estimate the magnitude of health risk before the stage of lead poisoning is reached.

One of the biochemical systems most sensitive to lead effects is the heme biosynthetic pathway. Owing to that the indicators showing lead effects on hemoglobin synthesis are the parameters of choice for biological monitoring of both adults and children. This paper deals with their applicability for biological monitoring of the children living near a lead smelting plant.

SUBJECTS AND METHODS

The subjects examined were asymptomatic boys (N=59) of school age (6 to 10 years) living in several settlements near two lead smelting plants (M. and T.) at different geographical locations. For each exposed group a relevant control group was examined. The boys in the control groups were matched to the boys in the exposed groups with regard to age, socio-economic status and nutritional conditions.

In each subject hemoglobin (Hb), zinc protoporphyrin (ZPP), erythrocyte δ-aminolevulinic acid dehydratase (ALAD) activity and blood lead (Pb-B) were determined from heparanised venous blood preserved from light and kept at 4 °C. Hb was determined spectrophotometrically by cyanmethemoglobin method[1]. The concentration of ZPP was determined by means of Bell-Aviv hematofluorometer[2] calibrated in mmolZPP/mol Hb. For ALAD activity the European standard method[3] was

* This investigation was supported by the Environmental Protection Agency, Research Triangle Park, NC., under a special foreign currency program JF-2-570-2-Extention.

used. Pb-B was analysed by flameless atomic absorption spectrophotometry[4,5]. All analyses have been performed in duplicate within 24 hours of blood collection.

The increased lead exposure in both examined areas M. and T. was verified through the environmental survey showing higher lead contamination in the vicinity of the lead smelting plant T.

RESULTS AND DISCUSSION

The biochemical findings are summarised and presented separately as arithmetic means ($\bar{X}$) and standard errors (SE) for each exposed group of children in Tables 1 and 2.

TABLE 1
STATISTICAL PARAMETERS OF BIOLOGICAL DATA IN BOYS (School age) LIVING IN THE VICINITY OF THE LEAD SMELTING PLANT M. (N=28)

Statistical parameter	Hb g/100 ml	ZPP mmol/mol Hb	ALAD U/1E	Pb-B µg/100 ml
$\bar{X}$	14.42	0.77	14.20	54.94
SE	0.174	0.090	0.919	2.845

TABLE 2
STATISTICAL PARAMETERS OF BIOLOGICAL DATA IN BOYS (School age) LIVING IN THE VICINITY OF THE LEAD SMELTING PLANT T. (N=31)

Statistical parameter	Hb g/100 ml	ZPP mmol/mol Hb	ALAD U/1E	Pb-B µg/100 ml
$\bar{X}$	14.06	1.20	8.17	59.53
SE	0.142	0.106	0.705	1.954

The difference in the results between the exposed and the control groups in both examined areas was very significant ($p<0.001$) for ZPP, ALAD and Pb, but not for Hb ($p>0.50$). The increased lead absorption did not affect Hb concentration.

The boys living in the vicinity of the lead smelting plant T. had a higher lead absorption (higher average ZPP and Pb values and lower average ALAD and

Hb values) than the boys living near the lead smelting plant M. A statistical evaluation showed that the difference between the two exposed groups was very significant for ALAD ($p<0.001$), significant for ZPP ($p<0.01$) but not significant for Pb-B and Hb. The Pb-B values failed to show the expected difference, what could be explained by non-steady lead exposure in both groups.

The same level ($p<0.001$) of the statistical significance of the difference in ZPP, ALAD and Pb-B values between the boys in the exposed groups and those in comparable control groups makes these biological parameters equally useful for the assessment of lead absorption. All the three parameters could be used for biological monitoring of the children living near a lead smelting plant. However, having in mind that ZPP concentration seems to be the most representative indicator of lead body burden[6,7] ZPP determination should be a test of priority. To discriminate the increased lead absorption from iron deficiency anemia in which ZPP is also elevated, the ALAD activity test should be performed too. The Pb-B determination may be followed-up, but not necessarily. It reflects the current exposure[8] which is less relevant for the assessment of health risk especially in the condition of long-term nonsteady lead exposure. In addition to this Pb-B seems to be more prone to methodological difficulties compared to ZPP and ALAD. Therefore it may be concluded that for biological monitoring of children living in the vicinity of a lead smelting plant the most important is to examine the concentration of ZPP and the activity of ALAD, while Pb-B determination can be omitted.

REFERENCES

1. International Committee for Standardization in Haematology. (1967) Br. J. Haematol. (Suppl.), 13, 71-73.
2. Lamola, A.A., Eisinger, J., Blumbert, W.E., Kometani, T. and Burnham, B.F. (1977) J. Lab. Clin. Med., 89, 881-890.
3. Berlin, A. and Schaller, K.H. (1974) Z. Klin. Chem. Klin. Biochem., 12, 389-390.
4. Fernandez, T.T. (1975) Clin. Chem., 21, 558-561.
5. Prpić-Majić, D., Firm, J., Keršanc, A. and Matijević, B. (1975) Proceedings of the Fourth Yugoslav Congress of Occupational Health, Documenta, Belgrade, pp. 434-436.
6. Sassa, S., Granick, J.L., Kapas, A. and Levere R.D. (1973) Biochem. Med. 8, 135-148.
7. Zielhuis, R.L. (1975) Int. Arch. Occup. Hlth., 35, 13-35.
8. World Health Organization (1977) Environmental Health Criteria 3, Lead, WHO, Geneva, 1-160.

Mechanisms of Toxicity and Hazard Evaluation
B. Holmstedt, R. Lauwerys, M. Mercier, M. Roberfroid eds

STATISTICAL STUDY OF SOME PARAMETERS ABLE OF INFLUENCING BLOOD LEAD LEVELS

G. DUCOFFRE, P. BRUAUX, F. CLAEYS-THOREAU, A. LAFONTAINE
Institut d'Hygiène et d'Epidémiologie, 14 rue J. Wytsman, 1050 Bruxelles.
E. SCHIFFLERS, M. SMANS
Département de Mathématique, Facultés Universitaires N-D de la Paix, 5000 Namur.

INTRODUCTION

In another communication presented at this Congress[1], we gave the results of the first campaign of sampling for the implementation in Belgium of the Council Directive on Biological screening of the population for lead[2]. In the previous paper, we showed that there is a big difference in blood lead concentration (PbB) between men and women. This difference cannot be fully explained by the existent difference in hematocrites ($\pm$ 5 %)[3]. The present paper deals with some others factors able of influencing the PbB levels and with a few tentative hypotheses explaining the discrepancy between men and women.

MATERIAL AND METHODS

The populations' choice, the blood lead analysis and the quality control were treated in the previous paper[1]. The statistical studies[4] were performed by using three tests :

- "t" tests (difference of the means)
- chi square tests
- analyses of variance[5].

These tests were carried out separately for adults men and women.
On the whole, 479 women and 819 men were studied, out of the eleven comparable adults' populations.
As we have already shown, the distribution of PbB values is not a normal one, but the normality is reached by taking the logarithm of blood lead concentration. Therefore, the logarithmic data have been used for the analyses of variance.

RESULTS AND DISCUSSION

Five factors are significantly able of influencing the blood lead concentration in total population, including men and women : sex, age, year of house's building (presence of lead pipes in many houses built before 1945) smoking and drinking habits. In this work we have studied separately the four last ones in men and women.

Table I gives the means of blood lead concentrations in each population's group for each studied factor and the results of t tests and chi square tests. According to these tests, age is a factor significantly able of influencing PbB values but only for women. Age of house's building is a significant factor as well for women as for men, whatever test used. Smoking habits are significant factor for men but not for women. Drinking habits are significant factor for men but at the limit of significance for women (not significant with "t" test, significant with chi square test).

TABLE I
BLOOD LEAD LEVELS IN BELGIAN POPULATION

	WOMEN			MEN		
	$\bar{X}$ PbB µg/L	t test	X^2 test	$\bar{X}$ PbB µg/L	t test	X^2 test
AGE ≤ 40 years > 40 years	144 175	S	S	204 210	NS	NS
HOUSE BUILT > 1945 ≤ 1945	149 174	S	S	197 218	S	S
NON SMOKERS SMOKERS	162 166	NS	NS	197 219	S	S
NON DRINKERS DRINKERS *	159 172	NS	S	194 217	S	S

S : Significant for P < 0,05 NS : Not significant for P < 0,05
* : Wine - beer - alcohol

The figure 1 shows the linear regression lines for influence of age on PbB level in men and women.

Some analyses of variance among the most important ones gave the following results.

1. There is no interaction between age, smoking and drinking habits in both sexes.
2. In women the age has a high and significant influence on PbB level and this appears clearly in figure 2.

The smoking habits when corrected with regard to age are significant ($p < 0,05$) while drinking habits corrected with regard to smoking habits aren't significant at all.

3. For men the age has not significant influence on PbB level. Smoking habits, when corrected with regard to age are highly significant. Drinking habits when corrected with regard to smoking habits are also highly significant.

All these results have been confirmed by "t" tests and chi square tests.

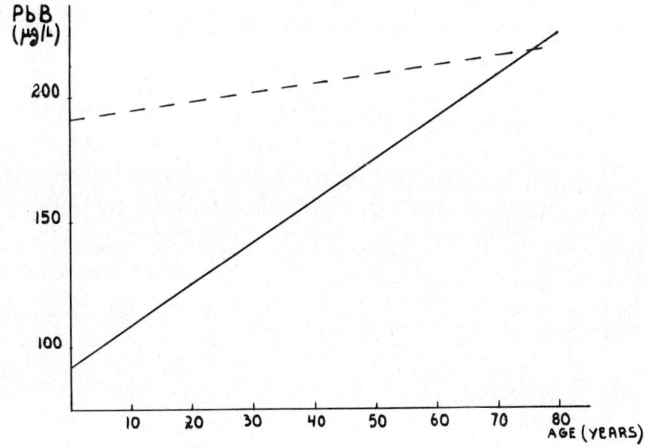

Fig 1 : REGRESSION LINE

--- MEN PbB = 0.035 X Age + 19.116 — WOMEN PbB = 0.166 X Age + 9.171

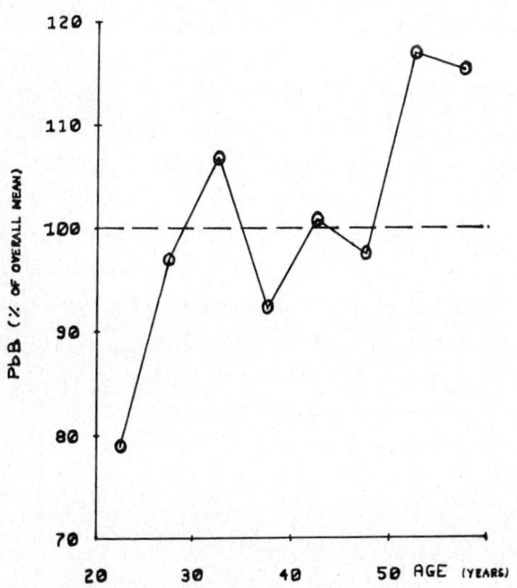

Fig 2 : PbB-Age WOMEN

Figure 3 displays the cumulative frequency of PbB values (logarithmic data) on probit scale for non smokers women, smokers women, non smokers men and women. The lines for smokers and non smokers are very close to each other in women but not in men. This illustrates the difference between influence of smoking habits in women and men. The figure 4 displays the same data for drinking habits and illustrates the difference between influence of those in women and men.

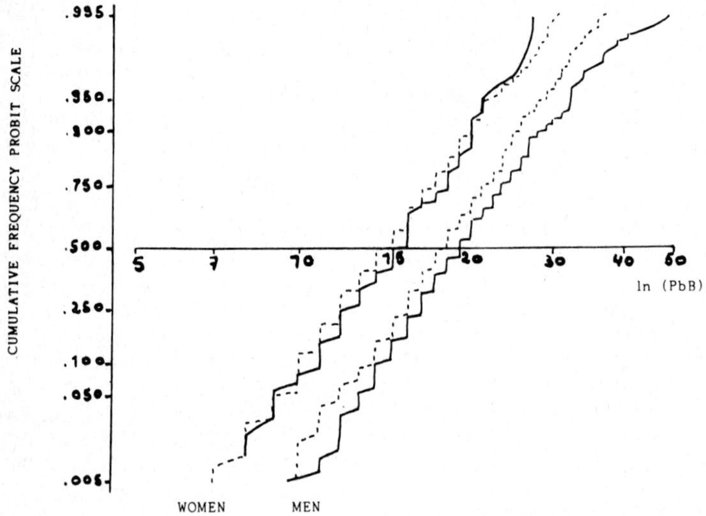

Fig 3 : SMOKING HABITS

--- NON SMOKERS — SMOKERS

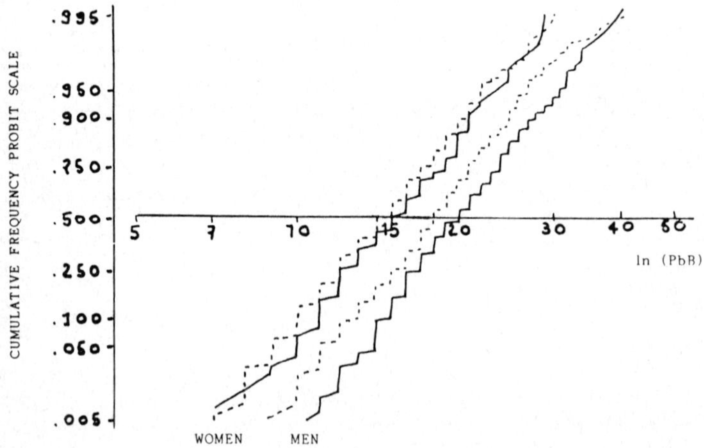

Fig 4 : DRINKING HABITS

--- NON DRINKERS — DRINKERS

SUMMARY AND CONCLUSIONS

In this work, we have studied some parameters able of influencing PbB levels. These are :

Sex : in women, the mean of blood lead concentration is about 40 µg/l lesser than in men.

Age : there is an increase of PbB values with age but mainly in women.

Year of house's building : the residents in houses built before 1945 have slightly higher PbB values than others.

Smoking and drinking habits : these are factors increasing the blood lead concentration but mainly in men.

Women seem to be less influenced, as well quantitatively as qualitatively, by some of these factors.

ACKNOWLEDGEMENTS

We are grateful to Miss J. WILMOTTE for her technical assistance.

REFERENCES

1. CLAEYS-THOREAU F., BRUAUX P., DUCOFFRE G., LAFONTAINE A. Exposure to lead of the belgian population. Second international Congress on Toxicology - Brussels, July 6-11 1980.
2. Council Directive of 29 march 1977 on biological Screening of the Population for Lead (77/312/EEC). Official Journal of the European Communities, 1977, 20, L105, 10-17.
3. GRADWOHL. Clinical Laboratory Methods and diagnosis, 6th edition, Frankel and Reitmen editors, 1963.
4. Sidney SIEGEL. Non parametric Statistics for the behavioral Sciences. International student edition, 1956.
5. GRAYBILL F.A. Theory and Application of Linear Model, 1976. Ed. Duxburi Press Massachussetts, 704, 575-582.

PESTICIDES AND MISCELLANEOUS

© 1980 Elsevier/North-Holland Biomedical Press
Mechanisms of Toxicity and Hazard Evaluation
B. Holmstedt, R. Lauwerys, M. Mercier, M. Roberfroid eds

TOXIC INTERACTIONS WITH DERMAL EXPOSURE TO ORGANOPHOSPHATE INSECTICIDES

SHELDON D. MURPHY
Division of Toxicology, University of Texas Medical School at Houston, P. O. Box 20708, Houston, Texas, 77025, U.S.A.

INTRODUCTION

Numerous studies[1,2] have demonstrated that the acute toxicity and anticholinesterase action of orally or parenterally administered organic phosphorothionate insecticides can be markedly altered by other compounds which modify their hepatic metabolism. Since occupational or incidental exposure of persons formulating or applying these insecticides is likely to be by the dermal route, it was considered important to determine if the metabolic and toxic interactions that have been identified in studies using other routes were similar in nature and degree when the insecticides were administered dermally.

The oral or i.p. toxicity of malathion [0,0-dimethyl-S-(1,2-dicarbethoxyethyl) phosphorothionate] is markedly potentiated by triorthotolyl phosphate (TOTP) and other compounds which inhibit tissue carboxylesterases that catalyze the detoxication of malathion[3]. Although the dermal toxicity of malathion to rats has been reported to exceed four g/kg[4], there is no information available concerning whether its dermal toxicity is potentiated under conditions that potentiate malathion toxicity by other routes.

Previous investigations have demonstrated that pretreatment of mice or rats with phenobarbital or other compounds that induce liver microsomal oxidases protects against the oral or i.p. toxicity of parathion (0,0-diethyl, 0-p-nitrophenyl phosphorothionate) and methyl parathion (0,0-dimethyl, 0-p-nitrophenyl phosphorothionate)[1,5,6]. Liver microsomal oxidases catalyze both activation (conversion of phosphorothionate to the phosphate which is the active anticholinesterase) and detoxication (oxidative cleavage to form p-nitrophenol and dialkyl thiophosphate) of these compounds[7]. Since induction of these oxidases protected against parathion and methyl parathion toxicity it appeared that the net effect of induction is detoxication. However, since extrahepatic activation of phosphorothionates has been demonstrated[8] it seemed possible that the relative importance on toxicity of inducing liver microsomal metabolism might depend upon the route of exposure. This hypothesis was examined by comparing the influence of phenobarbital pretreatment on the toxicity of parathion and methyl parathion given to rats by the oral and dermal routes.

MATERIALS AND METHODS

For most experiments technical grade (95 to 98% purity) samples of insecticides obtained from the manufacturers were tested. Young adult Holtzman rats (190-200g) were used. Males were used in the experiments with malathion, and females were used in the studies on parathion and methyl parathion.

TOTP was given to male rats either i.p. in corn oil (125 mg/ml) or by application to the skin as a solution in acetone 18 hr before dermal application of undiluted or acetone solutions of malathion or its oxygen analogue (malaoxon). Other rats were pretreated only with solvents and also given malathion dermally or were untreated (controls). For dermal dosing, rats were shaved in an area on the back of their neck ("neck") and, in some cases, on the back just forward of the tail ("tail"). An area of 3.5 cm^2 was circumscribed, and the TOTP or malathion solutions were carefully applied within that area. Rats were then caged individually. They were sacrificed and tissues removed for cholinesterase assays three hr after malathion, or for carboxylesterase at 18 hr after TOTP.

For the experiments with parathion and methyl parathion female rats were pretreated with phenobarbital by administering its sodium salt as a 0.1% solution in the drinking water[6] for one week prior to dosing with the insecticides. Parathion and methyl parathion were applied to shaved skin of the neck area as solutions in xylene adjusted so that the desired dose was contained in 0.5 ml/kg. Oral dosing was with corn oil solutions of the insecticides such that 1.0 ml/kg by gavage contained the proper dose. Controls were given corn oil only.

Cholinesterase activities of brain, submaxillary gland, diaphragm muscle, plasma or liver were measured by the colorimetric method of Ellman et al[9] as modified by Benke et al[10], using acetylthiocholine as substrate. Carboxylesterase was measured by determining the hydrolysis of alpha naphthol acetate[11] by 0.2 mg of liver and 10 mg of skin.

The end point of toxicity sought in most of these experiments was the dermal or oral dose of malathion, parathion or methyl parathion required to produce 50% inhibition of cholinesterase in control or pretreated rats. To determine this a range of doses of the insecticides were administered, and the animals sacrificed at a time after dosing that had been predetermined to correspond with the maximum degree of enzyme inhibition (3 hr after oral or dermal malathion; 1 hr after oral and 12 hr after dermal exposure to parathion and methyl parathion). Four or more animals were used at each pretreatment-challenge dosage combination. In some experiments with TOTP the ID_{50} for carboxylesterase was determined. The mean cholinesterase or carboxylesterase activities were used to calculate the percent inhibition as related to the mean activity of control animals. The percent inhibition was plotted against the log of the dose and from the dose response curves so constructed the ID_{50}'s were determined as described previously[11].

RESULTS AND DISCUSSION

Figure 1 illustrates the procedure used in this study to determine the dermal malathion ID_{50} for brain cholinesterase in rats pretreated with 125 mg/kg of TOTP i.p. The ID_{50} for control rats could not be determined since as much as 1000 mg/kg did not inhibit brain cholinesterase. Table 1 summarizes data obtained in a series of dose-response experiments. The dermal application of over 1 g/kg of either technical (95%) or highly purified (99+%) malathion did not appreciably inhibit brain acetylcholinesterase. However, considerably smaller doses of malathion inhibited brain cholinesterase in rats pretreated with TOTP by either the i.p. or dermal route. The data indicated that 250 mg/kg of TOTP applied dermally caused increased susceptibility of rats to dermal exposure of malthion by at least

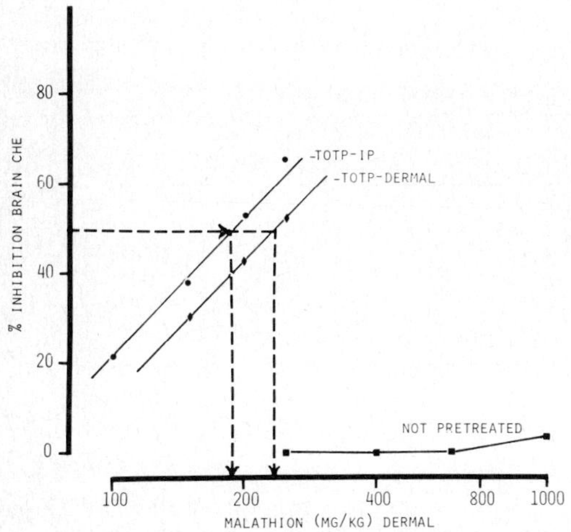

Fig. 1. Malathion ID_{50} after i.p. or dermal TOTP (125 mg/kg).

TABLE 1

ANTICHOLINESTERASE ACTION OF DERMALLY APPLIED MALATHION 18 HOURS AFTER TOTP IN RATS

Pretreatment	Brain CHE ID_{50} (mg/kg) 3 HR after Malathion	
	Malathion-95%	Malathion-99+%
0	>1000	>1200
TOTP - 125 mg/kg, i.p.	192	490
TOTP - 125 mg/kg, dermal	233	-
TOTP - 250 mg/kg, dermal	57	360

17-fold in the case of the technical grade sample of the insecticide and by at least 3-fold in the case of the highly purified sample. In other experiments the ID_{50} for brain cholinesterase for dermally applied malaoxon, the oxygen analogue of malathion, was 48 mg/kg in unpretreated rats and 12 mg/kg in rats pretreated with a dermal dose of 250 mg/kg of TOTP. A potentiation factor of 4-fold could therefore be calculated for this active metabolite of malathion. The results of another series of experiments, summarized in Table 2, indicate that doses of TOTP as low as 10 mg/kg applied dermally potentiated technical malathion by at least two-fold. Furthermore the degree of potentiation was

TABLE 2

INFLUENCE OF DERMAL SITE OF APPLICATION OF TOTP ON POTENTIATION OF DERMALLY APPLIED MALATHION (95%)

TOTP Pretreatment	CHE ID_{50} (mg/kg) for Malathion in:[a]	
	Brain	Submaxillary
250 mg/kg - neck	174	152
250 mg/kg - tail	175	-
10 mg/kg - neck	561	461
10 mg/kg - tail	481	395
0	>1000	>1000

[a]Malathion applied in all cases to the dorsal neck area 18 hr after TOTP and 3 hr before sacrifice. The same area was used for the neck application of both TOTP and Malathion.

essentially the same whether the malathion was applied to the same area of the skin as the TOTP or to a remote area.

Measurements of carboxylesterase in skin indicated that the activity of this tissue was only about 5 percent of the activity in liver. Nevertheless, TOTP whether given parenterally or dermally, inhibited the hydrolysis of alpha naphthol acetate in the liver and in the skin both at the site of application and remotely as shown in Table 3. These results suggest that TOTP is absorbed from its dermal site of application and exerts its potentiating action systemically.

The results of the experiments described above indicate that under conditions of reduced tissue carboxylesterase activity malathion may be unusually toxic by the dermal route. These experiments have demonstrated that marked potentiation of malathion toxicity by carboxylesterase inhibitors occurs by dermal as well as oral and parenteral routes of exposures.

TABLE 3

CARBOXYLESTERASE INHIBITION 18 HRS AFTER TOTP IN RATS

TOTP		ID_{50} (mg/kg for α- Naphthol acetate esterase)		
Route	Dose range tested mg/kg	Liver	Skin	
			Neck	Tail
Dermal (neck)	0.5-250	4.6	1.0	7.6
I.P.	10-250	10.0	35.0	-

Table 4 summarizes the results of a large number of dose response experiments to determine the effect of phenobarbital pretreatment on the anticholinesterase action of dermal and oral doses of parathion and methyl parathion in female rats. Inhibition of the cholinesterase activity of brain, diaphragm

TABLE 4

CHOLINESTERASE ID_{50}'S FOR PARATHION AND METHYL PARATHION IN FEMALE RATS WITH OR WITHOUT PHENOBARBITAL PRETREATMENT

			ID_{50} (mg/kg)[a]		
Insecticide	Route	Tissue	A Phenobarb. Pretreated	B Unpretreated	Ratio A/B
Methyl Parathion	Dermal	Brain	24.6	8.9	2.76
		Diaphragm	11.7	6.9	1.70
		Plasma	14.1	10.4	1.36
		liver	5.0	9.4	0.53
Methyl Parathion	Oral	Brain	4.00	2.75	1.45
		Diaphragm	4.50	2.49	1.81
		Plasma	2.56	2.08	1.23
Parathion	Dermal	Brain	15.45	2.90	5.33
		Diaphragm	15.40	3.50	4.40
		Plasma	3.29	1.45	2.27
		Liver	1.16	1.70	0.68
Parathion	Oral	Brain	13.00	1.73	7.51
		Diaphragm	10.16	1.65	6.16
		Plasma	2.32	1.15	2.02

[a]ID_{50} = Dose of insecticide required to produce 50% inhibition of cholinesterase activity.

muscle and plasma was determined in the experiments with oral dosing, while for the dermal exposure experiments a fourth tissue, liver, was also assayed for cholinesterase activity.

Comparison of the ratios of ID_{50} values in phenobarbital pretreated rats to ID_{50}'s in unpretreated rats permits a quantitative comparison of the influence of an inducer of liver microsomal oxidases. Phenobarbital pretreatment protected against the anticholinesterase action of parathion to a greater extent than methyl parathion irrespective of the route of exposure. The relatively smaller effect of phenobarbital on methyl parathion's anticholinesterase action may reflect the fact that an alternate pathway of detoxification, not dependent on microsomal oxidases (i.e. demethylation by cytoplasmic glutathione transferase[12]) is available to the dimethyl compound. It is also of interest to note that the protective effect of phenobarbital is most striking against brain and diaphragm cholinesterase activity. Inhibition of liver cholinesterase by dermal application of the insecticides was actually increased by phenobarbital pretreatment. This may be explained on the basis that phenobarbital induces in the liver the oxidative metabolism of the thiophosphates to their oxygen analogues which can immediately react with esterases in the liver. However, the oxygen analogues are also very susceptible to metabolic detoxication in the liver and may not escape to inhibit acetylcholinesterase in extrahepatic tissue. Thus the net effect of liver microsomal oxidase induction is protection against parathion and methyl parathion, and, as demonstrated in this study, this effect is qualitatively and quantitatively similar by both the oral and dermal routes of exposure.

In summary, on the basis of the results of the limited studies reported here it appears that it may be concluded that acute toxic interactions involving organophosphate insecticides are qualitatively similar by dermal exposure, oral or parenteral exposure.

ACKNOWLEDGEMENTS

Mr. Kenneth Cheever and Mr. Gary Bond contributed to the large number of experiments that are summarized here. This research was supported in part by research grants ES00084 and ES-01831 from the U.S. National Institute of Environmental Health Sciences.

REFERENCES

1. DuBois, K.P. (1969) Can. Med. Ass. J., 100, 173-179.
2. Murphy, S.D. (1969) Residue Rev., 25, 201-221.
3. Cohen, S.D. and Murphy, S.D. (1971) J. Pharmacol. Exp. Ther., 176, 733-742.
4. Gaines, T.B. (1969) Toxicol. Appl. Pharmacol., 14, 515-534.
5. Kamienski, F.X. and Murphy, S.D. (1971) Toxicol. Appl. Pharmacol., 18, 883-894.

6. Alary, J.G. and Brodeur, J. (1969) J. Pharmacol. Exp. Therap., 169, 159-167.

7. Neal, R.A. (1967) Biochem. J., 103, 183-191.

8. Norman, B.J. and Neal, R.A. (1976) Biochem. Pharmacol., 25, 37-45.

9. Ellman, G.L., Courtney, K.D., Andres, V. Jr., and Featherstone, A.M. (1961) Biochem. Pharmacol., 7, 88-95.

10. Benke, G.M., Cheever, K.L., Mirer, F.E. and Murphy, S.D. (1974) Toxicol. Appl. Pharmacol., 28, 97-109.

11. Murphy, S.D., Cheever, K.L., Chow, A.Y.K. and Brewster, M. (1976) Proc. Europ. Soc. Toxicol., Vol. XVII, 292-299.

12. Benke, G.M. and Murphy, S.D. (1975) Toxicol. Appl. Pharmacol., 31, 254-269.

© 1980 Elsevier/North-Holland Biomedical Press
Mechanisms of Toxicity and Hazard Evaluation
B. Holmstedt, R. Lauwerys, M. Mercier, M. Roberfroid eds

BIOCHEMICAL CHANGES IN THE RAT CEREBELLUM FOLLOWING CYPERMETHRIN ADMINISTRATION

EDWARD A LOCK AND PAMELA N BERRY
Biochemical Mechanisms Section, Imperial Chemical Industries Limited, Central Toxicology Laboratory, Alderley Park, Nr Macclesfield, Cheshire SK10 4TJ, UK

INTRODUCTION

Cypermethrin (± α cyano-3-phenoxybenzyl(±)cis.trans 3(2,2 dichlorovinyl)2,2-dimethyl cyclopropanecarboxylate) is a recently developed synthetic pyrethroid insecticide[1]. The toxic action of cypermethrin in the rat is similar to that described for decamethrin[2,3]. The first signs of poisoning are excessive salivation rapidly followed by continuous irregular jerking movements of the limbs progressing to sinuous writhing. Decamethrin has been reported to produce a marked increase in brain cyclic GMP content in animals showing signs of severe toxicity[4]. In this study we have examined the concentration of cyclic AMP, cyclic GMP, glucose, lactate and ammonia in the cerebellum of rats at various stages of cypermethrin toxicity.

MATERIALS AND METHODS

Cypermethrin (40% cis:60% trans) 91% pure was supplied by Plant Protection Division, ICI Limited, Jealott's Hill Research Station. Male rats (160-180 g) were given cypermethrin iv as a 50 mg/ml solution in dimethylformamide (DMF). Control animals received the same volume of DMF alone. Atropine was given ip as a 2 mg/ml solution in isotonic saline 15 min prior to cypermethrin. Animals were killed at various stages of intoxication by microwave irradiation focussed to the head. The cerebellum was removed, homogenised in perchloric acid (0.5 M) containing 2 mM EGTA, protein removed and the acid soluble fraction neutralised. The concentration of metabolites in the cerebellar extract were determined by fluorimetric-enzyme assays. Blood glucose and lactate were measured on blood collected from the trunk after decapitation and perchloric acid extraction. Cyclic nucleotides were measured by the competitive binding technique with [^{3}H]-cyclic AMP, [^{3}H]cyclic GMP and specific binding proteins using assay kits from the Radiochemical Centre, Amersham, Bucks, UK. Results are expressed as means ± SE with number of observations in brackets.

RESULTS

A single iv injection of cypermethrin (25 mg/kg), produced the following signs of toxicity: initially chewing and licking followed by salivation which was profuse by about 10 min. The first motor signs, continuous irregular jerking movements of the limbs, developed by 15-20 min, followed by clonic convulsions at about 30 min. This progressed to sinuous writhing movements which were continuous by about 40 min. Animals were killed at three different stages of toxicity: at profuse salivation, at the first convulsion and at the continuous writhing stage.

Cypermethrin caused no significant differences in the concentration of cerebellar cyclic AMP when compared with control animals (Table 1). The concentration of cyclic GMP was, however, increased at all times studied. Pretreatment with atropine, which blocked salivation, did not appear to alter the effect of cypermethrin on the cyclic GMP concentration (Table 2). The concentration of cerebellar lactate was increased at all times studied, whilst glucose was only significantly increased at the onset of the first convulsion (Table 1). Cypermethrin caused a progressive rise in blood glucose, lactate and ammonia, the glucose and lactate elevation being significant at the time of profuse salivation and the elevation in ammonia by the onset of the first convulsion (Table 3).

TABLE 1

EFFECT OF CYPERMETHRIN (25 mg/kg) ON CEREBELLAR METABOLITES

Metabolite	Control	Profuse Salivation	First Convulsion	Sinuous Writhing
Glucose[b]	1.52±0.07(24)	1.76 ±0.15 (8)	2.06[a]±0.11 (9)	1.82 ±0.07(6)
Lactate[b]	2.05±0.08(24)	2.46[a]±0.10 (9)	3.65[a]±0.50 (9)	6.34[a]±0.61(6)
Ammonia[b]	0.51±0.14 (4)	-	-	1.08 ±0.26(7)
Cyclic AMP[c]	8.2 ±0.5 (4)	8.7 ±0.9 (6)	9.8 ±1.4 (6)	-
Cyclic GMP[c]	4.1 ±0.4 (13)	23.8[a]±3.5 (13)	64.1[a]±6.2 (12)	76.0[a]±9.8 (6)

[a]Significantly different from control $P<0.05$. [b]µmol/g wet wt of cerebellum.
[c]pmol/mg protein.

DISCUSSION

Cypermethrin produces a sharp rise in blood glucose. This may be the result of an adrenal medullary reaction causing mobilisation of liver glycogen and an increase in oxidative metabolism. Brain glucose was elevated at the time of onset of the first convulsion. This is unusual as agents which produce convulsions or seizures usually decrease brain glucose[5,6]. In this case the increase

TABLE 2

EFFECT OF ATROPINE ON THE CYPERMETHRIN-INDUCED INCREASE IN CEREBELLAR CYCLIC GMP

Treatment	Time killed after cypermethrin or dimethylformamide (min)	Cyclic GMP (pmol/mg protein)
Saline-DMF	10	4.8±1.0(3)
	20	4.0±0.6(6)
Saline-Cypermethrin	10	17.6±5.5(6)
	18	23.9±6.2(8)
Atropine[a]-DMF	10	4.5±0.6(4)
	20	5.2±0.7(6)
Atropine[a]-Cypermethrin	10	12.4±2.0(7)
	18	25.9±6.6(9)

[a]Atropine (10 mg/kg) was given ip 15 min prior to DMF or cypermethrin (25 mg/kg) iv.

TABLE 3

EFFECT OF CYPERMETHRIN (25 mg/kg) ON BLOOD GLUCOSE, LACTATE AND AMMONIA

Metabolite	Control	Profuse Salivation	First Convulsion	Sinuous Writhing
Glucose[b]	5.8±0.4(15)	9.1[a]±0.9(8)	9.2[a]±1.5 (8)	11.2[a]±0.6(6)
Lactate[b]	1.5±0.1(15)	2.5[a]±0.4(8)	3.6[a]±0.3 (8)	11.3[a]±2.8(6)
Ammonia[c]	47.0±7.5(12)	52.7 ±6.0(6)	87.4[a]±16.8(6)	305[a]±73 (6)

[a]Significantly different from control $P<0.05$.
[b]μmol/ml blood.
[c]nmol/ml plasma.

produced by cypermethrin may be related to the marked hyperglycaemia. Associated with the increased in blood glucose is a marked increase in blood and brain lactate. At later times the increase in muscular activity may have contributed to the marked lactic acidosis. These increases in blood glucose and lactate are similar to those produced by a structurally related pyrethroid, decamethrin[3].

The elevation of cyclic GMP but not cyclic AMP in the cerebellum produced by cypermethrin seems not to be due to the convulsive state of the animals, since it is increased prior to convulsions when only salivation is observed. Various agents which cause hyperactivity, tremors or convulsions in rats increase the cyclic GMP content of the brain, particularly the cerebellum, without affecting cyclic AMP[4,7-9]. The cyclic nucleotide content of the postsynaptic cells in neural tissue is regulated by transmitters released from nerve terminals impinging on cells[10]. An increase in cyclic GMP in the cerebellum might be correlated with stimulation of the muscarinic cholinergic receptor, but atropine, a well known muscarinic cholinergic blocker, did not appear to reduce the cypermethrin induced release of cyclic GMP in the cerebellum. Atropine did, however, block cypermethrin-induced salivation indicating a cholinergic stimulation. Decamethrin increases cerebellar cyclic GMP concentrations in animals showing sinuous writhing[4], and at this time cerebellar acetylcholine is decreased rather than increased. All these findings seem to indicate that the elevated cyclic GMP may not be due to interference with muscarinic cholinergic neurotransmission.

ACKNOWLEDGEMENTS

The authors would like to thank Mr E Howard for technical assistance.

REFERENCES

1. Elliott, M. (1976) Environ. Health Perspect. 14, 3-13.
2. Barnes, J.M. and Verschoyle, R.D. (1974) Nature 248, 711.
3. Ray, D.E. and Cremer, J.E. (1979) Pestic. Biochem. Physiol. 10, 333-340.
4. Aldridge, W.N., Clothier, B., Forshaw, P., Johnson, M.K., Parker, V.H., Price, R.J., Skilleter, D.N., Verschoyle, R.D. and Stevens, C. (1978) Biochem. Pharmacol. 27, 1703-1706.
5. Sacktor, B., Wilson, J.E. and Tiekert, C.G. (1966) J. Biol. Chem. 241, 5071-5075.
6. Nahorski, S.R., Roberts, D.J. and Stewart, G.G. (1970) J. Neurochem. 17, 621-631.
7. Mao, C.G., Guidotti, A. and Costa, E. (1974) Brain Res. 79, 510-514.
8. Biggio, G., Costa, E. and Guidotti, A (1977) J. Pharm. Exp. Therap. 200, 207-215.
9. Mattsson, H., Brandt, K. and Heilbronn, E. (1977) Nature 268, 52-53.
10. Lee, T.P., Kuo, J.F. and Greengard, P. (1972) Proc. Natn. Acad. Sci. USA 69, 3287-3291.

Mechanisms of Toxicity and Hazard Evaluation
B. Holmstedt, R. Lauwerys, M. Mercier, M. Roberfroid eds

HEXACHLOROBENZENE (HCB) AND SOME OF ITS SULFUR-CONTAINING METABOLITES: TISSUE RETENTION AND EXCRETION ROUTES IN MICE

I. BRANDT[1], A. LYDÉN[1], P. SLANINA[2] and L. ALBANUS[2]
[1]Dept. of Pharmacology, Faculty of Veterinary Medicine, SLU, BMC, and
[2]Toxicology Laboratory, National Food Administration, Uppsala (Sweden)

HCB as well as some other environmental pollutants such as PCB and DDE are metabolically transformed to several sulfur-containing compounds, which appear in tissues and excreta of wild and experimental animals[1-3]. Although some of these compounds are stable enough to be retained in the food chain, little information is still available about the metabolic fate and biological significance of these metabolites. In the present investigation the distribution of HCB and some of its sulfur-containing metabolites was studied in pregnant and nonpregnant mice.

MATERIALS AND METHODS

Series of female C57Bl mice, some of them at late stage of pregnancy, were i.v. injected with HCB-^{14}C (I), methylthiopentachlorobenzene-^{14}C (II), 1,4-bis(methylthio)-2,3,5,6-tetrachlorobenzene-^{14}C (III) and methylsulfonylpentachlorobenzene-^{14}C (IV), respectively. One mouse was i.v. injected with 1,2,4-tris(methylthio)-3,5,6-trichlorobenzene-^{14}C (V). The animals were killed at intervals ranging between 20 min and 32 days after injection, mounted in an aqueous gel of carboxymethyl cellulose, frozen, sectioned onto tape in a cryostat microtome and submitted to autoradiography according to Ullberg[4]. At the time of killing the pregnant animals were on the 17th day of gestation; the day after the mating was called day 0. The compounds studied had the spec. act. 16.4 Ci/mol and were ≥99 % pure except for IV and V, which were ≥96 % and 81 % pure, respectively. Each animal generally received 5 µCi in 20 µl DMSO.

RESULTS

The autoradiograms of mice injected with HCB-^{14}C showed a strong uptake of radioactivity in the adipose tissues persisting for more than one month after the administration. Elevated concentrations of the labelled substance were also observed in the nasal discharge and adrenal cortex. The radioactivity of the blood exceeded that of the liver and kidneys under the whole period of investigation. As shown in figure 1, the labelled substances penetrated the placenta and the blood and liver concentrations in the fetus equalled those of the mother. As expected from the low rate of metabolism of HCB[2], the concentrations of radioactivity in the bile and intestinal contents of the injected animals were consistently low.

On the other hand the distribution patterns of all the sulfur-containing derivatives (II-V) were characterized by a pronounced concentration of label in the bile and intestinal contents, to a lesser extent in the urine and by an initially high but subsequently decreasing concentration in the fat (fig 2). As seen in the autoradiograms the concentration of radioactivity in the gastro-intestinal tract appeared to increase with increasing numbers of methylthio-groups in the molecule. All the metabolites gave rise to a similarly high concentration of label in the fetal intestine.

The administration of the methylsulfonylpentachlorobenzene-^{14}C (IV) resulted, in addition to the above mentioned sites, in a significant accumulation of radioactivity in the grey matter of the cerebellum and cerebrum (fig 3a) as well as in the adrenal cortex and corpus luteum. A similar, although much weaker, uptake in the brain was observed in the autoradiograms of mice injected with II. No accumulation of IV was observed in the fetal brain, which was almost void of radioactivity (fig 3b). After 4 days none of the labelled metabolites could be detected in the body of the experimental animals.

DISCUSSION

In contrast to the slowly metabolized HCB[2], its sulfur-containing derivatives seem to leave the body rapidly via biliary and renal excretion. The excretion pattern of the HCB-metabolites thus appear to differ from those of e.g. PCB-methylsulfones which are retained in the body to a considerably higher degree[1,5].

TEXT TO FIGURES

Fig. 1. Autoradiogram of a pregnant mouse 4h after injection of HCB-^{14}C (I) showing a strong accumulation in the adipose tissues.

Fig. 2. Autoradiogram of a pregnant mouse 4h after injection of methylthiopentachlorobenzene-^{14}C (II). Note the high concentration of labelled substance in the bile and intestinal contents. The radioactivity in the fat is low compared to fig 1.

Fig. 3. Details of autoradiograms of a pregnant mouse 1h after injection of methylsulfonylpentachlorobenzene-^{14}C (IV) showing the pronounced accumulation of label in the grey matter of the brain (a). The fetal brain is void of radioactivity, but a strong labelling is observed in the fetal intestine (b).

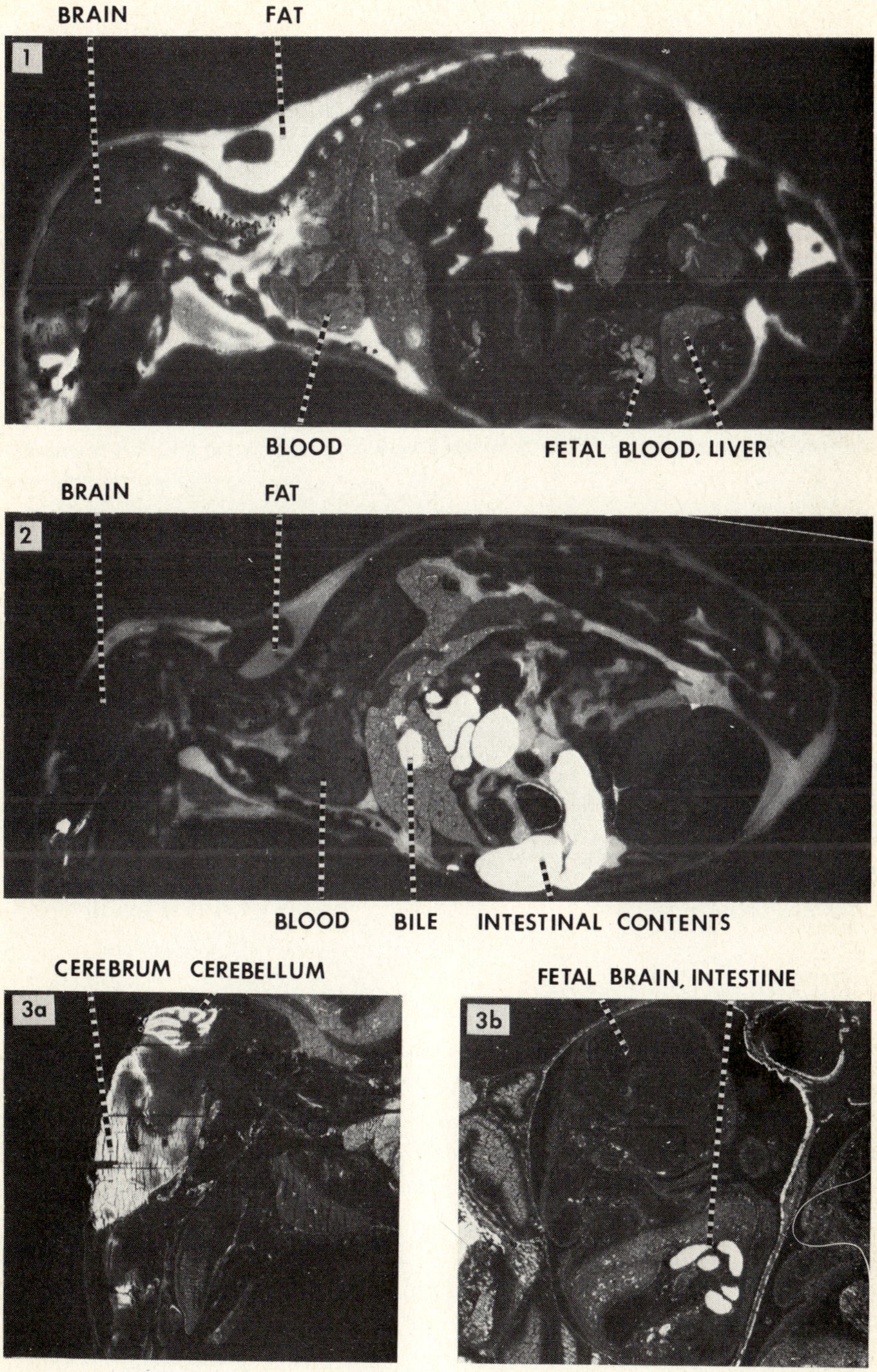
BRAIN
FAT
1
BLOOD
FETAL BLOOD, LIVER
BRAIN
FAT
2
BLOOD
BILE
INTESTINAL CONTENTS
CEREBRUM
CEREBELLUM
3a
FETAL BRAIN, INTESTINE
3b

The metabolic route leading to the sulfur-containing metabolites of HCB may as has been suggested for propachlor[6] and PCB[7], involve conjugation with glutathione (GSH). This assumption is strengthened by the identification of the pentachlorophenylmercapturic acid in the urine of rats treated with HCB[8]. The pronounced biliary excretion of II-V, as seen in the present investigation, also indicates a rapid transformation of these hydrophobic HCB-derivatives to more polar metabolites, presumably GSH-conjugates and other conjugates. As in the case of the metabolism of propachlor to methylsulfones[6] the formation of the methylthio-metabolites of HCB may involve cleavage of the GSH-conjugates, possibly by the intestinal flora, to unpolar compounds which could be subsequently reabsorbed, further metabolized and excreted in the bile. One implication of such enterohepatic circulation is the formation of metabolites with new biological properties[9], in this case possibly methylsulfonylpentachlorobenzene (IV) which accumulates in the grey matter of the brain. The weak uptake of II in the brain, however, indicates that the oxidation of II to IV is too limited to be visible in the autoradiograms, perhaps because of a more rapid metabolism of II to III. In contrast to IV, which so far has been found to be formed only after experiments *in vitro*, III has been shown to be present in the faeces of rats treated with HCB[2-3]. When searching for IV *in vivo*, analysis of brain tissue should be considered.

ACKNOWLEDGMENTS

The labelled compounds II-IV were kindly prepared by Dr. Åke Bergman, Wallenberg Laboratory, University of Stockholm, Stockholm. Economic support was given by the National Swedish Environment Protection Board.

References

1. Jensen, S. and Jansson, B. (1976) Ambio, 5, 257-260.
2. Jansson, B. and Bergman, Å. (1978) Chemosphere, 7, 257-268.
3. Koss, G. et al (1979) Arch. Toxicol., 42, 19-31.
4. Ullberg, S. (1954) Acta radiol., suppl 118, 1-110.
5. Brandt, I. and Bergman, Å. unpublished results.
6. Bakke, J.E. et al (1980) Science, in press.
7. Bergman, Å. et al (1980) Chem.-Biol. Interact., in press.
8. Renner, G. et al (1978) Chemosphere 7, 663-668.
9. Chasseaud, L.F. (1976) in Glutathione: metabolism and function Ed. Arias, I.M. and Jakoby, W.B. Raven Press. N.Y. pp 77-114.

© 1980 Elsevier/North-Holland Biomedical Press
Mechanisms of Toxicity and Hazard Evaluation
B. Holmstedt, R. Lauwerys, M. Mercier, M. Roberfroid eds

TOXICOLOGY OF TRIMETHYL- AND TRIETHYL PHOSPHOROTHIOATES

R.D. VERSCHOYLE, W.N. ALDRIDGE AND J.R.P. CABRAL
Toxicology Unit, Medical Research Council Laboratories,
Carshalton, Surrey, United Kingdom.

Trimethyl- and triethyl phosphorothioates are actual and potential impurities in many organophosphorus insecticides. The trimethyl phosphorothioates are potent potentiators of the toxicity of malathion in the rat[1] and are found in technical formulations of this insecticide[2]. In addition, they produce in the rat a delayed death not normally seen following poisoning with organophosphorus compounds[1].

The four organophosphorus compounds examined in this study, OOS-trimethyl phosphorothioate (I), OSS-trimethyl phosphorodithioate (II), OOS triethyl phosphorothioate (III) and OSS triethyl phosphorodithioate (IV) were prepared by Dr. J.W. Miles, Bureau of Tropical Diseases, Centre for Disease Control, Atlanta, U.S.A. and have purities $>$98%.

Female Porton derived Wistar rats (aged 8-10 wks, 160-180g) and LACA mice (aged 8-14 wks,approx 20-30g), fed ad lib on 41B diet were used throughout. Animals were deprived of food overnight prior to oral dosing. Intravenous injections were given via the lateral tail vein, glycerol formal was used as the solvent for both oral and intravenous dosing.

The acute LD_{50} values are shown in Table 1. Preliminary examination suggests that the toxicity to the male hamster is similar to the mouse.

After an LD_{50} dose, all four compounds produced an initial cholinergic response of fasciculations, salivation and urinary incontinence. However, these signs lasted less than 24 hr and deaths at this time were only seen with compound (IV); doses, 2-6 times the LD_{50}, were needed to cause early deaths with compounds (I), (II) and (III). Rats dosed at or near the LD_{50} with these latter compounds recovered from the initial mild cholinergic response. However, by day 3 they had lost weight and were panting with laboured respiration; all deaths were between days 3-6.

Although weight loss was reduced by force feeding with Vivonex (a complete liquid diet) survival was unchanged.

TABLE 1: ACUTE TOXICITY OF TRIMETHYL- AND TRIETHYL PHOSPHOROTHIOATES

		LD_{50} and confidence limits mg/kg			
Species	Route	Compound (I)	Compound (II)	Compound (III)	Compound (IV)
Rat	Oral	60 (51-71)	26 (20-35)	27 (21-34)	140 (122-160)
Rat	I.V.	45 (36-56)	42 (30-60)	38 (21-66)	95 (no con.lim.)
Mouse	Oral	134 (106-169)	198 (168-233)	170 (151-191)	126 (95-167)
Mouse	I.V.	123 (97-155)	149 (126-177)	90 (70-116)	83 (65-105)

Therapy with atropine, pyridine-2-aldoxime methyl methanesulphonate, (P_2S) or a combination of the two, following dosing of rats with (II) was unsuccessful, both when given on day 1 (1, 5 and 24 hr) (Table 2) and on day 3.

TABLE 2: TREATMENT WITH ATROPINE AND/OR P_2S OVER THE INITIAL 24 HOURS AND THE ORAL LD_{50} OF (II)

Species	Route	No Therapy	Atropine[a]	P_2S[a]	Atropine & P_2S[a]
Rat	Oral	26 (20-35)	20 (14-29)	25 (20-31)	28 (25-32)

a. Intraperitoneal injections of atropine 3 x 10 mg/kg, P_2S 3 x 100 mg/kg or atropine 3 x 10 mg/kg plus P_2S 3 x 100 mg/kg were given at 1,5 and 24hr after dosing.

Brain acetylcholinesterase, plasma cholinesterase and plasma carboxylesterase (hydrolysis of phenyl butyrate) were inhibited *in vivo* by compounds (I), (II) and (IV). Enzyme levels after (III) were not determined. Maximum inhibition occurred over the first 24 hr., corresponding to the time of death with compound (IV). However, deaths after (I) and (II) occurred at a time when activity of all enzymes had increased and was at least 50% of the control value.

Pretreatment with phenobarbitone caused a 5 fold decrease in the intraperitoneal toxicity of (II) and (III) to rats (Table 3).

TABLE 3: PRETREATMENT OF RATS WITH PHENOBARBITONE AND THE INTRAPERITONEAL LD_{50} OF (II) AND (III).

Compound	No Pretreatment	Phenobarbitone[a] Pretreatment
(II)	38 (32 - 45)	200 (126 - 318)
(III)	20 (17 - 25)	96 (84 - 109)

[a]Sodium phenobarbitone (500 mg/litre) was given in the drinking water for 7 days. Compounds (II) and (III) were given on the 8th day.

Following an LD_{50} dose of (II) (25 mg/kg) to rats there was little change in water content for either lung or thymus apart from a small increase in the lung on day 3 (Table 4). However, by day 3-4 lung weight had doubled and this increase was paralleled by the dry weight and persisted until day 10, even though survivors appeared normal.

Thymus weight decreased to about 50% between days 3 and 6 but was normal by day 10.

After all four compounds at oral LD_{50} doses lung showed a progressive diffuse interstitial thickening, maximal on day 4, leading to loss of alveolar space due to cellular proliferation and consolidation of large areas of all lobes. In rats surviving to day 8 the lesion had regressed and lung structure was normal, although lung wet and dry weight was still increased. Acute cellular depletion was seen in the cortical layer of the thymus between days 3 and 6.

DISCUSSION

The acute toxicity of the trimethyl- and triethylphosphorothioates in the rat falls into two distinct phases. The first is within 1-2 hr of an oral dose when cholinergic signs are seen; although deaths at this stage are only seen with compound (IV), when the LD_{50} is dominated by this effect.

With compounds (I), (II) and (III) no early deaths are seen unless doses much greater than the LD_{50} are given. The second phase is seen from days 3 to 6, maximal on day 4 and recognisable by weight loss and

TABLE 4: EFFECT OF (II) (ORAL 25 mg/kg) ON LUNG AND THYMUS WEIGHT AND WATER CONTENT.

Days After Dosing	Rat Wt. (g)	Lung Wet Wt. (mg)	Lung Dry Wt. (mg)	H_2O (%)	Thymus Wet Wt. (mg)	Thymus Dry Wt. (mg)	H_2O (%)
Control	168 (6)[a] ±1.8	968.7 ±80.7	187 ±7	80.4 ±.81	495 ±21.5	99.9 ±4.8	79.8 ±.67
1	159.8(5) ±2.0	1059.9 ±45.8	212 ±9.6	80.0 ±.37	460.9 ±23.8	96.6 ±4.9	79.0 ±1.1
3	149.8(5) ±0.7	1876[b] ±112	329[b] ±11.5	82.3 ±.42	238[b] ±17.4	47.8[b] ±3.4	79.9 ±.70
4	151.0(5) ±10.6	2049.6[b] ±184.8	372.9[b] ±16.9	81.5 ±.87	235.6[b] ±56.4	50.6[b] ±11.6	78.5 ±.59
5	161.5(4) ±15.4	1773[b] ±209.6	334.6[b] ±32.2	81.0 ±.39	261.0 ±108	56.5 ±21.9	77.4 ±1.0
6	162.7(4) ±5.5	1768[b] ±146	339[b] ±24.4	80.8 ±.34	257[b] ±98.5	55.1 ±20.7	78.3 ±.24
10	194.5(4) ±4.5	1665[b] ±70.55	339[b] ±14.5	79.9 ±.15	478 ±13.3	100.2 ±2.0	79.0 ±.23

a Figures in parenthesis are the number of rats.
b Significant with respect to the control $P < 0.05$.

laboured respiration; deaths occur in this period. Although deaths with compound (IV) occur in phase 1, in surviving animals, some lung damage is also demonstrable on days 3-6.

These compounds are less toxic to the mouse and hamster and both the anticholinesterase effect (phase 1) and the lung toxicity (phase 2) contribute to the LD_{50}.

The lung toxicity (phase 2) in the rat characterised by a massive increase in lung wet and dry weight associated with interstitial thickening and loss of alveolar space, but with rapid recovery, has not previously been described following poisoning with organophosphorus compounds.

REFERENCES

1. Aldridge, W.N., Miles, J.W., Mount, D.L. and Verschoyle, R.D. (1979). Arch. Toxicol., 42, 95-106.
2. Umetsu, N., Grose, F.H., Allahyari, R., Abu-El-Haj, S. and Fukuto, T.R. (1977). J. Agric. Food Chem., 25, (4) 946-953.

Mechanisms of Toxicity and Hazard Evaluation
B. Holmstedt, R. Lauwerys, M. Mercier, M. Roberfroid eds

IN VIVO STUDIES ON ADRIAMYCIN-INDUCED LIPID PEROXIDATION AND EFFECTS OF FERROUS IONS

H. KAPPUS, H. MULIAWAN and M.E. SCHEULEN[+]
Abteilung für Pharmakologie, Med. Institut für Umwelthygiene, Universität Düsseldorf, Gurlittstraße 53, D 4000 Düsseldorf 1, F.R.G.
[+]Innere Klinik und Poliklinik (Tumorforschung), Westdeutsches Tumorzentrum, Universität Essen, D 4300 Essen 1, F.R.G.

INTRODUCTION

It has been assumed that the antitumor drug adriamycin provokes lipid peroxidation in vivo[1-5]. This could explain its highly toxic effects on cardiac tissues, which have been observed in man and animals[5,6]. However, most of the data on adriamycin-induced lipid peroxidation are based on in vitro results, are obtained in vivo with controversial methods or are of indirect and speculative nature. Furthermore, quelamycin, a complex of adriamycin with iron ions which are well known to induce lipid peroxidation in vitro, has recently been introduced in clinical trials[7], although its toxicity is fairly high[8].

As an index of in vivo lipid peroxidation we used the method of determination of ethane expired by animals[9,10]. We were interested whether adriamycin can induce ethane formation in vivo and whether iron ions injected additionally influence ethane formation as well as toxicity.

MATERIALS AND METHODS

Male Wistar rats of 180 - 200 g body weight were injected with adriamycin (Adriblastin[R], Farmitalia) or $FeCl_2 \cdot 4H_2O$ or both intraperitoneally. They were placed separately in special gas-tight chambers for 6 h as described previously[10]. Sampling of the air of the chambers and the gas chromatographic analysis of ethane were the same as already described[10]. After 6 h they were removed from the chambers and were reexamined on the following days.

RESULTS AND DISCUSSION

Adriamycin itself is unable to induce ethane production of rats when treated with a dose of 20 mg/kg i.p.. The results shortly summarized here are reported elsewhere in detail: Compared to con-

TABLE

ETHANE EXPIRATION OF RATS TREATED WITH Fe^{2+}-IONS OR WITH ADRIAMYCIN AND Fe^{2+}-IONS (1 h LATER)

Start of sampling (Hours after last treatment)	Treatment (nmoles ethane / kg body weight / 6 h)		
	Controls [a]	Fe^{2+} [b]	Adriamycin and Fe^{2+} [c]
0	2.88 ± 0.88 (n = 4)	7.12 ± 0.80 (n = 4)	4.10 ± 0.31 (n = 8)
24	2.51 ± 0.13 (n = 4)	5.25 ± 0.63 (n = 4)	14.38 ± 3.25 (n = 6)
48	2.50 ± 0.11 (n = 4)	3.13 ± 0.52 (n = 4)	12.75 ± 2.49 (n = 4)
72	2.13 ± 0.25 (n = 4)	2.63 ± 0.36 (n = 4)	8.75 (n = 2)

[a]Animals received two i.p. injections of saline.

[b]Animals received an i.p. injection of saline and 1 h later 50 mg Fe^{2+}/kg (as $FeCl_2$) dissolved in saline i.p..

[c]Animals received an i.p. injection of 20 mg adriamycin/kg dissolved in saline and 1 h later 50 mg Fe^{2+}/kg (as $FeCl_2$) dissolved in saline i.p..

Mean values ± SD are shown.

trols a difference of ethane expiration of rats was not observed, neither immediately after treatment nor on the second or third day afterwards[11]. Only the very high doses of 45 and 65 mg adriamycin per kg, where most of the animals died within 72 h after treatment, induced slight increased ethane formation of rats[11].

The data of the Table which show the results of ethane expiration of rats treated with adriamycin and ferrous ions agree with this. The combined treatment rather inhibits than stimulates the amount of ethane formation measurable immediately after treatment. However, the ethane production measured 24 h afterwards without further treatment was increased in the animal group treated with both agents when compared to the ferrous-ion treated group (Table). The ethane expiration was still increased 48 h and to a lesser extent 72 h after treatment (Table). As can be seen from the numbers of the Table most of the animals died due to the combined treatment with adriamycin and Fe^{2+}, whereas all others survived.

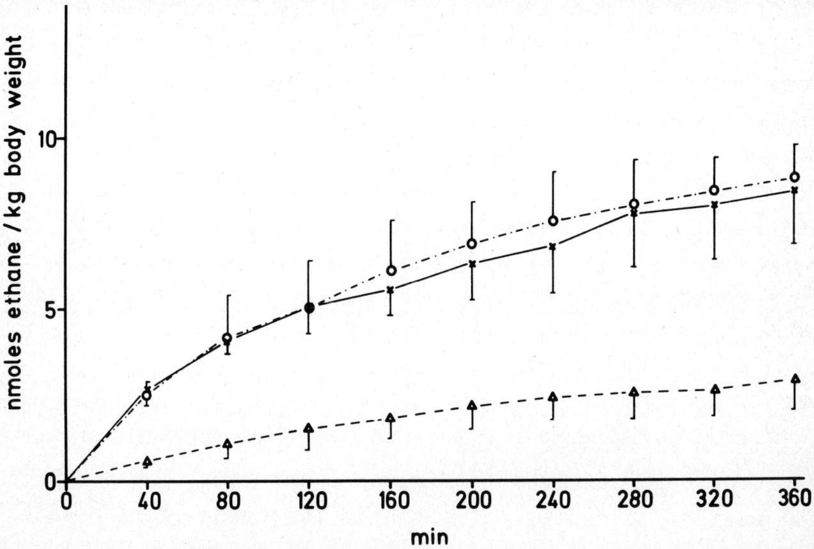

Figure 1. Ethane expiration of rats after the following treatment: Δ---Δ Control animals (n = 4) received saline i.p. and 24 h later once more saline. o-.-o Animals (n = 4) received saline i.p. and 24 h later 50 mg Fe^{2+}/kg (as $FeCl_2$) dissolved in saline i.p.. x——x Animals (n = 7) received 20 mg adriamycin/kg dissolved in saline i.p. and 24 h later 50 mg Fe^{2+}/kg (as $FeCl_2$) dissolved in saline i.p.. Sampling started immediately after the last treatment.

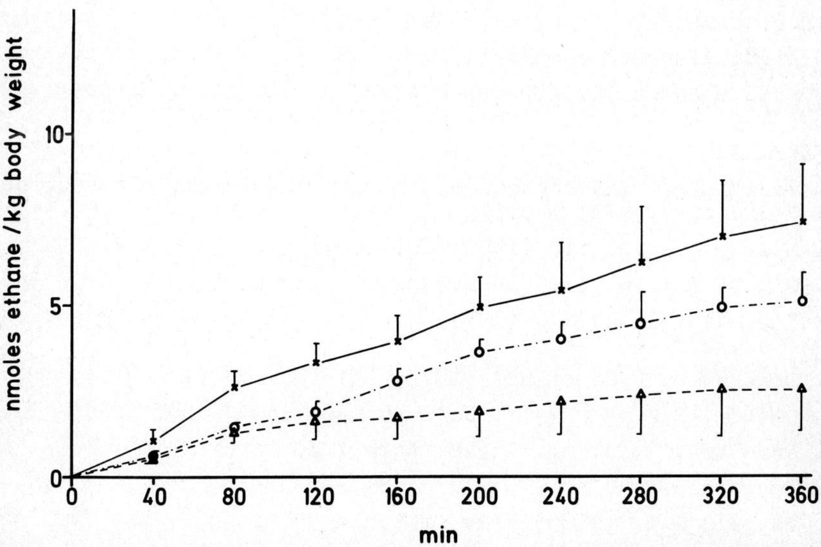

Figure 2. Ethane expiration of the same rats shown in Figure 1: Δ---Δ Control (n = 4), o-.-o Fe^{2+} (n = 4) and x——x adriamycin-Fe^{2+} (n = 3). Sampling started 24 h after the last treatment.

In order to explain this delay of stimulation of ethane formation which could not be found after treatment with the same doses of either compound[11] (Table), we changed the schedule of treatment. Because we found that the pretreatment of rats with adriamycin led to a higher mortality due to Fe^{2+}-ions than observed with Fe^{2+}-ions alone (data not shown), we injected adriamycin to rats which received just 24 h later Fe^{2+}-ions. Figure 1 shows that their ethane expiration was not increased due to the pretreatment with adriamycin over the value obtained with Fe^{2+} alone. Only a slight difference was observed when we measured ethane an additional period of 24 h later (Figure 2). In contrast to this, some animals treated with both compounds died within 24 h after the last treatment (compare the numbers of Figures 1 and 2), whereas all animals which received either compound survived[11] (Figures 1 and 2).

Our results indicate that a single injection of rats with 20 mg adriamycin per kg cannot induce lipid peroxidation in vivo. On the other hand, the combined treatment with adriamycin and ferrous ions leads to increased lipid peroxidation and toxicity. This effect is not due to adriamycin-induced damages which would make the organism more susceptible to ferrous ion-catalyzed lipid peroxidation. The mechanism responsible for this increase remains unclear.

In conclusion, we suggest that acute treatment with adriamycin in man might also not result in increased lipid peroxidation, whereas it could enhance lipid peroxidation and toxicity of other agents.

REFERENCES

1. Goodman, J. and Hochstein, P. (1977) Biochem. Biophys. Res. Commun., 77, 797 - 803.
2. Myers, C.E. et al. (1977) Science, 197, 165 - 167.
3. Stuart M.J. et al. (1978) Amer. J. Hematol., 5, 297 - 303.
4. Yamanaka, N. et al. (1979) Cancer Chemother. Pharmacol., 3, 223 - 227.
5. Donehower, R.C. et al. (1979) Life Sci., 25, 1 - 14.
6. Carter, S.K. (1975) J. Natl. Cancer Inst., 55, 1265 - 1274.
7. Gosalves, M. et al. (1978) Europ. J. Cancer, 14, 1185 - 1190.
8. Brugarolas, A. et al. (1979) Cancer Treat. Rep., 63, 909 - 913.
9. Tappel, A.L. (1980) Free Radicals in Biology Vol. IV, Academic Press, New York, pp. 2 - 48.
10. Köster, U. et al. (1977) Toxicol. Appl. Pharm., 41, 639 - 648.
11. Muliawan, H. et al. (1980) Cancer Letters, in press.

© 1980 Elsevier/North-Holland Biomedical Press
Mechanisms of Toxicity and Hazard Evaluation
B. Holmstedt, R. Lauwerys, M. Mercier, M. Roberfroid eds

THE USE OF BIOCHEMICAL METHODS FOR DETECTING CHANGES IN CELL POPULATION OF RAT BONE MARROW

ANDREW F WRIGHT AND MICHAEL S ROSE
Biochemical Mechanisms Section, Imperial Chemical Industries Limited, Central Toxicology Laboratory, Alderley Park, Nr Macclesfield, Cheshire SK10 4TJ, UK

SUMMARY

The *in vitro* incorporation of ^{14}C-glycine into haem, and ^{35}S-sulphate into macromolecules have been investigated as biochemical measurements with the potential to reflect the proportion of certain erythroid and myeloid cells within rat bone marrow.

Erythroid hyperplasia caused an increase of haem synthesis and a concomitant decrease in ^{35}S-sulphate incorporation.

Erythroid hypoplasia reduced haem synthesis and increased ^{35}S-sulphate incorporation.

The measures of haem synthesis and ^{35}S-sulphate incorporation thus provide useful tools for detecting specific changes in cell populations in rat bone marrow suspensions.

INTRODUCTION

Bone marrow is of increasing importance in toxicology with respect to the occurrence of chemically induced aplastic anaemia, pancytopaenia and leukaemia. The current routine methods of morphological examination of bone marrow in experimental animals are both subjective and time-consuming. This study was carried out to determine whether biochemical methods can be used to detect changes in population size of the major cell types within rat bone marrow.

The synthesis of haemoglobin is a process unique to the erythroid cell line and therefore haem synthesis was used as a measure of the maturing erythroid precursors[1].

The incorporation of ^{35}S-sulphate into bone marrow cells has been investigated as a process predominantly carried out within the myeloid cell series[2,3,4]. ^{35}S-sulphate is incorporated into sulphated glycosaminoglycans during granule formation predominantly in promyelocytes and metamyelocytes.

In order to evaluate these measurements, bone marrow cell suspensions were produced that were enriched or depleted with respect to myeloid or erythroid cells. Phenylhydrazine was used to induce erythropoiesis, whereas hypertransfusion of red blood cells was used to suppress erythropoiesis.

METHODS

Bone marrow cell suspensions were prepared in suspension culture medium (pH 7.3) and consisted of femoral bone marrow from at least five control or treated rats. The total and nucleated cell counts were determined using a Coulter Electronics cell counter.

The rate of haem synthesis was determined by measurement of the *in vitro* incorporation of 2-^{14}C glycine into haem, and expressed relative to nucleated cell number.

The incorporation of ^{35}S-sulphate was determined in the perchloric acid insoluble fraction of bone marrow cell suspensions. Previous experiments have shown this process to be dependent on oxidative metabolism and protein synthesis

RESULTS

Linear incorporations of ^{14}C-glycine (up to 90 min) and ^{35}S-sulphate (up to 30 min) were obtained in control bone marrow cell suspensions.

Red blood cell hypertransfusion

Three days after hypertransfusion there was a large reduction (30% of control) in the rate of haem synthesis with a corresponding increase (140% of control) in the rate of ^{35}S-sulphate incorporation (Figure 1). By day 7 the

FIGURE 1

THE EFFECTS OF RBC HYPERTRANSFUSION ON HAEM SYNTHESIS AND ^{35}S-SULPHATE INCORPORATION IN BONE MARROW SUSPENSIONS

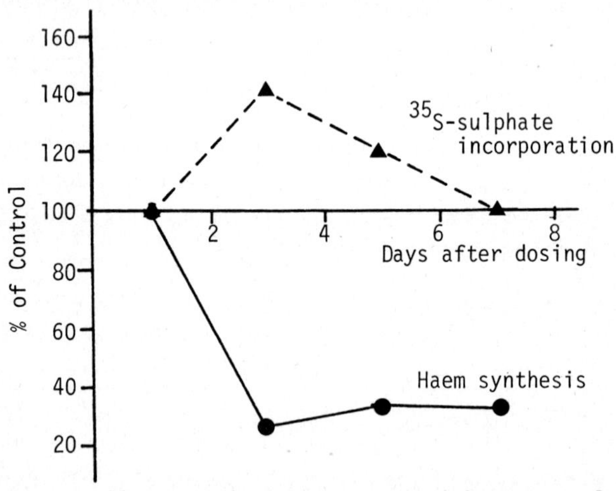

Femoral bone marrow cell suspensions were prepared from control rats and rats hypertransfused with RBC (equivalent to 50% blood volume). The initial rates of incorporation of 2-^{14}C glycine into haem and ^{35}S-sulphate into perchloric acid precipitates were expressed relative to the number of nucleated cells. Differences between mean rates were tested for significance using Student's 'T' test.

rate of ^{35}S-sulphate incorporation had returned to control levels whilst the rate of haem synthesis was still markedly reduced (Figure 1).

Phenylhydrazine

(a) Single dosing regime: After one dose of 40 mg phenylhydrazine/kg, haem synthesis was increased (135% of control) and remained at this level for at least 7 days after dosing (Figure 2). There were no changes in the rate of ^{35}S-sulphate incorporation.

FIGURE 2

THE EFFECTS OF 40 MG PHENYLHYDRAZINE/KG ON HAEM SYNTHESIS AND ^{35}S-SULPHATE INCORPORATION IN BONE MARROW SUSPENSIONS

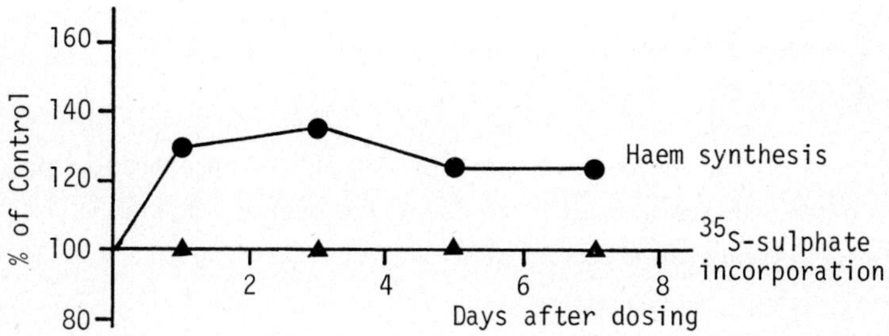

Femoral bone marrow cell suspensions were prepared from control rats and rats dosed subcutaneously with 40 mg phenylhydrazine/kg. The initial rates of incorporation of 2-^{14}C glycine into haem and ^{35}S-sulphate into perchloric acid precipitates were expressed relative to the number of nucleated cells. Differences between mean rates were tested for significance using Student's 'T' test.

(b) Multiple dosing regime: Three days after completion of five daily doses of 32 mg phenylhydrazine/kg, the number of nucleated cells obtained in the marrow suspensions was reduced (43% of control, Table 1). The rate of haem synthesis however expressed relative to nucleated cells was increased (127% of control) whilst the rate of ^{35}S-sulphate incorporation was reduced (56% of control, Table 1).

DISCUSSION

When erythropoiesis was suppressed by hypertransfusion of red blood cells a marked reduction in haem synthesis was observed (Figure 1). When erythropoiesis was stimulated by phenylhydrazine, an increase in haem synthesis was observed. It is therefore apparent that the measurement of haem synthesis to some degree reflects the erythropoietic state of the bone marrow.

Treatments designed to affect erythropoiesis altered ^{35}S-sulphate incorporation (Figure 1, Table 1). Available evidence suggests that ^{35}S-sulphate incor-

TABLE 1

THE EFFECTS OF PHENYLHYDRAZINE (3 DAYS AFTER 5 DAILY DOSES OF 32 MG/KG) ON HAEM SYNTHESIS AND ^{35}S-SULPHATE INCORPORATION IN BONE MARROW SUSPENSIONS

	Haem Synthesis	^{35}S-sulphate Incorporation	Nucleated Cells
% of Control	127±16(3)	56±15(3)	43±3(3)

Femoral bone marrow suspensions were prepared from control rats and rats dosed subcutaneously with 5 daily doses of 32 mg/kg and killed 3 days after the last dose. The initial rates of incorporation of 2-^{14}C glycine into haem and ^{35}S-sulphate into perchloric acid precipitates were expressed relative to the number of nucleated cells. Figures are mean % of control ± SEM with the number of experiments in parentheses.

poration is into a non-erythroid cell compartment. These treatments therefore appear to alter the non-erythroid cells of the marrow. Possible explanations are (1) the existence of a common stem cell pool leading to competition for particular cell lines, or (2) stimulation of non-erythroid cells as a consequence of transfusion of "foreign cells". Thus haem synthesis and ^{35}S-sulphate incorporation vary independently and may provide useful tools for detecting changes in the cell populations of bone marrow.

ACKNOWLEDGEMENTS

The authors acknowledge the technical assistance of Mr Kim Roser and Mr John Taylor and the valuable advice of Dr N M Blackett.

REFERENCES

1. Denton, M.J., Spencer, N. and Arnstein, H.R.V. (1975) Biochem. J. 146, 205.
2. Lajtha, L.G., Ellis, F. and Oliver, R. (1953) Brit. J. Cancer 7, 401.
3. Odell, T.T. (Jr), Tausche, F.G. and Gude, W.D. (1955) Am. J. Physiol. 180, 491.
4. Payne, D.N. and Ackerman, G.A. (1977) Blood 50, 841.

© 1980 Elsevier/North-Holland Biomedical Press
Mechanisms of Toxicity and Hazard Evaluation
B. Holmstedt, R. Lauwerys, M. Mercier, M. Roberfroid eds

RATE OF SKIN PENETRATION OF ORGANOPHOSPHATES MEASURED IN DIFFUSION CELLS

C. van HOOIDONK[x], B.I. CEULEN[x], H. KIENHUIS[x] and J. BOCK[xx]
Prins Maurits Laboratory TNO[x] and Medical Biological Laboratory TNO[xx],
P.O. Box 45, 2280 AA RIJSWIJK (Z.H.), The Netherlands

INTRODUCTION

Organophosphorus chemistry has attracted much attention since Schrader's discovery[1] of the biological activity of phosphorus acid derivatives with the basic formula $R_1R_2OP(O \text{ or } S)X$, where R_1 and R_2 may be alkyl, alkoxy or amino and X may be fluoride, cyanide, thiophenoxy, thiolate or dialkylphosphate.

The extensive use of this type of compounds as insecticides[2] and a possible use as chemical warfare agents[3] can lead to intoxications via percutaneous absorption. To quantify the risks and to develop skin decontamination methods quantitative penetration data are required.

Penetration experiments *in vivo* present difficulties concerning the determination of the amount of agent percutaneously absorbed. Analyses of the blood, urine, faeces or expired air are complicated and do neither quantify the amount of agent penetrated into the body nor the rate of penetration due to absorption in tissues or organs, metabolic degradation or a breakdown during passage through the skin.

Penetration data from model experiments *in vitro* with isolated skin in diffusion cells can be directly correlated with properties of the penetrant, vehiculum and species.

For two highly toxic organophosphates, VX (R_1=methyl, R_2=ethyl and X= S-(2-diisopropylaminoethyl)) and Soman (R_1=methyl, R_2=pinacolyl and X=fluoride), labelled with ^{35}S and ^{32}P respectively, the rate of penetration (v_{pen}) and the delay time (t_d) were determined for guinea pig skin and human skin.

MATERIALS AND METHODS

Materials. ^{35}S labelled VX and ^{32}P labelled Soman were synthesized in the Prins Maurits Laboratory TNO and had specific activities of 7.4 and 4.2 mCi/g. The radiochemical purities were shown to be better than 95%.

Skin. The abdominal skin of male and female guinea pigs was clipped and shaved 24 hours prior to testing. After being sacrificed, each animal was skinned and samples of 3 x 3 cm were mounted in the diffusion cell. Human skin removed during mastectomy was disposed from subcutaneous fat and stored at -20°C until required.

Diffusion cell. In a Teflon diffusion cell (Fig.1) a piece of skin is mounted on sharp needles to approx. the natural tension of the skin. Therefore, the skin of the living animal was marked with a stamp, then excised after sacrifice, and placed with the inkmarkings on the needles. Beneath the skin there is a continuous flow of a physiological salt solution and the passage of the agent from the epidermal side to the fluid is measured. Every 30 minutes a sample of 4 ml is collected using a fraction collector. The contamination was applied with a microsyringe. The penetration was followed for 24 hours. Four experiments can be done simultaneously (Fig.2). The rates of penetration are quantified by radioactive and enzymatic measurements. The first-mentioned method gives the sum of intact VX or Soman penetrating plus the radiolabelled degradation products. The enzymatic method quantifies exclusively the intact agent.

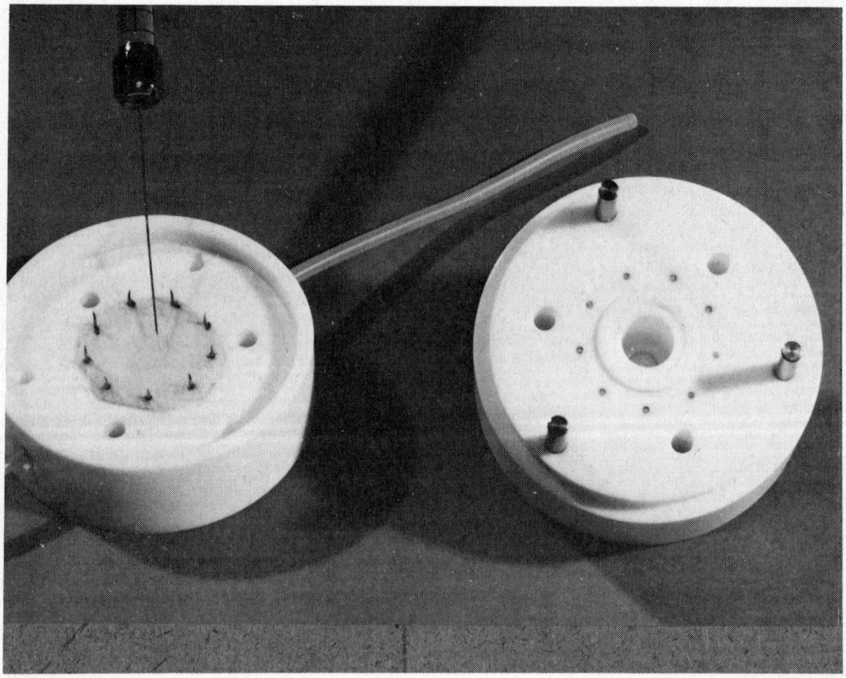

Fig.1 Diffusion cell

Radioactive assay. Radioactivity was measured with a Philips Liquid scintillation analyser PW 4540 with automated external standard quench correction.

Enzymatic assay. The assay is based on the inhibition of the enzyme butyrylcholinesterase by organophosphates. The partly inhibited enzyme shows a lower hydrolytic activity towards the substrate acetylthiocholine resulting in a diminished liberation of thiocholine which is assayed according to the method of Ellman[4]. In an automized procedure the inhibition reaction, the addition of substrate and the colorimetric determination of thiocholine was carried out. Concentrations down to 10^{-7} M can be assayed accurately.

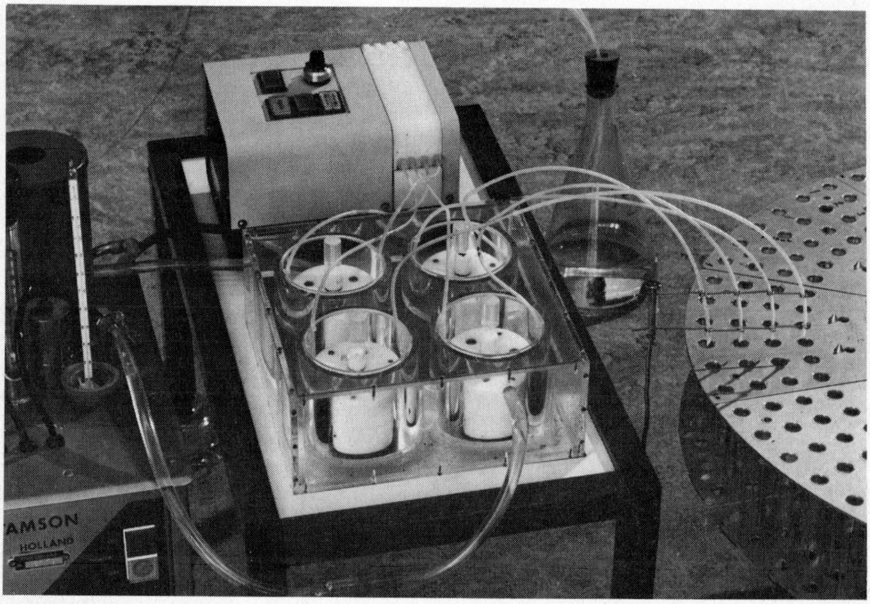

Fig.2. Thermostated holder with diffusion cells and fraction collector.

RESULTS

A typical example of a penetration curve is given in Fig.3. The cumulative amounts of agent penetrated through the skin and assayed radiologically and enzymatically are plotted vs. time. The curves are characterised by an initial rise from zero to a more or less constant penetration rate ("steady-rate"), v_{pen}, during some hours followed by a flattening of the curve due to exhausting agent. The intercept with the horizontal axis of the tangent to the curve is the delay time t_d.

Fig.3 shows that during the passage of Soman through guinea pig skin degradation occurs to a considerable extent. We observed percentages of degradation between 30 and 60. The differences are certainly due to biological variations.

Human skin degrades Soman to at least 80%. On the other hand, VX is not degraded by human skin and slightly degraded by guinea pig skin. Hence, the rates of penetration obtained from the radiological and enzymatic assay are identical. Further, we observed that the permeability of guinea pig skin is 2-3 times that of human skin. A compilation of all data is given in Table I.

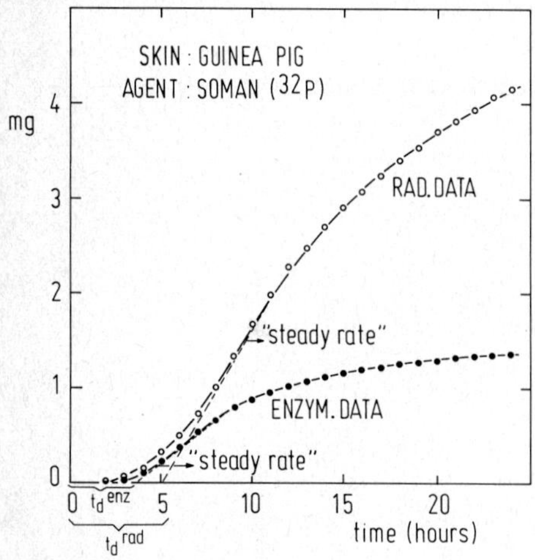

Fig.3.

The amount of Soman penetrated vs. time as measured radiologically and enzymatically. Contamination density 5 mg/0.8 cm^2, temp. 30°C.

TABLE I

SKIN PENETRATION DATA FOR VX AND SOMAN

HUMAN SKIN					GUINEA PIG SKIN			
Agent	t_d^{rad}	v_{pen}^{rad}	t_d^{enz}	v_{pen}^{enz}	t_d^{rad}	v_{pen}^{rad}	t_d^{enz}	v_{pen}^{enz}
VX[a]	3.8[b]	2.8[c]	3.7[d]	2.8[d]	2.7	8.6	2.7	8.1
SOMAN[a]	5.2	3.5	5.0	1.4	5.0	6.9	3.5	3.5

[a] 5 mg/0.8 cm^2

[b] radiologically measured (hours)

[c] radiologically measured (µg/cm^2.min)

[d] enzymatically "

REFERENCES

1. Schrader, G. (1963) Die Entwicklung neuer insektizider Phosphorsäure-ester, Verlag Chemie GmbH., Weinheim.
2. Perkow, W. (1968) Die Insektizide, Dr.Alfred Hüthig Verlag, Heidelberg.
3. Lohs, K. (1967) Synthetische Gifte, Deutscher Militärverlag, Berlin.
4. Ellman, G.L. "et al." (1961) Biochem.Pharmacol., 7, 88-95.

© 1980 Elsevier/North-Holland Biomedical Press
Mechanisms of Toxicity and Hazard Evaluation
B. Holmstedt, R. Lauwerys, M. Mercier, M. Roberfroid eds

THE EFFECT OF HYDRALAZINE ON COLLAGEN BIOSYNTHESIS AND SECRETION IN ISOLATED EMBRYONIC CHICK TENDON CELLS

Reza I. Bashey*, Sergio A. Jimenez*, and Tibor Balazs**
University of Pennsylvania*, Philadelphia; Food and Drug Administration**, Washington, D.C.

INTRODUCTION

Although hydralazine has been shown to be an effective antihypertensive agent, its clinical application has been limited because of the development of a systemic lupus erythematosus-like condition in some patients receiving this drug. The mechanisms responsible for development of this auto-immune disease are not known. It is possible that hydralazine may result in synthesis of an abnormal unhydroxylated collagen by chelating Fe^{++}, a cofactor necessary for synthesis of hydroxyproline and hydroxylysine (1,2). Alternatively, hydralazine or its metabolic products may bind to certain proteins including collagen and increase their antigenic properties (3). In attempts to clarify this problem we studied the effects of hydralazine on collagen biosynthesis and molecular structure using isolated chick embryo tendon fibroblasts.

MATERIALS AND METHODS

Fibroblasts were isolated from 17 day old chick embryo tendons as described by Dehm and Prockop (4). Subsequently 10^7 cells were incubated at 37°C in Kreb's medium containing various concentrations of hydralazine. After 20 min preincubation, ^{14}C-proline (1 μCi/ml) was added and the cells were incubated for 3 hr. The cells were separated from the media by centrifugation. Aliquots of media and cells were used to measure total ^{14}C-proline incorporation, ^{14}C-hydroxyproline synthesis and to characterize the labeled proteins as described previously (5-7).

RESULTS AND DISCUSSION

When cells were incubated in presence of hydralazine, no differences were observed in total ^{14}C-proline incorporation (Table 1). However, the drug markedly affected the secretion of labeled proteins into the media. In control fibroblasts, about 60% of the total ^{14}C-proline was secreted while in the treated cells, there was a dose-dependent inhibition of secretion of labeled molecules. At 0.5 and 1.0 mM hydralazine only 24 and 20% of the ^{14}C-proteins were found in the media respectively.

TABLE 1

Effect of Hydralazine on ^{14}C-proline Incorporation by Tendon Fibroblasts

Hydralazine added (mM)	^{14}C-proline incorporation (CPM x 10^{-6})			Secretion * (%)
	Cells	Medium	Total	
None	2.16	3.63	5.79	62.7
0.1	3.30	3.94	7.24	54.5
0.2	2.96	2.23	5.19	43.0
0.5	3.80	1.21	5.01	24.2
1.0	5.28	1.32	6.60	20.0

* Medium CPM/total CPM x 100

Table 2 shows that ^{14}C-hydroxyproline synthesis was not affected by 0.1 mM hydralazine, but greater concentrations caused profound decrease in this parameter. At concentrations of 0.5 and 1.0 mM, ^{14}C-hydroxyproline formation was inhibited. The degree of hydroxylation of media ^{14}C-proteins decreased from 43% in control cultures to less than 1% at 1 mM hydralazine. The degree of ^{14}C-proline hydroxylation of cell associated molecules showed decrease from 14% in control cells to less than 1% in cells incubated with increasing hydralazine concentrations.

TABLE 2

Effect of Hydralazine on ^{14}C-hydroxyproline Synthesis by Tendon Fibroblasts

Hydralazine added (mM)	^{14}C-hydroxyproline synthesis (CPM x 10^{-5})			Hydroxylation * (%)	
	Cells	Medium	Total	Cells	Medium
None	3.01	15.81	18.82	13.9	43.6
0.1	4.01	16.80	20.81	12.1	42.6
0.2	2.20	4.42	6.62	7.4	19.8
0.5	0.76	0.39	1.15	2.0	3.1
1.0	0.47	0.09	0.56	0.9	0.7

* CPM ^{14}C-hydroxyproline/total ^{14}C-proline CPM x 100

To characterize the nature of the ^{14}C-proteins synthesized in the presence of hydralazine, aliquots of cells and media were chromatographed under denaturing conditions as described previously (5,6). The chromatograms of labeled proteins from media (Fig. 1) and from cells (Fig. 2) are shown below:

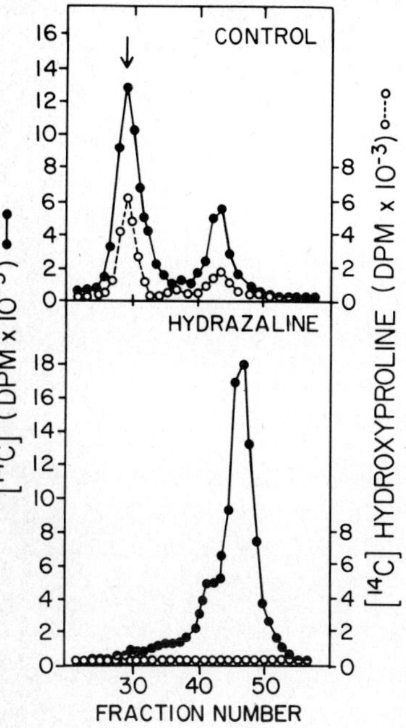

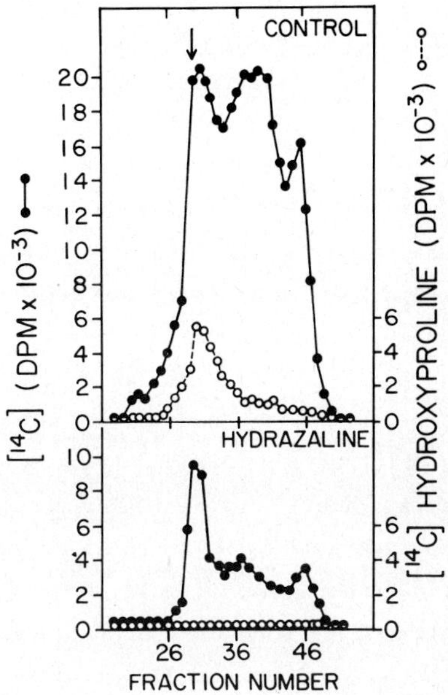

Fig. 1. SDS-agarose chromatography of media from control and hydralazine treated (1 mM) fibroblasts

Fig. 2. SDS-agarose chromatography of intracellular proteins from control and hydralazine treated (1 mM) fibroblasts

Arrow indicates elution position of reduced tendon procollagen.

It can be seen that in media from control experiments, about 70% of non-dialyzable ^{14}C-proline and about 90% of ^{14}C-hydroxyproline appeared in a sharp peak eluting in a position corresponding to normal procollagen. The degree of hydroxylation of these molecules was about 45%, a value consistent with fully hydroxylated procollagen. In contrast, media from cells treated with 1 mM hydralazine did not show any ^{14}C-procollagen and all the non-dialyzable radioactivity was recovered as low molecular weight peptides representing degradation products. None of the fractions contained ^{14}C-hydroxyproline. Characterization of the intracellular labeled molecules showed that in control cells, a substantial amount of radioactivity eluted in the position of procollagen but the majority was in smaller molecules. Only the procollagen fractions were shown to contain any ^{14}C-hydroxyproline. In the hydralazine treated cells, a large accumulation of ^{14}C-proline in the region of procollagen was demonstrated and only two minor small molecular weight peaks were found. None of the fractions contained ^{14}C-hydroxyproline suggesting that the major ^{14}C-proline peak represented unhydroxylated procollagen.

These results demonstrate that hydralazine interfered with collagen biosynthesis through inhibition of proline hydroxylation. Hydralazine caused a marked inhibition in secretion of labeled molecules which correlated with their degree of hydroxylation. When ^{14}C-hydroxyproline synthesis was completely abolished at 1 mM hydralazine, maximum reduction in secretion of ^{14}C-proline was observed.

Significant differences in the molecular size of the proteins synthesized in the presence and absence of hydralazine were demonstrated. Hydralazine caused a complete absence of radioactivity eluting in the region of procollagen and most of the ^{14}C-radioactivity appeared in the region of low molecular weight peptides which were probably degradation products. These changes were accompanied by a dramatic intracellular accumulation of unhydroxylated procollagen. These findings may be due to the fact that procollagen synthesized by the hydralazine treated cells could not achieve sufficient amount of triple helicity to be secreted and therefore accumulated inside the cells. Our findings indicate that synthesis of collagen molecules with an abnormal conformation and with increased susceptibility to proteolytic attack may be responsible at least in part, for the auto-immune effects of hydralazine.

ACKNOWLEDGEMENTS

This research has been partially supported by a contract from the F.D.A.; and a grant from the Eastern Pennsylvania Chapter of the Arthritis Foundation and partially subsidized by the Pew Memorial Trust.

REFERENCES

1. Bhatnagar, R.S., Rapaka, R.S., Liu, T.Z. and Wolfe, S.M. (1972) Biochim. Biophys. Acta, 271, 125-132.
2. Rapaka, R.S., Parr, R.W., Liu, T.Z. and Bhatnagar, R.S. (1977) Teratology 15, 185-193.
3. Paz, M.A. and Seifter, S. (1972) Amer. Jour. Med. Sci., 263, 281-290.
4. Dehm, P. and Prockop, D.J. (1971) Biochim. Biophys. Acta, 240, 358-369.
5. Jimenez, S.A., Dehm, P., Olsen, B.R. and Prockop, D.J. (1973) J. Biol. Chem. 248, 720-729.
6. Jimenez, S.A. and Yankowski, R. (1978) J. Biol. Chem. 253, 1420-1426.
7. Bashey, R.I. and Jimenez, S.A. and Perlish, J.S. (1977) J. Molec. Med. 2, 153-161.

Mechanisms of Toxicity and Hazard Evaluation
B. Holmstedt, R. Lauwerys, M. Mercier, M. Roberfroid eds

A SENSITIVE EXPERIMENTAL MODEL FOR THE ASSESSMENT OF HEPATOTOXICITY BY HALOGENOCOMPOUNDS: PROLACTIN BINDING TO THE SPECIFIC RECEPTORS

R. DI CARLO, G. MUCCIOLI, D. LANDO, O. BROSSA*, E. BURDINO*, I. CHIAPPINO*, O. DANNI*, S. MINA* and G. UGAZIO*
Institute of Pharmacology and Institute of General Pathology*,
University of Torino, Corso Raffaello 30, I-10125 Torino (Italy)

INTRODUCTION

Carbon tetrachloride (CT) is one of the most largely used halogenated solvents[1,2] and then one of the most important environmental and occupational pollutants[3]. Its toxic effects on man[4,5] and experimental animal[6,7,8] are reported. Further, CT poisoning represents a suitable experimental model for the quantitative assessment of the biological damage caused by halogenocompounds.

With the aim to achieve a more sensitive evaluation of liver injury after poisoning, the behaviour of the binding of prolactin (PRL) to microsomal receptors in rat liver was compared with that of the parameters used routinely. In the rat, liver is an important target organ for PRL which controls several metabolic functions of this tissue[9,10,11,12].

MATERIALS AND METHODS

Female Wistar rats (150-180 g b.wt) were given CT either by mouth (6 up to 100 μl per 100 g b.wt) or by inhalation[13] (2 h at either 50 or 100 ppm), and then killed by decapitation 24 or 48 h later. The animals were deprived of food 12 h prior to both intoxication and sacrifice. Liver and serum samples were harvested. Microsomal fraction was prepared by differential centrifugation[14] from 20% liver homogenate in 0.3 M sucrose.

Membrane binding assay for PRL was carried out by conventional competitive protein-binding techniques, as described by Shiu et al.[15] with some modifications, using ^{125}I-labelled ovine prolactin (30-50 μCi/μg) iodinated according to the procedure of Bolton and Hunter[16]. PRL receptors were quantitatively assayed by determining specific binding as the difference between binding in the absence and the presence of an excess of unlabelled PRL (1 μg). Specific binding was expressed as percentage of total radioactivity added to the incubation mixture and referred to 0.1 mg protein[17]. Scatchard analysis[18] was also evaluated by transformation of binding data from competition studies with increasing concentration of unlabelled hormone mixed with a known amount of tracer.

Hepatic triglycerides were determined colorimetrically[19] after extraction of lipids according to Folch et al.[20] and purification[21]. Serum concentration of sorbitol dehydrogenase (SDH), glutamate-oxalacetate transaminase (GOT) and glutamate-pyruvate transaminase (GPT) was assayed with the kits supplied by Boehringer (Boehringer Mannheim GMBH, FRG).

Statistical significance of the differences was evaluated by using the Student t-test at the confidence level of 95%.

RESULTS AND DISCUSSION

CT, given orally, affects all the parameters investigated in this research with a severity progressively increasing according to the dose (6 up to 100 μl per 100 g b.wt). A maximum loss in binding properties of PRL receptors occurs already when 25 μl are administered. This finding points out that the alteration of PRL binding is a very sensitive parameter under these rather severe experimental conditions (table 1).

The results obtained after a rather mild CT treatment (inhalation at 50 ppm) outline the higher sensitivity of SDH test and PRL binding assay as compared with the commonly used methods. In these experimental conditions, liver triglyceride content (HTG), GOT and GPT serum levels result to be unchanged or modified only 48 h after treatment (table 1).

Scatchard analysis of PRL binding shows that oral CT, even at the lowest dose (6 μl), reduces the amount of specific receptors and causes the appearance of an additional class of binding sites with higher capacity and lower affinity.

In vitro experiments are in progress with the aim to ascertain at which extent this biological damage possibly depends on a lipoperoxidative mechanism.

Since SDH test and PRL binding assay appear to be very sensitive methods, in our opinion they can be offered as suitable tools in the assessment of liver injury caused by halogenated pollutants provided with lower toxicity than CT.

TABLE 1

PARAMETERS SHOWING LIVER INJURY AFTER CARBON TETRACHLORIDE POISONING

Values are expressed as mean ± S.E., * difference significant vs controls

Treatments	h[a]	PRL[b]	SDH[c]	GPT[c]	GOT[c]	HTG[d]
Controls[e]		3.12 ± 0.88	2.5 ± 0.3	8.4 ± 0.7	128 ± 10	19.7 ± 1.3
6 µl[f]	48	1.50 ± 0.61*	259.0 ± 42.0*	60.0 ± 19.0*	510 ± 44*	51.0 ± 8.0*
25 µl	48	0.45 ± 0.29*	561.0 ± 87.0*	- -	- -	158.0 ± 18.0*
100 µl	48	0.70 ± 0.46*	966.0 ± 147.0*	- -	- -	342.0 ± 72.0*
50 ppm[g]	24	2.36 ± 0.62*	4.9 ± 1.3*	6.7 ± 1.2	147 ± 12	18.2 ± 1.3
50 ppm	48	1.77 ± 0.41*	7.7 ± 1.8*	7.3 ± 0.7	151 ± 9	32.1 ± 4.2*
100 ppm	24	2.43 ± 0.72*	124.0 ± 34.0*	38.0 ± 14.0*	388 ± 73*	36.4 ± 7.6*
100 ppm	48	1.26 ± 0.42*	135.0 ± 23.0*	22.0 ± 3.7*	237 ± 14*	55.7 ± 4.9*

[a] hours after poisoning 5 up to 7 rats per experimental group
[b] specific binding of ^{125}I-ovine PRL as % of total radioactivity added and per 0.1 mg protein
[c] mU per ml
[d] mg in the liver per 100 g body weight
[e] unpoisoned animals: 18 rats
[f] µl CT per 100 g body weight, given by mouth
[g] concentration of CT vapour in air administered by inhalation for 2 hours.

ACKNOWLEDGEMENTS

This work was supported, in part, by grants from Consiglio Nazionale delle Ricerche (Roma) and from Regione Piemonte (Torino), in part, by Research Fellowships to O.B., I.C. and S.M. from Regione Piemonte (Torino).

The authors are indebted to NIAMDD Pituitary Hormone Distribution Program and to Dr A.F. Parlow for the gift of ovine prolactin.

REFERENCES

1. Lovelock, J.E., Maggs, R.J. and Wade, R.J. (1973) Nature (London), 241, 194-196.
2. Singh, H.B., Fowler, D.P. and Peyton, T.O. (1976) Science, 192, 1231-1234.
3. Lovelock, J.E. (1974) Nature (London), 252, 292-294.
4. Hashimoto, S., Glende, E.A. Jr, and Recknagel, R.O. (1968) N. Engl. J. Med., 279, 1082-1085.

5. Korenke, H.D. and Pribilla, O. (1969) Arch. Toxikol., 25, 109-126.

6. Recknagel, R.O. (1967) Pharmacol. Rev., 19, 145-208.

7. Burdino, E., Gravela, E., Ugazio, G., Vannini, V. and Calligaro, A. (1973) Agents and Actions, 4, 244-253.

8. Slater, T.F. (1972) Free radical Mechanisms in Tissue Injury, Pion Ltd., London.

9. Chen, H.W., Hamer, D.H., Heininger, H. and Meier, H. (1972)Biochim.Biophys. Acta, 287, 90-97.

10. Richards, J.F. (1975) Biochem. Biophys. Res. Comm., 63, 292-299.

11. Thomson, M.J. and Richards, J.F. (1978) Life Sci., 22, 337-344.

12. Francis, M.J.O. and Hill, D.J. (1975) Nature (London), 255, 167-168.

13. Ugazio, G., Burdino, E., Danni, O. and Milillo, P.A. (1973) Biochem. Soc. Trans., 1, 968-972.

14. Posner, B.I., Kelly, P.A., Shiu, R.P.C. and Friesen, H.G. (1974) Endocrinology, 95, 521-531.

15. Shiu, R.P.C., Kelly, P.A. and Friesen, H.G. (1973) Science, 180, 968-971.

16. Bolton, A.E. and Hunter, W.M. (1973) Biochem. J., 133, 529-539.

17. Lowry, O.H., Rosebrough, N.J., Farr, A.L. and Randall, R.J. (1951) J. Biol. Chem., 193, 265-275.

18. Scatchard, G. (1949) Ann. N. Y. Acad. Sci., 51, 660-672.

19. Van Handel, E. and Zilvermit, D.B. (1957) J. Lab. Clin. Med., 50, 152-157.

20. Folch, J. Lees, M. and Sloane Stanley, G.H. (1957) J. Biol. Chem., 226, 497-509.

21. Ugazio, G., Congiu, A.M., Masala, B.L. and Serra, M.V. (1971) Studi Sassaresi, 49, 213-222.

AUTHOR INDEX

SUBJECT INDEX

A

B

Q

R

S

T